ENCYCLOPEDIA OF CANCER AND SOCIETY

CONTENTS

List of Articles

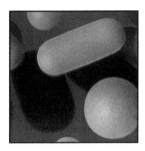

List of Contributors

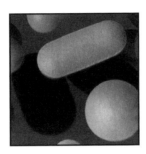

Achutan, Chandran
National Institute for Occupational Safety and Health

Afzal, Amber
Independent Scholar

Ahmed, Haitham
Dartmouth Medical School

Ahmed, Ayah
Kuwait University

Akter, Farhana
Kings College London

Alam, Sharita
Cornell University

Alavanja, Michael
National Cancer Institute

Ali, Muhammad Zeshan
Independent Scholar

Ali, Syed Mustafa
University of Health Sciences

Anthony, Navin
Providence Hospital

Ashing-Giwa, Kimlin
Independent Scholar

Auerbach, Karl
University of Rochester

Baharanyi, Hasani
Yale University

Bajaj, Sheetal
University of Southern California

Baker, Jin
Health and Food Institute

Bala, Poonam
University of Delhi

Bausch-Goldbohm, Sandra
TNO Quality of Life, Netherlands

Bax, Michael
Stanford University

Bazhenova, Lyudmila
University of California, San Diego

Blair, Mary
Independent Scholar

Boffetta, Paolo
International Agency for Research on Cancer

Boslaugh, Sarah
Washington University School of Medicine

Branagan, Andrew
Columbia University Medical Center

Brandt, Piet van den
Maastricht University, Netherlands

Brownson, Ross C.
Independent Scholar

Carethers, John
University of California San Diego

Carpenter, Catherine
Center for Human Nutrition David Geffen School of Medicine at UCLA

Castelao, Jose Esteban
University South Carolina Norris Cancer Center

Chan, R. V. Paul
Weill Medical College of Cornell University

Chen, Stephen
University of Toronto

Chen, Susanna
Western University of Health Sciences

Chen, Wendy
Harvard University

Chow, Jimmy
University of California, San Diego

Cipa-Tatum, Jillian
Independent Scholar

Clark, Cecily
Michigan State University

Clerkin, Cathleen
University of California, Berkeley

Clerkin, Michael
Sacramento City College

Clerkin, Paul
Sacramento City College

Connolly, Gregory
Harvard School of Public Health

Corfield, Justin
Geelong Grammar School, Australia

Coughlin, Steven
Centers for Disease Control and Prevention

Crammer, Corinne
American Cancer Society

Curry, Christine
Independent Scholar

Davidson, Michele
George Mason University

De Vocht, Frank
International Agency for Research on Cancer

Ding, Eric
Harvard School of Public Health

Dunne, Eileen
Centers for Disease Control and Prevention

Edenfield, Heather
Brigham and Women's Hospital

Eren, Gülnihan
Ege University Faculty of Medicine Turkey

Ezra, Navid
David Geffen School of Medicine at UCLA

Fernandes, Rochelle
Canadian College of Naturopathic Medicine

Ferrer, Rizaldy
Independent Scholar

Field, R. William
University of Iowa

Friedman, Carol
Centers for Disease Control and Prevention

Freudenheim, Jo
State University of New York, Buffalo

Frye, Stacy
Michigan State University College of Human Medicine

Gago-Dominguez, Manuela
University of Southern California Norris Cancer Center

Garg, Sonia
Brown Medical School

Garland, Cedric
University of California, San Diego

Garland, Frank C.
University of California, San Diego

Garshick, Eric
Harvard School of Public Health

Ghafoor, Sana
Independent Scholar

Gladwin, Rahul
University of Health Sciences, Antigua

Goldstein, Bradley
Lake Erie College of Osteopathic Medicine

Goode, Ellen
Mayo Clinic College of Medicine

Gorham, Edward D.
University of California, San Diego

Grant, William, B.
Sunlight, Nutrition, and Health Research Center

Gruenbaum, Benjamin
University of Connecticut

Gruenbaum, Shaun
Columbia Medical School

Gupta, Nakul
Ross University School of Medicine

Gushchin, Anna
University of Pittsburgh

Hale, Gregory
St. Jude Children's Research Hospital

Hall, Irene
Centers for Disease Control and Prevention

Hand, Gregory
University of South Carolina

Handy, Susan L.
University of California, Davis

Haque, Omar Sultan
Harvard Medical School

Harlston, Lois
Tennessee State University

Harris, Melanie
Lander College for Women

Hartge, Patricia
National Institutes of Health

Hebert, James
University of South Carolina

Hellawell, Jennifer
Cornell University School of Medicine

Herrera, Fernando A., Jr.
University of California, San Diego

Hoffmeister, Laura
Harvard University

Hohman, Donald
Kern Medical Center

Hu, Stephanie
Harvard Medical School

Huang, Sherry
University of California, San Diego

Ilyas, Sadia
University of Missouri, Kansas City

Ireton, Renee
Fred Hutchinson Cancer Research Center

Jaggers, Jason R.
University of South Carolina

Jeng, H. Anna
Old Dominion University

Jourabchi, Natanel
Independent Scholar

Jung, Barbara
University of California, San Diego

Kalipeni, Ezekiel
University of Illinois at Urbana-Champaign

Kawachi, Ichiro
Harvard School of Public Health

Kasow, Kimberly
St. Jude's Children Research Hospital

Khanijoun, Harleen K.
University of Alabama

Kilfoy, Briseis
Yale University

Kim, Daniel
Harvard University

Kim, Youngmee
American Cancer Society

Kolonel, Laurence
University of Hawaii

Krueger, Gretchen
University of California, Berkeley

Laden, Francine
Harvard Medical School

La Flair, Lareina
Harvard Medical School

Land, Charles
National Institutes of Health

Lawson, Herschel
Centers for Disease Control and Prevention

Lee, Simon
National Cancer Institute

Lee, Won Jin
Korea University

Leung, Sonia
University of Michigan

Liu, Simin
UCLA School of Public Health

Loscalzo, Mathew J.
University of California, San Diego

Lyerly, G. William
University of South Carolina

Malone, Ruth E.
University of California, San Francisco

Mariani, Lisa
Centers for Disease Control and Prevention

Markowitz, Lauri
Centers for Disease Control and Prevention

Marshall, James
Roswell Park Cancer Institute

Maruti, Sonia
Harvard University

Masood, Quratulain
National University of Sciences and Technology

McElroy, Lisa
Michigan State University

Mendelsohn, Jacquelyn
University of Arkansas

Mernitz, Heather
Tufts University

Messmer, Bradley
University of California, San Diego

Mikulski, Marek
University of Iowa

Mills, Paul
Cancer Registry of California

Mishra, Mark
National Cancer Institute

Mitra, Anirban
University of Southern California

Moadel, Alyson
Albert Einstein College of Medicine

Modelska, Sabina
Western University of Health Sciences

Mohr, Sharif B.
University of California, San Diego

Mokaya, Kemunto
Yale University School of Medicine

Moore, Jonathan
University of South Carolina

Nguyen, Tu-Uyen Ngoc
University of South Carolina

Nijhawan, Rajiv I.
Independent Scholar

Nnama, Obianuju
Michigan State University

Novak, Shawna
Independent Scholar

Novogradec, Ann
York University, United Kingdom

Olsson, Ann
International Agency for Research on Cancer

Ouma, Veronica
Hofstra University

Padula, Alessandra
University of L'Aquila, Italy

Pandit, Rahul
St. Petersburg State Medical Academy, Russia

Parascandola, Mark
National Institute of Health

Park, Crystal
University of Connecticut

Patel, Alpa
American Cancer Society

Patel, Krunal
Independent Scholar

Patel, Shalu
Independent Scholar

Prabakar, Cheruba
University of Connecticut School of Medicine

Peethambaram, Prema P.
Mayo Clinic College of Medicine

Quinn, John
University of Illinois, Chicago

Radhakrishnan, Priya
Catholic Healthcare West

Ranft, Elizabeth
Western University of Health Sciences

Rattan, Rishi
University of Illinois, Chicago

Reid, Mary E.
Roswell Park Cancer Institute

Riedmueller, Lauren
St. Edward's University

Rodriguez, Jorge
Ponce School of Medicine

Rozenfeld, Boris
Independent Scholar

Saleh, Kamal
Independent Scholar

Salem, Aliasger K.
University of Iowa

Salem, Husein, K.
University of Manchester, United Kingdom

Salem, Murtaza K.
University of Nottingham, United Kingdom

Saraiya, Mona
Centers for Disease Control and Prevention

Sathya, Chethan
University of Toronto, Canada

Scott-Connor, Carol
University of Iowa

Seely, Dugald
Canadian College of Naturopathic Medicine

Shahverdian, Edwin
Independent Scholar

Shen, John
Washington University School of Medicine

Sherry, Mark
University of Toledo

Shultz, Jennifer
Independent Scholar

Siano, Maria
Ramapo College of New Jersey

Singh, Navneet
University of Toronto, Canada

Smith, Carmela M.
New Mexico State University

Song, Zirui
Harvard Medical School

Stechschulte, Sarah
Independent Scholar

Stefanek, Michael
American Cancer Society

Steinmaus, Craig M.
California Environmental Protection Agency

Sukerkar, Preeti
Northwestern University

Sullivan, Jaron
Texas A&M Health Science Center

Tapya, Sara
University of Iowa

Tavassoly, Iman
Mazandaran University of Medical Sciences, Iran

Tavassoly, Omid
Tarbiat Modares University, Iran

Thomas, Christopher
Centers for Disease Control and Prevention

Thun, Michael
American Cancer Society

Tsigelny, Igor
University of California, San Diego

Walsh, John
Shinawatra University, Thailand

Wang, Xiang-Dong
Tufts University

Wang, Sophia
National Institutes of Health

Wang, Y. Claire
Harvard University

Waskey, Andrew
Dalton State College

Wellisch, David K.
University of California, Los Angeles

Wills, Richard
Independent Scholar

Wilkens, Lynne R.
University of Hawaii

Wingo, Phyllis
Harvard University

Winograd, Claudia
University of Illinois at Urbana-Champaign

Wright, Clark J.
University of South Carolina

Yeh, James
Boston University

Yonekawa, Yoshihiro
Weill Medical College of Cornell University

Young, Sara
Canadian College of Naturopathic Medicine

Zelterman, Daniel
Yale University

Zeltser, Marina
Independent Scholar

Atlas of Cancer

Normal Appearance vs. Appearance with Spread of Cancer	A1
Brain Surgery: Removal of Brain Tumor and Cyst	A2
Bladder Cancer	A2
Breast Cancer	A3
Breast Cancer with 45 percent Mortality	A3
Cervical Cancer Progression	A4
Colon Cancer	A4
Lung Cancer with Metastasis to Lymph Nodes and Liver	A5
Metastasis	A6
Chemotherapy and Radiation	A6
Neck Tumor	A7
Ovarian Cancer Progression	A8
Prostate Cancer Progression	A9
Rectal Cancer Progression	A9
Skin Cancer Melanoma Progression	A10
Stomach Cancer	A10
Uterine Cancer Progression	A11
Testis Cancer, Metastatic	A12
Pelvic Cancer, Widespread	A13
Abdominal Tumor Mass	A14
Bilateral Nasal Cancer with Surgical Removal	A15
Brain Tumor with Compression of Adjacent Structures	A16

Normal Appearance vs. Appearance with Spread of Cancer

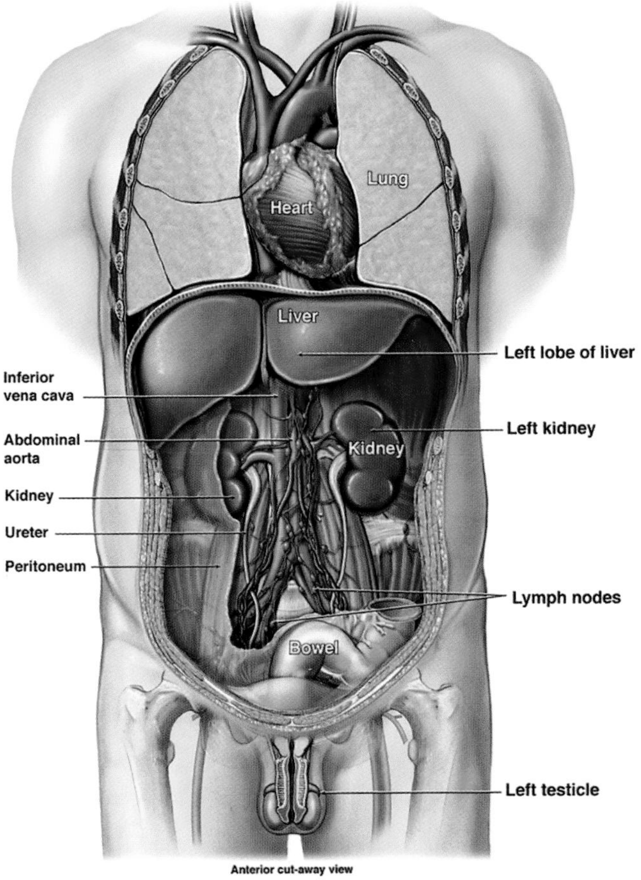

Lung
Heart
Liver
Left lobe of liver
Inferior vena cava
Left kidney
Abdominal aorta
Kidney
Kidney
Ureter
Peritoneum
Lymph nodes
Bowel
Left testicle

Anterior cut-away view

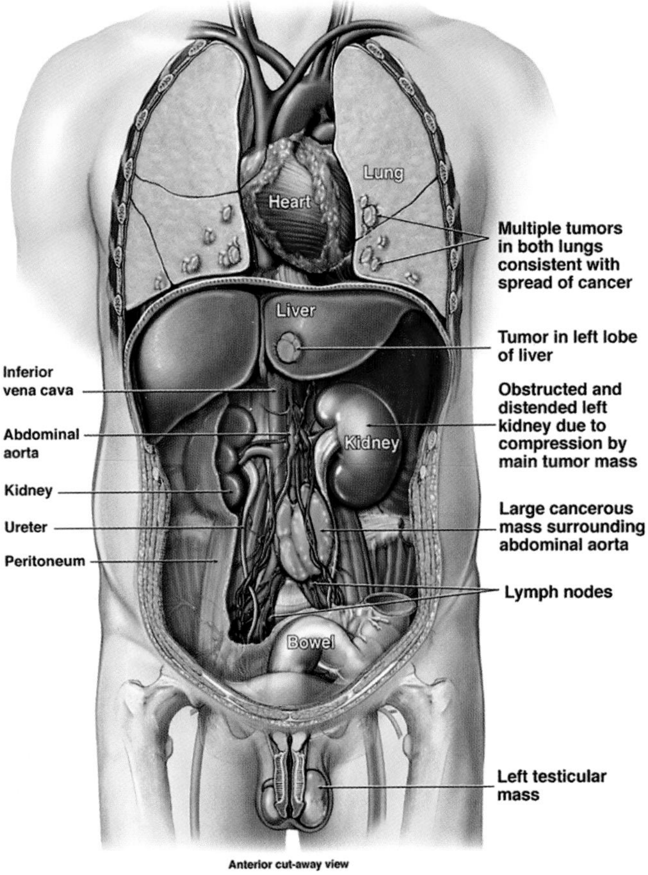

Lung
Heart
Multiple tumors in both lungs consistent with spread of cancer
Liver
Tumor in left lobe of liver
Inferior vena cava
Obstructed and distended left kidney due to compression by main tumor mass
Abdominal aorta
Kidney
Kidney
Ureter
Large cancerous mass surrounding abdominal aorta
Peritoneum
Lymph nodes
Bowel
Left testicular mass

Anterior cut-away view

Brain Surgery: Removal of Brain Tumor and Cyst

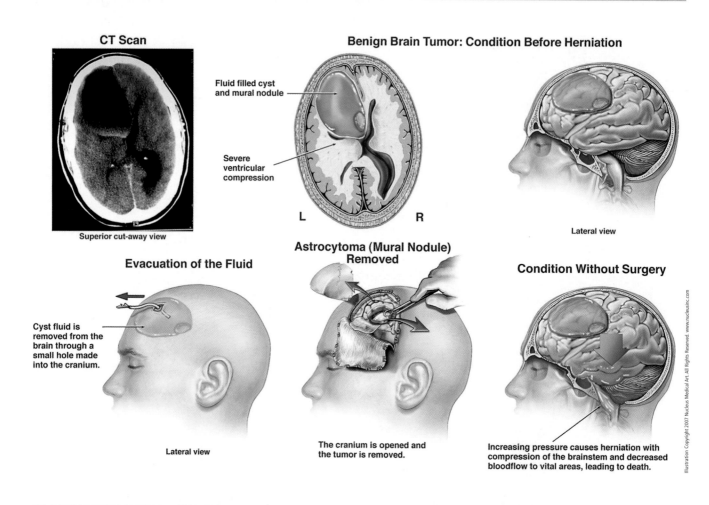

CT Scan

Superior cut-away view

Benign Brain Tumor: Condition Before Herniation

Fluid filled cyst and mural nodule

Severe ventricular compression

L   R

Lateral view

Evacuation of the Fluid

Cyst fluid is removed from the brain through a small hole made into the cranium.

Lateral view

Astrocytoma (Mural Nodule) Removed

The cranium is opened and the tumor is removed.

Condition Without Surgery

Increasing pressure causes herniation with compression of the brainstem and decreased bloodflow to vital areas, leading to death.

Bladder Cancer

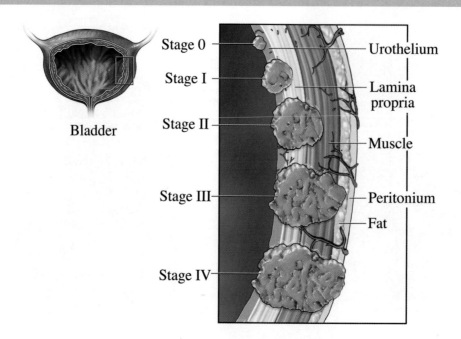

Bladder

Stage 0 — Urothelium

Stage I — Lamina propria

Stage II — Muscle

Stage III — Peritonium

Stage IV — Fat

Breast Cancer

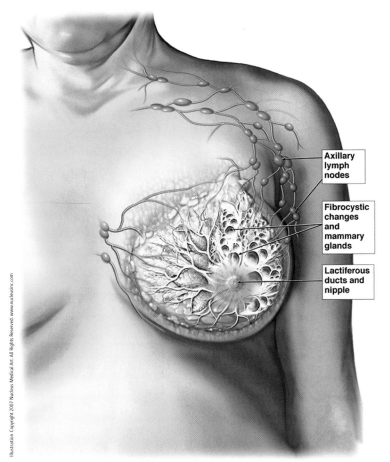

Axillary lymph nodes

Fibrocystic changes and mammary glands

Lactiferous ducts and nipple

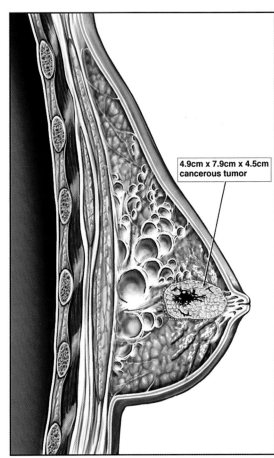

4.9cm x 7.9cm x 4.5cm cancerous tumor

Breast Cancer with 45 percent Mortality

Front view of breast

Side view cut section of breast

Carcinoma

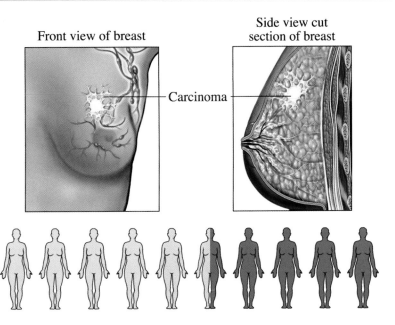

Cervical Cancer Progression

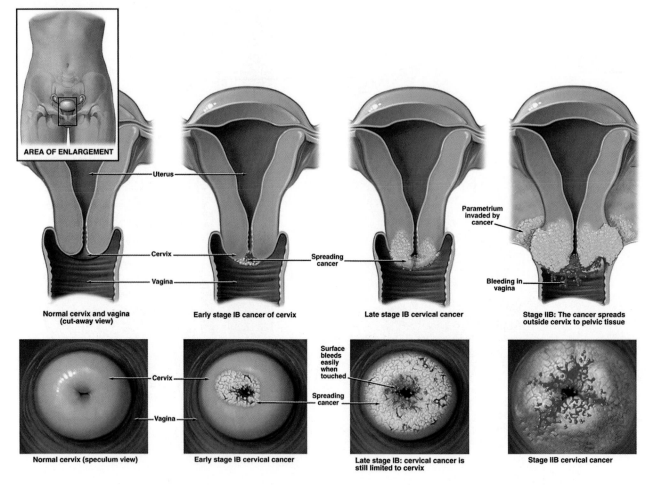

AREA OF ENLARGEMENT

Uterus

Cervix

Vagina

Spreading cancer

Parametrium invaded by cancer

Bleeding in vagina

Normal cervix and vagina (cut-away view)

Early stage IB cancer of cervix

Late stage IB cervical cancer

Stage IIB: The cancer spreads outside cervix to pelvic tissue

Cervix

Vagina

Surface bleeds easily when touched

Spreading cancer

Normal cervix (speculum view)

Early stage IB cervical cancer

Late stage IB: cervical cancer is still limited to cervix

Stage IIB cervical cancer

Colon Cancer

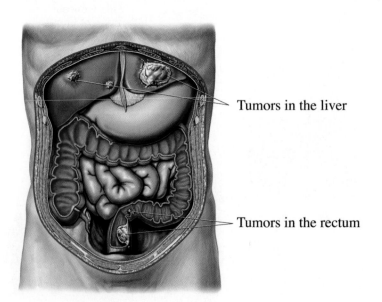

Tumors in the liver

Tumors in the rectum

Lung Cancer with Metastasis to Lymph Nodes and Liver

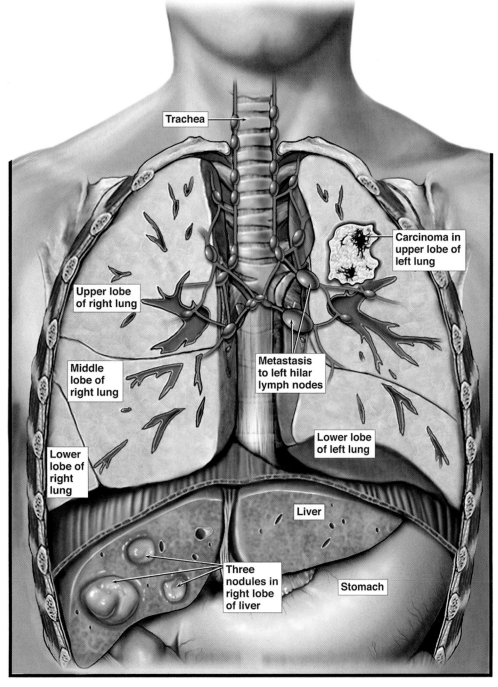

Anterior cut-away view

Metastasis

Chemotherapy and Radiation

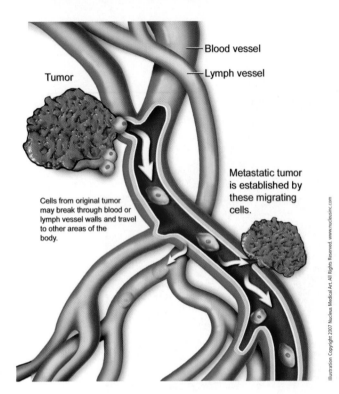

Tumor

Blood vessel

Lymph vessel

Cells from original tumor
may break through blood or
lymph vessel walls and travel
to other areas of the
body.

Metastatic tumor
is established by
these migrating
cells.

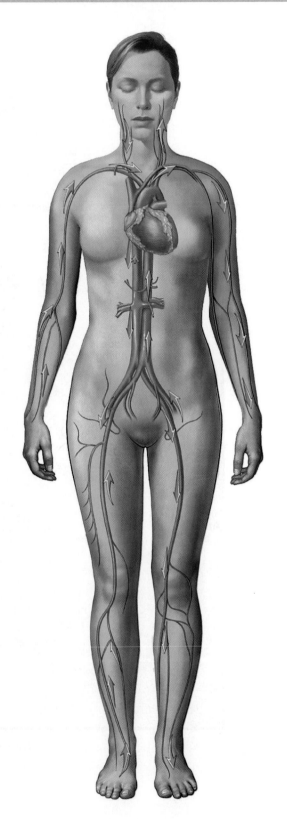

Neck Tumor

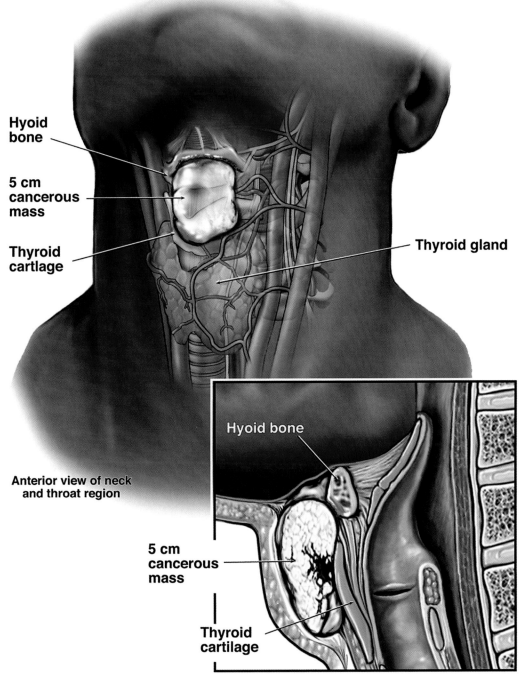

Hyoid bone

5 cm cancerous mass

Thyroid cartlage

Thyroid gland

Anterior view of neck and throat region

Hyoid bone

5 cm cancerous mass

Thyroid cartilage

Sagittal view of neck and throat region

Ovarian Cancer Progression

Progression of Ovarian Cancer

Condition

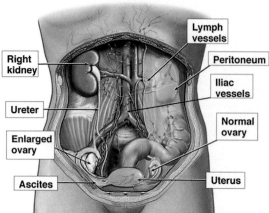

Right kidney

Ureter

Enlarged ovary

Ascites

Lymph vessels

Peritoneum

Iliac vessels

Normal ovary

Uterus

Anterior view of deep abdominal structures

"Serum pregnancy test should certainly be ordered for correlation with fluid around the right ovary and an enlarged appearance. If this is negative, follow up sono could be performed in one month to recheck the size of the right ovary. Endovaginal sono is recommended at this time."

"An endovaginal transducer is utilized to evaluate the uterus and ovaries. The left ovary measures 3.5 cm in greatest dimension. The right ovary, however is enlarged in appearance measuring 5 cm in greatest dimension. Ill defined echogenic area is seen probably hemorrhagic cyst. A mass in the ovary cannot completely be excluded and follow up is recommended to assure resolution to normal size."

Condition

Anterior view of deep abdominal structures

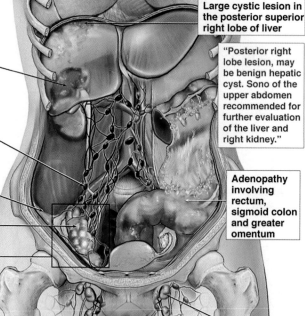

Right sided hydronephrosis consistent with partial obstruction of the right ureter secondary to tumor

Extensive bilateral iliac adenopathy and moderate retroperitoneal adenopathy

Ascites

Multiple lobulated 3-6 cm mass in the pelvis consistent with extensive metastatic disease.

Large cystic lesion in the posterior superior right lobe of liver

"Posterior right lobe lesion, may be benign hepatic cyst. Sono of the upper abdomen recommended for further evaluation of the liver and right kidney."

Adenopathy involving rectum, sigmoid colon and greater omentum

Bilateral adenopathy involving obdurator nerve

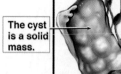

The cyst is a solid mass.

Prostate Cancer Progression

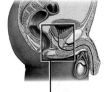

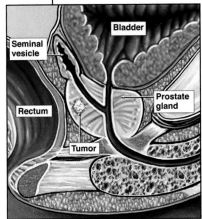

Early Stage Prostate Cancer

Bladder
Seminal vesicle
Rectum
Tumor
Prostate gland

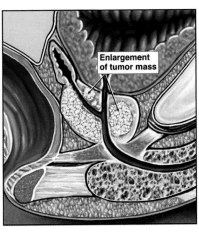

Subsequent Condition

Enlargement of tumor mass

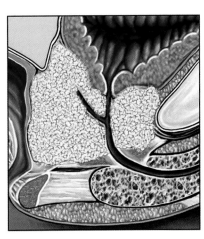

Eventual Condition

Sagittal views

Rectal Cancer Progression

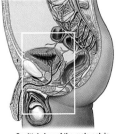

Sagittal view of the male pelvis

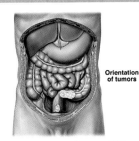

Orientation of tumors

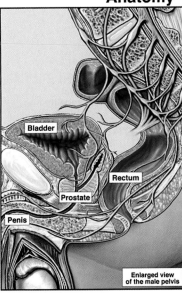

Normal Anatomy

Bladder
Prostate
Rectum
Penis

Enlarged view of the male pelvis

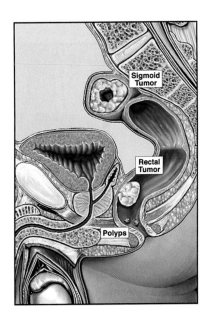

Subsequent Condition

Sigmoid Tumor
Rectal Tumor
Polyps

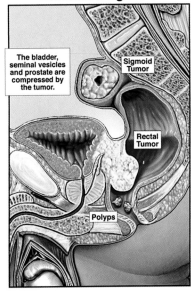

Eventual Diagnosis

The bladder, seminal vesicles and prostate are compressed by the tumor.

Sigmoid Tumor
Rectal Tumor
Polyps

Skin Cancer Melanoma Progression

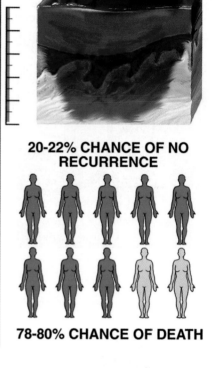

DIAGNOSIS OF SLIDE at least 0.5mm DEPTH

0.5mm

ENLARGED SECTION OF SKIN WITH MOLE IN SITU

90-95% CHANCE OF CURE

5-10% CHANCE OF DEATH

DIAGNOSIS OF SLIDE 2.5mm TO 2.6mm DEPTH

2.5-6mm

33% CHANCE OF NO RECURRENCE

67% CHANCE OF DEATH

DIAGNOSIS OF SLIDE 4.9mm DEPTH

4.9mm

20-22% CHANCE OF NO RECURRENCE

78-80% CHANCE OF DEATH

Stomach Cancer

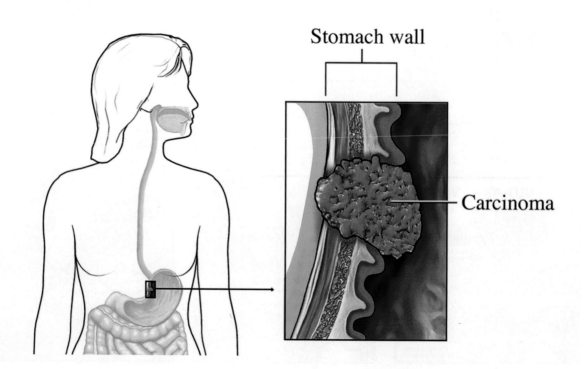

Stomach wall

Carcinoma

Uterine Cancer Progression

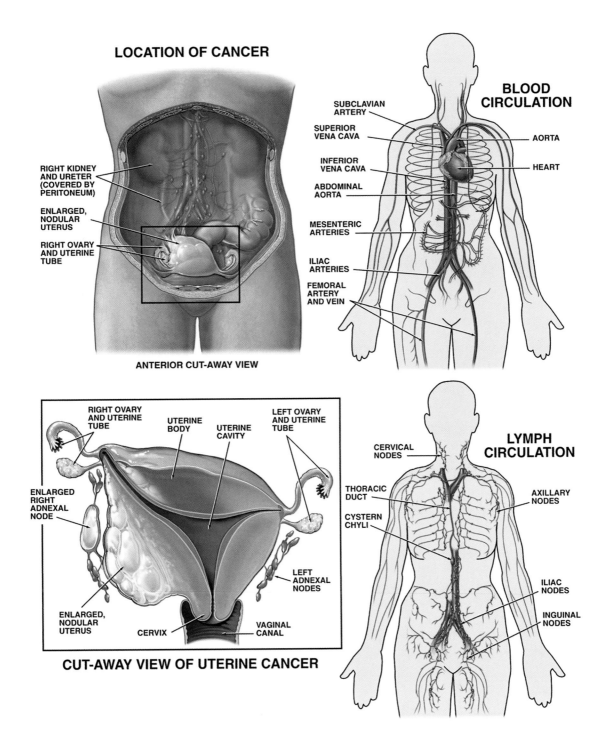

LOCATION OF CANCER

RIGHT KIDNEY AND URETER (COVERED BY PERITONEUM)

ENLARGED, NODULAR UTERUS

RIGHT OVARY AND UTERINE TUBE

ANTERIOR CUT-AWAY VIEW

BLOOD CIRCULATION

SUBCLAVIAN ARTERY

SUPERIOR VENA CAVA

INFERIOR VENA CAVA

ABDOMINAL AORTA

MESENTERIC ARTERIES

ILIAC ARTERIES

FEMORAL ARTERY AND VEIN

AORTA

HEART

RIGHT OVARY AND UTERINE TUBE

UTERINE BODY

UTERINE CAVITY

LEFT OVARY AND UTERINE TUBE

ENLARGED RIGHT ADNEXAL NODE

LEFT ADNEXAL NODES

ENLARGED, NODULAR UTERUS

CERVIX

VAGINAL CANAL

CUT-AWAY VIEW OF UTERINE CANCER

LYMPH CIRCULATION

CERVICAL NODES

THORACIC DUCT

CYSTERN CHYLI

AXILLARY NODES

ILIAC NODES

INGUINAL NODES

Testis Cancer, Metastatic

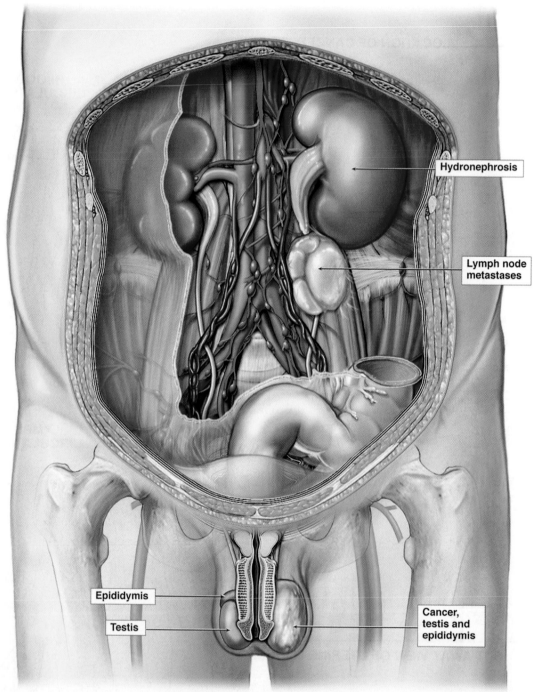

Hydronephrosis

Lymph node metastases

Epididymis

Testis

Cancer, testis and epididymis

Anterior cut-away view of abdomen and pelvis

Pelvic Cancer, Widespread

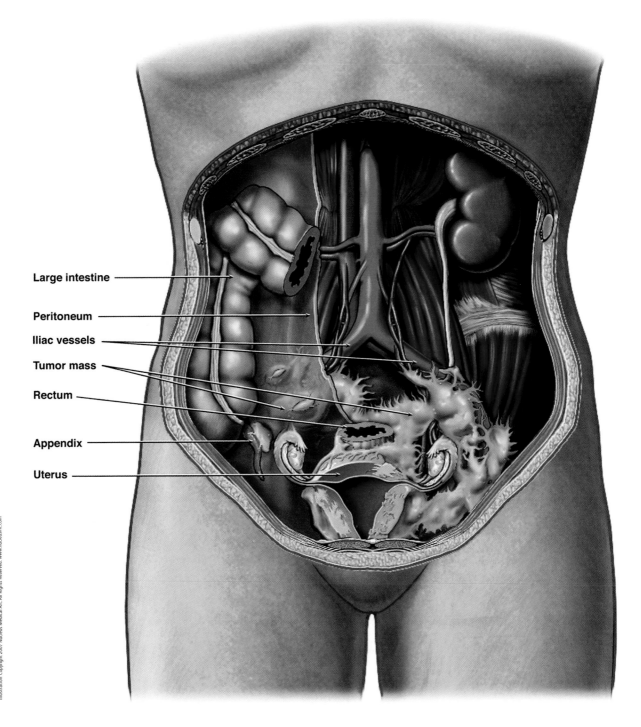

Large intestine

Peritoneum

Iliac vessels

Tumor mass

Rectum

Appendix

Uterus

Abdominal Tumor Mass

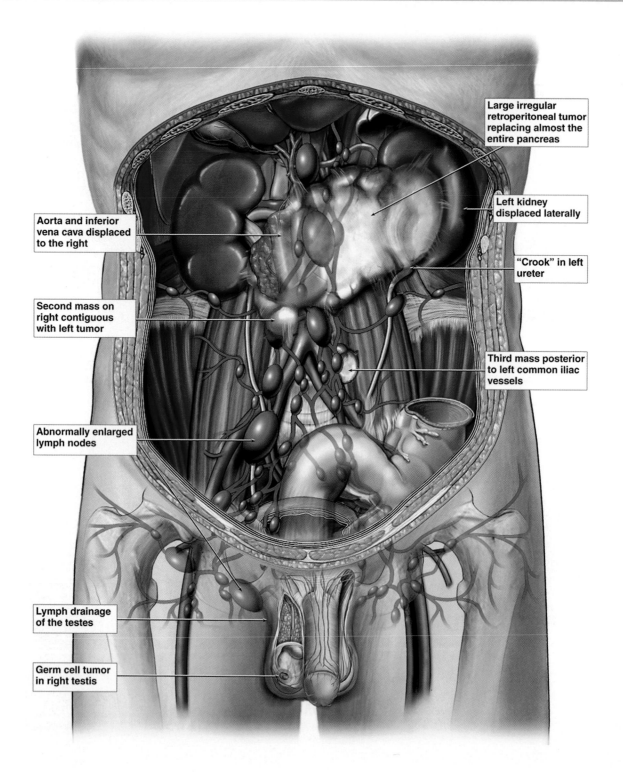

Large irregular retroperitoneal tumor replacing almost the entire pancreas

Left kidney displaced laterally

Aorta and inferior vena cava displaced to the right

"Crook" in left ureter

Second mass on right contiguous with left tumor

Third mass posterior to left common iliac vessels

Abnormally enlarged lymph nodes

Lymph drainage of the testes

Germ cell tumor in right testis

Bilateral Nasal Cancer with Surgical Removal

Pre-operative Condition

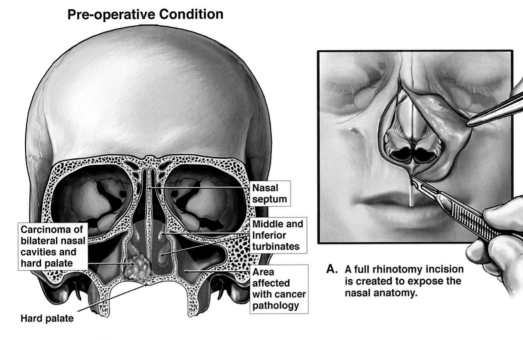

Nasal septum

Carcinoma of bilateral nasal cavities and hard palate

Middle and Inferior turbinates

Area affected with cancer pathology

Hard palate

Anterior cut-away view

A. A full rhinotomy incision is created to expose the nasal anatomy.

B. The nasal septum is resected along with the bilateral medial maxillectomies.

C. A saw is used to remove the hard and soft palates and the remaining tumor.

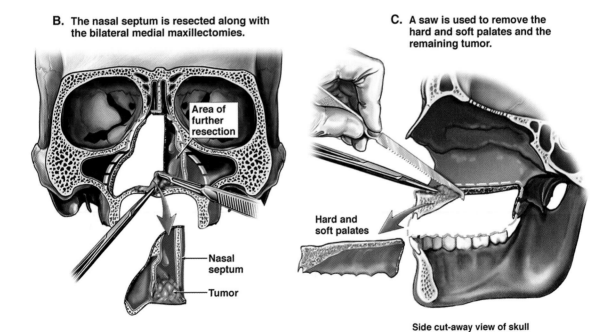

Area of further resection

Nasal septum

Tumor

Hard and soft palates

Side cut-away view of skull

Brain Tumor with Compression of Adjacent Structures

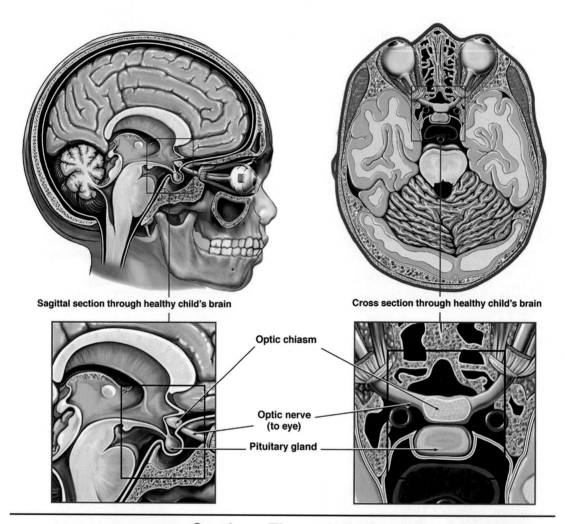

Sagittal section through healthy child's brain

Cross section through healthy child's brain

Optic chiasm

Optic nerve
(to eye)

Pituitary gland

Sections Through Brain

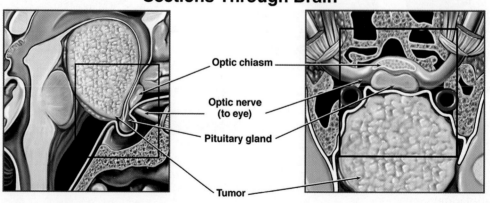

Optic chiasm

Optic nerve
(to eye)

Pituitary gland

Tumor

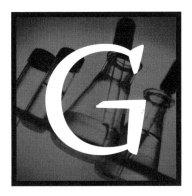

Gallbladder Cancer

CANCER OF THE gallbladder is considered to be a highly fatal cancer that caused approximately 3,200 deaths in the United States in 2006. Most cases are incidentally found and are in an advanced stage on discovery. Early detection by monitoring risk factors, symptoms, and diagnostic workups can influence treatment options and outcomes of this aggressive cancer.

Gallbladder cancer is the seventh most-common gastrointestinal tumor. It affects women two to six times more than men, and the incidence increases with age. Caucasians have a 50 percent greater incidence compared with African Americans. It tends to be a disease of the elderly, with a median age of diagnosis of approximately 65 years. The rates of gallbladder cancer are highest in South American countries and among the Native American population. The lowest incidences are in the United States and Singapore.

A number of risk factors are associated with the development of gallbladder cancer. The presence of long-term inflammation, such as gallstones (cholelithiasis), can increase the likelihood of tumors. It is thought that gallstones can promote mutations in the cells of the gallbladder that progress into cancer. Although the incidence of gallstone formation is common, only 0.3 percent to 3 percent of patients with gallstones develop gallbladder cancer. Long-term infections with different types of bacteria (i.e., *Salmo-*

nella, E. coli, and *H. pylori*) can increase the risk of cancer. The gallbladder can also have growths extending from its surface, called polyps, that can be malignant. A condition known as porcelain gallbladder, in which the wall of the gallbladder becomes covered with calcium deposits, has been associated with cancer in 20 percent of patients. Other causes include obesity, oral contraceptives, and chemicals from the rubber industry.

Although the risk factors may be quite specific, the patient may present with symptoms that are quite vague. Clinical symptoms usually include abdominal pain, weight loss, loss of appetite, nausea, and vomiting. Some patients develop jaundice (yellowing of the skin, tissues, or body fluids), abdominal distension, and itching. Early cancer may not show any symptoms and could be an incidental finding. An important issue that arises with gallbladder cancer is that often when symptoms develop, the cancer is in a noncurable state.

DIAGNOSIS AND TREATMENT

Various studies can be used to diagnose the presence of gallbladder cancer. Ultrasound is the usual diagnostic study when gallstone-related disease is suspected. Ultrasound can show thickened walls and masses, but it may not give a conclusive diagnosis of gallbladder cancer. Computed tomography (CT) scan gives a better picture of the extent of tumor growth and spread. Magnetic resonance cholangiopancreatography (MRCP) is used to visualize the local anatomy of the gallbladder and to differentiate between benign and malignant lesions. Biopsy of the gallbladder prior to surgery is not suggested due to the increased risk of the tumor's spreading to other areas.

Treatment of gallbladder cancer is dependent on the stage of the cancer. Staging determines the extent to which the cancer has grown or spread from the primary site. Treatment options run the gamut from simple cholecystectomy (removal of the gallbladder) to radical cholecystectomy (removal of the gallbladder, excision of specific bile ducts, removal of regional lymph nodes, and removal of parts of the liver) or to radiation therapy, chemotherapy, palliative care, or a combination of these options.

Cancer of the gallbladder has been shown to have a dismal prognosis in its advanced stages. Patients who have risk factors, as mentioned above, may benefit from examination of the gallbladder wall. Early diagnosis is the key to improving survival and cancer-related complications.

SEE ALSO: Anticancer Drugs; Bile Duct Cancer, Extrahepatic; Radiation Therapy; Surgery.

BIBLIOGRAPHY. A. Jemal, et al., "Cancer Statistics, 2006," *CA: A Cancer Journal for Clinicians* (v.56/106–130, 2006); S. Misra, et al., "Carcinoma of the Gallbladder," *The Lancet Oncology* (v.4/167–176, 2003); National Cancer Institute, "Surveillance Epidemiology and End Results," http://seer.cancer.gov (cited xxx); G. Leonard and E. O'Reilly, "Biliary Tract Cancer," in *Bethesda Handbook of Clinical Oncology* (Lippincott Williams & Wilkins, 2005); D. Bartlett, "Gallbladder Cancer, 2000," *Seminars in Surgical Oncology* (v.19/145–155, 2000); H. Wanebo and D. Savarase, "Gallbladder Cancer," www.uptodate.com (cited September 2005).

NAVIN ANTHONY, M.D.
PROVIDENCE HOSPITAL

Gasoline

GASOLINE IS A naturally occurring organic compound used to fuel gasoline engines. It is called gasoline in the United States, but it is called benzene, petrol, or other names in other countries. After the development of

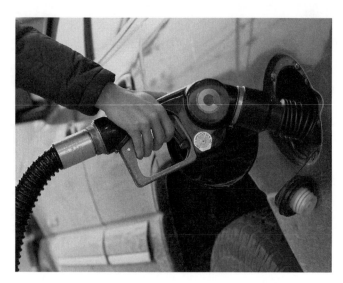

Many of the additives in gasoline, such as the antiknocking additives, have been classified as Group B2 carcinogens.

the internal combustion engine by German engineer Karl Benz in 1885, many carriage companies became "horseless carriage" companies and began to produce automobiles as an alternative form of transportation to the horse and buggy, and the railroads. The 1911 U.S. Circuit Court of Appeals decision allowed Ransom E. Olds, Henry Ford, and others to use four-cycle engines to build automobiles. This court decision opened the door to an explosion in the production of cars, especially after Henry Ford mastered the assembly-line process of production. Ford's Model A and Model T automobiles soon made automobiles affordable to most Americans and great numbers of people overseas. The nearly simultaneous discoveries of vast oil fields in Texas, Oklahoma, California, and many other places provided a steady supply of oil that could be refined into gasoline. During the 20th century the development of the global oil industry was driven by a quest for oil to be refined into gasoline.

Gasoline engines use a mixture of air and fuel. The mixture is exploded in sealed chambers, which may number one to eight or more. In automobiles, the number is between four and eight. The piston chambers may be arranged at an angle in V-6 or V-8 engines, for example, or they may be arranged perpendicular to the ground as straight piston motors.

The gasoline in a piston will not explode spontaneously, so a spark from a spark plug is used. The spark is produced in a gap between the plug and a metal flange. The result is an explosion inside the cylindrical chamber. The gasoline-and-air mixture is already compressed, so the explosion creates a very hot pressurized gas that pushes the piston out in a stroke that turns a crankshaft to accomplish work. The readiness of gasoline to ignite is measured by its octane rating. More specifically, the octane rating measures the resistance of the gasoline to premature ignition.

Millions of tons of gasoline are used in automobiles every year. The combustion of gasoline is a major cause of smog and other forms of air pollution. Much of the waste is carbon dioxide; however, many other compounds are in the exhaust fumes. These exhaust fumes pollute the atmosphere and can create numerous health problems.

Chemically, gasoline is C_8H_{14} plus other radicals that can or may be attached. It can be manufactured from anything containing carbon and hydrogen. Gasoline is found with the natural gas that accompanies petroleum. Natural gasoline is usually called casinghead gasoline. It is mixed with the enormous quantities of gasoline manufactured in oil refineries.

When crude oil is refined, gasoline is one of the products. Gasoline is made from the refracting process. Crude oil contains a complex mixture of hydrocarbons and at times other chemicals. In some few cases crude oil is almost pure enough to be taken from the ground and put into the lubricating system of an automobile. Quite often, however, it contains contaminants such as sulfur and metals.

Gasoline sold commercially contains more than just gasoline. The oil companies make gasoline tailored to meet the characteristics of climate and gasoline engines. An assortment of more than 25 compounds can be mixed with gasoline to make different kinds of fuels. One reason for the additive chemicals is that gasoline burns differently in different types of engines.

Certain types of gasoline may lead to engine misfires. The pistons in different types of gasoline engines have different compression and firing characteristics. Just simple gasoline put into most engines will not work well because the engine may misfire, knock, or ping. Gasoline composed of a straight chain of carbon atoms tends to knock badly when fired in a cylinder. High-compression engines and low-compression engines experience knocking or pinging from premature firing if the gasoline-and-air mixture is not suited to that type of engine.

Knocking occurs in an engine when the gasoline vapors and air in the cylinders explode spontaneously rather than burn at a uniform rate. When knocking occurs, it causes a loss of power in the engine. It can be prevented by using a gasoline mixture that does not explode spontaneously as the temperature and pressure in the engine increase.

Gasoline composed of many branched carbon chains or those with rings has a greatly reduced tendency to knock. Straight-chained hydrocarbons have low octane ratings. Ring-type hydrocarbons have intermediate octane ratings. High-branched alkanes and benzene-ring-shaped (aromatic) hydrocarbons have the highest octane ratings. Refiners have mastered the process for making gasoline blends composed of the branched and ringed forms of gasoline.

The antiknocking characteristics of hydrocarbons used in gasoline are designated by an octane rating. The octane rating is a number that indicates the tendency of a gasoline to knock in a high-compression engine. The higher the octane rating is, the lower is the tendency for an engine to knock. Iso-octane is a form of gasoline with an excellent antiknocking quality. It is used as a standard. Its rating is 100. By contrast, n-heptane has a 0 rating because it knocks so badly. If a gasoline has a rating of 90, it has a 90 percent mixture of iso-octane and a 10 percent mixture of n-heptane.

LEAD AND GASOLINE ADDITIVES

Lead is a soft metal that has been found to be useful in gasoline as an additive that prevents preignition or knocking. Although lead is not highly poisonous, it can be rendered toxic when it combines with acids or oxides. The lead in gasoline expelled from exhaust pipes poses a major health hazard. A common form of lead additive is lead tetraethyl: $Pb(c2H5)4$.

In the 1970s lead pollution was recognized by state and federal governments. Steps were taken to eliminate the use of lead in gasoline. By the 1980s most of the gasoline in the United States was no longer sold as leaded gasoline, allowing the amount of air pollution caused by automobiles to be reduced. Many other countries followed suit.

Gasoline additives are used to increase the octane rating, to inhibit corrosion, to act as lubricators, and to allow for greater compression ratios. The goal is to increase the efficiency of the burn in the piston cylinder. Several types of additives are used.

Metal deactivators are used to neutralize metal ions. The metal ions are usually present in the fuel because acids in the fuel system corrode the metal parts. The metal deactivators are especially aimed at lead and copper. A common metal deactivator is N,N'-disalicylidene-1,2-propanediamine, which, like other metal deactivators, blocks metal contaminants from oxidizing with hydrocarbon to form precipitates or gummy residue in the engine.

Corrosion inhibitors are additives that stop or slow corrosion of metal engine parts. Hydrazine has been used, but it is a carcinogen, so its use is being discouraged.

Oxygenates are additives that add oxygen to the explosive reaction that takes place when the fuel mixture in the piston is ignited. Some common fuel oxygenates are methyl tert-butyl ether, tert-amyl methyl ether, diisopropyl ether, ethyl tert-butyl ether, tert-amyl alcohol, and tert-butyl alcohol. Antioxidants inhibit free radicals.

CARCINOGENIC ADDITIVES IN GASOLINE

Many of the additives in gasoline, such as the antiknocking additives, are carcinogenic. Contemporary gasoline formulas have been classified by the U.S. Environmental Protection Agency as Group B2 carcinogens—possible human carcinogens. Experiments with aerosolized gasoline in laboratory animals produced tumors.

MTBE (methyl tertiary butyl ether) is an oxygenate that is a carcinogen. Perhaps more important than its residue as exhaust fumes or its industrial handling is its presence in groundwater. Gasoline left in underground storage tanks that later leaked into the ground and migrated into the local groundwater system contaminated drinking water. Considerable controversy has surrounded MTBE as a carcinogen. The International Agency for Research on Cancer has not found it to be a carcinogen; however, it has motivated politicians and courts in the United States to action.

Ethylbenzene is another common additive to gasoline. It has been classified by the IARC as a possible carcinogen because test results on laboratory animals showed likely cancerous cells following exposure.

SEE ALSO: Automobiles; Chemical Industry; Pollution, Air.

BIBLIOGRAPHY. L. Fishbein and I. K. O'Neill, eds., *Environmental Carcinogens: Methods of Analysis and Exposure Measurement, Benzene and Alkytated Benzenes* (International Agency for Research on Cancer, 1988); Art F. Diaz and Donna L. Drogos, eds., *Oxygenates in Gasoline: Environmental Aspects* (American Chemical Society, 2002); Magda Lovei, *Phasing out Lead from Gasoline: Worldwide Experience and Policy Implications* (World Bank Publications, 1998); Casare Maltoni, et al., eds., *Carcinogenesis Bioassays and Protecting Public Health: Commemorating the Life Work of Casare Maltoni and Colleagues* (New York Academy of Sciences, 2002); Ellen E. Moyer and Paul T. Kostecki, eds., *MTBE Remediation Handbook* (Kluwer Academic Publishers, 2004).

ANDREW J. WASKEY
DALTON STATE COLLEGE

Gastric (Stomach) Cancer

GASTRIC CANCER, ALSO commonly referred to as stomach cancer, is a malignancy (nonbenign, invasive, and spreading tumor) that develops in the stomach, one of many organs in the abdomen. Risk factors include smoking; men are more likely to develop stomach cancer, and infection with *H. pylori* also increases risk. Gastric cancer has the potential to metastasize (spread from its original spot to new body sites) throughout the stomach and to nearby organs, mainly the small intestine and esophagus. More aggressive gastric cancers may also spread to nearby lymph nodes and other organs, such as the colon, liver, pancreas, ovaries, and lungs.

The most common form of gastric cancer is adenocarcinoma, which is a malignant tumor arising from glandular tissue. In gastric cancer, cells that normally repair and reproduce in a controlled fashion begin to divide and grow uncontrollably, forming a lump (tumor) in the inner lining of the stomach. Sometimes these cancer cells form a diffuse tumor that spreads along the stomach lining without forming a distinct lump.

SCREENING AND DIAGNOSIS

Gastric cancer is often poorly diagnosed because its effects are asymptomatic or cause mainly nonspecific symptoms in the early stages of the disease. By the time noticeable symptoms manifest, the cancer has

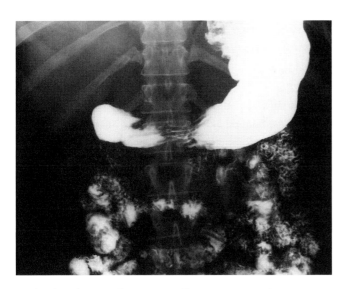

By the time that gastric cancer manifests symptoms, the cancer may have had a chance to metastasize to other parts of the body.

had a chance to metastasize to other parts of the body, resulting in relatively poor prognosis. Early signs and symptoms include heartburn, indigestion, and loss of appetite. These symptoms may eventually develop into abdominal pain, nausea and/or vomiting (possibly with blood), diarrhea or constipation, fatigue, weight loss, and bloody stool.

In screening for gastric cancer, the physician will ask about the patient's general medical history, perform a physical exam, and order laboratory tests. The initial screening test may be a fecal occult blood test (FOBT), looking for hidden blood in the feces, followed by a gastroscopic exam to visualize the upper part of the gastrointestinal (GI) tract and an upper-GI series to X-ray images of the esophagus and stomach, although computed tomography (CT) scanning and positron-emission tomography (PET) scanning may be used for more advanced cases. Abnormal tissue found will be biopsied and sent to a pathologist for histological examination and microscopic anatomical inspection, examining for the presence of cancerous cells.

Treatment for gastric cancer, like that for any other form of cancer, is tailored to the specific needs and general health of each individual, as well as the size, location, and stage of tumor spread. Therapy and management of stomach cancer may include surgery, chemotherapy, and/or radiation therapy, although new treatment options are being studied in clinical trials.

According to the National Cancer Institute, nearly 760,000 cases of gastric cancer are diagnosed worldwide each year. In the United States, gastric cancer represents only 2 percent (24,000 cases) of all new cancer cases each year, with a mortality rate of 12,400 per year. Worldwide incidence of gastric cancer has declined rapidly over recent decades, possibly due to better control of certain risk factors such as *Helicobacter pylori* bacterium and other dietary and environmental considerations, such as refrigeration of food. Only a very small percentage of gastric cancers is thought to be genetic, with studies currently in process.

SEE ALSO: Colon Cancer; Esophageal Cancer; Gastric (Stomach) Cancer, Childhood; Gastrointestinal Carcinoid Tumor.

BIBLIOGRAPHY. Daniel T. Dempsey, "Stomach: Malignant Neoplasms of the Stomach," in *Schwartz's Surgery* (McGraw-Hill, 2006); Paul C. Schroy, "Clinical Features and Diagnosis of Gastric Cancer," UpToDate Online, 2006.

NATANEL JOURABCHI
INDEPENDENT SCHOLAR

Gastric (Stomach) Cancer, Childhood

WITH STOMACH OR gastric cancer, cells of the stomach become abnormal and divide without control or order. Gastric cancer can develop anywhere in the stomach and spread into the esophagus or small intestine. It can also spread to nearby lymph nodes and to organs such as the liver, pancreas, colon, lungs, and ovaries.

INCIDENCE AND RELATED DISORDERS

Although the incidence of gastric carcinoma is on the decline, it remains the second-most frequently occurring cancer in the world. In the United States, African Americans, Hispanic Americans, and Native Americans are 1.5 to 2.5 times more likely to have gastric carcinoma than are whites. The disease is rare before the age of 40, but its incidence increases steadily until it peaks in the 70s. Men are twice as likely to develop gastric cancer as women.

In children, the risk of gastric cancer is greater among lower socioeconomic classes. An environmental exposure, probably beginning early in life, is related to the development of gastric cancer, with dietary carcinogens considered to be the most likely factor. Other factors contributing to this disease are overcrowding, poor sanitation, inadequate preservation of food, and poor nutrition.

The most common gastric or small-bowel cancer in children is lymphoma or lymphosarcoma. Abdominal pain that comes and goes, an abdominal mass, and a celiaclike picture may be present.

Helicobacter pylori infection, which causes gastritis and peptic ulcers, is also associated with the development of gastric cancer. Approximately 50 percent of the world population is infected with *H. pylori*, with the highest incidence in developing countries. *H. pylori* infection can be treated by antimicrobial therapy combined with a proton pump inhibitor, but no treatment regimen is 100 percent effective. Multiple drugs, frequent dosing, and length of treatment often contribute to poor patient compliance, and antibiotic eradication therapy is associated with increasing drug resistance. Carcinoid tumors, another type of cancer found in the stomach, are usually benign and most often an incidental finding in the appendix following appendectomy. Metastasis (spreading) is rare but can result in the carcinoid syndrome (flushing, sweating, hypertension, diarrhea, and vomiting), associated with serotonin secretion.

Cancer of the stomach is difficult to cure unless it is found in an early stage (before it has begun to spread). Unfortunately, because early stomach cancer causes few symptoms, the disease is usually advanced when the diagnosis is made. Early diagnosis is often impeded in socioeconomically deprived communities that lack readily available medical care and treatment. Still, even advanced stomach cancer can be treated, and its symptoms can be relieved. Treatments for stomach cancer may include surgery, chemotherapy, and/or radiation therapy. Investigations and clinical trials continue in the search for new treatments (e.g., biological therapy) and improved ways of using established therapeutic modalities. A patient may be given a single type of treatment or a combination of therapies.

SEE ALSO: Cancer Therapy Evaluation Program (CTEP); Chemotherapy; Childhood Cancers; Gastric (Stomach) Cancer; Gastrointestinal Carcinoid Tumor.

BIBLIOGRAPHY. Daniel Dempsey, *Schwartz's Surgery: Malignant Neoplasms of the Stomach* (McGraw-Hill, 2006); Robert Mayer, *Gastrointestinal Tract Cancer: Tumors of the Stomach* (McGraw-Hill, 2006); A. J. Shepherd, et al., "Childhood *H. pylori*: Disappearing Disease or Chronic Infection?" *British Journal of Community Nursing* (v.9/5, May 2004).

NAVID EZRA
DAVID GEFFEN SCHOOL OF MEDICINE AT UCLA

Gastrointestinal Carcinoid Tumor

GASTROINTESTINAL CARCINOID TUMORS are rare, slow-growing, enigmatic neoplasms that arise from the neuroendocrine cells of the gastrointestinal tract. The tumors have diverse presentation, characterized by hyperchromatic nuclei, necrosis, high mitotic activity, hormonal secretion, and malignant potential. Gastrointestinal carcinoids comprise 2 percent of all gastrointestinal tumors. The incidence of these tumors is approximately 2.5 in 100,000 people per year.

TUMOR CHARACTERISTICS

Neoplastic proliferations of neuroendocrine cells may occur throughout the entire gastrointestinal tract. They can affect the stomach and duodenum (foregut carcinoid tumors), appendix and ileum (midgut carcinoid tumors), and rectum (hindgut carcinoid tumors).

Foregut tumors may arise due to deletions and mutations of the MEN1 (Multiple Endocrine neoplasia type 1) gene. Midgut carcinoid tumors may display genetic aberrations on chromosome 18.

The majority of tumors arise from enterochromaffin cells of Kulchitsky, which are neural crest cells situated at the base of the crypts of Lieberkühn. These are glands found in the epithelial lining of the small intestine. Appendiceal tumors, however, may arise from Schwann-cell-related neuroendocrine cells in the submucosa layer.

Autocrine stimulation of EGF-R (epidermal growth factor receptor) by coexpression of TGF-alpha (transforming growth factor-alpha) is suggested as a possible cause for the development of hindgut carcinomas. Other risk factors for developing the disease include presence of other diseases, such as chronic atrophic gastritis associated with pernicious anemia and AIDS.

The tumors produce a variety of endocrine substances such as plasma CgA (chromogranin A), which can act as biochemical markers and are useful during diagnosis. Foregut carcinoids produce serotonin (5-hydroxytryptamine), gastrin, and somatostatin. Midgut carcinoids, often presenting with high metastatic tumor burdens, produce high levels of serotonin, serotonin breakdown products, tachykinins, and urinary 5-hydroxyindoleacetic acid. The hindgut carcinoids present with a wide spectrum of hormonal peptides, including insulin. Excessive levels of serotonin secreted by the carcinoids may exceed the capacity of the enzyme monoamine oxidase present in the liver and lung to metabolize serotonin, resulting in the carcinoid syndrome. This causes facial flushing, asthmatic wheeze, diarrhea, impotence, endocardial fibrosis, and tricuspid stenosis. Carcinoid syndrome is often the only clinical pattern diagnostic of carcinoid tumor.

Many techniques are available to help identify stage and differentiate the tumors. The use of endoscopic ultrasonography, computerized tomography, and magnetic resonance imaging, traditionally used to detect localized tumors, has been supplemented with techniques such as somatostatin receptor scintigraphy, a nuclear medicine imaging technique that uses the radioactive drug octreotide. The drug is similar to somatostatin in structure; thus, it attaches to tumor cells expressing receptors for somatostatin and, hence, enables detection of the location of tumor cells. Newer techniques such as positron emission tomography may challenge its position in the future.

The optimal curative therapy for carcinoid tumors is surgical excision, used to avert local manifestations and decrease hormone secretion. Surgically treated patients also have an increased survival rate, particularly those with carcinoids in the appendix and rectum.

Long-term therapy focuses on alleviating symptoms and stabilizing tumor growth, particularly for metastatic disease, using techniques such as radiofrequency catheter ablation to destroy cancerous cells.

Metastatic disease is associated with a poor overall prognosis of survival; however, many gastrointestinal tumors are localized and thus, long-term survival for the tumors is possible.

SEE ALSO: Carcinoid Tumor, Childhood; Radiation Therapy; Surgery.

BIBLIOGRAPHY. Icon Health Publications, T*he Official Patient's Sourcebook On Gastrointestinal Carcinoid Tumors: Directory For The Internet Age* (Icon Health Publications, 2004); I. M. Modlin, et al., "Therapeutic Options for Gastrointestinal Carcinoids," *Clinical Gastroenterology & Hepatology (v.4/5, 2006).*

FARHANA AKTER
KINGS COLLEGE, LONDON

Genentech (United States)

GENENTECH IS A medical biotechnology company headquartered in San Francisco, California. This well-known corporation has the distinction of being the first company to use living organisms and biological techniques to produce products that improve human health, and it is considered to be the first established biotechnology company. Since its conception, Genentech has designed numerous biologic-based therapies for the treatment of serious and life-threatening diseases that are now commercially available. Genentech is particularly invested in cancer research and has developed several highly successful anticancer therapeutic agents.

Genentech was incorporated in April 1976 by Robert A. Swanson and Dr. Herbert W. Boyer, a biologist at the University of California, San Francisco. Boyer, along with Stanley N. Cohen of Stanford University, described the first recombinant DNA technique in 1973. The groundbreaking discovery of recombinant DNA technology allowed scientists to exploit the fast-growing and replicative properties of bacteria to create large quantities of specific proteins. The name *Genentech* was chosen to signify the phrase *genetic engineering technology.*

Initially, the company sought out ways to harness these recombinant DNA techniques to engineer copies of important human molecules and develop new therapeutics. Synthesis of insulin (the first human protein to be synthesized), for example, was accomplished by a joint effort of Genentech and City of Hope National Medical Center.

Throughout the following decades, as advances in the fields of molecular biology, immunology, and others uncovered a deeper understanding of human disease at the genetic level, Genentech used the latest technology to research new methods of exploiting and interrupting abnormal molecular pathways involved in disease states. Several types of drugs created by Genentech are now approved treatments for diseases ranging from immunological and tissue growth and repair disorders to cancer.

The branch of Genentech devoted to research and production of cancer therapies is known as Genentech BioOncology™ and develops novel biologic-based therapeutic agents. Genentech BioOncology focuses primarily on four areas of human physiology affecting tumor pathogenesis: angiogenesis (new blood vessel growth); apoptosis (programmed cell death); B-cell biology (immune system lymphocytes); and human epidermal growth factor receptor (HER) signaling, a family of cell surface proteins involved in the regulation of cellular growth and development. Together, these and other molecular pathways that may facilitate the growth and survival of cancerous cells are targeted in the creation of novel antitumor drugs.

Genentech has created several therapeutic agents demonstrated to be highly effective in treating cancers. Noteworthy examples of Genetech's contribution to clinical oncology are Rituxan®, Avastin®, and Tarceva®.

Rituxan (rituximab) was the first in a class of treatments known as monoclonal antibody therapy (biologic therapy that stimulates a patient's own immune system to attack tumor cells) to be approved by the U.S. Food and Drug Administration for the treatment of cancer and is effective in several types of lymphoma.

Avastin (bevacizumab), another monoclonal antibody therapy, targets a protein known as VEGF that is involved in tumor blood vessel growth and maintenance; it is effective in certain cases of colorectal cancer and lung cancer.

Tarceva (erlotinib) is a small-molecule therapy that targets one of the HER proteins, HER1, and is active in certain types of lung cancer and pancreatic cancer.

In addition, several experimental cancer therapies are currently being evaluated for safety and efficacy at various stages of clinical development.

SEE ALSO: Biologic Therapy; Gene Therapy; Technology, New Therapies.

BIBLIOGRAPHY. Genentech, "First Successful Laboratory Production of Human Insulin Announced: September 6, 1978," www.gene.com (cited December 2006); Nicholas Wade, "Gene Splicing Company Wows Wall Street," *Science* (v.210, 1980).

ANDREW R. BRANAGAN
BEN-GURION UNIVERSITY OF THE NEGEV AND
COLUMBIA UNIVERSITY MEDICAL CENTER

Gene Therapy

GENE THERAPY PROVIDES new approaches in the treatment of many hereditary and acquired diseases. This emerging field offers novel potential therapeutic modalities. Recombinant DNA technology has brought the idea of treating gene-related diseases such as cancers by meddling with the gene structures. The term *gene therapy* indicates a spectrum of therapeutic procedures that includes using genetic materials to affect cells to reach an effective cure. We also can define gene therapy as a novel form of drug delivery that uses the patient's cells to produce agents with therapeutic effects. These procedures can be ex vivo or in vivo. Many preclinical studies have demonstrated the usefulness and efficacy of gene therapy.

Cancer has been the subject of many gene-therapy studies for several reasons. First, the increased knowledge of cancer molecular biology has revealed much information about genetic alterations causing different cancers. Also, many known genetic alterations give rise to cancers that can be targets for gene therapy. As a matter of fact, there are many options for designing a trial to test gene therapy on different cancers. The complex nature of the mechanisms behind genetic causes of cancers, however, has made gene therapy for cancer more difficult than for simple hereditary diseases. The emerging science of systems biology can solve this problem, as it considers all the factors causing cancer as a system. Second, the initial tools used in gene therapy, such as viruses, are being exploited as oncolytic agents by themselves. Finally, the lack of an efficient treatment option for many kinds of cancers has persuaded researchers to look at gene therapy as a possible novel approach in the treatment of cancer. Immunotherapy, oncolytic virotherapy, and gene transfer are the main approaches in cancer gene therapy, although the presence of RNA interference (RNAi) technology has introduced a new approach.

Candidate diseases considered for gene therapy include monogenic disorders such as hemophilia and many complex disorders, such as autoimmune disorders and cancers. For simple genetic diseases due to a mutation in a special gene, the process of gene therapy is to insert a normal functional gene into a target cell or tissue to replace the missed or defective gene. For polygenic disorders, the process of gene therapy involves insertion of genes stimulating the immune response, genes inducing cell death, genes affecting cellular information or processes, or genes producing a protein with special therapeutic properties. The case of nonhereditary diseases like cancers is like the latter. The aim of all gene-therapy methods is to reach an effective and stable expression of the modified genes in target cells or tissues for as long as needed. This aim must also imply the minimum side effects.

In general, there are two different ways to perform gene therapy. In the case of in vitro or ex vivo gene therapy, specific cells isolated from a subject are purified and, after genetic modification, are administered to the subject again. In the case of in vivo gene therapy, the genetic modification is performed by gene transferring into a subject's tissue using a vector. Although there are still many concerns regarding safety, social, and ethical issues, many clinical trials are being done to establish the efficacy of gene therapy in different diseases such as cancers. Many in vitro trials have used different gene-therapy models and have shown significant results.

Cancer gene therapy is a fast-growing field in medicine, and it will be one of the therapeutic modalities in cancer treatment in the near future. The available cancer therapeutic modalities have many negative side effects. Cancer gene therapy can play an important role in managing different kinds of cancers. In the lung-cancer model, for example, gene therapy has provided cancer vaccines with high efficacy; it also has increased survival benefits by introducing normal genes into cells to replace defective ones. Some tests have been done in preclinical studies on gliomas, liver cancer, and pancreatic cancers.

On September 14, 1990, researchers from the American National Institutes of Health started the first trial of gene therapy for treatment of a rare genetic disease named severe combined immunodeficiency (SCID). At that time, advances in molecular biology and genetic engineering had made it possible to sequence the human genome and clone it. This progress, plus the availability of methods and tools for modifying genetic materials, provided scientists the possibility to think about novel treatment of diseases at the genome level.

A 4-year-old girl named Ashanti Delsilva, who suffers from SCID as a genetic disease, was the first patient who underwent the first approved gene therapy. In a patient with SCID, the immune system does not work properly, and the patient is vulnerable to infections. The result of the first gene-therapy trial was hopeful, and Ashanti's immune system achieved higher performance after gene therapy, allowing her a normal life for some months. In this trial, some of Ashanti's white blood cells were isolated and grown in vivo. Then the defective gene causing SCID was replaced by a functional gene via gene transfer. The gene transfer was done with the help of genetic-engineering advances. Then the genetically modified white blood cells were infused into Ashanti's blood. Although this treatment worked for just a few months, it was the start of a new era of gene-therapy clinical trials.

In 1999 a patient participating in a gene-therapy trial died, and this event raised many questions about gene therapy and its use as a treatment.

METHODS OF GENE THERAPY

It is possible to perform gene therapy on both somatic cells (most of the cells of the body) and germ-line cells (such as sperm and ova). So far all the attempts to study the efficacy of gene therapy have been about gene therapy of somatic cells, because a complex procedure is required for gene therapy of germ-line cells. Germ-line-cell gene therapy involves many arguments about biomedical ethics, too.

Gene therapy of somatic cells is performed in vivo and ex vivo. In the in vivo type, the therapeutic interfering with genes is done on the cells in the body. In the ex vivo type, this process is done on the cells isolated from the body, and after gene modification, these cells are introduced to the body again for therapeutic results.

Vectors are tools for transferring genes into target cells or tissues. Although direct injection of naked DNA encoding a specific protein with a therapeutic role seems to be easy work, in practice it is necessary to upgrade this method by using other molecules and procedures. Vectors play an important role in this case. They can transfer genes into the nuclei of target cells while protecting genes from degradation and ensuring the final transcription of the transferred genes.

Vectors must be easy to use in clinical studies; however, it must be possible to produce and purify them in large amounts and at high concentrations inexpensively. Some kinds of vectors for gene therapy have all the properties explained.

Viral vectors such as retroviral, adenoviral, and adeno-associated viral vectors are common vehicles for gene transfer. The process of gene transfer into cells by viral vectors is called gene transduction. Nonviral vectors such as plasmids and liposomes are used as gene-transferring tools in a process called gene transfection.

Both viral and nonviral vectors have advantages and disadvantages. Although no complete and ideal vector has been introduced, viral and nonviral vectors are widely used in gene-therapy trials.

Other kinds of vectors used in cancer gene therapy are bacterial vectors, which have the advantage of targeting the gene therapy. The most recent generation of vectors includes hybrid vectors.

Viruses can easily introduce their DNA into cells with very high efficacy. This characteristic is used for making viral vector systems. Insertion of a therapeutic gene into the genome of a virus by genetic-engineering technology and using the properties of the virus to deliver this gene with high efficacy in target cells is the general feature of a viral vector system.

Viral vectors are developed by genetic modifications of a variety of viruses, including retroviruses, adenoviruses, poxviruses, parvoviruses (adeno-associated viruses, or AAV), herpes viruses, and others. The viruses used as vectors are engineered to be different from wild types. In fact, viral vectors do not have the ability to replicate and infect because they are supposed to deliver a therapeutic gene into target cells without any other viral activity. After the genetic-engineering process, the viral vector looses some of its genes to loose reproducing ability in target cells. The engineered viral vector can replicate only in a cell line that supplies the deleted function. Loosing the replication ability provides a safety condition in which the virus is just a vehicle for transferring a gene without any other activity, but it is necessary to produce very high amounts of viral vectors. For this reason, packaging cell lines have been developed. These

special cell lines can replace a function of a deleted viral gene for the production of recombinant viruses.

Sometimes the interaction of viral vector and a host-cell genome is inevitable because of the reactivation of the virus. In the process of recombination, the therapeutic vector can get the loosed gene and achieve its pathologic properties again. It means that the new reactivated vector may miss the therapeutic gene and can be a source of infection in the target cells. This is one of the limitations that must be noted in using viral vectors.

Adenoviruses are double-strand DNA viruses that do not have an envelope. Their genome size is about 36kb encoding 50 viral polypeptides. Adenoviruses are the most common vectors that are best described and widely used. There are different serotypes of adenoviruses, but the most commonly used serotypes are type 2 and type 5. Adenoviruses are associated with many human disorders, which has made them suitable for use as gene-therapy vectors in different diseases. Although adenoviruses have been shown to have useful capabilities to be powerful vectors, there are some disadvantages for their application as vectors, such as their complexity, stability, and wide cell specificity.

Retroviruses are small RNA viruses. Their replication is via a DNA intermediate. These viruses are among the first viral vector systems for gene therapy. The genome of a retrovirus includes few genes, and it is possible to replace the pathologic viral genes with the therapeutic genes. This process will make the virus unable to replicate. It is a good point for using retroviruses as viral vector systems. Like other kinds of vectors, retrovirus vectors have some limitations, such as low transfection efficacy.

Adeno-associated viruses are kinds of parvoviruses. These viruses are single-strand DNA viruses that do not have any virus envelope. The most common AAV vector is made from serotype 2 of these viruses. The viruses can infect a wide range of human and other mammalian cells, and they can ensure a long-lasting expression of therapeutic transferred genes. AAV gene-delivery systems have been used successfully in gene therapy for some disorders, including cystic fibrosis and hemophilia A. Preclinical application of these vector systems has had hopeful results for treatment of myocardial infarction, liver cirrhosis, and colon and pancreatic cancers. Lack of a host cellular immune response has made AAV

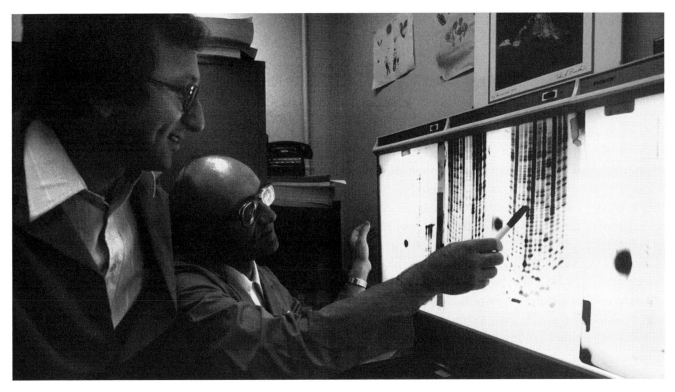

Research scientists examining the genetic code in the DNA. Cancer gene therapy is a fast-growing field in contemporary gene therapy. Immunotherapy, oncolytic virotherapy, and gene transfer are the main approaches in cancer gene therapy.

vector systems a very efficient and promising delivery system in gene therapy.

The herpes simplex virus (HSV) is a double-strand DNA virus with no envelope. Gene transfer vectors are based on HSV type-I (HSV I). The most important benefit of HSV-based vectors is their high cloning capability for foreign genes because of the big genome of these viruses. In fact, there are many genes in the virus genome to be deleted and replaced by a big therapeutic gene or several small therapeutic genes.

Poxviruses, which are derived from vaccinia virus, are other viruses for making viral delivery systems. They can be engineered by insertion of the therapeutic gene directly into the vaccinia genome; it is not necessary to delete or inactivate any gene in the virus genome. The cloning ability of these vectors is high, but the replication ability is a problem that can cause side effects.

There are other viruses that are used in gene therapy as delivery systems. All the viral vector systems have both significant benefits and disadvantages. Development of more efficient viral vectors depends on the progress in genetic engineering to increase the advantages and decrease the disadvantages of these vectors.

Nonviral vector systems are other tools for gene transferring. These vectors are safer than viral vectors and can be more easily used. It is possible to produce these vectors in large amounts. This property and their low host immunogenicity have made them more applicable than viral vectors.

A nonviral vector is a molecule of DNA with the therapeutic gene; its expression is dependent on the host-cell transcription and translation system. The advantages of using nonviral vectors include low toxicity, virtually unlimited clone capacity, low immunogenicity, and capability of repeated application.

Oligodeoxynucleotides, lipoplexes, and polyplexes are common nonviral vectors. Naked plasmid DNA is the simplest nonviral vector. Naked plasmid DND has been used in many clinical and preclinical trials as DNA vaccination.

Synthetic oligodeoxynucleotides are one of the nonviral vectors; they inhibit the expression of the genes responsible for a disease. Lipoplexes are a combination of plasmid DNA and lipids. In fact, in lipoplex plasmid DNA is covered by lipids into organized structure like liposomes or micelles. This facilitates the effective transfer of DNA into target cells while keeping it intact from any degradation. Vectors made from a combination of polymers and DNA are called polyplexes. Polylysine is an example of polyplexes. Although nonviral vectors are safer than viral vectors, the improvement of their safety is important. The idea of omitting the sequences that have no relation to therapeutic sequence can help increase their safety.

As viral and nonviral vectors have their own advantages and disadvantages, a new generation of vectors has been made using both technologies.

Virosomes are the most common types of hybrid vectors. They are made by fusion of lipoplex with inactivated HVJ (hemaglutinating virus of Japan) or influenza virus. In hybrid vector technology, the main aim is to use the advantages of both viral and nonviral vectors while decreasing their limitations.

Bacterial vectors are used in cancer gene therapy. Hypoxia is a good indicator of a tumor area. Some kinds of anaerobic bacteria can colonize selectively in a hypoxic area. This ability is very useful for using these kinds of bacteria as vectors for targeting gene therapy. Bacterial vectors can transfer therapeutic genes, genes encoding toxins, protein stimulating the immune response, and cytokines into tumor tissue in the course of cancer gene therapy.

Two groups of bacterial vectors have had significant results in tests. The first group consists of the strictly anaerobic bacteria, including the *Clostridium* and *Bifidobacterium* species, which have been used during in vivo trials and showed positive results. The second group consists of attenuated auxotrophic strains of *Salmonella typhimurium*. The bacteria in this group need tumor-specific nutrition factor for selective replication in tumor tissue. They use these nutrients for their own metabolism and inhibit the cancer cells to use them and grow.

Cancer gene therapy is a fast-growing field in contemporary gene therapy. Several cancer vaccine treatments are in last-stage trials, and gene-transfer technology shows hopeful hints for increasing the efficacy of current chemotherapy regimens. Progresses in oncolytic virotherapy are increasing, giving hopes for passing current obstacles. The completed clinical trials and ongoing clinical trials will provide us the information we need to evaluate the use of gene therapy as a formal cancer therapeutic modality. Clinical-trials data will reveal the significance of preclinical studies' results.

The most important challenge in cancer gene therapy is the impact of gene therapy on noncancerous cells. In other words, there are still unsolved problems in targeting cancer cells while keeping other tissues intact. It is one of the necessities for practicing gene therapy in clinical settings. In fact, the specificity of cancer gene therapy is still an item to be noted. Regarding this problem, we should be able to discriminate cancer cells from normal cells when performing gene therapy based on the properties of cancer cells.

There are some unique characteristics in the microenvironment of cancer. Properties such as hypoxia and presentation of necrotic areas are useful items for this purpose. These kinds of properties of a cancer microenvironment are good indicators of cancer tissues. It is possible to apply hypoxia-sensitive elements in a vector so that the gene on the vector can be expressed only in target cancer cells.

Another way to limit the effects of gene therapy in cancer cells is to use toxin precursors that are capable of being activated in a hypoxic condition. In other word, it is possible to administer agents with the ability to induce tumor-specific toxicity. This form of gene therapy is possible by using bacterial systems as vectors for transferring genes in target tumor tissues.

APPLICATION OF IMMUNOTHERAPY

For the past 100 years, the idea of stimulating or boosting the immune system to target cancer cells has existed as a method of cancer treatment. The main challenge for putting this idea in practice has been the ability of cancer cells to escape immune-system detection via some complex mechanisms. New gene-therapy techniques can help overcome this problem.

Creating recombinant DNA vaccines is a common procedure in gene therapy. These vaccines differ from vaccines used for infectious diseases because they are used to cure the disease, not to prevent the disease. In fact, these vaccines boost the patient's immune system to detect cancer cells by presenting it highly antigenic and immunostimulatory cellular debris.

In making a recombinant vaccine for cancer treatment, cancer cells are first isolated from the patient as autologous cells or from the established cancer cell lines as allogenic cells. Then these cells go under the genetic-engineering processes to be more easily detected by the immune system of the patient. To make the cells more recognizable by the immune system, one or more genes, which are often cytokine genes, are added to the cells. These new genes produce proinflammatory immune-stimulating molecules. The engineered cells are grown in vitro and then are killed. Their cellular contents are used to prepare a recombinant vaccine.

Another option in immunotherapy is to transfer immunostimulatory genes such as cytokines to the tumor tissue in vivo.

A very interesting procedure in immunotherapy is the direct change in a patient's immune system to be sensitive to cancer cells via gene therapy. One approach applies mononuclear circulating blood cells or bone marrow gathered from the patient. The selected cell type is altered by adding a tumor antigen. The modified cells can cause an immune reaction to the cancer cells, leading to the eradication of cancer. In other methods, the gene can added in vivo by a vector.

There are some clinical trials on immunotherapy for different cancers. These ongoing clinical trials are testing immunotherapy and cancer vaccines for prostate cancer, pancreatic cancer, kidney cancer, melanoma, and lymphoma. It seems that cancer vaccines will be among the cancer treatment options in the future, as early preclinical cancer-vaccine models have shown positive significant results.

One of the challenges in using immunotherapy is the very low response of cancer self-antigen. Although vaccines used for infectious diseases generally lead to antigen-specific T-cell precursors in the range of 10 percent, the response for self-antigens of cancer is often less than 1 percent. Even if a successful immune response is achieved in a clinical trial, maintaining it may be difficult. For more efficacy, the next generation of cancer vaccines must deal with this problem.

Recently, the idea of using cancer vaccines in combination with other therapeutic modalities has been developed so that cancer vaccines can be used as an adjuvant therapy after surgery or chemotherapy.

Emerging gene therapy made it possible to put a 100-year-old idea into clinical practice. Before the birth of gene therapy, oncolytic agents had been proposed as the agents capable of targeting cancer cells and destroying them. In cancer gene therapy, these oncolytic vectors are genetically engineered viral viruses that can destroy cancer cells while not meddling with normal tissue. These oncolytic vectors first infect cancer cells and then induce cell death via propagation of the virus, expression of cytotoxic proteins, and cell lysis.

Vaccinia, adenovirus, HSV type I, reovirus, and Newcastle disease virus are common oncolytic vectors in cancer gene therapy. These viruses have two useful characteristics that made them candidates to be selected as oncolytic vectors: They have the ability to target cancer tissues, and they can be easily modified by genetic-engineering techniques.

Oncolytic therapy is a powerful gene-therapy method based on performed trials; it has been used in animal models for treatment of bladder cancer, colon cancer, and osteosarcoma with significant positive results. Although this method works well in animal models, its applications in humans is still facing some limitations. In the human body, antibodies for the viral vectors are used as oncolytic agents, and the immune system of the patient can easily destroy the vector before it can affect the cancer cells. The use of the replication-competent viral particles often needs a very high safety measurement; for this reason, performing a clinical trial using oncolytic therapy is expensive and hard. This obstacle will be passed by development of powerful new vector systems.

So far, there have been some ongoing clinical trials using oncolytic therapy. The most notable adenovirus therapy undergoing clinical trial for intractable cancer is the ONYX-015 viral therapy. ONYX-015 is an adenovirus engineered to lack the viral E1B protein. The other type of oncolytic therapy undergoing clinical trials uses HSV type I (HSV-1). Two vectors, G207 and NV1020, are currently in phase I and phase II trials for treatment of intractable cancers. The technology of oncolytic therapy is a growing field, and there are still many challenges to overcome regarding using this technology.

Gene transfer is one of the most common methods in gene therapy that has been used widely against cancers. The main aim of this method is to replace a defective or missed gene with a functional one. It is possible to insert normal functional genes into cells or tissues to replace a target abnormal gene. For insertion of genes into host cells, a number of different vectors are available. The type of the vector is determined by the desired specificity of the gene-transfer therapy and also the time needed for the gene to be functional in the host cell and have an effective result.

Gene-transfer technology consists of a very wide spectrum of modalities. Many initial trials have established the efficacy of this method in different cancer treatments, and many clinical trials are being done on different kinds of cancers using the gene-transfer procedure. Rexin-G for prostate cancer, HDVtk for glioblastoma, p53 for head and neck cancers, MDA-7 for melanoma, and TNF-α for pancreatic cancer are the genes that are being used in ongoing clinical trials of gene-transfer technology.

As many genes are involved in the development of a cancer, transferring one gene into cancer cells to replace a defective one may not have high efficacy, which is one of the limitations of using gene-transfer technology. As the scenario behind cancer is a very complex phenomenon, and one single genetic alteration seems to be insufficient to describe all the processes of cancer development, we need to study the genetic factors causing cancers in a systems-level approach. In this approach, we will understand the whole system leading to a cancer, and with this understanding, it will be easy to design more accurate gene-therapy methods.

Recently, the technology of RNAi has affected a great deal in the field of gene therapy. In RNAi technology, double-strand RNA is used to inhibit the expression of a specific gene. For targeting messenger RNA (mRNA) and performing a posttranscriptional gene therapy, short interference RNA (siRNA) or silencing RNA is used. RNAi is a short oligonucleotide of about 19 to 23 nucleotides with a high specificity for target genes. Application of siRNA in cancer gene therapy has had very good results so far, and many trials are being done to test this technology for different kinds of cancers.

Despite the powerful abilities of siRNA, there are still many challenges ahead in using it to fight cancers. The mode of delivery, the precise sequence of the siRNA used, and cell-type specificity are some of the main challenges.

CANCER SYSTEM BIOLOGY

Gene therapy is a method that interferes with genes. In many complex diseases, such as cancers, many genes play roles, and these genes have many complex interactions, so it is not wise to hope for a significant result when we deal with only one gene in gene therapy. Systems biology is the science of studying biologic systems as a whole; its aim is to explore the complexity of interactions in biologic systems. As in the case of gene therapy, cancers have been among the most interesting cases to be studied by this new science. Study of cancer as a complex disease in systems biology will reveal the exact mechanisms of gene expressions and gene-networks interactions, which will lead to improvements in the techniques and targets used in gene therapy.

ETHICAL AND SOCIAL ISSUES

From the birth of gene therapy, there have been different questions from the perspective of ethical and social issues. The debates about these items gave birth to a new field that focuses on preparing research protocols for genetic engineering and gene therapy. Differences between somatic-cell and germline-cell gene therapy constituted a cornerstone in distinguishing between appropriate and inappropriate types of genetic interventions. It is believed that somatic-cell gene therapy is not a real intervention in genes, but a kind of extension of former therapeutic methods. For this reason, there are limited ethical challenges regarding using it. It seems that this idea is generally accepted, as somatic-cell gene therapy will help producing the same medications as conventional therapies. In SCID, for example, we can infuse the enzyme ADA, which is missed because of a gene defect in the bloodstream of the patient, as a conventional therapy. When we perform gene therapy for SCID, we help the white blood cells of the patient produce ADA by themselves. Then this gene therapy is similar to conventional therapy.

Most concerns about the ethical issues of gene therapy are about germ-line-cell genetic engineering, which is believed to be a kind of modification of the blueprint of human beings. Also, one of the early debates in somatic-cell gene therapy was about the possible effect of engineered genetic materials on germline cells such as sperm and ova and their precursors inherited by the patient's offspring. But by selecting vectors and methods of somatic-cell gene therapy in a careful manner, this problem is solved.

Although there have been limited arguments recently about using somatic-cell gene therapy, the debate over germ-line gene therapy has not been solved yet.

Despite the many benefits of gene therapy, its possible harms must be noted, and there should be studies evaluating these matters. The conclusion is that as genetic knowledge such as the knowledge of gene therapy grows, the wisdom of using it in a proper way must be increased with regard to social and ethical fundamentals.

FUTURE PERSPECTIVE

There has been much interest in using gene therapy for treatment of different cancers because cancer is a leading cause of death around the world. Cancer gene therapy is still in its infancy, but it is growing fast, giving hope for exciting results in the future. Development of new and safer methods of gene therapy is of high importance. Designing better new vectors will improve the easy design of gene-therapy methods for cancers. As cancer is a complex disease, the systems and integrative-biology approach will create a new understanding of the gene interactions causing cancers. This is vital for improving cancer-gene-therapy efficacy because understanding the mechanisms causing cancers at systems level will lead to an efficient and accurate designation of gene-therapy methods.

The new technology of RNAi or gene silencing can play an important role in cancer gene therapy in the near future. With the growing attention to gene therapy as an emergent treatment for cancer, social and ethical challenges are being raised. There is a real need for study of the social and ethical issues regarding gene therapy and the questions surrounding it.

SEE ALSO: Biologic Therapy; Drugs; Future of Cancer; Technology, New Therapies; Vaccines.

BIBLIOGRAPHY. Denna Cross, "Gene Therapy for Cancer Treatment: Past, Present and Future," *Journal of Clinical Medicine and Research* (v.4/3, 2006); Helen M. Blau and Matthew L. Springer, "Molecular Medicine, Gene Therapy: A Novel Form of Drug Delivery," *The New England Journal of Medicine* (v.333/18, 1995); Kevin C. Kelley, *Treatment of Hemophilia Monograph Series, Number 17* (World Federation of Hemophilia, 2000); Leland H. Hartwell, et al., *Genetics: From Genes to Genomes* (McGraw-Hill Higher Education, 2000); Robert M. Sade and George Khushf, "Gene Therapy: Ethical and Social Issues," *Journal of South Carolina Medical Association* (v.94/9, 1998); Ruben Hernandez-Alcoceba, et al., "Gene Therapy of Liver Cancer," *World Journal of Gastroenterology* (v.12/38, 2006); Roman Gardlik, et al., "Vectors and Delivery Systems in Gene Therapy," *Journal of Medical Sciences Monitor* (v.11/4, 2005); Wei Lv, et al., "RNAi Technology: A Revolutionary Tool for the Colorectal Cancer Therapeutics," *World Journal of Gastroenterology* (v.12/29, 2006).

IMAN TAVASSOLY
MAZANDARAN UNIVERSITY OF MEDICAL SCIENCES, IRAN
OMID TAVASSOLY
TARBIAT MODARES UNIVERSITY, IRAN

Genetics

EVER SINCE THE domestication of plants and animals began some 15,000 years ago, humans have wondered why and how the characteristic traits of parents are transmitted to their offspring. The earliest theories put forward by Greek philosophers were based on conjecture and superstition. These theories were acceptable until modern genetics entered the arena in the late 19th century, following the experiments of Austrian monk Gregor Mendel.

Genetics is a branch of biology that deals with genes and their inheritance. Genes may be considered to be pieces of biological information that parents pass to their offspring and are present in all living organisms. All things in nature—such as a person's height, the color of a rabbit's fur coat, the shape of a leaf, and the taste of a fruit—are dictated by genes.

The major challenge facing geneticists is understanding how all this information is stored in cells, how is it transmitted from one generation to the next, and why a slight variation in genetic code changes an organism's growth or even causes disease and death. Modern geneticists are beginning to understand genetic variability and heredity while also participating in and benefiting from rapid progress in other fields, such as molecular biology, biochemistry, and cell biology. Genetic engineering, a branch of modern genetics, is a technique used by geneticists to modify the very genes of an organism. Although genetic engineering has been a boon to the advancement of medicine and science, it has also been covered in the news media due to various ethical and legal issues.

DNA AND RNA

Although all humans have the same set of genes, a slight variation in alleles can make each person genetically unique. The basic vehicle for transmitting genes from one generation to the next is DNA, also known as deoxyribonucleic acid. DNA is stored as a supercoiled molecule called a chromosome found inside the nuclei of cells. Segments of DNA that contain all the information required for synthesis of a product (polypeptide chain or RNA molecule) and that include both the coding and noncoding sequences are called genes. Genes dictate the synthesis of proteins, which carry out all life's functions in a living cell.

Today, genetics is playing an increasing role not only in healthcare, but also in other areas of society. Fruits have been genetically modified so that they taste and look better, and can last longer. Certain fruits and vegetables are being modified to carry vaccinations inside them so that in the near future, getting vaccinated against hepatitis B would simply be a matter of eating a genetically altered potato. Additionally, these vaccine fruits and vegetables could be transported to remote areas in Third World countries that may lack health personnel to administer vaccine injections.

Milk-producing cows have been genetically altered to produce more milk during their lives, and cattle raised for food have been genetically modified to grow faster.

Furthermore, genetics is playing a crucial role in criminal investigations. DNA collected from blood, hair, semen, and skin samples at the crime scene is compared with the DNA from the suspect. Numerous court cases have been in the news lately, involving some unfortunate people who were wrongly convicted many years ago and are now been freed because their DNA tests came back negative.

Genetics has also led to the development of the Human Genome Project, an international collaboration to sequence the complete human genome, defined as the total of all the genetic information encoded in every nucleated cell of the human body. The Human Genome Project is already revolutionizing genetics by providing insights into many diseases and promoting the development of better diagnostic tools, preventive measures, and therapeutic methods in the near future. Finally, genetics has led to the development of gene therapy, a relatively new experimental procedure during which abnormal diseased genes are replaced by healthier ones.

BASIC PRINCIPLES OF GENETICS

Most hereditary units of cells are located in the nucleus. These units are called genes, which direct cellular activities and control cellular structure. Human so-

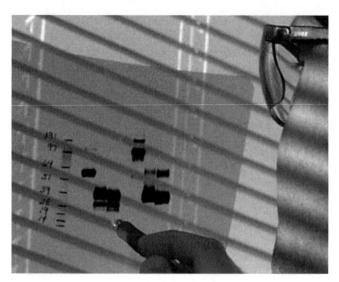

A researcher examining the genetic code sequence. There are 46 chromosomes, and each has a different sequence.

matic (body) cells have 46 (23 pairs) of chromosomes; 23 are inherited from each parent. Each chromosome is a long molecule of DNA that is coiled together by several proteins. This complex of DNA, proteins, and some RNA is called chromatin. The total of all genetic information in a cell is called a genome.

DNA is also contained within mitochondria in animal cells and chloroplasts in plant cells. It is very important for this genetic information to be transmitted from parents to offspring. Organisms cannot grow or function properly if this information is missing or defective. To convey genetic information to their descendants, living cells participate in two different types of cell division: mitosis and meiosis.

Mitosis (asexual reproduction) is used by prokaryotes, which are single-celled organisms. During mitosis, a cell doubles its DNA and then divides into two cells, evenly distributing DNA to each daughter cell.

Mitosis is a five-state process: prophase, metaphase, anaphase, telophase, and cytokinesis. During prophase, chromatin fibers condense into paired chromatids; the nucleolus and nuclear envelope disappear; and each centrosome moves to the center of the cell. In metaphase, the centromeres of chromatid pairs line up at the metaphase plate. In anaphase, the centromeres split; identical sets of chromosomes move to opposite poles of the cell. In telophase, the nuclear envelopes and nucleoli reappear; chromosomes resume chromatin form; and mitotic spindles disappear. Finally, in cytokinesis, a contractile ring forms a cleavage furrow around center of the cell, dividing the cytoplasm into separate and equal portions.

Meiosis (sexual reproduction) involves halving the number of chromosomes in a gamete cell; then the sperm and egg unite to form a zygote, which contains the full number of chromosomes. Meiosis occurs in two substages: meiosis I and meiosis II. Meiosis I is composed of prophase I, prometaphase I, metaphase I, anaphase I, and telophase I. Meiosis I is preceded by interphase I, during which DNA is replicated. Synapsis occurs during prophase I; the two homologs are joined by a complex of proteins that forms a tetrad, or bivalent, consisting of two homologous chromosomes with two sister chromatids each.

During prometaphase I, the nuclear lamina disintegrates, and the nuclear envelope breaks into small vesicles, permitting the fibers of the spindle to invade the nuclear region. Later, Golgi breaks down into vesicles. During metaphase I, the kinetochores arrive at the equatorial plate, and chromosomes are fully condensed and have distinguishable shapes.

The homologous chromosomes separate in anaphase I, while individual chromatid pairs are pulled to the poles, with one homolog of a pair going to one pole and the other homolog going to the opposite pole.

Meiosis II is similar to mitosis, but one difference is that DNA does not replicate before meiosis II. The number of chromosomes in the resulting cells is, therefore, half that found in diploid mitotic cells. In meiosis II, sister chromatids are not identical, and there is no crossing over. Thus, meiosis ensures that sexual reproduction will produce a zygote that has received one set of chromosomes from the male parent, and the other set from the female parent, to form a full set of chromosomes.

MENDEL'S LAWS

Mendel's experiments with pea plants revealed two fundamental principles of heredity: the law of segregation and the law of independent assortment. Mendel crossed white flowers with purple flowers and noted that the offspring had only purple flowers. He crossed the purple offspring among themselves, and the third generation came out to be 75 percent purple-flowered plants and 25 percent white-flowered plants.

Mendel concluded that the alleles for a character (which in this case is flower color) are packaged in separate gametes. In conclusion, purple flower is a dominant trait, and white flower is a recessive trait. This separation of alleles into separate gametes is summarized as Mendel's Law of Segregation.

Mendel's experiments that followed the inheritance of flower color or other characters focused on only a single character via monohybrid crosses. He conducted other experiments involving the inheritance of two different characters—a dihybrid cross.

In one dihybrid-cross experiment, Mendel studied the inheritance of seed color and seed shape. Mendel crossed true-breeding plants that had yellow, round seeds (YYRR) with true-breeding plants that had green, wrinkled seeds (yyrr). One possibility was that the two characters were transmitted from parents to offspring as a package; however, this was not the case in practicality. An alternative hypothesis was that the two pairs of alleles segregated independently—that is, the presence of one specific allele for one trait has no impact on the presence of a specific allele for the second trait. This hypothesis came out to be true.

Mendel concluded that each character appeared to be inherited independently. This independent assortment of each pair of alleles during gamete formation is called Mendel's Law of Independent Assortment.

EXCEPTIONS TO MENDEL'S LAWS

In the mid-1860s, Mendel was the first and only scientist to come up with a theory of inheritance; therefore, he faced little or no criticism from the scientific community. Slowly through research, however, scientists have come to understand that nature doesn't always conform to Mendel's simple laws. Here are some new theories that explain contradictions to Mendel's Laws:

Codominant. If both the alleles are partly expressed in a single organism, the alleles are termed codominant.

Incomplete dominance. When a phenotype caused by a heterozygous genotype is different from the phenotype seen in both homozygous genotypes, and its severity is seen in both, the phenotype is described as incompletely dominant.

Multiple alleles. Some traits are controlled not by one or two alleles but by a complex combination of multiple alleles. Blood type in humans, for example, is controlled by three alleles—namely, I_A, I_B, and i. These three alleles appear in six different combinations: I_AI_A, I_BI_B, ii, I_Ai, I_Bi, and I_AI_B. These six combinations give rise to four different blood types in humans: A, B, AB, and O.

CONTROVERSY AND CRITICISM

Despite heavy contributions of genetics to health and science, there has been some criticism from the community. Some observers think that genetically modified organisms could harm the environment in the long run. Some also feel that genetic therapy may affect other genes in unknown ways. Recent methods such as cloning and stem-cell research have been brought into the media spotlight for being unethical despite giving hope for treatment of disabilities deemed untreatable by other methods. These and other theories have forced the geneticists to draw the line between science and social responsibility.

SEE ALSO: Education, Cancer; Gene Therapy.

BIBLIOGRAPHY. Robert Nussbaum, et al., *Genetics in Medicine* (Thompson & Thompson, 2001); Gerard J. Tortora and Bryan H. Derrickson, *Principles of Anatomy and Physiology* (John Wiley & Sons, Inc., 2003).

RAHUL GLADWIN
UNIVERSITY OF HEALTH SCIENCES,
ANTIGUA SCHOOL OF MEDICINE

Genzyme (United States)

GENZYME CORPORATION, HEADQUARTERED in Cambridge, Massachusetts, is one of the world's largest biotechnology companies, reporting $2.7 billion in revenue and spending $503 million on research and development (R&D) during 2005. Genzyme employs over 8,500 people worldwide in 32 countries and currently is marketing over 25 drugs approved by the U.S. Food and Drug Administration (FDA), in addition to running 9 genetic-testing labs. It is traded on the NASDAQ exchange under the symbol GENZ. Current areas of research include lysosomal storage disorders, renal disease, orthopedics, transplant and immune disease, genetics, and oncology. Cerezyme (imiglucerase), which replaces the function of glucocerebrosidase in patients with Type 1 Gaucher's disease, has

been the company's largest revenue generator since the mid-1990s, but since the purchase of Ilex Oncology, Inc., of San Antonio, Texas, in December 2004, oncology has become a major focus for the company.

Henri A Termeer, president and CEO of Genzyme since 1985, has stated that he expects that in the future, Genzyme will be known primarily for cancer treatments. Currently, Genzyme markets two anticancer drugs—Campath (alemtuzumab) for the treatment of chronic B-cell lymphocytic leukemia and Clolar (clofarabine) for refractory lymphoblastic leukemia—as well as Thyrogen (thyrotropin) for the detection of thyroid cancer.

Genzyme began as a small startup firm in 1981, specializing in creating drugs to replace deficient enzyme function in patients with lysosomal storages diseases such as Gaucher's disease and Fabry's disease. Lysosomal storage diseases, which result from genetically inherited deficiencies of a single enzyme, are extremely rare. Each individual disease afflicts less than 10,000 people worldwide. Because the potential market is so small, large pharmaceutical companies have avoided investing in R&D to develop new drugs for these and other rare diseases.

In an effort to spur research dollars into these so-called orphan diseases, defined as those with less than 200,000 patients in the United States, Congress passed the Orphan Drug Act in 1983. This law allowed companies like Genzyme to tax-deduct a portion of clinical-trial costs and granted a seven-year exclusive license to the first drug approved by the FDA for any of the orphan diseases. The first Genzyme product to pass clinical trial was the recombinant protein Ceredase, approved by the FDA in 1991 for the treatment of Gaucher's disease. This was followed by Cerezyme in 1994, a second-generation version of Ceredase that was much cheaper and easier to produce in large quantities.

Because Genzyme has a monopoly on treatment for Gaucher's disease, the company has been able to generate a tremendous amount of revenue from the very small patient population. A year of biweekly Cerezyme injections costs about $200,000, and the drug must be taken for life. Similarly, Genzyme's other lysosomal storage disorder treatments Fabrazyme and Aldurazyme cost between $175,000 and $200,000. These extremely high prices have generated criticism, most notably a series of articles in *The New York Times*.

It is Genzyme's policy to give away drugs to patients without insurance, especially patients in developing nations. These giveaways account for 10 percent of the 4,500 patients taking Cerezyme. In 2005, Genzyme donated a total of $64 million in free pharmaceuticals and donated another $10 million in cash to various charities.

SEE ALSO: Biologic Therapy; Chemotherapy; Cost of Therapy.

BIBLIOGRAPHY. Genzyme corporate website, genzyme. com; Sara Calabro, "The Price of Success?", *Pharmaceutical Executive* (March 2006); Jeffrey Krasner, "Genzyme Banks Its Future on Cancer Drugs," *Boston Globe* (January 4, 2005); Alex Berenson, "A New Cancer Drug Shows Promise, At a Price That Many Can't Pay," *New York Times* (February 15, 2006).

JOHN PAUL SHEN
WASHINGTON UNIVERSITY SCHOOL OF MEDICINE

Georgia

THIS CAUCASIAN REPUBLIC was part of the Russian empire until 1922, when it became a constituent of the Union of Soviet Socialist Republics. It became an independent nation in 1991. It has a population of 4,694,000 (2004) and has 436 doctors and 474 nurses per 100,000 people. An example of cancer incidence rates in Georgia includes 171.4 cases of cancer in males per 100,000, according to the International Agency for Research on Cancer.

While Georgia was part of the Soviet Union, health care was extensive, and many people from elsewhere in the Soviet Union went to Georgia for rest cures. Many sanatoriums treated people suffering from cancer, which as a cause of death was low. The National Cancer Centre of Georgia is a member of the International Union Against Cancer. In 1950 there were 149 beds for cancer patients in Georgia, rising to 375 in 1960 and 410 in the following year.

During the 1960s, although most research into curing cancer was conducted in Moscow or Leningrad (St. Petersburg), there was some important research in the Georgian republic, most of it coordinated by the Research Institute of Oncology of the Ministry of Health at Tbilisi. One study, by K.D. Eristavi, et al., was on morphohistochemical characteristics of chemical blastomogenesis in the lungs of monkeys. Another study involved G.E. Georgadze, et al., working on thyroid tumors with J-131 and chemical carcinogens.

At the Institute of Experimental and Clinical Surgery of the AMS. in Tibilisi, L.K. Sharashidze, et al., worked on histochemical indices of enzyme activity in neurons of the central nervous system accompanying induced skin cancer. T.G. Natadze of the Medical Institute of Tibilisi was also involved in cancer research, in his case on vasodilator factors of tumors in animals and men.

Other studies at the Research Institute of Oncology at Tibilisi included one by G.K. Gersamia into the state of histochemical features of genetical and plastic substances of tumor cells in mice before and after radiation; one by R.A. Chitiashvili into intravital radiography used for the diagnosis of cervix uterine cancer; one by B.B. Adamia and G.E. Georgadze into the reversibility of the intraepithereal cervix uterine cancer; and a large project by T. Khatiashvili, et al., into the results of transvaginal X-ray therapy of cancer in the cervix of the uterus and the treatment ascertainment by the cytological and cytochemical method. In a related area, L.J. Charkviani worked with V.D. Tokua on the cancerogenic properties of smegma.

In the area of breast cancer, G.V. Bilanishvili worked on the compensatory-adaption ability of the lymphatic system of the breast, and K.K. Madich worked on skin-cancer epidemiology. In addition, D.D. Ghogheliani, et al., from the Institute of Oncology in Tibilis worked on the clinical classification of the carcinoma cervix; D.R. Chkeidze, et al., worked on the effects of hormonal controls in carcinogenesis; and R.G. Khujadze and K.K. Madich studied the effectiveness of the application of various cytostatic preparations in the course of combined treatment of mammary cancer.

ENVIRONMENTAL CONCERNS

In recent years, there has been an increase in smoking in Georgia, with a consequent rise in lung cancer. A study in 1991 showed cases of adult T-cell leukemia in an HTLV-1 infected family in Georgia.

There has also been worry about nuclear waste from Soviet-era nuclear sites. In one scare in February 1997, some 11 Georgian soldiers started to develop radiation burns, with others gradually being diagnosed with cancers. This led a Georgian commission of inquiry to identify 352 contaminated sites in November 1997.

SEE ALSO: Breast Cancer; Cervical Cancer; Nuclear Industry; Radiation; Smoking and Society.

BIBLIOGRAPHY. L.S. Kavtaradze and K.F. Vepkhvadze, "Razvitie onkologicheskof pomoshchi nasleniiu Gruzinskof SSR za gody sovetskof vlasti," *Voprosy Onkologii* (v.16, 1970); *Lancet* (v.338, 1991); Diego Llumá, "Former Soviet Union: What the Russians Left Behind," *Bulletin of the Atomic Scientists* (v.56/3, 2000).

JUSTIN CORFIELD
GEELONG GRAMMAR SCHOOL, AUSTRALIA

Germ Cell Tumor, Extracranial, Childhood

GERM CELLS ARE in the developing embryo and give rise to the testes in males and the ovaries in females. If these cells migrate to other areas of the body, such as the chest or abdomen, they can become cancerous.

A tumor is an uncontrollable growth of cells or tissues, and extracranial refers to locations other than the brain. Three main branches of this type of tumor are sacrococcygeal, mediastinal, and retroperitoneal. Some research indicates that germ cell tumors that occur in early childhood more often arise in the sacrum and the coccyx (sacrococcygeal), whereas those found in adolescence and young adulthood are often in the chest (mediastinal). These tumors can be benign and noncancerous or malignant and cancerous. They can occur with unknown risk factors or cause and mostly become evident before or during adolescence.

Germ cell tumors present in different regions of the body and have different symptoms, and diagnosis is difficult. Symptoms may be very specific, such as pain in the affected area, or very general, such as constipation, urine retention, and breathing difficulty. Furthermore, the diagnosis and determination of whether the tumor has spread, or metastasised, will depend upon multiple diagnostic tests.

An ultrasound may be used for morphological identification of a tumor for a developing fetus, as well as an alphafetoprotein (AFP) test. A computerized tomography (CT) scan can also be used. Last, a biopsy of a suspicious tumor can offer definitive proof with histological examination in identifying germ cell tumors.

GERM CELL STAGES

Staging helps define the nature of the cancer, such as where it is located, where it has spread, and whether it is affecting the functions of other organs. Doctors use diagnostic tests to determine the cancer's stage; however, sometimes the exact stage of the cancer is not known until the time of surgery. Knowing the stage helps the doctor decide what kind of treatment is best and can help predict a patient's prognosis (chance of recovery).

There are different stage descriptions for different types of cancers. According to the National Cancer Institute, the following stages are used for extracranial germ cell tumors:

Stage I: The tumor can be completely surgically removed and has not spread.

Stage II: Cancer has spread to surrounding tissues or lymph nodes. Surgery may not remove all cancer cells from surrounding tissues.

Stage III: Cancer has spread to surrounding tissues, has affected several lymph nodes, and is found in fluid in the abdomen, and surgery cannot remove the entire tumor from the surrounding tissue.

Stage IV: Cancer has spread to other organs, generally, the lungs, liver, or brain.

Recurrent: Recurrent disease means that the cancer has recurred (come back) after it has been treated. It may recur in the original site of the tumor or in another place.

TREATMENT OF CHILDREN

Clinical trials are the standard of care for the treatment of children with cancer. In fact, about 75 percent of children with cancer are treated as part of a clinical trial. Clinical trials are research studies that compare standard treatments (the best treatments available) with newer treatments that may be more effective or less toxic. Cancer in children is rare, so it can be hard for doctors to plan treatments unless they know what has been most effective in other children. Investigating new treatments involves careful monitoring using scientific methods, and all participants are followed closely to track their progress.To take advantage of these newer treatments, all children with cancer should be treated at a specialized pediatric cancer center or program. Doctors at these centers have extensive experience in treating children with cancer and have access to the latest research. Many times, a team of doctors treats children with cancer. Pediatric cancer centers often have extra support services for children and their families, such as nutritionists, social workers, and counselors. Special activities for kids with cancer may also be available.

The treatment of extracranial germ cell tumors depends on their size and location, whether the cancer has metastasized and to what extent, and the patient's overall health before diagnosis. Currently, surgery and chemotherapy are the most effective treatment modalities. Radiation therapy can also be performed. Often, these treatments are applied in unison, with chemotherapy given before surgery to reduce the tumor before surgery. The goal of surgery is to remove the tumor, along with some surrounding tissue, to make sure that the entire tumor is removed.

Chemotherapy is the use of drugs to kill cancerous cells. Chemotherapy may be given before surgery to shrink the tumor or after surgery to destroy any remaining cancer. It also may be combined with radiation therapy. Chemotherapy drugs can be given by mouth or injection. Because chemotherapy kills healthy cells as well as cancerous cells, it may cause side effects, which can include hair loss, vomiting, nausea, diarrhea, fatigue, infection, bleeding, and mouth sores. Side effects usually go away when chemotherapy is finished. The specific drugs that are commonly used for treating germ cell tumors include cisplatin (Platinol), etoposide (VePesid, Etopophos, Toposar), bleomycin (Blenoxane), and cyclophosphamide (Cytoxan, Neosar).

Through ongoing research, the medications used to treat cancer are constantly being evaluated in different combinations and to treat different cancers. Talking with the doctor is often the best way for patients to learn about medications, their purpose, and their potential side effects or interactions. Follow-up care and close physician monitoring, examinations, follow-up X-rays, and blood tests after completion of therapy are necessary to confirm no recurrence.

Cancer and cancer treatment can cause a variety of side effects; some are easily controlled, and others require specialized care. Following are some of the side effects that are most common to germ cell tumors and their treatments.

Diarrhea. Diarrhea is frequent, loose, or watery bowel movements. It is a common side effect of certain chemotherapeutic drugs or of radiation therapy to the pelvis, such as in women with uterine, cervical, or ovarian cancers. It can also be caused by certain tumors, such as pancreatic cancer.

Fatigue (tiredness). Fatigue is extreme exhaustion or tiredness and is the most common problem that people with cancer experience. More than half of patients experience fatigue during chemotherapy or radiation therapy, and up to 70 percent of patients with advanced cancer experience fatigue. Patients who feel fatigue often say that even a small effort, such as walking across a room, can seem like too much. Fatigue can seriously affect family and other daily activities, can make patients avoid or skip cancer treatments, and may even affect the will to live.

Hair loss (alopecia). A potential side effect of radiation therapy and chemotherapy is hair loss. Radiation therapy and chemotherapy cause hair loss by damaging the hair follicles responsible for hair growth. Hair loss may occur throughout the body, including the head, face, arms, legs, underarms, and pubic area. The hair may fall out entirely, gradually, or in sections. In some cases, the hair will simply thin—sometimes unnoticeably—and may become duller and dryer. Losing one's hair can be a psychologically and emotionally challenging experience and can affect a patient's self-image and quality of life. However, the hair loss is usually temporary, and the hair often grows back.

Infection. An infection occurs when harmful bacteria, viruses, or fungi (such as yeast) invade the body and the immune system is not able to destroy them quickly enough. Patients with cancer are more likely to develop infections because both cancer and cancer treatments (particularly chemotherapy and radiation therapy to the bones or extensive areas of the body) can weaken the immune system. Symptoms of infection include fever (temperature of 100.5 degrees F or higher); chills or sweating; sore throat or sores in the mouth; abdominal pain; pain or burning when urinating or frequent urination; diarrhea or sores around the anus; cough or breathlessness; redness, swelling, or pain, particularly around a cut or wound; and unusual vaginal discharge or itching.

Mouth sores (mucositis). Mucositis is an inflammation of the inside of the mouth and throat, leading to painful ulcers and mouth sores. It occurs in up to 40 percent of patients receiving chemotherapy treatments. Mucositis can be caused by a chemotherapeutic drug directly, by the reduced immunity brought on by chemotherapy, or by radiation treatment to the head and neck area.

Nausea and vomiting. Vomiting, also called emesis or throwing up, is the act of expelling the contents of the stomach through the mouth. It is a natural way for the body to rid itself of harmful substances. Nausea is the urge to vomit. Nausea and vomiting are common in patients receiving chemotherapy for cancer and in some patients receiving radiation therapy. Many patients with cancer say they fear nausea and vomiting more than any other side effects of treatment. When they are minor and treated quickly, nausea and vomiting can be quite uncomfortable but cause no serious problems. Persistent vomiting can cause dehydration, electrolyte imbalance, weight loss, depression, and avoidance of chemotherapy.

Follow-up care for this type of cancer depends on the location of the tumor and the therapy used. Generally, patients are monitored with examinations, X-rays, and blood tests for two years after completion of therapy to check for recurrence. After this time, it is unlikely that the cancer will recur, and the focus of the follow-up changes to potential late side effects of chemotherapy, including abnormalities of growth and development, and damage to specific body organs. Because of the effects of the drugs most commonly used to treat these tumors, regular tests of kidney function, lung function, fertility, and blood cell production may be required.

Doctors and scientists are always looking for better ways to treat patients with germ cell tumors. A clinical trial is a way to test a new treatment to prove that it is safe, effective, and possibly better than a standard treatment. Patients who participate in clinical trials are among the first to receive new treatments, such as new chemotherapy drugs, before they are widely available. However, there is no guarantee that the new treatment will be safe, effective, or better than a standard treatment. Patients decide to participate in clinical trials for many reasons. For some patients, a clinical trial is the best treatment option available. Because standard treatments are not perfect, patients are often willing to face the added uncertainty of a clinical trial in the hope of a better result. Other patients volunteer for clinical trials because they know that this is the only way to make progress in treating germ cell tumors, such as finding new drugs. Even if they do not benefit directly from the clinical trial, their participation may benefit future patients with germ cell tumors.

To join a clinical trial, patients must complete a learning process known as informed consent. During informed consent, the doctor should list all the patient's options so that the person understands the standard treatments and how the new treatment differs from the standard treatment. The doctor must also list all the risks of the new treatment, which may or may not be different from the risks of standard treatment. Finally, the doctor must explain what will be required of each patient to participate in the clinical trial, including the number of doctor visits, tests, and the schedule of treatment.

Research involving more advanced diagnostic procedures and treatments for extracranial, extragonadal germ cell tumors is ongoing. Advancements may still be under investigation in clinical trials and may not be approved or available at this time. Patients should always discuss all diagnostic and treatment options with their doctors. Clinical trials are under way to investigate new combinations of chemotherapy drugs to treat extracranial, extragonadal germ cell tumors. One study is evaluating the use of cyclophosphamide with cisplatin, etoposide, and bleomycin in children newly diagnosed with this type of cancer.

SEE ALSO: Alternative Therapy: Pharmacological and Biological Treatment; Chemotherapy; Childhood Cancers; Germ Cell Tumor, Extragonadal.

BIBLIOGRAPHY. D. Billmire, et al., "*Malignant* Mediastinal Germ Cell Tumors: An Intergroup Study," *Journal of Pediatric Surgery* (v.36/1, 2001); L.A. Ries, et al., "*Cancer* Incidence and Survival Among Children and Adolescents 1975–1995" (National Cancer Institute SEER Program, NIH Pub. No. 99-4649, 1999); www.childhoodcanceralliance.org/acc/Main (cited December 20, 2006).

JOHN M. QUINN
UNIVERSITY OF ILLINOIS AT CHICAGO

Germ Cell Tumor, Extragonadal

THE TERM *EXTRAGONADAL* means outside the reproductive organs. Germ cells refer to the reproductive cells, such as the sperm and the eggs, which are initially located in the yolk sac outside the embryo. During development, the germ cells normally migrate to the embryo into the pelvis to become ovarian cells or into the scrotal sac as testicular cells. However, extragonadal germ cell tumors develop when these germ cells migrate to other parts of the body and become cancerous.

Extragonadal germ cell tumors (EGCT) are rare among germ cell tumors and can be either benign (noncancerous) or malignant (cancerous). Benign EGCT are called benign teratomas, which are often large and more common than malignant EGCT. Most of these benign tumors occur in children, and the great majority of these tumors can be treated with surgery alone. Although benign tumors do not spread, they may cause other problems, such as pressing on nearby organs.

Malignant EGCT can be divided into two types: nonseminoma (for example, embryonal carcinoma, yolk-sac tumor, and mixed germ cell tumors) and seminoma (or germinoma in females). Although the malignant type is much more common in males, extragonadal tumors can occur in females with equal frequency as in males for the benign type.

Nonseminomas tend to grow and spread more quickly than seminomas. As a result, they usually are large and cause symptoms. If untreated, malignant EGCT may metastasize to the lungs, lymph nodes, bones, liver, or other parts of the body.

EGCT can be diagnosed via a variety of tests and investigations, such as biopsy (removing a sample of tumor for examination under microscope); complete blood count and other blood tests; and medical imaging modalities such as computed tomography scan (CT), magnetic resonance imaging (MRI), x-ray, and ultrasound. In addition, EGCT often produce proteins known as tumor markers that can be measured from the blood. These markers are alpha-fetoprotein (AFP) and human chorionic gonadotrophin (HCG), and their levels are checked in the diagnosis of EGCT as well as being monitored throughout the treatment.

There are different treatments available for EGCT patients, depending on factors such as the type, size, and location of the tumors; levels of tumor markers in the blood; extent of metastasis; and initial response to treatment and recurrence. Typically, patients are given good prognosis if they have nonseminoma EGCT carrying tumor in the back of the abdomen with slightly higher tumor marker levels in the blood and no sign of spread of tumor to other organs.

By contrast, patients have poor prognosis if they have nonseminoma EGCT carrying tumor in the chest with high level of tumor markers and metastasis of tumor cells to organs other than the lungs.

There are three standard treatments available: radiation therapy, chemotherapy, and surgery. For seminoma, treatments often involve radiation therapy for small tumors in one area. Chemotherapy is administered if the tumors are larger or have spread, and surgery may be required if there is a large tumor remaining after chemotherapy. For nonseminoma, chemotherapy followed by surgery is often performed to remove any remaining tumor.

SEE ALSO: Chemotherapy; Germ Cell Tumor, Extracranial, Childhood; Surgery.

BIBLIOGRAPHY. Raymond E. Lenhard, Jr., et al., eds., *Clinical Oncology* (American Cancer Society, 2001); Mark H. Beers, et al., eds., *The Merck Manual of Diagnosis and Therapy*, (Merck Research Laboratories, 2006).

STEPHEN CHEN
UNIVERSITY OF TORONTO

Germany

GERMANY HAS A population of 82,425,000 (2004) and has 350 doctors and 957 nurses per 100,000 people. An example of cancer incidence rates in Grmany includes 317.7 cases of cancer in males per 100,000, according to the International Agency for Research on Cancer.

There was early work in Germany on cancer, but the first person who made significant discoveries was Wilhelm Fabry, a surgeon who left extensive case notes and was involved in the dissection of axillary lymph nodes in patients suffering from breast cancers.

During the 19th century great advances were made in the study of cancer in Germany. Rudolf Ludwig Carl Virchow founded a journal on anatomy and suggested that one cause of cancer was local irritation. Arthur Nathan Hanau was involved in successfully transplanting cancer in mammals.

Other cancer specialists of the period included Ludwig Rehn, who noted the frequent appearance of papilloma and carcinoma of the bladder found in men employed in the aniline dye industry; Ernst August Franz Albert Frieben, who reported the carcinogenic effect of X-rays in men and women; David Paul von Hansemann, who originated the theory of anaplasia; S. W. Goldberg and Efim Semenovic, who recorded the first successful use of radium in the treatment of cancer; and Carl Oluf Jensen, who carried the rat sarcoma through 40 generations of rodents without any change in microscopic structure.

Martin Benno Schmidt supported the theory of the hematogenous origin of carcinoma metastases, and Jacob Wolff wrote a four-volume history of cancer research that was published by Fischer in Jena. Moritz Wilhelm Hugo Ribbert believed in the theory of the embryonal origin of cancer. Fritz Brenner, who had completed a medical degree at the University of Heidelberg, described Brenner's tumor, a rare ovarian tumor that is usually benign.

Adolph Hannover wrote *Das Epithelioma*, published in Leipzig in 1852, and coined the word epithelioma. He did not recognize the malignant character, however, believing that metastases were produced by cancer cells arriving through the bloodstream.

Carl Thiersch, a professor of surgery at Erlangen, was the inventor of the skin graft that bears his name; he managed to disprove Virchow's theory on the connective-tissue origin of cancer. Bernard Langenbeck from Gottingen proposed a new theory of cancer metastasis in 1840, which was later proved to be fundamentally correct.

Other people who contributed to cancer treatment in Germany at this time included Julius Friedrich Cohnheim, a German–Jewish pathologist from the University of Berlin; Karl Thiersch, a surgeon from Munich; Richard von Volkmann, a prominent surgeon and poet from Leipzig; and Wilhelm von Waldeyer, an anatomist from Braunchsweig. Mention should also be made of prominent U.S. oncologist Leo Loeb, who was born in Germany in 1869 and emigrated to the United States in 1897, where he contributed much to experimental pathology.

In 1887 Crown Prince Frederick of Germany, the son of Kaiser Wilhelm I, was diagnosed with throat cancer by German physicians. The prince had been a heavy smoker for many years. By contrast, the eminent British physician Sir Morell Mackenzie, basing his opinion on a biopsy made by Rudolf Virchow, claimed that what was found was only a throat lesion and that an operation for cancer was unnecessary. As a result, the operation was canceled. Mackenzie was knighted by Queen Victoria in September 1887 and awarded the Grand Cross of the Hohenzollern Order soon afterward. In November, however, the tumor was confirmed as being cancerous. The Crown Prince became Emperor Frederick III on March 9, 1888, and died on June 15. German doctors accused Mackenzie of being inept, and the German press was extremely critical of him. He then wrote his book *The Fatal Illness of Frederick the Noble* (Sampson Low, 1888). As it contained confidential information on a patient, Mackenzie was censured by the Royal College of Surgeons.

Victoria, Princess Royal, daughter of Queen Victoria and consort to Frederick III, died of cancer of the spine.

During the period of Nazi rule, German scientists worked extensively on the prevention of lung cancer. Adolf Hitler never smoked, and this fact was used in the campaign to persuade others not to smoke. Much work was undertaken by Karl Astel, director of the Institute of Tobacco Hazards Research at the University of Jena, who banned smoking by students on campus and was known for snatching cigarettes from the mouths of students. The institute also supported the research of pathologist Eberhard Schairer and a young colleague, Erich Schöniger, who published a paper in 1943 that compared the rates of lung cancer in men and women, and between rural and urban populations.

In 1939 the Nobel Prize for Physiology or Medicine was awarded to Gerhard Domagk, a bacteriologist and pathologist from Brandenburg who discovered, in 1932, the antibacterial effects of Prontosil, the first of the sulfonamide drugs. Domagk was unable to accept the Nobel award because of Nazi policy, but in 1947 he received the gold medal and a diploma.

After World War II, Germany was divided, and two separate cancer treatment systems were established. A nationwide cancer registry was established in East Germany in 1949. A comparison of cancer deaths in

Würtemberg in 1910 and in 1970, performed in 1970, managed to show the effect of environmental pollution and the use of chemicals on the increase of cancer in the intervening 60 years. Extensive work was done on cancer treatment from the 1950s, but the increasing life expectancy rate meant that cancer rates in the country were high.

Rainer Schrage of the University of Frauenklinik studied the results of 700,000 preventive gynecological examinations. Other studies in West Germany included many studies of cervical cancer, breast cancer, lung cancer, oral cancer, stomach cancer, and cancers of the neck and head.

There was also research in East Germany on cancer treatment. Günter Pasternak and Luise Pasternak of the Institute of Cancer Research, Experimental Section of the German Academy of Sciences, studied the immunologic studies on the presence of a leukemia virus and virus-induced antigens in leukemic and nonleukemic tissues. Bodo Teichmann of the same institute worked on a test for chemotherapeutics by the diffusion chamber method. P. Langen worked on the inhibitors of the degradation of the carcinostatic nucleosides 5-fluroeoxyurdine and 5-Iododeoxyuridine.

Heinz Fischer of the Geschwulstkilinik der Medizinischen Fakultat (Charité), East Berlin, published the cytogenic studies in carcinoma cells. G. Marx and W. Widow from the Zentralinstitut für Krebsforschung der Akademie der Wissenschaften der D.D.R. studied the role of radical mastectomy in the treatment of breast cancer. Many prominent Germans died of cancer. Johannes Brahms, composer and pianist, died of cancer in Vienna. Friedrich Engels, social philosopher and collaborator with Karl Marx, suffered from cancer in his later years, finally succumbing to the illness. Hans Fritzsche, journalist and broadcaster, died of cancer. Willy Brandt, chancellor of West Germany from 1969 until 1974, died of cancer in 1992. Franz von Eckert, a musician, died of stomach cancer. Regine Hildebrandt was a biologist who went into politics for the Greens and later died of cancer.

The longtime leader of East Germany, Erich Honecker, was arrested after the collapse of communism in East Germany but was released as he was ill from liver cancer, to which he succumbed in Santiago, Chile.

SEE ALSO: Bladder Cancer; Breast Cancer; Cervical Cancer; Dyes and Pigments; Smoking and Society; X-Rays.

BIBLIOGRAPHY. "Eponym: Brenner's Tumor," *Cancer Bulletin* (v.18, 1966); John Cornwell, *Hitler's Scientists: Science, War and the Devil's Pact* (Viking, 2003); D. Panzer and G. P. Wildner, "Zur Geschichte der Krebsstatistik in Deutschland bis 1949," *Zeitschrift fur Arztliche Fortbildung* (v.79, 1985); L. J. Rather, "Lagenbeck on the Mechanism of Tumor Metastasis," *Clio Medica* (v.10, 1975); R. Schmautz and M. Holm-Hadulla, "Cancer Mortality in Würtemberg, 1910 and 1970," *Zentralblatt fur Krebsforschung* (v.87, 1976); Jan A. Witkowski, "Experimental Pathology and the Origins of Tissue Culture: Leo Loeb's Contribution," *Medical History* (v.27, 1983).

JUSTIN CORFIELD
GEELONG GRAMMAR SCHOOL, AUSTRALIA

Gestational Trophoblastic Tumor

GESTATIONAL TROPHOBLASTIC TUMOR (GTT) is a disease that affects women of childbearing age. It occurs when conception leads to tissue growing in the uterus in which cancer cells also form. The disease is also referred to as molar pregnancy, gestational trophoblastic disease, and other names. It is a comparatively rare disease.

The disease takes two principal forms. In the first form, the molar pregnancy occurs with the union of sperm and egg cells without development into a fetus. Instead, cysts form. These cysts do not spread outside the uterus. The second form occurs when a fetus does develop, and the cancer cells are created in the uterus, where they remain and grow further after the pregnancy ends as a result of birth or abortion. This is a choriocarcinoma and can develop from the remnants of a molar pregnancy or, more unusually, at the point of attachment of the placenta. This disease may spread to other parts of the body.

GTT is not generally easy to diagnose in its early stages and will appear as a regular pregnancy. Physicians will check for vaginal bleeding or any signs of abnormal movement.

Tests include manual examination of the uterus to search for growths, as well as ultrasound and blood tests to search for the presence of GTT. In the case of blood tests, the presence of the hormone beta-HCG indicates the disease.

It is possible to treat GTT in a variety of ways and with a variety of degrees of success, depending on the general state of health of the patient, the extent (if any) to which the disease has spread, and the formation of the disease.

If the cancer is metastatic—has spread to other parts of the body—the diagnosis depends on a variety of factors, including the length of time since the latest pregnancy, the areas of the body to which the cancer has spread, the beta-HCG level, and whether chemotherapy has previously been received.

Treatment options include surgery, chemotherapy, and radiation therapy. Surgery involves cutting the cancerous tissue from the body, perhaps as a hysterectomy. Chemotherapy uses drugs to try to kill the cancerous cells. Radiation therapy is most commonly used when the GTT has metastatized to other parts of the body where this treatment is more appropriate. The treatment may be delivered either externally or internally.

Even successful procedures require careful subsequent monitoring, as it is possible for the cancer to recur in places where it has already struck. Physicians will construct suitable regimes for checking patients and promoting well being during and after treatment.

SEE ALSO: Chemotherapy; Radiation Therapy; Surgery; Women's Cancers.

BIBLIOGRAPHY. Isaac Blickstein and Louis G. Keith, *Multiple Pregnancy: Epidemiology, Gestation, and Perinatal Outcome* (Informa Healthcare, 2005); Steven A. Vasilev, ed., *Perioperative and Supportive Care in Gynecologic Oncology: Evidence-Based Management* (Wiley-Liss, 2000).

JOHN WALSH
SHINAWATRA UNIVERSITY

Ghana

THIS WEST AFRICAN gained its independence July 1, 1960, and becoming the Republic of Ghana. It has a population of 20,757,000 (2004) and has 6.2 doctors and 72 nurses per 100,000 people. An example of cancer incidence rates in Ghana includes 89.1 cases of cancer in males per 100,000, according to the International Agency for Research on Cancer..

During the time the Gold Coast was a British colony, formal health care in hospitals and clinics was used mainly by Britons, Europeans, and the wealthy elite. Most people had no access to the hospital system and tended to rely on herbal and tribal practices to deal with tumors. These practices were usually unsuccessful, because the most prevalent type of cancer contracted in the Gold Coast was liver cancer. Dr. Michael Vane, in his account of his time in nearby Sierra Leone, wrote that in his experience, cancer was extremely rare in British West Africa except for liver cancer, because most people did not live long enough to contract the disease.

Although there are cases of cancers recorded from the early 1900s, treatment started in earnest only in the 1950s. After independence, the health care system in the country was considerably enlarged. The Faculty of Medicine at the University of Ghana, Accra, and the School of Medical Sciences at the University of Science and Technology, Kumasi, both have cancer treatment programs. Also, much research has been undertaken at the School of Allied Health Sciences, College of Health Sciences, University of Ghana, Korle-Bu.

The best-known form of cancer in Ghana is Burkitt's tumor. During the 1960s, J. Kovi and W. N. Laing from the National Institute of Health and Medical Research at the Ghana Academy of Sciences and the Central Clinical Laboratories in Accra researched endocrine-gland involvement in Burkitt's tumor. The human T-cell leukemia–lymphoma virus is also prevalent in Ghana.

There was no major review of cancer mortality patterns in Ghana between 1953 and the study conducted by Edwin K. Wiredu and Henry B. Armah in 2006, although there had been studies of individual cancers. Some of the information on prostate cancer was used to work out similarities with prostate-cancer sufferers in the United States. Retrospective review of the autopsy records of the Department of Pathology, as well as medical certificates for all deaths at the Korle-Bu Teaching Hospital in Accra from 1991 until 2000, showed that cancer represented 15.4 percent of deaths.

The man who led Ghana to independence, Kwame Nkrumah, president of Ghana from 1960 to 1966, suffered for some years from cancer and went to Bucharest, Romania, seeking treatment in August 1971. His death in April 1972 focused much medical attention in Ghana on cancer treatment. Several Britons connected with Ghana succumbed to lung cancer, including Granville George Leveson-Gower, a British politician who urged Britain to take over Dutch possessions on the Gold Coast.

SEE ALSO: Liver Cancer, Adult (Primary); Liver Cancer, Childhood (Primary); Prostate Cancer.

BIBLIOGRAPHY. David Birmingham, *Kwame Nkrumah* (Cardinal, 1990); Dennis Burkitt, "A Sarcoma Involving the Jaws in African Children," *British Journal of Surgery* (v.46, 1958–1959); S. B. Naaeder and E. Q. Archampong, "Cancer of the Colon and Rectum in Ghana: A 5-Year Prospective Study," *British Journal of Surgery* (v.81.3, 1994); K. David Patterson, *Health in Colonial Ghana: Disease, Medicine and Socio-economic Change, 1900–1955* (Crossroads Press, 1981); Michael Vane, *Black Magic and White Medicine* (W. R. Chambers Ltd., 1957); Edwin K. Wiredu and Henry B. Armah, "Cancer Mortality Patterns in Ghana: A 10-Year Review of Autopsies and Hospital Mortality," *BMC Public Health* (v.6, 2006).

JUSTIN CORFIELD
GEELONG GRAMMAR SCHOOL, AUSTRALIA

Glass Industry

GLASS IS A supercooled liquid form of silicon dioxide (SiO_2) combined with some other materials. Glass is made from raw materials such as sand, especially quartz sand. It has almost the same chemical composition as crystal quartz.

Glass is not affected by living organisms, so it is a biologically inert material. It is fragile in thin plates and can shatter easily. If rolled into thick plates, however, it may be strong enough to withstand severe blows, even resisting in bullets in bulletproof glass. When glass is mixed with other selected materials it can attain great strength. Other properties can be added by heat treating. Color can be added with the addition of iron oxides to form greens and browns. Manganese oxides can give deep amber to glass or can be used to make an amethyst color. Manganese can also be a decolorizer. Cobalt oxide will color clear glass deep blue, whereas gold chloride will produce a ruby red. Reds can be produced from selenium compounds, and ambers and browns from carbon oxides or by mixing sulfur compounds. Copper compounds used in glassmaking will produce light blue colors or red. Mixing manganese, cobalt, and iron will make black, but using antimony oxides or tin compounds will turn glass white. Uranium oxides combined with glass will produce a glowing yellowish green.

HISTORY OF GLASSMAKING

Glassmaking began at least as early as the ceramic coating on some ancient forms of pottery produced 5,000 years ago. About 2,800 years ago the ancient Phoenicians discovered a process for making glass. From them, it spread to other regions, including the Far East.

After 1300 the Venetians began to dominate European glassmaking. Since the 1500s, when the manufacture of Bohemian glass was begun, there have been many manufacturers of fine glass products. Many of these products are well known to collectors as Waterford crystal, Wistar or Leerdam glass, and many others.

By the 17th century large quantities of low-cost glass were used to make bottles. In England, bottles were dark brown or green. The color was due to the presence of iron in the sand used in glassmaking. In addition, sulfur in the coal burned to heat the sand to a molten condition added another impurity that affected color. Other natural impurities were eventually discovered to be the source of different colors. In 1679 gold chloride was used for the manufacture of clear glass. These techniques included using

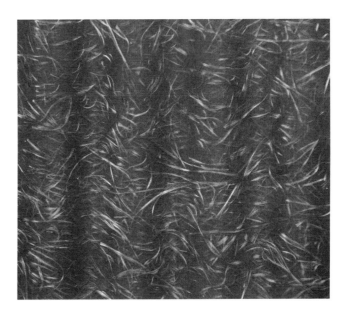

Regulators do not regard fiberglass to be a human carcinogen, but some agencies do list it as an animal carcinogen.

manganese dioxide and cerium oxide to remove iron and sulfur impurities.

The modern glass industry uses many techniques, special effects, and chemicals to produce a wide variety of glass. Iridescent glass (iris glass), for example, can be made by adding a variety of metallic compounds. Spraying the surface of glass with stannous chloride, lead chloride, or other compounds is the preparatory step before reheating the glass to a high temperature in a reduced atmosphere to achieve stunning effects. When glass is iridescent, it appears to emit a variety of colors and is called dichroic glass. As the glass is moved to different angles, or as light strikes at different angles a glass that is held in a fixed position, the glass emits a variety of colors. Iridescence can also be achieved with the use of thin coatings of metals such as gold or silver.

SHAPING GLASS

The manufacturing of glass can be accomplished by craftsmen or craftswomen who may use one of four methods for shaping glass.

Blown air stretches the glass into desired shapes. This method can be performed by using hand techniques and by forcing air into a mass of molten glass that can then be forced into a mold.

The use of molds to shape glass is the second widely used technique for shaping molten glass. Usually called casting, this method is often used to make large glass objects such as the lenses for the great observation telescope on Mount Palomar. Art glass and architectural glass can also easily be made with this method, which usually pours the molten glass from a ladle or directly from a tilted furnace.

Glass can also be shaped by drawing it into tubes, fibers, thin plates, or other shapes. Plate glass is often made by liquefying it on top of a bath of molten tin. Because the melting point of glass is higher than that of tin, the glass plate can be easily drawn from the molten-tin bath with a very smooth surface on both sides.

Pressed glass is the fourth technique for shaping glass. It can be done in a number of ways. One way is for molten glass to be dropped into a mold. The molten glass is then pressed into the mold with a plunger, which forces the molten glass to assume the shape of the mold. Many useful products are made with this method, including ashtrays, bowls, baking dishes, and dinner plates. Pressed glass can be made by hand or with machines that press the

molten glass into molds. Glass can also be shaped after it has cooled. A variety of methods include reheating the glass object and then twisting, drawing, cutting, or in some other way shaping it into the desired final form.

ANNEALING, TEMPERING, AND DECORATING

Usually after glass has been put in its desired shape, it is reheated and then gradually cooled in a process called annealing. The process removes stresses from the glass that could cause it to shatter because it cooled unevenly when it was first shaped.

Tempering glass is a process in which glass is reheated after it has been shaped and then suddenly cooled rapidly with blasts of cool air or a dip into a bath of cool oil or chemicals. Tempering adds strength to the glass.

Glass can be decorated via a number of techniques, including etching with hydrofluoric acid, sandblasting, cutting, and fired decorations.

CARCINOGENS

There are several ways in which glass can become a carcinogenic agent. The most common and widespread way is through fiberglass, which is also called glass wool. Fiberglass is used in an enormous number of products, including thermal insulation of industrial buildings and homes. It is also used as acoustic insulation or as fireproofing. It has been found to add significant strength to plastics, cement, and textiles. It is used in a variety of gadgets, seals, and car parts; in lubricating fluids in automobiles; and in as many as 30,000 commercial products.

Studies of laboratory animals have found that the animals acquired cancer from exposure to fiberglass. In these studies, the fiberglass was implanted in the lungs of the subject animals. Attempts to create the same effects through simple inhalation did not produce the same results. To date, similar findings of cancer in humans have not occurred. Neither do scientists agree on the likelihood that fiberglass can cause lung cancer.

Since the 1940s it has been known that miners and others who work where there are high levels of silicon dust can develop siliconosis. This ailment of the lung can cause irritations that can turn into tuberculosis or lung cancer. The International Agency for Research on Cancer and the National Toxicology

Program consider fiberglass to be an animal carcinogen but do not classify it as a human carcinogen. On the other hand, the U.S. Occupational Safety and Health Agency does not regard fiberglass to be a carcinogen. The U.S. Environmental Protection Agency lists it as an animal carcinogen.

The Canadian government, after a review of the scientific evidence, found fiberglass unlikely to be a human carcinogen. The same finding was made by the United Kingdom, the Netherlands, and the European Union in a 1997 study of fiberglass.

At risk of getting glass-induced lung cancer are glass workers who grind lenses or other types of glass. Special-purpose glass fibers are considered to be carcinogenic in animals. Glass workers who add color to glass are exposed to much higher levels of carcinogenic risk than others. Some workers are exposed to chromium and arsenic compounds, which are known carcinogens.

SEE ALSO: Industry; Lung Cancer, Non-Small Cell; Lung Cancer, Small Cell.

BIBLIOGRAPHY. Robert H. Doremus, *Glass Science* (John Wiley & Sons, 1994); Joan E. Kaiser and Raymond E. Barlow, *The Glass Industry in Sandwich* (Schiffer Publishing, 1999); J. E. E. Shelby, *Introduction to Glass Science and Technology* (Springer-Verlag, 2005); Christopher W. Sinton and William M. Carty, *Raw Materials for Glass and Ceramics: Sources, Processes, and Quality Control* (John Wiley & Sons, 2006); Jane Shadel Spillman, *The American Cut Glass Industry: T. G. Hawkes and His Competitors* (Antique Collector's Club, 2006); Quentin R. Skrabec, *Michael Owens and the Glass Industry* (Pelican Publishing Co., 2007).

ANDREW J. WASKEY
DALTON STATE COLLEGE

GlaxoSmithKline (United Kingdom)

THE MISSION OF GlaxoSmithKline, Inc. (GSK), is to "improve the quality of human life by enabling people to do more, feel better and live longer." Headquarters are in the United Kingdom; GSK also has a U.S.-based business. In 2007, GSK employees worked in 116 nations. The World Health Organization has named three priority diseases: HIV/AIDS, malaria, and tuberculosis. As of 2007, GSK is the only pharmaceutical company that produces medications for all three of these diseases. GSK recognizes its position in the global community; to this end, the company offers medications at a discounted rate to those nations that cannot afford the full price.

GSK research and development focuses on six disease fields: asthma, diabetes, digestive disorders, infections, mental health, and virus control. Products in these fields include treatments for migraines, heart failure, and cancer, as well as vaccines for hepatitis A, hepatitis B, and whooping cough. Additional products manufactured by GSK include dental-care products, over-the-counter medications, nutritional drinks, and smoking-cessation products.

The GSK history began in London, England, in 1715, when Silvanus Bevan established Plough Court Pharmacy, which would become Allen and Hanburys, Ltd. In America in 1830, John K. Smith opened a drugstore in Philadelphia, Pennsylvania. His brother, George, joined him 11 years later, and the business became known as John K. Smith & Co. The company then changed names to Smith and Shoemaker, which hired Mahlon Kline as a bookkeeper in 1865. Ten years later, the company name became Smith, Kline and Co. In 1873, the parent company of Glaxo was founded by Joseph Nathan in New Zealand. More than a century and many new formations and mergers later, Glaxo Wellcome united with SmithKline Beecham in 2000 to form GlaxoSmithKline.

Two entities oversee operations at GSK: a board of directors and a corporate executive team. The board of directors is made up of executive directors and directors; this 11-member board manages the business aspects of GSK. The corporate executive team is led by a chief executive officer.

SEE ALSO: Clinical Trials; Experimental Cancer Drugs; Pharmaceutical Industry.

BIBLIOGRAPHY. Ahmed F. Abdel-Magid and Stephane Caron, *Fundamentals of Early Clinical Drug Development: From Synthesis Design to Formulation* (Wiley-Interscience, 2006); Anne Clayton, *Insight into a Career in Pharmaceutical Sales* (Pharmaceuticalsales.com Inc.,

2005); Rick Ng, *Drugs—From Discovery to Approval* (Wiley-Liss, 2004); Adriana Petryna, et al., *Global Pharmaceuticals: Ethics, Markets, Practices* (Duke University Press, 2006).

CLAUDIA WINOGRAD
UNIVERSITY OF ILLINOIS AT URBANA-CHAMPAIGN

Government

GOVERNMENT PLAYS A major role in cancer control. Besides financing and delivering cancer screening and treatment services, governments contribute to the prevention of cancer through the provision of information to the public, the use of economic incentives to influence cancer-related behaviors, and legislation.

Government decisions to intervene must be weighed against issues such as consumer acceptance, administrative costs, industry concerns, and the potential impact of policies on health equity. The history of tobacco control suggests that no single government action is likely to succeed by itself in eliminating cancer risks, particularly when vested interests stand to gain from the sales of products (e.g., cigarettes) that are the targets of intervention.

GOVERNMENT INTERVENTION

Libertarians often point out that products such as cigarettes and cheeseburgers are legally manufactured and distributed. Under what circumstances are governments justified in intervening in the market for these products?

According to standard economic analysis, there are two situations in which government has a legitimate interest in intervention. The first situation is information failure. Because children are not rational consumers, they are unlikely to be cognitively equipped to weigh the consequences of behaviors before initiating them. In the case of addictive products, such as cigarettes, habits formed in early life may have lasting consequences and prove to be irreversible. Government, therefore, has a responsibility to step in to restrict the distribution of cigarettes to minors and to restrict advertising directed toward children. Manufacturers of consumer products also tend to underprovide information to consumers (even decisionally

competent adults) unless they are forced to do so by laws such as the Federal Cigarette Labeling and Advertising Act (1965) and the Nutrition Labeling and Education Act (1990).

The second situation in which governments have a legitimate interest in intervening in the marketplace is when there are externalities. The costs of treating illnesses caused by smoking and obesity, for example, are borne by taxpayers through Medicare and Medicaid. Governments are justified in attempting to recover these external costs by imposing excise taxes on cigarettes. Although economic analyses suggest that smokers already pay their way at prevailing levels of excise tax in the United States, these calculations do not often take into account the additional costs of treating illnesses caused by passive smoking (another instance of negative externality).

Governments may be additionally justified in raising the excise tax on addictive products such as cigarettes to discourage consumption by youth. Obesity similarly imposes external costs to taxpayers through excess cases of cancer, cardiovascular disease, diabetes, and other illnesses. These provide a rationale for governments to raise excise taxes on foods and beverages that contribute to the risk of obesity, although many questions remain about which foods should be targeted, as well as what the level of tax ought to be.

The hierarchy of strategies available to governments to reduce cancer risk can be ranked in order of effectiveness: (a) the provision of information to the public; (b) the use of economic incentives to influence behaviors; and (c) the passage and enforcement

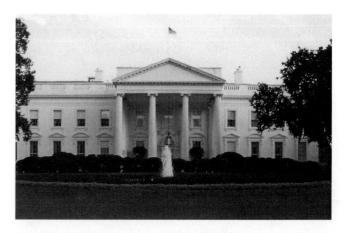

The U.S government's policy toward cancer often stems from whomever is the current occupant of the White House.

of regulations and legislation governing the manufacture, distribution, advertising, and use of products that increase cancer risk.

The provision of information to the public is exemplified by mandating health warnings on cigarette packs and labeling of nutrition content on foods. Educational strategies are the least paternalistic of government interventions and, hence, are likely to be met with the highest levels of consumer acceptance as well as the least industry resistance. Although indispensable among the menu of options available to governments, informational strategies also have their drawbacks.

First, to be effective, the provision of information requires consumers to absorb the new knowledge and to act on it consciously. Often, those who are able to act on the information will do so (e.g., quit smoking), leaving behind the rest, who are unable to change their behavior.

From a health equity perspective, educational strategies have a tendency to widen disparities in cancer outcomes. Before the widespread knowledge that smoking is a cause of cancer, for example, educational disparities in tobacco use were quite modest. However, following the 1964 Surgeon General's Report on Smoking and Health (as well as subsequent mass-media campaigns), better-educated Americans succeeded in stopping smoking in far greater numbers than less-educated Americans, contributing to a widening of cancer disparities by educational level. Providing effective educational messages is also not a straightforward matter when it comes to food labeling. It is unclear how best to transmit information about the nutrition content of foods in ways that are easily understood by children and adolescents. The key lesson is that governments must go beyond providing information to consumers.

In contrast to informational strategies, economic incentives bypass conscious consumer decision making. By the law of supply and demand, raising the price of commodities via an excise tax will tend to reduce levels of consumption; conversely, subsidizing products will increase demand.

Raising the excise tax on cigarettes has proved to be a highly effective strategy of tobacco control worldwide. An advantage of cigarette taxes is that youth as well as lower-income groups tend to be more price elastic (i.e., they respond more to a given increase in price). Taxing cigarettes will thus tend to reduce socioeconomic disparities in cancer risk.

On the other hand, taxes are also a blunt instrument in the sense that they cannot distinguish between beneficial and harmful consumption. Thus, the proposal to tax certain foods to curb the obesity epidemic is complicated by the difficulty of identifying which foods ought to be taxed. Some foods may be high in saturated fats, for example, but they may also provide valuable nutrients in other respects. Evidence concerning the price elasticity of demand for foods (as opposed to cigarettes) also remains sparse. If consumers are price inelastic (e.g., if low-income consumers prefer fried foods no matter what the price), raising taxes will be regressive unless the tax increases are matched by subsidies on nutritious and attractive alternatives.

Within the hierarchy of government interventions, regulation and legislation tend to be associated with the most far-reaching and long-lasting effects. Examples in tobacco control include restrictions on advertising cigarette products, as well as banning smoking in workplaces and public settings.

Among tobacco-control experts, the introduction of restrictions on indoor smoking is widely acknowledged to be among the most effective strategies for reducing the prevalence of smoking. The reason is because such restrictions not only encourage smokers to stop, but also because legislation changes societal norms about the acceptability of smoking. It should be noted that carried to extremes, such legislation can end up stigmatizing people who smoke, so legislators must weigh the claims of personal freedom against the rights of nonsmokers not be to harmed.

Several governments have also enacted a total ban on cigarette advertising and promotion (e.g., New Zealand, Norway, Finland, and Canada), which resulted in a roughly 7 percent drop in consumption, according to econometric studies. Several countries also currently restrict the marketing of foods on television aimed at children. Australia bans food advertisements targeted at children under the age of 14, and Sweden bans the use of cartoon characters to sell foods to children under 12.

A recent Institute of Medicine study concluded that the preponderance of evidence suggests that television marketing of foods to children influences their consumption. Although television advertising of cigarettes has been banned in the United States since

1965, commercials during children's viewing hours in this country are still rife with food advertisements.

CONCLUSIONS

Governments have at their disposal a wide range of instruments to prevent cancer at the population level. No single magic bullet is likely to suffice in making a decisive difference to cancer control. A combination of educational, economic, and legislative strategies is likely to prove most effective in the long term. Moreover, solid grounds exist for justifying government intervention in the marketplace for consumer products that contribute to cancer risk. The obesity epidemic is unlikely to be solved by the actions of consumers and markets alone. The history of tobacco control illustrates several effective strategies by which governments have succeeded in reducing the burden of cancer. Although the evidence base for effective interventions is still incomplete, the prevention of obesity has emerged as another target for government action.

SEE ALSO: Diet and Nutrition; Obesity; Prevention, Health and Exercise; Tobacco Smoking.

BIBLIOGRAPHY. Daniel Kim and Ichiro Kawachi, "Food Taxation and Pricing Strategies to 'Thin' Out the Obesity Epidemic: A Research and Policy Perspective," *American Journal of Preventive Medicine* (v.30/5, 2006); John M. McGinnis, et al., eds., "Food Marketing to Children and Youth: Threat or Opportunity?" (National Academies Press, 2006); Michelle D. Mello, et al., "Obesity—The New Frontier of Public Health Law," *New England Journal of Medicine* (v.354/24, 2006); U.S. Department of Health and Human Services, "Reducing the Health Consequences of Smoking: 25 Years of Progress, A Report of the Surgeon General" (DHHS Publication No. 89-8411, 1989).

Ichiro Kawachi, Ph.D.
Harvard School of Public Health

Greece

WITH A WELL-DOCUMENTED history and literary tradition stretching to the ancient world, Greeks dominated many parts of the eastern Mediterranean.

This country was occupied by the Turks in stages from 1354 to 1460 until it proclaimed its independence in 1829. In 1864 the British handed over their colony, which covered the Ionian islands. Greece has a population of 10,648,000 (2004) and has 392 doctors and 257 nurses per 100,000 people. An example of cancer incidence rates in Greece includes 234.9 cases of cancer in males per 100,000, according to the International Agency for Research on Cancer.

Cancer was known in ancient Greece. The ancient Greek doctor Hippocrates identified some medical problems having to do with hard swellings and ulcers that tended to become fatal. He felt that cancers came from an imbalance in fluids, particularly an eruption of black bile—a theory that had much superficial logic. Certainly, he realized that a tumor was often a systemic problem and that mere surgery would not always work. Because of the appearance of tumors, Hippocrates called the disease *karkinos,* the word for *crab,* which remains the symbol for cancer (as well as a sign of the zodiac). The famous Roman medical writer Galen later built on Hippocrates' theories for his own views on cancer.

During the period of Ottoman rule over Greece, there were few developments in cancer treatment. After independence, there was some work on cancer—especially, in recent years, on environmental cancer from pollution.

The prominent U.S. oncologist Georges Nicholas Papanicolaou was born in Greece; he was responsible for establishing the Papanicolaou Cancer Research Center in Miami, Florida. John Christodouloupoulos, head of the Gastroenterology Section at Metaxas Memorial Cancer Hospital in Piraeus during the 1960s, worked on serum gamma-glutamyl transeptidase. B. Lissaios, et al., also from the same hospital, worked on the adjunctive chemotherapy in head and neck cancer. Constantin G. Papvasiliou from Alexandra University Hospital, Athens, worked on cancer of the nasopharynx in Greece during the 1970s.

I. Gorgas and Gr. Skalkeas from King Paul's Hospital at the University of Athens researched carcinoma of the breast in young women. S. Skamnakis and A. Lemonidis of the Department of General Surgery at the Hippocration General Hospital, Thessaloniki, worked on problems concerning malignant melanoma.

In recent years, there have been many cancer trials in Greece, including particularly important ones on colorectal cancer, largely under the aegis of the Panhellenic Association for Continual Medical Research; on clinical treatment of oral cancer at Athens General Hospital; and on endometrial cancer, which is much less common in Greece than in other countries.

The Hellenic Cancer Society and the Hellenic Society of Oncology are both members of the International Union Against Cancer.

Many important Greeks and people connected with Greece have died from cancer. Princess Anastasia of Greece, the wife of Prince Christopher of Greece and Denmark, died from cancer. Sophocles Venizelos, prime minister in 1950, died from a lung tumor. Mary Challens, who wrote on ancient Greece under the name Mary Renault, died of cancer. Melina Mercouri, a singer and politician, smoked throughout her life and died from lung cancer. Xan Fielding, a British writer on Crete and translator, died from cancer.

SEE ALSO: Breast Cancer; Chemotherapy; Colon Cancer; Pollution, Air; Women's Cancers.

BIBLIOGRAPHY. Erskine Carmichael, "Dr. Papanicolau and the Pap Smear," *The Alabama Journal of Medical Science* (v.21, 1984); James S. Olson, *Bathsheba's Breast: Women, Cancer and History* (Johns Hopkins University, 2002); Ronald W. Raven, *The Theory and Practice of Oncology* (Parthenon Publications, 1990); V. G. Valaoras, et al., "Lactation and Reproductive Histories of Breast Cancer Patients in Greater Athens, 1965–67," *International Journal of Cancer* (v.3, 1969); Apostolos Xilomenos, et al., "Colorectal Cancer Screening Awareness Among Physicians in Greece," *BMC Gastroenterology* (v.6, 2006).

JUSTIN CORFIELD
GEELONG GRAMMAR SCHOOL, AUSTRALIA

Green, Adele

A PROFESSOR AT the Queensland Institute of Medical Research, Australia, Adele Green has been active in the development and use of sunscreen to protect people against skin cancer. As well as highlighting this to adults, her work has led to many "sun-smart" programs in primary schools. Adele Chandler Green graduated M.B.B.S. with first-class honors from the University of Queensland in 1976; she completed her Ph.D. in 1984 and M.Sc. in 1985 from the London School of Hygiene and Tropical Medicine. She then returned to Australia and became deputy director and laboratory head of the Cancer & Population Studies Group at the Queensland Institute of Medical Research and conjoint professor at the University of Queensland. A member of the council of the National Health and Medical Research Council (NHMRC) of Australia, she was chairperson of the Health Advisory Committee of the NHMRC from 2000 to 2003. In 2004 she was made a Companion of the Order of Australia "for services to medical research through significant advances made in the field of the epidemiology of skin cancer and ovarian cancer, to public health including Indigenous health, and for leadership in the wider science community."

SUNSCREEN RESEARCH

One of her major pieces of research involved getting the residents of Nambour, a town 65 miles north of Brisbane, Queensland, to test the use of sunscreen. This research involved 800 people chosen randomly from the electoral roll who applied SPF 15-plus sunscreen every day for five years; the remainder of the subjects used sunscreen as they had done normally, which tended to be only when they were sunbathing or in the sun for recreational purposes. The research rapidly showed that melanomas can appear in people who do not regularly use sunscreen, especially in occupational exposure to the sun. This situation occurred in part because many white-skinned Australians had precancerous cells in their skin called initiated cells, which may have developed in childhood, adolescence, or young adulthood.

Continued exposure to sunlight resulted in the appearance of melanomas. As a result, a number of young adults in their late 20s and early 30s were found to have basal-cell carcinomas. The overall conclusion of Green's research was that using sunscreen heavily as an adult, even for five years, was no substitute for using it as a child to prevent the emergence of precancerous cells; thus, it is particularly important for children to use sunscreen and stay out of direct sunlight as much as possible.

SEE ALSO: Australia; Skin Cancer (Melanoma); Sun Exposure (Australia).

BIBLIOGRAPHY. *Medical Directory of Australia* (Australasian Medical Publishing Co., 2006); *Who's Who in Australia* (Crown Content, 2006).

JUSTIN CORFIELD
GEELONG GRAMMAR SCHOOL, AUSTRALIA

Gregoire, Christine

THE DEMOCRATIC GOVERNOR of the U.S. state of Washington, Christine Gregoire became famous for her battle against breast cancer a year before her election as governor. She has regularly referred to this situation in many speeches and has used it to encourage many women to have regular screenings for breast cancer.

Christine O'Grady was born on March 24, 1947, in Auburn, Washington. She grew up on a small farm, attending the University of Washington, from which she graduated with a B.A. in 1969. She specialized in

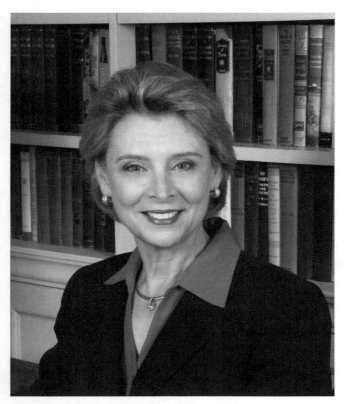

Washington state governor Christine Gregoire became a famous anti-cancer advocate after her bout with breast cancer.

speech and sociology. She worked as a clerk and typist with the Washington State Department of Social and Health Services, where she met Mike Gregoire, whom she subsequently married. She attended law school at Gonzaga University in Spokane, graduating J.D. *cum laude* in 1977.

Gregoire then worked as an assistant attorney general in the office of Slade Gordon, the state attorney general. From 1988 until 1992, she was director of the Washington Department of Ecology and was then elected attorney general, being twice reelected. During this time she was involved in a lawsuit against the tobacco industry, winning the state a $4.5 billion share of the settlement, including a $500 million bonus for her role.

In 2003 Gregoire was diagnosed with breast cancer after a routine checkup and a mammogram showed some cancer cells in her left breast—ductal carcinoma in situ, which could prove fatal if not treated. The checkup followed her decision to run for governor. She later said that she got the checkup largely because if she were asked about her health during the election campaign in which she was to stand as a candidate for governor, she wanted to be able to state that truthfully she had a clean bill of health. The cancer had been caught early, and she had surgery, which was successful. Initially, she thought of resigning from politics but was encouraged by her doctor to seek treatment and then decide on her career. By September 2003, Gregoire was recovering, still working as attorney general and very much a candidate in the race.

Gregoire's battle with cancer was much publicized in the media, and since she was elected governor in 2004, she has been a supporter of cancer charities. At the Susan G. Komen Breast Cancer Foundation's Race for the Cure in Seattle in 2005, she said, "I'm racing for the cure so that none of our sons and daughters, nieces and nephews, ever have to hear the words 'You have cancer.'"

She said that she briefly considered keeping quiet about her operation, but then decided that it would be a great opportunity to show the advances in medicine and encourage more women to have mammograms on a regular basis. Gregoire has gained much support from many citizens of Washington state for her attack on the tobacco industry. Indeed, Tobacco-Free Kids Action Fund campaigned for her in recognition of her support for tobacco control.

SEE ALSO: Breast Cancer; Tobacco Industry; United States.

BIBLIOGRAPHY. *Who's Who in America* (Marquis Who's Who, 1993–2005); *Who's Who of American Women* (Marquis Who's Who, 1993–2000); *Who's Who in American Politics* (R. R. Bowker/Marquis Who's Who, 1993–1999); *Who's Who in the West* (Marquis Who's Who, 1994–2002).

JUSTIN CORFIELD
GEELONG GRAMMAR SCHOOL, AUSTRALIA

Guatemala

THIS CENTRAL AMERICAN country, located south of Mexico, was a Spanish colony until it gained its independence on September 15, 1821. It has a population of 14,280,596 (2004) and has 93 doctors and 27 nurses per 100,000 people. An example of cancer incidence rates in Guatemala includes 146.1 cases of cancer in males per 100,000, according to the International Agency for Research on Cancer.

During the Spanish period, health care remained underdeveloped, with only the wealthy managing to get surgical treatment for cancer; others relied on herbal infusions. Many people did not live long enough to develop symptoms from cancer, so awareness was not very good, and treatment was extremely poor.

Many cancers in Guatemala are from environmental factors such as pollution and bad diet, but lung cancer remains a major cause of death for men, and there is also a rising number of people suffering from skin cancer. Currently, women outnumber men in terms of people diagnosed with cancer at a ratio of 2.7 to 1.

The main form of cancer for women of reproductive age, and the second major cause of cancer for women of all ages in Guatemala, is uterine or cervical cancer. To increase knowledge of cervical cancer, the Pan-American Health Organization has assisted the Guatemalan government. To encourage women to have screenings for cervical cancer, Sue Patterson founded the Women's International Network for Guatemalan Solutions in 2001; it operates out of Antigua, the old capital, and has been successful in raising awareness in the general community. Other common cancers for women include breast cancer, skin cancer, and stomach cancer. For men, stomach cancer is extremely common, followed by skin cancer, lung cancer, and prostate cancer. There is also the prevalence of human T-cell leukemia–lymphoma virus in some black former slave communities in Guatemala.

The main cancer organizations in the country are the Instituto de Cancerología (Cancer Institute) and La Liga Nacional Contra el Cáncer (The National League against Cancer). The Liga Nacional Contra el Cáncer Guatemala/Piensa is a member of the International Union against Cancer. The official medical research center for the country is the Academia de Ciencis Medicas, Fisicas y Naturales de Guatemala. There are also a faculty of medicine at the Universidad de San Carlos de Guatemala and a school of medicine at the Universidad Francisco Marroquin, both in Guatemala City.

SEE ALSO: Cervical Cancer; Lung Cancer, Non-Small Cell; Lung Cancer, Small Cell; Prostate Cancer; Skin Cancer (Melanoma); Skin Cancer (Non-Melanoma).

BIBLIOGRAPHY. Dr. Carlos Salazar, "Oncologia: Viviendo con el Cáncer," www.infovia.com.gt/vidamedica/oncologia.htm (cited November 2006); Instituto Nacional de Estadística, *Mortalidad de 1992 a 1996* (Instituto Nacional de Estadística, 1999); "Knowledge and Use of Tobacco among Guatemalan Physicians," *Cancer Causes and Control* (v.13.9, 2002); Pan-American Health Organization, "Assessment of Guatemala's Efforts for Cervical Cancer Prevention and Control," http://ncd.bvsalud.org/portals/cervicalCancer/docs/en/GuatemalaCC.doc (cited November 2006); Roxana Valdés-Ramos, et al., "Can the Degree of Concordance with Recommendations for a Cancer Prevention Diet and Lifestyle Be Assessed from Existing Survey Information Data," *American Journal of Clinical Nutrition* (v.74.6, 2001).

JUSTIN CORFIELD
GEELONG GRAMMAR SCHOOL, AUSTRALIA

Guinea

THIS WEST AFRICAN country was a French colony until it gained its independence on October 2, 1958. Guinea has a population of 9,246,000 (2004) and has 13 doctors and 56 nurses per 100,000 people. An example of cancer incidence rates in guinea includes 95 cases of cancer in males per 100,000, according to the International Agency for Research on Cancer.

During the French colonial period, most people in French Guinea did not live long enough to suffer from cancer, with both Europeans and Africans dying at early ages, mainly from tropical diseases. There were some early cases of Africans suffering from liver cancer, with no cure at the time, although herbal infusions were often used. Apart from the main hospital in Conakry, the capital, medical care remained underdeveloped.

In 1938, the postal authorities in French Guinea issued a semipostal stamp commemorating the fourth anniversary of the death of Marie Curie. It served to raise awareness of cancer, and also cancer treatment, among the Europeans in Guinea. After independence, there were major upgrades of hospitals and medical care facilities throughout the country. In spite of these upgrades, the rates of liver cancer have remained high. As many as a third of men who die from cancer succumb to liver cancer. Prostate cancer and stomach cancer, by contrast, account for only 8.1 percent and 6.2 percent of male cancer deaths, respectively. For women, the main cause of death from cancer is cervical cancer (46 percent), followed by liver cancer (12.5 percent) and breast cancer (10.9 percent). There is also the prevalence of human T-cell leukemia–lymphoma virus in Guinea. Medical care in the country centers on the faculty of medicine at the Université Gamal Abdel Nasser de Conakry.

SEE ALSO: Breast Cancer; Cervical Cancer; Liver Cancer, Adult (Primary); Liver Cancer, Childhood (Primary); Prostate Cancer.

BIBLIOGRAPHY. M. Koulibaly, et al., "Cancer Incidence in Conakry, Guinea: First Results from the Cancer Registry 1992–1995," *International Journal of Cancer* (v.70/1, 1997); A. Soyannwo and S. D. Amanor-Boadu, "Management of Cancer Pain—A Survey of Current Practice in West Africa," *The Nigerian Postgraduate Medical Journal* (v.8/4, 2001).

JUSTIN CORFIELD
GEELONG GRAMMAR SCHOOL, AUSTRALIA

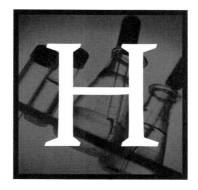

H. Lee Moffitt Cancer Center & Research Institute, University of South Florida

THE H. LEE Moffitt Cancer Center & Research Institute (Moffitt) in Tampa, Florida, opened in 1986 and was named a National Cancer Institute Comprehensive Cancer in 2001. It is named for H. Lee Moffitt, a Florida state representative who was a cancer survivor himself and was instrumental in the creation of Moffitt and in securing funding from the Florida state legislature. Construction for the initial facility came primarily from the state cigarette tax.

The purpose of Moffitt is to fight cancer through patient care, education, and research. As of 2006 Moffitt was licensed for 162 hospital beds; it employed over 2,800 staff members, 300 physicians, and 600 research faculty and research support staff. In 2006 Moffitt had over 6,000 inpatient admissions and over 200,000 outpatient visits. Research funding as of January 2005 was over $52 million, almost $43 million of that in peer-reviewed grants.

Patient care at the Moffitt Cancer Center is provided through an interdisciplinary team approach and is organized into several areas: Blood & Marrow Transplantation, Comprehensive Breast Cancer, Cutaneous Oncology, Gastrointestinal Malignancies, Genitourinary Oncology, Gynecologic Oncology, Head & Neck Oncology, Internal & Hospital Medicine, Malignant Hematology, Neuro-oncology, Psychosocial & Palliative Care, Sarcoma, and Senior Adult Oncology (for patients age 70 and older). The Blood & Marrow Transplantation program is the largest of its type in the southeastern United States.

The Lifetime Cancer Screening & Prevention Center is a freestanding facility that provides clinical screening, diagnostic services, educational programs, and research. Specific programs include genetic screening and counseling, smoking-cessation programs, clinical research trials, and community education.

Specialized services have been developed for high-risk patients, including the Genetic Counseling and Testing Program (the first such program in the region). The Tobacco Research and Intervention Program conducts research on psychosocial and behavior factors that contribute to tobacco use; provides smoking-cessation and tobacco education; and conducts training programs at the undergraduate, graduate, and postdoctoral levels.

Moffitt offers support services for cancer patients, survivors, and their families. The Integrative Medicine program offers acupuncture treatments, yoga classes, meditation and guided-imagery sessions, nutritional services, pharmaceutical counseling, and relaxation massage. In addition, the Arts in Medicine program promotes the role of the creative arts—including music, visual arts, dance, and writing—in influencing well being and recovery for cancer patients, family members, caregivers, and hospital staff.

Clinical social workers are available to help patients and their families assess their situations and develop effective ways of managing the emotional and practical effects of having cancer. Several support groups are available at Moffitt, including groups for breast cancer, lung cancer, brain tumors, prostate cancer, laryngectomies, families and friends of cancer patients, and children and parents who have a family member with cancer.

EDUCATION AND RESEARCH

Moffitt provides educational resources for the general public through its website, including information on different types of cancer, common treatments, and clinical trials. Links to other sources of information are also provided.

The Patient Education Research Center (PERC) at Moffitt is a library providing up-to-date cancer information for patients, family members, caregivers, and the public. Available resources at the PERC include health and medical reference books, pamphlets and brochures, consumer health magazines and newsletters, computer software, and audiotapes and videotapes. Cancer Answers—a toll-free telephone service staffed by registered nurses who provide information about types of cancer, treatments, and clinical trials—handles over 12,000 calls per year.

The Graduate Medical Education Office at Moffitt offers oncology fellowship training for physicians in several areas, including Blood & Marrow Transplant, Hematology and Medical Oncology, Neurosurgery, OB/GYN, Surgical Pathology, Psychosocial & Palliative Care, Urology, Breast Oncology, Radiation Oncology, and Musculoskeletal Oncology. *Cancer Control Journal*, a peer-reviewed journal indexed in Medline, is published four times per year by Moffitt.

The Moffitt Research Institute (MRI) supports the cancer center's mission to contribute to cancer prevention and cure. Research at the MRI is organized into three major areas and six scientific programs. The Basic Research area includes the Molecular Oncology, Immunology, and Drug Discovery programs. The Cancer Prevention and Control area includes the Health Outcomes and Behavior and the Risk Assessment, Detection, & Intervention programs. The Clinical Investigations area includes the Experimental Therapeutics program.

The goals of the Molecular Oncology program are to understand the molecular basis of oncogenesis and ultimately to develop new and better therapies for cancer. Research in the Molecular Oncology program focuses on signal transduction and gene regulation, both of which lend themselves to translation studies and collaboration with other programs within Moffitt.

The goals of the Immunology program are to discover the nature of the host–tumor relationship and to harness these discoveries to improve clinical care. Specific areas of study within the Immunology program include innate immunity, adaptive immunity, molecular mechanisms controlling gene mechanisms in immune cells, and translation of research findings into immunotherapy.

The Drug Discovery Program conducts research on many levels, from basic research in topics such as the study of signal conduction pathways to conducting clinical trials, with the ultimate goal of creating efficacious and safe anticancer drugs.

The Health Outcomes & Behavior program has three specific aims: to understand the determinants of behaviors that lead to cancer prevention and early detection, and to develop methods to promote those behaviors; to improve the quality of life of cancer patients; and to improve the quality of cancer care. Tobacco research is a particular focus, and research currently in progress includes basic research into factors that influence tobacco use and development of improved smoking-cessation and relapse-prevention programs, in particular for subgroups such as pregnant women.

The Risk Assessment, Detection & Intervention program focuses on preventing cancer mortality though improved methods of early detection, clinical prevention for high-risk individuals, and improved understanding of etiology. It has three specific aims: to identify factors (such as genetic, lifestyle, or viral) associated with cancer risk; to evaluate new cancer-prevention clinical interventions; and to identify and validate new approaches to early detection of cancer, including nanotechnology, molecular markers, and imaging.

SEE ALSO: Education, Cancer; National Cancer Institute; Smoking and Society; Smoking Cessation (nicotine replacement); Tobacco Smoking.

BIBLIOGRAPHY. *Cancer Control Journal* website, www. moffitt.org/moffittapps/ccj/index.html (cited December

2006); H. Lee Moffitt Cancer Center & Research Institute website, www.moffitt.org (cited December 2006).

SARAH BOSLAUGH
WASHINGTON UNIVERSITY SCHOOL OF MEDICINE

H. Lundbeck (Denmark)

H. LUNDBECK A/S of Denmark is an international pharmaceutical company "engaged in the research and development, production, marketing and sale of drugs for the treatment of psychiatric and neurological disorders." It specializes in drugs for cancer, depression, schizophrenia, Alzheimer's disease, and Parkinson's disease.

Based in Copenhagen, H. Lundbeck was founded in 1915 by Hans Lundbeck as a trading company involved in the sale of many items from overseas to Denmark, including aluminum foil, photographic equipment, and machinery.

In 1924 it started selling pharmaceutical products and cosmetics. By the late 1930s the company started to produce its own pharmaceuticals, and, building up its own research department, it started production, which was interrupted during World War II when Denmark was occupied by Germany. Since the end of World War II, H. Lundbeck has grown massively. In 2003 the company's revenue was 9.9 billion Danish kroner (U.S. $1.7 billion).

H. Lundbeck is best known in oncological circles for its recent development of the drug Siramesine, which was originally envisaged as a treatment for anxiety. During clinical trials, however, the drug turned out to be able to kill resistant cancer cells. This situation led to collaboration between Lundbeck and the Danish Cancer Society. It was discovered that Siramesine could kill cancer cells by affecting the lysosomes. With Siramesine-treated tumor cells displaying some increased levels of reactive oxygen species, lysosomal membrane permeabilization, chromatin condensation, and shrinkage, this could lead to the detachment of cancer cells. The drug has been tested in mice, and clinical trials in humans are planned to commence soon. Its particular use is for people for whom radiation or chemotherapy is not an option, but also to prevent the cancer cells from building up any resistance against other drugs.

SEE ALSO: Clinical Trials; Drugs; Pharmaceutical Industry.

BIBLIOGRAPHY. *Lundbeck* Magazine, www.materials.lundbeck.com/lundbeck/88/ (cited May 2007). Lundbeck web site. www.lundbeck.com/ (cited May 2007); *H. Lundbeck A/S: International Competitive Benchmarks and Financial Gap Analysis* (Icon Group International, Inc. 2000); *H. Lundbeck A/S: Labor Productivity Benchmarks and International Gap Analysis* (Icon Group International, Inc. 2000).

JUSTIN CORFIELD
GEELONG GRAMMAR SCHOOL, AUSTRALIA

Haematology Society of Australia and New Zealand

THE HAEMATOLOGY SOCIETY of Australia and New Zealand (HSANZ) is a not-for-profit organization created in 1998 through the combination of the Haematology Society of Australia and the New Zealand Society for Haematology.

Hematology is the branch of medical practice concerned with conditions of the blood. These conditions range from the common iron deficiency anemia, to cancers originating in the blood, to rare forms of abnormal blood coagulation.

The blood as an "organ" literally affects all other organs as it flows through the body and therefore abnormalities in the blood can cause malfunctioning in all other organs. The aims of the HSANZ are to promote the study of hematology, promote improved standards of research, foster interest in hematology among other regional and international bodies, and promote scientific communication among scientists and other experts in hematology by facilitating visits of such people to Australia and arranging for Australian experts to travel abroad. The HSANZ secretariat is located in Sydney, Australia.

MEETINGS AND MEMBERSHIP

HSANZ holds an annual scientific meeting. The 2006 meeting was held in Hobart, Tasmania, in conjunction with the Australia and New Zealand Society of Blood Transfusion and the Australasian Society of Thrombosis and Haemostasis. HSANZ also holds branch scientific meetings in Australia and New Zealand, and it maintains a list of hematology-related conferences and courses on its website.

Ordinary membership in HSANZ is reserved for medical graduates who have worked in hematology for at least three years and for medical and other graduates who have worked at least three years in research relevant to hematology. Trainee membership is available to hematologists engaged in clinical or laboratory training. Associate membership is available to people who have made a significant contribution to hematology but are not otherwise eligible for membership.

RESEARCH AWARDS AND RESOURCES

HSANZ, together with the Clinical Oncology Society of Australia and the Medical Oncology Group of Australia, grants the Haematology and Oncology Targeted Therapies fellowship, which promotes translation and clinical research in hematology in Australia. Two research grants of $50,000 are awarded annually to support research initiatives. The Celgene/HSANZ Educational Grants of $3,000 are awarded annually to four trainees to allow them to attend and present at an international meeting. The Baikie Award is awarded annually to the best presentation at the HSANZ annual scientific presentation by a HSANZ member age 35 or younger; it includes a $2,000 award and the Baikie Medal. The HSANZ Travel Grant is awarded to allow recipients to present at the HSANZ annual scientific meeting. The Schering/HSANZ Young Investigator Scholarship and the Amgen/HSANZ Young Investigator Scholarship are awarded annually to a recent medical or science graduate committed to a career in hematology, and provide $30,000 to be used for study at a clinical or laboratory center of excellence, preferably overseas.

The HSANZ website includes several resources of interest to hematologists. Resources available to nonmembers include a list of hematology-related recommended readings, abstracts from previous HSANZ annual meetings, and links to hematology-related websites. HSANZ members can access further resources, including discussion forums and a list of members.

SEE ALSO: Australia; Australia and New Zealand Society of Blood Transfusion; New Zealand.

BIBLIOGRAPHY. Haematology Society of Australia and New Zealand, www.hsanz.org.au (cited May 2007); Eric Bogdanich and Eric Koli, "2 Paths of Bayer Drug in 80's: Riskier One Steered Overseas," *New York Times* (May 22, 2003).

SARAH BOSLAUGH
WASHINGTON UNIVERSITY SCHOOL OF MEDICINE

Haemophilia Society of Malaysia

THE HAEMOPHILIA SOCIETY of Malaysia is the national hemophilia organization for Malaysia, providing information and resources about hemophilia in English and Malay. As of 2006 the president of the society was Mohamed Aris Hashim Mohamed. The society offices are located within the National Blood Centre in Kuala Lumpur, Malaysia. Over 1,200 hemophiliacs were registered with the society as of December 2001.

Basic information about hemophilia and other clotting disorders is available in English and Malay from the society's website, as are reports on society activities and information about the history and state of hemophilia care in Malaysia. The society also sponsors workshops and seminars for medical professionals and the general public. In March 2006 a hemophilia treatment seminar attended by 87 medical staff members from across Malaysia was jointly organized by the society, the Ministry of Health, the Physiotherapy Department of Kuala Lumpur General Hospital, and the National Blood Bank. This seminar emphasized a multidisciplinary approach to modern hemophilia care, including the roles of dentists, nurses, physiotherapists, laboratory workers, and psychological counselors. It was followed by a three-day physiotherapy workshop led by a guest lecturer from the World Federation of Hemophilia (WFH).

TWINNING PROGRAMS

The society recently took part in the twinning program of the World Federation of Hemophilia, in which hemophilia treatment centers and patient organizations in a developed country are paired with their counterparts in a developing country for the purpose of sharing knowledge and best practices.

The Haemophilia Society of Malaysia was paired with the Pakistan Hemophilia Patients' Welfare Society, a relationship so successful that it was awarded the "Twin of the Year Award 2005" organization award from the World Federation of Hemophilia at the WFH Congress in Vancouver, Canada.

The accomplishments of this relationship included establishing chapters of the national hemophilia organization in all provinces in Pakistan, conducting patient assessments throughout the country, and establishing a national office in Islamabad. The program has created models that can be used with Haemophilia Societies in other developing countries.

The society provided information about the number of hemophiliacs in Malaysia and the number infected with HIV through blood transfusions as part of an investigation of a tainted blood product sold in Malaysia and other Asian countries in the 1980s. The product, Factor VIII concentrate, is used by hemophiliacs to prevent bleeding or stop bleeding episodes.

The investigation revealed that after a method of heat-treating blood to kill the AIDS virus was commonly used in the creation of Factor VIII, older stocks that potentially carried the AIDS virus were sold in Malaysia and other Asian countries by Cutter Biological, a division of Bayer.

SEE ALSO: Education, Cancer; Hepatitis C; Malaysia.

BIBLIOGRAPHY. Eric Bogdanich and Eric Koli, "2 Paths of Bayer Drug in 80's: Riskier One Steered Overseas," *New York Times* (May 22, 2003); Chan Chee Khoon, "Blood Money: Bayer, Haemophiliacs, and AIDS," www.aliran.com/oldsite/monthly/2003/5f.html; Hemophilia Society of Malaysia website, www.hemofilia.org.my/v1.

SARAH BOSLAUGH
WASHINGTON UNIVERSITY SCHOOL OF MEDICINE

Haemophilia Society of the United Kingdom

THE HAEMOPHILIA SOCIETY of the United Kingdom is the national charity for people with hemophilia and related bleeding disorders. It was founded in 1950 and has a network of 17 local groups and over 2,000 members. The society offices are located in London.

The Haemophilia Society provides information, advice, and support services for patients and their families, and serves as an advocate for them to receive optimal care and treatment. It also provides services for hemophiliacs infected with Human Immunodeficiency Virus (HIV) and hepatitis C.

The society is also concerned with advancing services and care to people with bleeding disorders worldwide and is a founding member of the World Federation of Hemophilia, created in 1963. A research funding program run by the Haemophilia Society provides small grants (usually 5,000 to 10,000 pounds) for medical and psychosocial research aimed at improving treatment for individuals with bleeding disorders. Some of the research is commissioned directly by the society, and some is awarded through a competitive grant process. A grant application and information about the research currently and previously funded by the Haemophilia Society are available from the society website.

As of 2006 the society was advocating for a public inquiry into the use of contaminated blood and blood products in the 1970s and early 1980s by the National Health Service, which resulted in thousands of people becoming infected with HIV and hepatitis C.

PUBLICATIONS AND RESOURCES

The society produces several publications, including fact sheets, booklets, press releases, magazines, and newsletters, and it makes available through its website some materials produced by other organizations. Most publications are available free of charge and can be downloaded from the society's website.

Newsletters and magazines produced by the society and available online include *HQ*, the official magazine of the Haemophilia Society, published three times per year; *HQ News*, a newsletter published twice per year; *H3*, a newsletter published three times per year for people affected by hemophilia, hepatitis C, and/or HIV; *HQ Too!*, a magazine published for young people with bleeding disorders; and *Female Factors*, a magazine published for women affected by bleeding disorders.

Basic information about hemophilia and other bleeding disorders is available on the society's website. Fact sheets on topics such as benefits rights, career issues, and travel insurance for people with bleeding disorders may also be downloaded from the website or ordered from the society. The website also includes a directory of hemophilia centers and comprehensive-care centers in the United Kingdom, as well as discussion forums on topics related to bleeding disorders.

SEE ALSO: Education, Cancer; Hepatitis C; United Kingdom.

BIBLIOGRAPHY. The Haemophilia Society www.haemophilia.org.uk; Lorna Martin, "Left to Die: The Hidden Victims of an NHS Blunder," www.observer.guardian.co.uk (cited November 2006).

SARAH BOSLAUGH
WASHINGTON UNIVERSITY SCHOOL OF MEDICINE

Hair Dye

THERE ARE SEVERAL reasons why we should be concerned about hair dyes in relation to cancer risk: the widespread use of hair dyes; findings of an increased cancer risk in hairdressers and barbers; findings from animal studies showing that the main components of hair dyes, a class of chemicals known as aromatic amines, are carcinogenic; findings from human studies showing an increased risk of cancer in users of permanent hair dyes; and the U.S. Food and Drug Administration's Food, Drug, and Cosmetic Act, which exempts hair dyes from the certification process used for other cosmetic colors.

Hair dyes are used widely in developed nations, both to change natural hair color and to cover gray hair. In the United States, 40 percent of women age 18 to 60 use hair dyes regularly. Thus, any increase in risk of cancer with use of hair dyes can have important public health implications due to the high prevalence of this exposure.

Hairdressers have been known to experience higher risk of bladder cancer than the general population. In 1993, the International Agency for Research on Cancer concluded that "occupation as a hairdresser or a barber entails exposures that are probably carcinogenic."

The main components of hair dyes are aromatic amines, which have been found to be mutagenic in vitro and cause cancer in laboratory animals. Aromatic amines, also called arylamines, were the first established human bladder carcinogens identified from occupational settings. Industrial use of these dyes has been under strict regulation for more than 50 years in the United States, but in addition to cigarette smoking, which is a major source of arylamine exposure in the United States today, long-term use of hair dyes represents a source of arylamines in humans.

Paraphenylenediamine (PPD), an arylamine, is the main component of permanent hair dyes, used in almost every product on the market today, regardless of brand. The available data suggest that PPD and hydrogen peroxide—a combination used in all permanent hair dyes—form a genotoxic carcinogen. A recent re-evaluation by the European Commission's Scientific Committee on Cosmetic Products and Non-Food Products intended for consumers concerning p-phen-

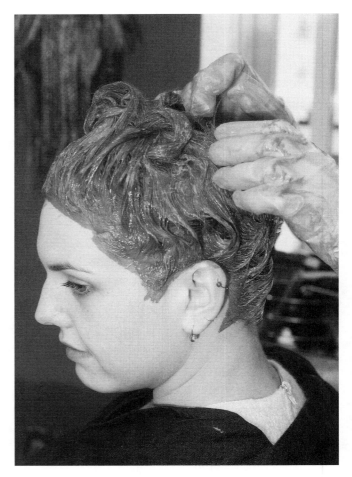

Hair dyes have an exemption from any regulation in the U.S. 1938 Food, Drug, and Cosmetic Act.

ylenediamine, adopted during the 19th plenary meeting of February 27, 2002, considered the results from animal studies to be supportive of the carcinogenic potential of PPD together with hydrogen peroxide.

In human studies, use of personal hair dyes has been associated with cancers of the bladder and non-Hodgkin's lymphoma. A limited number of studies have examined the association between personal use of hair dyes and bladder cancer, and results have been inconsistent. One recent meta-analysis found the pooled relative risk for users of hair dyes was only 1.01 for bladder cancer. The main difficulties in evaluating this association are exposure assessment; potential confounding by lifestyle factors; and small sample size, especially small sample size of subjects with intensive exposure, mainly women. Information is also limited on the various types of hair dyes and genetic susceptibility.

In a study conducted in Los Angeles, an excess bladder cancer risk was found among permanent-hair-dye users, not among users of other types of dyes, and the risk was higher among permanent-hair-dye users with a N-acetyl-transferase 2 (NAT2) or cytochrome-P450 (CYP1A2) slow phenotype. In a second meta-analysis, sensitivity analyses revealed a 22 percent to 50 percent increase in bladder cancer risk for hair-dye users.

Studies have examined the association between personal use of hair dyes and blood or hematopoietic cancers, and the overall evidence suggests an increased risk of this type of cancer among hair-dye users. A recent meta-analysis found that the pooled relative risk for users of hair dyes was 1.15 for all blood cancers. The risk appeared to vary by subtype of blood cancers, with a significantly increased risk observed for non-Hodgkin's lymphoma and lymphocytic leukemia but not for other types.

REGULATION

Currently, hair dyes fall under a 1938 exemption in the Food, Drug, and Cosmetic Act. This Depression-era provision exempts hair dyes from the certification process required of other cosmetic colors. It requires the dyes only to carry warnings about skin irritation or eye injury.

California recently passed the country's first state cosmetics regulatory act, the California Safe Cosmetics Act, which will require manufacturers to report the use of potentially hazardous ingredients to the state Department of Health Services. Following the release of the Los Angeles bladder report, which concluded that the long-term use of these chemicals could cause bladder cancer, the European Commission banned 22 hair-dye substances. The commission had asked the hair-dye producers to provide safety files for the 115 chemicals used in hair dyes to prove that these substances do not pose a health risk for consumers. The ban concerns 22 chemicals in hair dye for which the industry has not submitted any safety files.

Risk of cancer from hair dye appears to differ by gender, type of hair dye, shade or color, frequency, duration and lifetime cumulative use, calendar time period of use, interactions with other risk factors (such as smoking) and genetic influences.

Gender. Most studies found an increased cancer risk from hair dyes among women, but not among men. This is not surprising, because women use hair dyes more often than men do, and the lack of exposure–disease association among male subjects is likely the result of a low exposure rate leading to low study power to detect the anticipated association.

Hair-dye type. Distinction among different types of hair dyes in epidemiologic studies is potentially important, given the distinct chemical properties and content of dyes. Among users, permanent (oxidation) dyes constitute about 85 percent of the dyes; semipermanent, 10 percent; and temporary rinses, 5 percent.

Permanent-dye precursors are mixed with hydrogen peroxide and chemical couplers such as resourcinol to create a colored oxidation product within the hair shaft. They are called permanent because the dyes formed do not readily diffuse onto the hair during subsequent shampooing.

Semipermanent and temporary dyes deposit color directly on the outer cuticle or surface of each hair and wash out after one to a few dozen shampooings. Earlier studies did not examine personal-hair-dye use by the three major categories of dyes—permanent, semipermanent, and temporary—but recent studies did. When the different hair-dye types were examined, an association with increased bladder and blood cancer risk was found only for permanent dyes, not for semipermanent or temporary hair color.

Shade or color. The color produced by each dye is determined by the proportional composition of chemicals. The greater the concentration of the chemical is, the darker the color. Other factors affecting the color are hair-color shade, texture, and mode of application. Higher risks of blood cancers have been observed for users with the longest duration and the greatest number of applications of permanent and/or dark hair dyes.

Frequency, duration, and cumulative lifetime use. The Los Angeles report showed that the more hair dyes a person uses, the higher that person's risk of bladder cancer. This study found not only a frequency-dependent but also a duration-dependent association between personal use of permanent hair dyes and bladder cancer risk. Thus, women who used permanent dyes at least once a month for a year or longer were twice as likely to develop bladder cancer as women who did not use permanent hair dyes. Those women who used permanent dyes monthly for 15 years or more were more than three times as likely to develop bladder cancer as non-dye users.

Calendar time period of use. From 1978 to 1982, the formulations of hair-coloring products were modified to eliminate or replace some carcinogenic compounds. Consistent with those changes, a study conducted in Connecticut and another study in Europe observed that the increase in lymphoma risk is found only among people who used dyes before 1980. It is unknown at present whether this detected difference in risk means that hair dyes made after 1980 are safe or whether it reflects a latency period (i.e., that people may have not used the new products long enough to get cancer).

Although the hair-dye industry has replaced several ingredients found to cause cancer in animals, some of the cancer-causing compounds have been replaced by similarly structured chemicals, and some scientists feel that the similar structures of these ingredients make it likely that their cancer-causing potential will not differ much from that of the chemicals they are replacing. In addition, the most common ingredient used in hair-dye formulations, PPD, has remained unchanged for the past 50 years.

Interactions with other risk factors. A study has found an additive interaction between hair dyes and smoking in bladder cancer development. This may be relevant because such an additive interaction could mask the effect of hair dyes on bladder cancer in smokers, therefore exposing the need to study a non-smoking population.

Genetic influences. The Los Angeles report found that the risk of cancer from hair dyes appears to differ by polymorphisms in chemical (arylamine) metabolizing genes. It appears that certain women may be more susceptible to bladder cancer associated with the use of permanent hair dyes than other women, depending on their genetic makeup.

The body is able to detoxify arylamines, the chemicals in hair dyes, but because of humans' genetic makeup, some people detoxify these compounds more efficiently than others. It has been proposed that the people that cannot efficiently detoxify arylamines are the ones most at risk from hair dyes. The body's efficiency in removing such toxins depends on whether someone possesses the fast or slow version of these arylamine detoxifying genes.

In the Los Angeles study, women whose bodies could eliminate carcinogenic arylamines only slowly had a higher risk of bladder cancer than women whose bodies eliminated the carcinogens more rapidly. Thus, in women with certain slow arylamine detoxifying genes, such as the NAT2 slow and the CYP1A2 slow phenotypes, exclusive use of permanent hair dye was associated with a nearly tripled risk of developing bladder cancer.

To establish definitively whether hair dyes pose a risk of cancer, further studies are warranted, conducted primarily in women, with detailed information on hair-dye type; color; frequency, duration, and cumulative lifetime use; calendar years of use; smoking; dyeing methods; and genetic susceptibility.

SEE ALSO: Bladder Cancer; Cosmetics; Dyes and Pigments; Tobacco Smoking.

BIBLIOGRAPHY. M. Gago-Dominguez, et al., "Use of Permanent Hair Dyes and Bladder-Cancer Risk," *International Journal of Cancer* (v.91, 2001); M. Gago-Dominguez, et al., "Permanent Hair Dyes and Bladder Cancer: Risk Modification by Cytochrome P4501A2 and N-Acetyltransferases 1 and 2," *Carcinogenesis* (v.24, 2003); B. Takkouche, et al., "Personal Use of Hair Dyes and Risk of Cancer: A Meta-Analysis," *The Journal of the American Medical Association* (v.293, 2005); M. Huncharek and B. Kupelnick, "Personal Use of Hair Dyes and the Risk of Bladder Cancer: Results of a Meta-Analysis," *Public Health Reports* (v.120, 2005).

MANUELA GAGO DOMINGUEZ, PH.D.
JOSE ESTEBAN CASTELAO, PH.D.
USC NORRIS CANCER CENTER

Haiti

THIS NATION, LOCATED in the Caribbean, occupies the western part of the island of Hispaniola, the other part being occupied by the Dominican Republic. It was a French colony based on slavery and sugar plantations until a revolution resulted in Haiti's achieving independence on January 1, 1804.

Since then Haiti has been one of the poorest countries in the world. It has a population of 7,656,000 (2004) and has 8.4 doctors and 11 nurses per 100,000 people. An example of cancer incidence rates in Haiti includes 202 cases of cancer in males per 100,000, according to the International Agency for Research on Cancer. Health services in Haiti have long been extremely under-resourced. In 1957, in the first election using universal suffrage, François "Papa Doc" Duvalier, a doctor who had earned a good reputation working with the poor, was elected. He proclaimed himself president for life in 1964, and when he died in 1971, he was succeeded by his son. During the rule of "Baby Doc," as Jean-Claude Duvalier was known, health services deteriorated further.

The low life expectancy meant that few people in the Duvalier era lived long enough to develop cancer, although prostate cancer, liver cancer, and cancers resulting from environmental problems did affect a small number of people. Indeed, François Duvalier's predecessor, Daniel Fignole, died from prostate cancer.

The human T-cell leukemia–lymphoma virus is prevalent in some communities in Haiti. One of the main opposition leaders in Haiti, Father Gérard Jean-Juste, has been diagnosed with leukemia; in January 2006 he was allowed to seek medical treatment in Miami, Florida. There are a faculty of medicine and pharmacy at the Université d'Etat d'Haiti (State University of Haiti), in Port-au-Prince.

SEE ALSO: Dominican Republic; Liver Cancer, Adult (Primary); Liver Cancer, Childhood (Primary); Prostate Cancer.

BIBLIOGRAPHY. E. J. Mitacek, et al., "Cancer in Haiti 1979–84: Distribution of Various Forms of Cancer According to Geographical Area and Sex," *International Journal of Cancer* (v.38.1, 1986).

JUSTIN CORFIELD
GEELONG GRAMMAR SCHOOL, AUSTRALIA

Head and Neck Cancer

HEAD AND NECK cancer refers to a number of malignancies (nonbenign, invasive, and spreading tumors) that may originate in the mouth (oral cavity), salivary glands, nasal cavity, paranasal sinuses, larynx (Adam's apple), throat (pharynx), cervical lymph nodes of the neck, or skin of the face and neck.

Most cancers of the head and neck manifest as squamous cell carcinomas, which are malignant tumors that develop in the epithelium tissue, lining the exterior and interior bodily cavities as well as the lumen of organs and blood vessels. These tumors have the potential to metastasize (spread from the original spot to new body sites) throughout the head and neck and to nearby organs if not found in time.

In head and neck cancer, cells that normally repair and reproduce in a controlled fashion begin to divide and grow uncontrollably, forming a lump (tumor) in the epithelial layer of the skin and/or various mucous membranes. This type of cancer is characterized by reddish and scaly skin that may eventually present as an open sore.

Head and neck cancers are among the few cancers that can be diagnosed properly, as specific causes for presenting symptoms can usually be identified. Individuals with head and neck cancer may present with symptoms such as a persistent pain in the throat, a sensation of pain or difficulty when swallowing, a change in voice, persistent pain in the ear, and/or bleeding in the mouth or throat.

In screening for head and cancer, the physician will ask about the patient's general medical history, perform a physical exam, and order laboratory tests if appropriate. Any suspected cancerous lesions or tumors will be biopsied and sent to a pathologist for histological examination and a microscopic anatomical inspection, examining for the presence of cancerous cells. Treatment for head and neck cancer, like that for any other form of cancer, is tailored to the specific needs and general health of each individual, as well as the size, location, and stage of tumor spread. Therapy and management of head and neck cancer may include surgery, chemotherapy, and/or radiation therapy, although new treatment options are being studied in clinical trials.

Head and neck cancer is a common disease worldwide. Some of the highest incidence rates are in parts of India and Southeast Asia, where chewing tobacco is a very common practice. Some forms of head and neck cancer are more prevalent in areas of the Middle East and North Africa, where the disease is more commonly associated with infection by the Epstein-Barr virus. Generally, occupational exposure, radiation, dietary factors, and genetics are also risk factors that may play a role.

SEE ALSO: Childhood Cancers; Oral Cancer, Childhood; Tobacco Related Exposures.

BIBLIOGRAPHY. Richard O. Wein, et al., "Disorders of the Head and Neck," in *Schwartz's Surgery* (McGraw-Hill, 2006); Kerstin M. Stenson, et al., "Overview of Head and Neck Cancer," UpToDate Online (cited 2006).

NATANEL JOURABCHI
INDEPENDENT SCHOLAR

Hepatitis B

HEPATITIS B VIRUS (HBV) infection is a major public health crisis globally. Approximately one-third of the world's population is exposed to HBV at some time in their lives; 300 million individuals worldwide are carriers of HBV; and over 1 million people die annually from complications due to liver failure and liver cancer. Appreciating the significant impact of HBV on human health involves understanding HBV; the pathogenesis of HBV infection and the human immune response; the efficacy and availability of the hepatitis B vaccine; and the clinical manifestations, both acutely and chronically, from HBV infection.

VIRUS COMPOSITION AND TRANSMISSION

HBV belongs to the *Hepadnaviridae* family of viruses and is composed of a central core particle made up of the nucleocapsid protein, which surrounds the viral genome (DNA) and the polymerase protein. The viral genome is made of partially double-stranded DNA (3,200 base pairs) and has four overlapping reading frames that encode for the envelope, core, polymerase, and X proteins.

Surrounding the nucleocapsid core is a lipid bilayer (envelope) derived from the host cell from which the HBV was produced. This envelope is studded with viral-encoded proteins (surface protein) involved in virus/hepatocyte (liver cell) attachment. After HBV binds to the hepatocyte cell membrane, the virus-envelope protein mediates the fusion of HBV with the cell membrane, allowing for the uncoating of the virion in the hepatocyte cytoplasm and the entry of the viral DNA into the nucleus, where the virus can remain latent or replicate to produce new virions.

At various points in the life cycle and pathogenesis of HBV, different proteins are expressed by the virus and detectable via blood and biopsy tests. Similarly, the presence of antibodies to viral antigens can help determine the stage of infection. Testing for these antigens and antibodies allows a healthcare provider to determine the stage of infection.

HBV is transmitted from person to person in several ways. Perinatal transmission, or infection at the time of birth is a common means of transmission in Southeast Asia and China, and worldwide this is the most common route of HBV infection. In the United States, Canada, and Western Europe, HBV is more commonly transmitted through sexual contact or intravenous drug use. In addition, HBV is a serious infectious occupational hazard for healthcare workers. HBV is not spread via contaminated food or water; neither is it spread through casual contact with infected individuals.

The most effective means of preventing HBV transmission is the HBV vaccine, which is given as a series of three intramuscular injections. This vaccine, first used in 1982, was the first vaccine to prevent development of a cancer (hepatocellular carcinoma). The vaccine is a recombinant subunit vaccine that contains a single viral protein: the surface antigen. Surface antigen can be produced in yeast, bacterial, or human cell lines, and multiple surface proteins spontaneously assemble into viruslike particles. The formation of viruslike particles appears to be important because vaccination with the monomeric capsid protein does not induce a protective immune response.

More than 95 percent of children vaccinated against HBV develop adequate antibodies in their blood (directed against the surface antigen of HBV). The vaccine is effective in preventing children and adults from developing acute hepatitis and, therefore, protects against chronic HBV infection and the sequlae. Over 116 countries worldwide include the HBV vaccine in their national vaccination programs, but price

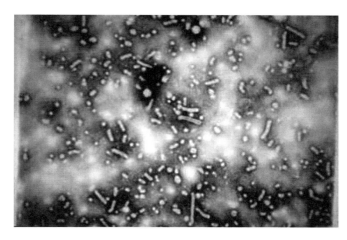

Hepatitis B virus (HBV) is composed of a central core particle made up of the nucleocapsid protein.

has been the main obstacle in providing vaccination in many parts of the developing world.

SYMPTOMS OF INFECTION

Infection with HBV can have an acute or chronic course. Symptoms are related to dysfunction of the liver's metabolic roles, and this destruction is partially mediated by the immune response to infected hepatocytes. Normally, the liver is involved in detoxification, production of bile (and subsequent fat absorption), production of clotting factors, storage of glycogen, production of proteins, and generation of cholesterols.

During the acute phase of infection, most individuals have subclinical hepatitis (70 percent); the remainder develop icteric hepatitis. There are prodromal symptoms that often precede acute hepatitis, such as a skin rash, painful swollen joints, and fever. Acute hepatitis produces symptoms such as anorexia, nausea, jaundice (yellowing of the skin), icterus (yellowing of the white part of the eyes), and abdominal pain. These symptoms can last two to four months.

Rarely—in less than 0.5 percent of adults infected with HBV—acute infection leads to fulminant liver failure. These patients are seriously ill, with encephalopathy (confusion or coma) and easy bruising or bleeding in addition to the symptoms described earlier in this section. This situation is likely caused by a massive lysis (destruction) of infected hepatocytes by cells of the immune system. The majority of patients are able to recover from acute hepatitis;

as discussed later in this article, however, some may progress to chronic infection.

Acute infection with HBV can lead to chronic infection. The age at which a person is infected with HBV is the primary determinant of progression to chronic infection. If HBV is acquired perinatally, 90 percent of individuals will have chronic HBV infection, whereas only 20 percent to 50 percent will have chronic infection if HBV is acquired between 1 and 5 years of age. Of adults who contract HBV, less than 5 percent will progress to chronic HBV infection.

Chronic infection is diagnosed only after six months have passed since the onset of acute hepatitis. This diagnosis can be difficult when the acute infection was subclinical. Most individuals with chronic HBV infection remain without symptoms for decades, with an occasional flare or reactivation of acute symptoms. Chronic hepatitis can eventually lead to cirrhosis of the liver, or a state of scarring and fibrosis. Patients are often fatigued and susceptible to infection, and may lose weight and become malnourished due to malabsorption. Poor absorption of vitamins A and D leads to vision impairment and osteopenia (thinning of bones), respectively. In addition, liver cirrhosis can lead to gynecomastia (swelling of breast tissue), atrophic testicles, and palmar erythema (red palms).

If cirrhosis progresses to advanced cirrhosis, or chronic liver failure, individuals may develop portal hypertension. This occurs when the liver becomes too fibrotic and scarred to filter and transport blood adequately, causing a backup of blood from the portal venous system into the systemic venous system. This condition can cause fluid retention and edema (swelling); ascites (fluid retention in the abdomen); and a backup of blood into veins around the umbilicus, rectum, and lower esophagus. If the backup of blood becomes severe enough, patients can experience severe bleeding, exacerbated by the lack of clotting factors secondary to cirrhosis. They may vomit blood or have rectal bleeding.

Because portal hypertension precludes sufficient detoxification of ammonia and other metabolites, patients can experience encephalopathy, leading to confusion and coma. The backup of blood into the spleen can cause splenomegaly (spleen enlargement) and, secondarily, spleen dysfunction, anemia (decreased red blood cells), leukopenia (decreased white blood cells), and thrombocytopenia (decreased platelets).

One of the most noticeable signs of liver failure is jaundice, or yellowing of the skin. The normal liver eliminates a compound caused bilirubin, but hepatic dysfunction leads to a backup of bilirubin into the circulation and to accumulation of this yellow compound in the skin, conjunctiva, and mucous membranes.

TREATMENT FOR CHRONIC INFECTION

Chronic HBV infection is sometimes treated with interferon or lamivudine, with the goal of treatment being suppression of viral reproduction and improvement of liver function tests. Treatment with interferon both directly inhibits viral replication and stimulates the immune system to fight HBV infection. Interferon treatment is effective in less than half of those treated and causes side effects such as fever, headache, fatigue, nausea, and vomiting.

Lamivudine is a nucleoside drug that interferes with the replication of the HBV genome and is effective at decreasing viral reproduction. Another method for treating chronic liver failure is liver transplantation. Both medical treatment and liver transplantation for cirrhosis are expensive and have variable success, and they are not available to most patients in the developing world.

Chronic HBV infection is also involved in the development of hepatocellular carcinoma (HCC), or cancer of the liver cells. Worldwide, HCC causes between 250,000 and 1 million deaths annually. Most cases of HCC occur in people between the ages of 35 and 65.

There are significant differences in incidence of HCC worldwide. High-incidence regions, with more than 15 cases annually per 100,000 people, include sub-Saharan Africa, China, Hong Kong, and Taiwan. There are fewer than three cases annually per 100,000 people in the Americas, Europe, Australia, and regions of the Middle East.

These differences are likely due to variations in age of exposure to HBV, exposure to other hepatitis viruses, and environmental contributions.

Additionally, men are more likely to develop HCC, with an average increased incidence of 3.7 compared with women. Factors that make people more likely to develop HCC include length of chronic liver disease, male gender, environmental toxins, chronic hepatitis C virus carrier, hereditary hemochromatosis, and other factors causing cirrhosis.

DIAGNOSIS AND PROGNOSIS

Most HCCs are initially suspected based on a history of chronic liver disease, computed tomography scans, or ultrasound evaluation of the liver. Definitive diagnosis of HCC is via liver biopsy and examination under a microscope. Blood tests to detect alpha-fetoprotein concentrations are also used in screening patients with chronic HBV or cirrhosis, but this protein is not specific for HCC. If the levels of alpha-fetoprotein increase in someone with chronic liver disease, it is suspicious for development of HCC.

People who have HCC in the developing world often die from the liver cancer within a few months of diagnosis. If the liver tumor is small, and the patient has access to a hospital with surgical facilities, surgery to remove the mass or liver transplantation may be curative. If the tumor is very large, if there are multiple tumors, or if the tumor has spread beyond the liver, treatment may consist of chemotherapy, embolization (clotting) of the hepatic artery, or radiation. These treatments may prolong life but are not curative.

SEE ALSO: Hepatitis C, Hepatocellular (Liver) Cancer, Adult (Primary); Hepatocellular (Liver) Cancer, Childhood (Primary).

BIBLIOGRAPHY. Johnson Y. Lau, *Hepatitis B and D Protocols: Detection, Genotypes, and Characterization* (Springer-Verlag, 2004); Johnson Y. Lau, *Hepatitis B and D Protocols: Immunology, Model Systems and Clinical Studies* (Springer-Verlag, 2004).

CHRISTINE CURRY
INDEPENDENT SCHOLAR

Hepatitis C

BY THE EARLY 1970s, it was clear that a large proportion of patients with acute and chronic hepatitis were not infected with the hepatitis A virus or hepatitis B virus (HBV). Initially, patients were described as having non-A, non-B hepatitis, but in 1989 the hepatitis C virus (HCV) was identified and cloned.

HCV is a major cause of chronic liver disease, with 170 million people, or 3 percent of the world's population chronically infected and an additional 3 million to

4 million people newly infected each year. The prevalence of HCV infection varies greatly among regions. In Egypt, for example, over 20 percent of the population is infected with HCV, whereas in Scandinavia the prevalence is less than 0.5 percent. Appreciating the burden of disease caused by HCV requires an understanding of the virology, pathogenesis, clinical manifestations, and consequences of chronic infection.

VIRUS COMPOSITION AND TRANSMISSION

HCV is an enveloped RNA virus in the *Flaviviridae* family and is not related to any known hepatitis viruses. The genome of HCV is composed of positive-sense RNA (9,500 nucleotides) with highly conserved, untranslated regions flanking a single open reading frame. From this single open reading frame a single, large polyprotein is generated, which undergoes posttranslational processing by enzymes from both the host hepatocyte (liver cell) and HCV. This processing yields the structural, nonstructural, and enzyme components of HCV. Because HCV is an RNA virus, its polymerase enzyme lacks proofreading ability, which leads to multiple errors in every round of viral replication. Often, it leads to nonfunctional genomes or incompetent viruses, but on occasion the mutated viruses survive and can replicate. This creates a very diverse population of HCV, which provides challenges in diagnosis, treatment, and vaccine development.

The variations created by the mutations during replication of HCV allow the virus to be separated into six major genotypes, with over 50 identified subtypes. The evolution of each genotype was likely influenced by infection patterns, human migration, and immune selection, yielding geographic distributions of the HCV genotypes.

HCV is also described as having quasispecies, meaning that there is hypervariability in rapidly changing or nonconserved portions of the genome. It is unclear what the clinical significance of this variability is, but there is evidence that the response to treatments is influenced by the genotype with which the person is infected. In addition, the rapidly changing genome prevents the development of conventional vaccines and can allow HCV to evade the host immune response.

Transmission of HCV is largely through direct contact with human blood. Most commonly, transmission is due to reuse of unsterilized needles, syringes, or other medical equipment; via needle sharing among users of intravenous drugs; transfusion with blood that is not screened for HCV; or secondary to transplantation of solid organs infected with HCV. Within the first six months of intravenous drug use, over 50 percent of users become infected with HCV, and almost 90 percent are infected in one year. Infection with HCV is also a serious concern for healthcare workers who frequently will come into contact with contaminated blood, fluids, and needles. The risk of acquiring HCV from a needle stick that is from a patient known to be infected with HCV is 2 percent on average and increases if the exposure is from a hollow-bore needle. HCV can also be transmitted through sexual contact or perinatally (during childbirth). Infrequent modes of transmission may include ear/body piercing, circumcision, or tattooing when inadequately sterilized equipment is used. HCV is not spread via casual contact or contaminated foods or water.

SYMPTOMS OF INFECTION

Individuals who contract HCV rarely experience symptoms of acute hepatitis. Less than 25 percent of acutely infected people will have jaundice (yellow skin), malaise, nausea, and abdominal pain. In addition, acute HCV infection rarely causes fulminant hepatic failure unless the person has an underlying infection with HBV.

The real danger from HCV infection is the development of chronic infection, and 80 percent to 100 percent of those infected with HCV have detectable HCV in their blood persistently. Chronic infection often remains asymptomatic for decades, and patients may have only nonspecific symptoms, such as fatigue, nausea, anorexia, myalgia (muscle pain), arthralgia (joint pain), weakness, and weight loss.

One of the complications seen most commonly from chronic HCV infection is cirrhosis. Cirrhosis is a state of scarring or fibrosis of the liver that prevents the hepatocytes from performing their normal metabolic roles. Normally, the liver is involved in glycogen storage, production of plasma proteins, aiding in digestion by producing bile, and detoxifying compounds in the bloodstream. Patients often lose weight and become malnourished secondary to malabsorption because the liver is not able to produce bile to aid sufficiently in fat digestion and absorption.

As the scarring in the liver progresses, individuals may develop portal hypertension. This situation occurs when the liver becomes too fibrotic and scarred to filter and transport blood adequately, causing a backup of blood from the portal venous system into the systemic venous system. This condition can cause fluid retention and edema (swelling); ascites (fluid retention in the abdomen); and a backup of blood into veins around the umbilicus, rectum, and lower esophagus.

If the backup of blood becomes severe enough, patients can experience severe bleeding, exacerbated by the lack of clotting factors secondary to cirrhosis. They may vomit blood or have rectal bleeding. Because portal hypertension precludes sufficient detoxification of ammonia and other metabolites, patients can experience encephalopathy, leading to confusion and coma. The backup of blood into the spleen can cause splenomegaly (spleen enlargement) and, secondarily, spleen dysfunction, anemia (decreased red blood cells), leukopenia (decreased white blood cells), and thrombocytopenia (decreased platelets).

One of the most noticeable signs of liver failure is jaundice, or yellowing of the skin. The normal liver eliminates a compound caused bilirubin, but hepatic dysfunction leads to a backup of bilirubin into the circulation and accumulation of this yellow compound in the skin, conjunctiva, and mucous membranes.

ANTIBODY DEVELOPMENT

Another complication of chronic HCV infection is the development of cryoglobulinemia, which is due to the accumulation of abnormal antibodies that are made in response to HCV infection. These antibodies can aggregate and deposit in small blood vessels and cause vasculitis (blood vessel inflammation). Symptoms include joint pain and swelling; a raised and purple skin rash; loss of protein from damaged kidneys, with subsequent swelling of the legs; and foot and nerve pain.

Patients may also develop Raynaud's phenomenon, which occurs when small blood vessels in the fingers and toes spasm in response to cold temperatures, leading to the fingers turning white and painful.

Subsequent to the development of cirrhosis, chronic infection with HCV leads to hepatocellular carcinoma (HCC). It seems that unlike in the case of HBV, cirrhosis seems to be a significant risk factor for HCC development secondary to HCV infection. Factors increasing the risk for HCC in HCV-infected individu-

als include advancing age, male gender, worsening of cirrhosis, greater hepatic inflammation, coinfection with hepatitis B, excessive alcohol use, iron overload (seen in hemochromatosis), infection with the human immodeficiency virus (HIV), and diabetes/obesity.

The HCV genotype 1b may be associated with a more severe course of liver disease and a greater risk of HCC. There are also geographic variables that influence the development of HCC, as individuals in Japan who are infected with HCV have a higher risk of developing HCC than those in the United States.

DIAGNOSIS AND TREATMENT

HCV infection is rarely diagnosed at the time of infection because few individuals are symptomatic. If HCV infection is suspected due to the presence of risk factors—or in individuals with hepatitis, cirrhosis, or HCC—several blood tests are available. These tests detect antibodies specific to HCV and test for circulating HCV RNA in the blood. HCV RNA can usually be detected within 1 to 3 weeks after infection, and the antibodies are detectable within 3 to 12 weeks.

Blood tests to detect alpha-fetoprotein concentrations are also used in screening patients with chronic HBC or cirrhosis, but this protein is not specific for HCC. If the levels of alpha-fetoprotein increase in someone with chronic liver disease, it is suspicious for development of HCC.

The goal of treatment for HCV is the elimination of viral infection, improvement of liver function tests, and the prevention of cirrhosis and HCC. Treatment often consists of interferon, which both reduces HCV replication and stimulates the immune system to fight HCV infection. Interferon is often given in combination with ribavirin, an antiviral drug that mimics nucleosides (the building blocks of DNA and RNA), thereby interfering with viral reproduction. Treatment of end-stage or advanced liver disease and cirrhosis caused by HCV infection is also possible with liver transplantation.

However, recurrence of HCV infection detectable in the bloodstream is almost universal after transplantation, and over 25 percent of patients will have a recurrence of hepatitis. All these treatment options are expensive, noncurative, and out of reach for the majority of those living in the developing world. For this reason, prevention of infection is important.

PREVENTIVE MEASURES

Because of the high mutation rate of HCV, the presence of multiple genotypes, and the lack of knowledge about protective immune responses against HCV, there is no vaccine available. To protect against HCV infection, there should be screening and testing of all blood and organ donors, as well as virus inactivation in plasma-derived products.

In addition, there must be strict infection-control practices in healthcare settings, with sterilization of equipment and no reuse of needles. Harm reduction for those who inject drugs involves counseling on not reusing needles, needle-exchange programs, and drug-recovery programs. If applied, these preventive methods could help reduce the spread of HCV and thereby decrease the incidence of hepatitis, cirrhosis, and HCC.

SEE ALSO: Hepatitis B; Hepatocellular (Liver) Cancer, Adult (Primary); Hepatocellular (Liver) Cancer, Childhood (Primary).

BIBLIOGRAPHY. M. Mori, M.C. Yoshida, N. Takeichi, and N. Taniguchi, eds., *LEC Rat: A New Model for Hepatitis and Liver Cancer* (Springer-Verlag, 1992); Edward Tabor, ed., *Viruses and Liver Cancer, Vol. 6* (Elsevier Science & Technology Books, 2002).

CHRISTINE CURRY
INDEPENDENT SCHOLAR

Hepatocellular (Liver) Cancer, Adult (Primary)

HEPATOCELLULAR CARCINOMA (HCC) is a cancer of liver hepatocytes, the main type of cells in the liver. The liver has a number of vital functions, including filtering harmful substances from the blood, producing bile to digest fats, producing clotting factors to stop bleeding, and storing glycogen.

Worldwide, HCC is a common cancer; it is associated with cirrhosis and with hepatitis B and C. It is usually diagnosed in its later stages, which can limit treatment options. HCC accounts for about 6 percent of all cancers worldwide and results in 250,000 to 1 million deaths annually. Eighty percent of HCC cases

are in developing countries in sub-Saharan Africa and Southeast Asia, where hepatitis B is endemic.

The most common causes of HCC in the developing world are hepatitis B and aflatoxin (a toxin produced by fungi) food contamination; in the developed world, the most common causes are hepatitis C and alcoholism, which causes cirrhosis (the irreversible scarring of liver tissue). Other risk factors include being male, family history of liver cancer, other causes of cirrhosis, smoking, vinyl chloride, and thorium dioxide.

Public health interventions and lifestyle changes, such as decreasing alcohol consumption, can decrease the incidence of HCC. A national hepatitis B vaccination program in Taiwan, for example, significantly decreased hepatitis B and HCC rates. Though there currently is no hepatitis C vaccine, decreasing risky behaviors (such as the use of contaminated needles and unprotected sex) and regulating blood products can decrease transmission of hepatitis C, which is transmitted via blood.

SYMPTOMS AND DIAGNOSIS

Symptoms of HCC are similar to those of chronic liver disease, making the diagnosis of HCC difficult, because most patients have liver disease. Signs and symptoms include jaundice, enlargement of the spleen, accumulation of fluid in the abdomen, upper abdominal pain, and weight loss.

In addition to physical examination and standard blood tests, diagnosis usually involves blood tests for alfa-fetoprotein (AFP), a tumor marker of HCC, and imaging studies, such as ultrasound and computed tomography (CT) scan or magnetic resonance imaging (MRI). In the appropriate clinical setting, a classic appearance on CT or MRI combined with an elevated AFP level is sufficient for establishing the diagnosis of HCC. Biopsy is performed when the imaging studies are inconclusive. Screening for HCC is generally recommended for high-risk groups—people with chronic hepatitis B, hepatitis C, and cirrhosis—and typically involves an ultrasound and blood test of AFP levels.

TREATMENT AND PROGNOSIS

Staging of cancers assists in determining treatment options and prognosis. A variety of HCC staging methods are available, most often classifying the cancer by size and spread. Multiple treatment modalities currently exist: surgical resection of tumor, liver transplantation, radiofrequency ablation, radiation therapy, and chemotherapy. Although the optimal treatment is surgical resection, the majority of patients are not eligible due to the advanced stage of the tumor or underlying liver disease.

In the United States, the five-year relative survival rate—the percentage of patients who are still alive five years after the cancer is diagnosed—is less than 10 percent. Survival in developing countries is even lower due to lack of access to healthcare.

Prognosis is affected by the stage of the cancer, underlying liver function, and the patient's general health.

SEE ALSO: Hepatitis B; Hepatitis C; Hepatocellular (Liver) Cancer, Childhood (Primary).

BIBLIOGRAPHY. M. Abeloff and A. James, et al., *Clinical Oncology* (Churchill Livingstone, 2004); J. Bruix and M. Sherman, "Management of Hepatocellular Carcinoma," *Hepatology* (v.42/5, 2005); National Cancer Institute, "Liver Cancer," www.cancer.gov (cited December 2006).

SONIA LEUNG
UNIVERSITY OF MICHIGAN MEDICAL SCHOOL

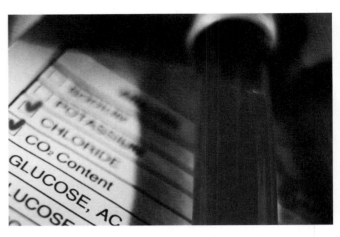

A blood test is often used to diagnose Hepatocellular carcinoma (HCC), a cancer of liver hepatocytes cells.

Hepatocellular (Liver) Cancer, Childhood (Primary)

CHILDREN'S HEPATOCELLULAR CARCINOMA (HCC), or hepatoma, is a rare cancer of the liver with an incidence of less than one per million children. A hepatoma is a primary tumor that develops in the liver, and in children it is usually seen in livers that have suffered infection (hepatitis B or hepatitis C) or metabolic disease.

HCC develops when hepatocytes of the liver become cancerous and can occur in children of any age between birth and age 19. Although HCC is one of the most prevalent solid-organ tumors worldwide, it is very rare in children, with less than 1 percent of all cases occurring in patients younger than 20. St Jude Children's Research Hospital reports that the incidence of childhood hepatoma is 0.7 per million children, with a mean age of onset between 12 and 14.

The causes of HCC are not completely understood, although genetic inheritance as well as several other influencing factors are thought to play a role in the tumor development. Hepatitis B and hepatitis C (viral liver infections) significantly increase the risk of development of hepatomas in children, whereas hepatitis B immunization may decrease this risk. In addition, congenital diseases that cause liver scarring, such as tyrosinemia and alpha-1 antitrypsin deficiency, may increase the risk for development of hepatomas in children. Chronic ethanol abuse and excessive use of anabolic steroids are also thought to increase risk for HCC, but these are less likely causes for hepatomas in children.

SYMPTOMS AND DIAGNOSIS

Early signs and symptoms of HCC are not always unique to liver disorders. Abdominal tenderness and distention (particularly in the right upper quadrant), nausea, and vomiting are common symptoms. Symptoms may also include fatigue, weight loss, and/or anorexia. As the tumor continues to grow, patients may suffer from jaundice, internal bleeding in the digestive tract, or fluid collection in the abdominal cavity.

Methods used to diagnose HCC include imaging studies, blood tests, and biopsies (most definitive of the diagnosis). Prognosis and treatment of the cancer depend on the staging (tumor size and whether it has spread to other organs) and the child's overall health.

TREATMENT

Surgery and possible chemotherapy are often successful treatments, depending on the size and spread of the cancer. Hepatomas that are small and have not spread outside the liver are usually surgically removed. In larger cancers that have not spread outside the liver, and where surgical removal of the tumor is not possible, a liver transplant may be a treatment option. To supplement surgical treatment, chemotherapy may be used to shrink larger cancers before surgery or to kill remaining cancer cells after surgery. Chemotherapy uses toxic drugs to kill the cancerous cells and is injected into the body through a needle in an artery or vein. Chemotherapy may be administered systemically to target cancer cells outside the liver in advanced-stage hepatomas or may be injected into the liver's main artery to target cancerous cells in the liver preoperatively or postoperatively. Unfortunately, HCC does not respond nearly as well to chemotherapy as other common cancer types do.

SEE ALSO: Chemotherapy; Childhood Cancers; Hepatitis B; Hepatitis C; Hepatocellular (Liver) Cancer, Adult (Primary); Liver Cancer, Childhood (Primary).

BIBLIOGRAPHY. Cincinnati Children's Hospital Medical Center, "Hepatocellular Carcinoma/Hepatoma—Childhood Liver Cancer," www.cincinnatichildrens.org (cited December 2006); St. Jude Children's Research Hospital, "Hepatocellular Carcinoma," www.stjude.org (cited December 2006).

HAITHAM AHMED
DARTMOUTH MEDICAL SCHOOL
SHARITA ALAM
CORNELL UNIVERSITY
AYAH AHMED
KUWAIT UNIVERSITY

Herbert Irving Comprehensive Cancer Center

THE HERBERT IRVING Comprehensive Cancer Center is a National Cancer Institute-designated Comprehensive Cancer Center, one of three located in New York City. The Irving Center is affiliated with New York-Presbyterian Hospital and Columbia University. Its mission is to provide the infrastructure and resources to promote laboratory, clinical, and population-based cancer research and to facilitate the application of this research to cancer prevention. The Irving Center also provides education and training in cancer research and prevention for scientists, clinical investigators, patients, and the general public.

The Irving Center was named after Herbert Irving, cofounder and former vice chairman of Sysco Corporation and a major contributor to cancer research at Columbia University and Presbyterian Hospital. Among their other gifts, Irving and his wife, Florence Irving, have funded five professorships at Columbia and oncology inpatient and outpatient units.

The Herbert Irving Comprehensive Cancer is one of two cancer centers affiliated with New York-Presbyterian Hospital: the other is the Weill Cornell Cancer Center. The Irving Center's specialty facilities include a Breast Center; a Prostate Center; an Infusion Center; dedicated programs for gynecological cancers, digestive cancers, and lung cancers; and a pediatric oncology inpatient unit located in the Morgan Stanley Children's Hospital of New York-Presbyterian Hospital.

Interdisciplinary research is a core emphasis at the Irving Center, in particular the use of concepts and methods in cellular and molecular biology to enhance understanding of the etiology and pathophysiology of cancer and to develop strategies for prevention, diagnosis, and treatment. Major research breakthroughs achieved by Irving Center investigators include identification of the virus associated with Kaposi's sarcoma and certain lymphomas; development of a DNA test for cervical center; identification of a gene implicated in brain, prostate, and breast cancer; and development of a combination drug regimen for prostate cancer.

FACILITIES

The Irving Center includes several core facilities that provide services required by many researchers at the center; some services are available to outside researchers also.

The Animal Facility offers animal-husbandry and veterinary services for investigators who use mice in their research. It includes a transgenic/chimeric mouse production service; a barrier facility for the maintenance and breeding of pathogen-free mice; and two laboratories for performing surgical and experimental procedures, including embryo transfers.

The Biomarkers Facility provides reception, handling, and storage for human samples (e.g., blood, urine, oral cells) collected for use in research studies. In some cases stored samples may be available to investigators other than those who collected the samples; demographic, questionnaire, and biomarker data from the original studies may also be available.

The Biostatistics Facility provides statistical expertise and support for research projects at the Irving Center. Specific services offered include collaborative research, consulting services, protocol review, data management, and biostatistical training. The Clinical Trials Facility makes available information about clinical trials conducted at the Irving Center, including a search facility for open trials that is accessible through the Irving Center website. The Optical Microscopy Facility provides microscope system for three-dimensional (3D) imaging and includes two full-time staff members trained in cell biology and 3D microscopy.

The DNA Analysis and Sequencing Facility performs DNA sequencing and provides three Molecular Dynamics Imaging instruments and two instruments for Real Time PCR for use by researchers.

The Experimental Molecular Pathology Facility provides services in three areas: tumor banking, experimental histopathology, and experimental molecular cytogenetics. The tumor-banking service collects, stores, and distributes human tissues collected after autopsies and surgical procedures for research purposes. The histopathology service processes human and nonhuman tissues for histopathology and histochemistry. The molecular cytogenetic service provides instruments for chromosome recognition technologies, which can provide karyotypic and molecular cytogenetic characterization of human and rodent tumor cells.

The Oncoinformatics Facility offers services to integrate information sharing across Irving Center facilities, including infrastructure, data modeling, analysis and mining, software tools, and training. The Radiation Research Facility offers devices that are sources of ionizing radiation (X-rays and gamma rays) and of low-frequency electric and magnetic fields. The facility also provides expertise in designing experiments and protocols.

The Flow Cytometry Facility provides flow-cytometry services, which use fluorescent probes that allow measurements of the characteristics of cells suspended in a fluid stream. The Recruitment Core facilitates recruitment of human research subjects and assists investigators in study design.

The Transgenic Mouse Facility produces transgenic and chimeric mice, and provides gene-targeting services to investigators. The facility also provides advice and consultation on matter such as the analysis and breeding of gene-targeted and transgenic mice and on design of gene-targeting vectors and transgenic constructs.

EDUCATION

The Division of Hematology and Medical Oncology within the Columbia University Department of Internal Medicine offers fellowships for physicians that include both direct patient care and research training in laboratory, clinical, and public health research. Epidemiology and population science research training is offered in conjunction with the Mailman School of Public Health at Columbia University.

The division includes over 30 faculty members. Faculty specialties include marrow and stem cell transplantation; breast cancer; gastrointestinal cancer; genitourinary cancer; geriatrics; hematology; leukemia, lymphoma, and myeloma; melanoma; respiratory, head, and neck cancer; and sarcomas and mesotheliomas.

The Irving Center participates in the Continuing Umbrella of Research (CURE) program, developed and funded by the National Institutes of Health. CURE is a national program that places minority high school students and four minority college students as paid summer interns in the state-of-the-art research laboratories.

SEE ALSO: AIDS-Related Cancers; Cervical Cancer; Education, Cancer; Prostate Cancer.

BIBLIOGRAPHY. The Herbert Irving Comprehensive Cancer Center website, www.ccc.columbia.edu (cited December 2006); New York-Presbyterian Cancer Centers website, www.nypcancer.org (cited December 2006).

SARAH BOSLAUGH
WASHINGTON UNIVERSITY SCHOOL OF MEDICINE

Herbicide

ACCORDING TO THE Merriam-Webster dictionary, an herbicide is "an agent used to destroy or inhibit plant growth." Any chemical or substance that inhibits or prevents the growth of weeds that are unwanted can be considered an herbicide.

By definition, herbicides (like all pesticides) are synthetic chemicals specifically designed to be toxic to several biological targets. They are deliberately released into the environment, yet their toxicity is not necessarily selective to one or even a few species of plants.

In the United States, although herbicides are commonly used for domestic purposes on lawns and gardens, the vast majority of herbicides are used in production agriculture, wherein more than 433 million pounds of herbicides are used each year.

The U.S. Environmental Protection Agency (EPA) reported that $31.7 billion was spent on all types of pesticides throughout the world in 2001. Herbicide expenditures comprised 44 percent of this total. In the United States, $6.4 billion was spent on pesticides, and the proportion spent on herbicides was even larger, at 58 percent. Within the United States in 2001, 78 percent of all expenditure for pesticides was for production agriculture. In terms of amount applied, of the 1.2 billion pounds of pesticide active ingredients used in the United States, 46 percent was herbicides. Therefore, potential for human exposure to these chemicals is considerable, and efforts to prevent or mitigate human contact are warranted because the health effects of exposure remain unknown.

TYPES OF HERBICIDES AND THEIR EFFECTS
Several chemical classes are commonly used as herbicides and may exert their effect through different mechanisms. The triazine herbicides (such as cyanazine, simazine, and atrazine) act by preventing photosynthesis; hence, they are considered to be preemergent herbicides.

The most heavily used herbicides in the United States are the glyphosphates (phosphonate chemicals commonly sold as Roundup), which are nonselective, postemergence, broad-spectrum herbicides. Other types of herbicides include the phenoxyacetic acids, such as 2,4-D, which are both pre- and postemergent herbicides.

Additional chemical classes include the phenoxy benzoic acids (such as Dicamba), the thiocarbamates (such as EPTC), the anilides (such as alachlor), and dipyridal compounds (such as paraquat).

The traditional marker of danger for adverse health effects in humans as regards cancer risk is evidence of genotoxicity of chemicals, such that evidence from laboratory studies demonstrates actual damage to DNA from exposure to the chemical. Although some herbicides may have genotoxic properties (e.g., sulfallate), there are other types of mechanisms by which the herbicides may exert their carcinogenic potential. Hormonal action induced by chemicals such as the triazine herbicides (e.g., atrazine), for example, may result in lengthening of the estrous cycle in which exposure to endogenous estrogen causes increases in mammary and uterine tumors in laboratory animals.

Additionally, alterations in immune function may result from exposure to other herbicides. The phenoxyacetic acid herbicide 2,4-D is associated with enhanced T-cell and B-cell immune response in murine (mouse) models and in humans, and it has been associated with reductions in lymphocyte subsets, including circulating helper and suppressor T cells and natural killer cells, all of which may increase cancer risk.

The phenoxyacetic acid herbicides are also associated with peroxisome proliferation, which may be another mechanism by which cancer risk may be heightened in humans.

The relationship between use and exposure to herbicides and cancer risk in humans is difficult to ascertain. Ironically, the primary approach used for evaluation of carcinogenic activity in humans relies upon bioassays in rodents (rats and mice) that are fed relatively high does of pesticidal active ingredients for relatively short periods (feeding studies). In this type of study (usually two years in length), rodents are fed high concentrations of the active ingredients of the pesticides; then they are sacrificed, and their tissues are pathologically examined for evidence of cancerous changes or numbers of tumors.

These studies are limited in several ways: It is impractical to conduct such studies on all pesticides in use; there are great uncertainties in making extrapolations from animals to humans; and the studies do not allow for identification of the mode of action of the chemical. They also fail to evaluate simultaneous exposure to multiple pesticides, which may be a more realistic model of human exposure.

There are tests that can be conducted at the cellular level, such as the Ames test (to detect mutagens), and other mammalian cell assays, such as the mouse lymphoma assay.

In addition, cytogenetic assays can be performed in which structural and numerical aberrations in chromosomes can be evaluated in cells exposed to the suspect chemical. However, the most direct method to evaluate human health risks is to study human populations.

CLASSIFICATIONS

Several scientific bodies, including the International Agency for Research on Cancer (IARC) and the EPA, have devised scoring methods to combine cellular-level tests, rodent studies, and human observations for several of the most commonly used herbicides in the United States and have assigned designations of their potential to cause cancer in humans.

Based on the results of these studies, pesticides (including herbicides) are classified in the latest EPA report (1999) as Carcinogenic to Humans; Likely to Be Carcinogenic to Humans; Suggestive Evidence of Carcinogenicity, But Not Sufficient to Assess Human Carcinogenic Potential; Data Are Inadequate for an Assessment of Human Carcinogenic Potential; and Not Likely to Be Carcinogenic to Humans.

This most recent scheme is not necessarily comparable to earlier schemes (in 1996 and 1986) that used alphanumeric classifications, including Groups A, B1, B2, C, D, and E. Examples of herbicides and their most recent classifications are 2,4-D (Group D-Not Classifiable as to Human Carcinogenicity), Alachlor (Likely to Be Carcinogenic to Humans [High Doses]), Amitrole (Group B2-Probable Human Carcinogen), Cyanazine (Group C-Possible Human Carcinogen), Dicamba (Group D-Not Classifiable as to Human Carcinogenicity), Glyphosphate (Group E-Evidence of Noncarcinogenicity for Humans), Metolachlor (Group C-Possible Human Carcinogen), Pendimethalin (Group C-Possible Human Carcinogen), Simazine (Group C-Possible Human Carcinogen), and Trifluralin (Group C-Possible Human Carcinogen).

EXPOSED POPULATIONS

Observations in human populations (i.e., epidemiological studies) have been conducted in which populations exposed to herbicides have been evaluated in regard to cancer risk. Because the most heavily exposed populations are farmers and farm workers, and because throughout the world nearly 50 percent of the entire labor force is engaged in agriculture, it seems reasonable to examine cancer risk in these populations first and to consider the health effects observed to be sentinel events that may predict events in the general population exposed to lower amounts of these chemicals.

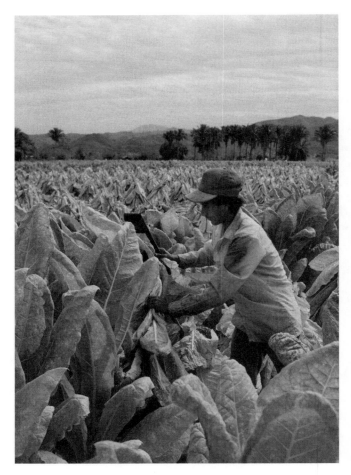

Tobacco harvest: Nearly 50 percent of the world labor force is engaged in agriculture. Most are exposed to herbicides.

HUMAN STUDIES AND CANCER RISKS

Several forms of cancer in humans are found to be excessive among farmers, and these are good candidates for cancers that may be associated with exposures to pesticides, including herbicides. The list includes stomach, prostate, brain, and testis cancers, as well as soft-tissue sarcoma, non-Hodgkin's lymphoma, multiple myeloma, and leukemia.

Several herbicides have been evaluated in relation to many of these cancers, and most studies have concentrated on the phenoxyacetic acid herbicide 2,4-D, the triazine herbicides (atrazine, simazine, and cyanazine), and the isopropylamine compound glyphosphate (found in Roundup). Risk of non-Hodgkin's lymphoma, soft-tissue sarcoma, prostate cancer, and other forms of cancer has been associated with use of the phenoxyacetic acid herbicide 2,4-D. Studies of atrazine initially found elevated risk of ovarian cancer, but more recent studies have not been able to replicate those findings, although an elevation in non-Hodgkin's lymphoma was found among people exposed to atrazine who had also been exposed to other pesticides. There is some limited evidence that glyphosphate is associated with multiple myeloma.

Perhaps the best evidence for determining human cancer risks associated with exposures to herbicides comes from the Agricultural Health Study (AHS)—a joint venture of the National Cancer Institute, the National Institute for Occupational Safety and Health, the EPA, and the National Institute of Environmental Health Science. In this study, thousands of farmers and licensed pest-control operators (and their spouses) living in Iowa and North Carolina were enrolled beginning in 1993. This type of study is referred to as a cohort study, and at its inception, almost 90,000 participants completed a detailed questionnaire in which they reported on past use of pesticides (including herbicides), as well as several other lifestyle characteristics, such as smoking history.

The cohort has been followed for several years; newly diagnosed cancers have been detected through the state cancer registries in Iowa and North Carolina, and several results have been released.

Lung-cancer risk in the AHS was found to be elevated fourfold to fivefold in those participants highly exposed to two herbicides, including metolachlor and pendimethalin; the result was not explained by known risk factors for lung cancer, such as smoking. The use of pentimethalin (commercially known as Prowl) was associated with an increase in cancer of the rectum. Those women in the AHS who had husbands exposed to 2,4,5-T (a phenoxyacetic acid herbicide) experienced a doubling in breast-cancer risk, although there were only 19 breast-cancer cases on which to base the analysis. A commonly used herbicide called alachlor was associated with leukemia and multiple-myeloma risk in the AHS such that there were a threefold increase in leukemia and a sixfold increase in multiple myeloma in exposed workers compared with the non-exposed. Associations were also observed in the AHS for the herbicide Dicamba, including elevated lung and colon cancer in the most heavily exposed workers.

Other studies of farm workers in the United States have been completed. Female Hispanic farm workers in California exposed to relatively high levels of the herbicide 2,4-D were found to be at higher risk of breast can-cer. In the same study, use of 2,4-D was associated with an increase in risk of non-Hodgkin's lymphoma. Farm working men exposed to the herbicide simazine experienced an increase in risk of prostate cancer as well.

The completion of the Human Genome Project, in which human genes have been identified, has opened new avenues of research for determining the health effects of human exposures to herbicides. In particular, differences in certain metabolizing genes, including those that activate and deactivate carcinogens found in the environment, may offer protection against adverse health effects or increase the impact of herbicides on cancer risk in humans. Of special interest are polymorphisms in the cytochrome p450 genes (CYP), the glutathione -S transferase genes (GST), and the paraoxonase (PON) genes. Current and ongoing epidemiologic research studies such as the AHS will be able to differentiate herbicide-associated cancer risks in subsets of the population who possess different polymorphisms in these metabolizing genes.

SEE ALSO: Breast Cancer; Chemical Industry; Pesticide; Prostate Cancer.

BIBLIOGRAPHY. Shelia Hoar Zahm, et al., "Pesticides and Cancer," *Occupational Medicine: State of the Art Reviews* (v.12/2, 1997); Michael Alavanja and Jane Hoppin, "Health Effects of Chronic Pesticide Exposure: Cancer and Neurotoxicity," *Annual Review of Public Health* (v. 25, 2004); Science Information Management Branch, Health Effects Division, Office of Pesticide Programs, *Chemicals Evaluated for Carcinogenic Potential* (U.S. Environmental Protection Agency, 2004).

PAUL K. MILLS
CANCER REGISTRY OF CALIFORNIA

Herbst, Roy

THE CHIEF OF the section of Thoracic Medical Oncology and associate professor of medicine, as well as co-director of the Phase I Clinical Trials Working Group at M.D. Anderson Cancer Center in Houston, Texas, Roy Herbst is one of America's leading authorities on research for the treatment of lung cancer.

Herbst spent much of his recent medical research efforts into looking into the synergistic effects of pairing erlotinib (Tarceva) and bevacizumab (Avastin), which he believed may be useful in treating patients who have advanced non-small cell lung cancer. Essentially, he used Avastin, which, as monoclonal antibody, would inhibit angiogenesis, starving the cancer tumor of the blood it needs to survive.

Herbst found that Avastin, combined with chemotherapy, was particularly successful, and when it was combined with the new agent ZD6474, early tests gave positive results. In an interview with *OncoLog*, he said, "The success with Avastin and Tarceva in combination is promising but, more importantly, it speaks to the need for more studies combining different biologic agents in lung cancer to attack different targets at the same time."

In 2005, Herbst and 13 other contributors put together the *Atlas of Lung Cancer*, published by Current Medicine in Philadelphia.

SEE ALSO: Clinical Trials; Lung Cancer, Non-Small Cell; United States.

BIBLIOGRAPHY. "Combining Biologic Agents for the Treatment of Lung Cancer: An Evolving Strategy—An Expert Interview with Dr. Roy S. Herbst," www.medscape.com/viewarticle/509023 (cited November 2006); Diane Witter, "Improving the Odds in Lung Cancer," *OncoLog* (v.51/1, 2006).

JUSTIN CORFIELD
GEELONG GRAMMAR SCHOOL, AUSTRALIA

Hirschowitz, Basil I.

A PROMINENT U.S. gastroenterologist, Basil I. Hirschowitz was the winner of the Charles F. Kettering Prize of the General Motors Cancer Foundation in 1987 for "the invention and development of the flexible fiber-optic endoscope, an instrument that revolutionized the diagnosis of many common cancers." Hirschowitz developed an improved optical glass fiber that allowed for the creation of the flexible endoscope. This device revolutionized the field of gastroenterology and allowed cancer surgeons to inspect areas of their patients more closely without invasive surgery. Hirschowitz was born in 1925 in South Africa, growing up on a farm. He graduated from the Medical School of the University of Witwatersrand, Johannesburg (B.Sc. in Physiology, 1943; M.B.B.Ch., 1947). He also completed a two-year residency at the school. There, he was greatly inspired by Robert Broom in palaeontology; Raymond Dart in anatomy and palaeontology; and Moses M. Suzman, whom he described as "a physician's physician."

After four years of graduate medical studies in London, one being in cardiology under Sir John McMichael at the Postgraduate Medical School, Hammersmith, and three years under Sir Francis Avery Jones at the Central Middlesex Hospital, he completed his doctorate with a thesis titled *The Physiology of Pepsinogen in the Human.*

In 1953 Hirschowitz moved to the United States and continued his G.I. fellowship at the University of Michigan, where he was a member of the faculty from 1954 until 1957. In 1955 he founded the Gastroenterology Research Group with Clinton Texter, and from 1957 until 1959 he was at Temple University in Philadelphia. He then moved to the School of Medicine at the University of Alabama, Birmingham, where he became the founding chief of gastroenterology, a position he held until 1988.

DEVELOPMENT OF FIBERSCOPE

In 1954 Hirschowitz started working on the fiberscope while he was on a fellowship with Marvin Pollard at the University of Michigan, Ann Arbor. He became interested after reading an article about it by H. H. Hopkins and N. S. Kapany, "A Flexible Fiberscope Using Static Scanning," published in *Nature* in 1954. After visiting the authors in Britain, he decided to try to merge the work on fiber optics with endoscopy.

At Ann Arbor, with physicist C. Wilbur Peters and his student Larry Curtiss, he devised a makeshift scheme. There were some early technical problems, but in late 1956 he managed to produce a glass-coated fiber with the optical qualities required for the fiber bundle of a gastroscope to enable doctors to look inside patients.

It was in February 1957, after much work on fiber-optic endoscopy, that Hirschowitz passed the first prototype instrument down his own throat; a few days later, he was able to test it on a patient. This endoscope is now preserved at the Smithsonian museum.

He then collaborated with American Cystoscope Manufacturing, Inc., to produce a saleable instrument. In October 1960 the first production model was made, and Hirschowitz was able to assert in *The Lancet* that "the conventional gastroscope has become obsolete on all counts."

The model developed by Hirschowitz was gradually developed and improved, allowing for the repositioning of lenses to allow for a wider field of vision, and later the addition of channels to work biopsy forceps and to take minute samples. The next stage involved the device's development to allow for suction, air, water, and a four-way controlled tip deflection.

HONORS AND ACTIVITIES

Hirschowitz is professor emeritus and professor of physiology at the University of Alabama, Birmingham. His work has appeared in more than 350 papers (the first appearing in *Gastroenterology* in 1951). He has conducted research on the effects of nonsteroidal anti-inflammatory drugs on the GI tract, Zollinger-Ellison syndrome, peptic ulcer, and esophagitis. He has been awarded the Schindler Medal of the American Society for Gastrointestinal Endoscopy, the Friedenwald Medal of the American Gastroenterological Association, the Distinguished Lecturer Award and the Distinguished Scientist Award of the American College of Gastroenterology, and the Markovitz Award of the Surgical Research Society of America. He has been elected Master of the American College of Physicians, a member of the Association of American Physicians, and a Fellow of the Royal College of Physicians (London) and the Royal College of Physicians (Edinburgh). He is an Honorary Fellow of the Royal Society of Medicine (London), and an Honorary Member of the British Society of Gastroenterology and the Italian Society of Gastroenterology.

SEE ALSO: Technology, New Therapies; United States; University of Alabama at Birmingham Comprehensive Cancer Center.

BIBLIOGRAPHY. *American Men and Women of Science* (R. R. Bowker/Gale Group, 1971–2003); Rodney B. Nelson, "History," in *Endoscopy in Gastric Cancer* (Springer-Verlag, 1979); *Who's Who in America* (Marquis Who's Who, 1974–2003); *Who's Who in Science and Engineering* (Marquis Who's Who, 1994–2001).

JUSTIN CORFIELD
GEELONG GRAMMAR SCHOOL, AUSTRALIA

History of Cancer

IN ALMOST ALL ancient civilizations, the practice of medicine represented an amalgamation of religion and magic, attributing disease diagnosis and therapeutics to the supernatural. Because religion and religious ideology dictated the practice of medicine, it almost seemed imperative that medical science would be dominated by magical charms, rituals, and appeasement of deities, which in turn were controlled by the state. Cancer is one affliction that set off a series of experiments and research that continues till the present day. What is this disease that has made man almost its slave, despite the tremendous leaps medicine has made over the past several centuries? What are the origins of this disease, as commonly accepted by scholars of the history of medicine?

The first written evidence of the existence of cancer (derived from *karcinos*, the Greek word for *crab*), as occurring in malignant and benign forms, is found in the medical papyri of Egypt dating to about 3,000 years ago, when cases of malignant neoplasms were revealed in Egyptian mummies. Most prominent among these papyri were the Edwin Smith and George Ebers papyri, both of which contain elaborate descriptions of cancer, aspects of surgery, and treatment of diseases through magic and medicinal drugs. Interestingly, the medical information contained in the two collections reflects heightened patronage from the pharaohs—a feature that bears close resemblance to medicine practiced in other ancient civilizations.

In India, the oldest repositories of ancient medicine, its art, and practice were found in the four Vedas (Rgveda, Samveda, Yajurveda, and Atharvaveda), written about 3,000 years ago. The Vedas contain lucid references to magical and religious incantations followed in the treatment of various ailments, until well into the 6th century B.C.E., when, with the rise of various schools of philosophy (Nyaya and Lokayata, for example), the transition in medical practice from magicoreligious to rational therapeutics altered the character of the medical profession. It provided a new outlook to a new class of physicians that began to question the scriptural declarations of the ruling religious ideologies. It is important to note that the medical profession in most ancient civilizations met the same fate of alteration, accommodation, suppression, and triumph with a change in the nature of the state. Although the exact causes and ways of dealing with cancer are still being unraveled by physicians, it is significant to note that some of the earliest medical schools described the "unconquered" disease in its entirety. The Hippocratic School, for example, described various kinds of cancer affecting the human body.

CHANGING PERSPECTIVES

Western societies in recent decades have focused their medical attention on identifying the exact diagnosis and treatment of cancer. Although most medical discoveries of the 17th and 18th centuries were regrouped only retrospectively to assess their relevance in the practice of medicine, the description of the origin of body cells and their function in the human body remained controversial until well into the early 19th century.

Repeated attempts were made to describe the onset of the disease as afflicting various organs of the human body. Quite often, there was a tendency to explain the cause of cancer as related to perceived abnormalities in lymph.

Credit for the discovery of the phenomenon of uncontrolled growth of cells went to Rudolf Ludwig Virchow, a pathologist who correlated the clinical aspects of disease with cell pathology. For him, the cellular abnormality in the human body led to cancer, thus calling for scientific research at the micro and macro levels of pathology. Thus, even in the aftermath of the surgical and anatomical discoveries of the earlier centuries, the cause and cure of cancer hitherto remain unexplained.

As medical procedures advanced, earlier men of science saw a dramatic change in the treatment followed for the treatment of cancer. This was more visible in the field of oncology and in later surgical procedures in which certain kinds of cancer were treated through surgical triumphs of the time.

The 19th century, then, was the most propitious time for research improvements in cancer. The marriage of surgery with biomedical sciences throughout the 19th century explained the success of medical men in getting close to dealing with cancer. Theodor Billroth, William Hasted, and Rudolf Virchow were some of the prominent figures who gave a new form of scientific character to the medical profession during the century.

As one moves into the 20th century, one notices a strengthening of the efforts by medical men in combating cancer. Institutional support in the form of specialized ways of dealing with the disease dominated the medical scene, such as the establishment of the Cancer Research Fund in London at the turn of the 20th century. Similar institutions were founded under the aegis of the rich elites in India. Tata Memorial Hospital, founded in Bombay in 1941, offers an example of the interest and efforts of the local elites, the Parsis, in facilitating further research into the disease.

Despite medical and scientific efforts in most diseases, in cancer, too, there was a shift toward the adoption of a social paradigm to explain the disease, contesting the dominant models of health and disease.

With inordinate amounts of money being invested in cancer research, it may seem that the alarming nature of the disease will call for justice in the way it is approached.

However, this is not always the case. Quite often, there has been a tendency to medicalize the approach to the study of cancer by health and medical educators, by epidemiologists, and by some health activists who identify most epidemiological hazards with race and class. Accordingly, the incidence of specific diseases tends to be related to specific groups or even individuals within those specific groups.

If scientific and medical knowledge is open to debates among scholars, the study of cancer provides an arena for this interaction. This is best seen in exploring the world of diagnosis and therapeutics beyond biomedicine. In recent years, there has been increasing interest in the promotion of alternative or complementary medical systems, especially in Western societies. Originating from some of the ancient civilizations of the world, traditional practices of China and India have gained considerable prominence at the popular level. Even at the political level, there has been a resurrection of governmental interest and intervention in perpetuating the newly acquired popular interest in alternative therapies.

Such trends have emerged from the need to focus on people's perspective of health and illness, providing a fresh outlook on the slow yet steady transition from the erstwhile biomedical model to a socioeconomic paradigm supporting lifestyles, culture recognition, and individual perceptions of disease and health. This transition is especially relevant in the light of chronic illnesses, which tend to change individual experiences of health and illness.

SEE ALSO: Cost of Therapy; Disease and Poverty; Hospitals.

BIBLIOGRAPHY. A. K. Dalal and S. Ray, eds., *Social Dimensions of Health* (Rawat Publications, 2005); Sarah Curtis and Ann Taket, *Health and Societies: Changing Perspectives* (Hodder Arnold, 1995); Phil Brown, "Popular Epidemiology, Toxic Waste and Social Movements," in Jonathan Gabe, ed., *Medicine, Health and Risk: Sociological Approaches* (Blackwell Publishers, 1995).

POONAM BALA
UNIVERSITY OF DELHI

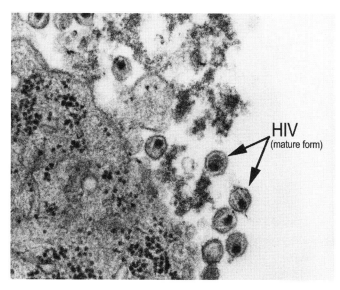

This image reveals the presence of mature forms of the human immunodeficiency virus (HIV).

HIV/AIDS-Related Cancers

WORLDWIDE, ABOUT 38 million people are living with human immunodeficiency virus (HIV) infection, and infection rates are still rising in many sub-Saharan countries, Eastern Europe, and Asia. About 50 percent of all people living with HIV worldwide are women. In the United States, there are more than 1 million cases of HIV, and about 40,000 new infections occur every year. The majority of persons with HIV in the United States are men (74 percent), but the proportion of women infected has risen in recent years.

HIGHLY ACTIVE ANTIRETROVIRAL THERAPY

Since the onset of the HIV epidemic in 1981, it has become apparent that persons infected with HIV have increased risk for certain cancers, such as non-Hodgkin's lymphoma and Kaposi's sarcoma. These cancers are referred to as AIDS-defining cancers because they are part of the constellation of malignant and nonmalignant conditions that define the syndrome. Since 1996, highly active antiretroviral therapy (HAART) has been used to suppress effectively the replication of HIV and to decrease morbidity and premature mortality. With the advent of HAART, the progression from diagnosis of HIV infection to development of acquired immunodeficiency syndrome (AIDS) and the progression from AIDS to death have slowed substantially. HAART and prolonged survival have been associated with increased risk for other chronic disease syndromes. Study findings indicate that HAART reduces the risk of Kaposi's sarcoma and possibly non-Hodgkin's lymphoma but may not alter the risk of other AIDS-related cancers. Studies using record linkage on population-based registries of persons with HIV/AIDS and cancer have

reported that the risk for cancer is higher for persons with AIDS than for the general population.

Risks for AIDS-related lymphoma and other malignant diseases may vary by demographic characteristics of population subgroup (e.g., gender, race, or ethnicity) or by pathological characteristics (tissue histology). Lymphoma, for example, consists of more than 30 different cancer types and subtypes. Much of what is known about the risks of AIDS-related lymphomas comes from epidemiological studies.

SPECTRUM STUDIES

In the Adult/Adolescent Spectrum of the HIV Disease Project, investigators abstracted medical records from 89 hospitals and clinics in nine U.S. cities from January 1994 through June 1997. Analyses of the data showed no decrease in the incidence of Hodgkin's disease or non-Hodgkin's lymphoma during that period.

In a study of the spectrum of AIDS-associated malignancies, population-based data from cancer registries and AIDS registries in the United States and Puerto Rico were linked. Cases of non-Hodgkin's lymphoma that occurred more than three years before the initial report on the AIDS registry were not regarded as AIDS defining. From 1986 through 1990, 1,793 cases of non-Hodgkin's lymphoma were identified among 40,733 person-years of observation. Among persons younger than 70 years of age, the risk (incidence) of non-Hodgkin's lymphoma was 113-fold higher among persons with AIDS than among those in the general population. The risk of Hodgkin's disease was 7.6-fold higher among persons younger than 70 years.

In 1984 and 1985, the Multicenter AIDS Cohort Study enrolled 1,813 gay men infected with HIV. The follow-up study reported that the incidence of non-Hodgkin's lymphoma in this group increased significantly, at 21 percent per year from the early 1990s through 1997. However, none of the more recently enrolled patients with non-Hodgkin's lymphoma had used potent antiretroviral therapies.

Analysis of data from the Swiss HIV Cohort Study showed that use of HAART may prevent most excess risk of non-Hodgkin's lymphoma and Kaposi's sarcoma but not Hodgkin's lymphoma and other non-AIDS-defining cancers. Unexpectedly, the risk of Hodgkin's lymphoma among HIV-infected persons treated with HAART was three times that among untreated patients. This finding suggests the need for further research and clarification.

Results from an International Collaboration on HIV and Cancer indicated that the overall incidence of non-Hodgkin's lymphoma declined from 6.2 percent to 3.6 percent between the periods 1992–96 and 1997–99.

INVASIVE CERVICAL CANCER

The increased incidence of specific types of malignant disease identified in patients with HIV infection includes invasive cervical cancer as well as non-Hodgkin's lymphoma and Kaposi's sarcoma. Invasive cervical cancer is an AIDS-defining malignant disease when it occurs in the presence of HIV infection. Overall, studies have not suggested that the introduction of HAART affected cervical-cancer rates.

In many studies on AIDS-related malignant diseases, few or no cases of invasive cervical cancer were reported. The Swiss HIV Cohort Study reported only six cases. No cervical cancers were reported in an analysis of data from the AIDS–Cancer Match Registry Study. In the Women's Interagency HIV Study of 2,628 women with HIV, from October 1994 to September 2001, only one case of cervical cancer was observed.

Several studies have examined the incidence, prevalence, or persistence of premalignant changes in the cervix (cervical squamous intraepithelial lesions) among HIV-infected women. In some but not all stud-ies of HIV-positive women, use of HAART has been related to partial regression of these lesions. Important preventive measures for both HIV-positive and HIV-negative women include use of the Papanicolaou (Pap) test in screening for cervical cancer, vaccination against infection with human papillomavirus (HPV), and use of safety measures during sexual activity.

OTHER CANCERS

Reports of increased risk for other HIV-associated malignant diseases are inconsistent. Survival of patients with HIV infection has been prolonged because of better methods for prevention and treatment of infectious complications and more effective antiretroviral therapies. One might expect an increase in incidence of cancers such as lung cancer or prostate cancer because patients are living longer.

In the Women's Interagency HIV Study, increased incidence of lung cancer was observed. Several studies have examined a possible link between HIV/AIDS and lung cancer, but no association has been confirmed. Increased risk of liver cancer has been reported among men infected with both HIV and hepatitis C during the HAART era.

SEE ALSO: Cervical Cancer; Kaposi's Sarcoma; Lymphoma, AIDS-Related; Sarcoma, Kaposi's.

BIBLIOGRAPHY. O.C. Baiocchi, et al., "Impact of Highly Active Antiretroviral Therapy in the Treatment of HIV-Infected Patients with Systemic Non-Hodgkin's Lymphoma," *Acta Oncology* (v.41, 2002); R.J. Biggar, et al., "Kaposi's Sarcoma and Non-Hodgkin's Lymphoma Following the Diagnosis of AIDS, Multistate AIDS/Cancer Match Study Group," *International Journal of Cancer* (v.68, 1996); F. Bonnet, et al., "Malignancy-Related Causes of Death in Human Immunodeficiency Virus-Infected Patients in the Era of Highly Active Antiretroviral Therapy," *Cancer* (v.101, 2004); G.M. Clifford, et al., "Cancer Risk in the Swiss HIV Cohort Study: Associations with Immunodeficiency, Smoking, and Highly Active Antiretroviral Therapy," *Journal of the National Cancer Institute* (v.97, 2005); C. Cooksley, et al., "HIV-Related Malignancies: Community-Based Study Using Linkage of Cancer Registry and HIV Registry Data," *International Journal of Sexually Transmitted Diseases and AIDS* (v.10, 1999); S.H. Ebrahim, et al., "AIDS-Defining Cancers in Western Europe, 1994–2001," *AIDS Patient Care and Sexually Transmitted Diseases* (v.18, 2004); M.

Frisch, et al., For the AIDS-Cancer Match Registry Study Group, "Human Papillomavirus-Associated Cancers in Patients with Human Immunodeficiency Virus Infection and Acquired Immunodeficiency Syndrome," *Journal of the National Cancer Institute* (v.92, 2000); A.E. Grulich, et al., "Rates of Non–AIDS-Defining Cancers in People with HIV Infection Before and After AIDS Diagnosis," *AIDS* (v.16, 2002); M. Herida, et al., "Incidence of Non–AIDS-Defining Cancers Before and During the Highly Active Antiretroviral Therapy Era in a Cohort of Human Immunodeficiency Virus-Infected Patients," *Journal of Clinical Oncology* (v.21, 2003); International Collaboration on HIV and Cancer, "Highly Active Antiretroviral Therapy and Incidence of Cancer in Human Immunodeficiency Virus-Infected Adults," *Journal of the National Cancer Institute* (v.92, 2000); L.P. Jacobson, et al., "Impact of Potent Antiretroviral Therapy on the Incidence of Kaposi's Sarcoma and Non-Hodgkin's Lymphomas Among HIV-1-Infected Individuals: Multicenter AIDS Cohort Study," *Journal of Acquired Immune Deficiency Syndrome* (v.21/S1, 1999); J. L. Jones, et al., "Effect of Antiretroviral Therapy on Recent Trends in Selected Cancers Among HIV-Infected Persons: Adult/Adolescent Spectrum of HIV Disease Project Group," *Journal of Acquired Immune Deficiency Syndrome* (v.21/S1, 1999); M. Maiman, et al., "Cervical Cancer As an AIDS-Defining Illness," *Obstetrics and Gynecology* (v.89, 1997); A. Newnham, et al., "The Risk of Cancer in HIV-Infected People in Southeast England: A Cohort Study," *British Journal of Cancer* (v.92, 2005); J. Palefsky, "Human Papillomavirus-Related Tumors in HIV," *Current Opinion in Oncology* (v.18, 2006).

Steven S. Coughlin, Ph.D.
H. Irene Hall, Ph.D.
Mona Saraiya
Centers for Disease Control and Prevention

Holden Comprehensive Cancer Center at The University of Iowa

THE HOLDEN COMPREHENSIVE Cancer Center at the University of Iowa (UI) was established in 1980 by the board of regents of the state of Iowa. The Holden Center, located in Iowa City, coordinates all cancer-related patient care, education, and research at the UI and at the UI hospitals and clinics.

The mission of the Holden Center is to reduce the pain and suffering caused by cancer in Iowa, surrounding communities, and the world through improved cancer prevention and treatment. This mission is embodied in three areas of endeavor: promotion of cancer research; provision of high-quality cancer care, including prevention, detection, and treatment; and education about cancer for the general public and cancer professionals.

In 2000 the Holden Center became a National Cancer Institute (NCI) Cancer Center and shortly thereafter was designated an NCI Comprehensive Cancer Center; the latter designation was renewed in 2005. The name Holden Cancer Center was adopted in 2000 in recognition of a $25 million gift from the Holden family of Williamsburg, Iowa; the current name was adopted when the center was granted Comprehensive Cancer Center status by the NCI.

PATIENT CARE AND SUPPORT SERVICES

In 2005, over 26,000 patients with a primary diagnosis of cancer were treated at the Holden Center, and over 4,000 were admitted as inpatients. Most patients are seen at the Cancer Center Clinic of the John and Mary Pappajohn Clinical Cancer Center, which includes an outpatient clinic, procedure rooms, a chemotherapy suite, laboratories, and a breast-imaging center. A few Holden Center units are located in separate parts of the UI hospitals. The Adult Blood and Marrow Transplant Unit is housed in the Carver Pavilion; the Pediatric Blood and Marrow Transplant Unit is in the Colloton Pavilion; and Radiation Oncology is located in the Pomerantz Pavilion.

The Holden Center provides support services to cancer patients and their families. Psychiatric evaluation and counseling is available for patients experiencing emotional or psychiatric symptoms that interfere with their daily functioning, quality of life, or treatment completion. Social workers are available to assist patients in issues relating to emotional and social support. Cancer support groups meet regularly at the center. An online cancer support group is also available, and outreach support groups (which are sponsored by the Holden Center but meet elsewhere) are held regularly in Fort Madison Hospital, Keokuk Area Hospital, Washington County Hospital, and Henry County.

The Patient Representative Program provides services for patients and visitors, including advocacy, assistance, information, crisis help, and complaint resolution. The Helen K. Rossi Guest House provides low-cost accommodations for patients receiving treatment at the UI hospitals and clinics, and their families. Translation and interpretation services are available in 26 languages. Palliative care—including pain and symptom management, support in dealing with emotional and social issues, and spiritual support—is provided by the UI Hospitals and Clinics Palliative Care Service.

Pain-management services are available through the UI Pain Management and Support Group Program, which offers multidisciplinary assistance in pain management.

The Cancer Information Service of the Holden Center maintains a toll-free telephone line and e-mail address through which patients, family members, healthcare providers, and the general public may receive information about cancer. The Holden Center website also provides a link to the Iowa Consortium for Comprehensive Cancer Control, a web portal providing access to information about cancer and cancer resources, focusing on resources within Iowa.

CLINICAL TRIALS AND RESEARCH PROGRAMS

The Holden Center received over $55 million in research funding in 2005. During that year, 249 clinical trials were open at the center, with 3,173 patients enrolled in them.

The Holden Center has six research programs: Cancer Immunology and Immunotherapy, Cell Signaling and Development Pharmacology, Free Radical Cancer Biology, Tumor Imaging, Cancer Epidemiology, and Cancer Genetics and Computational Biology. These research programs are supported by 17 core facilities, including Biostatistics, Central Microscopy Research, Flow Cytometry, Radiation and Free Radical Research, Gene Transfer Vector, and Small Animal Imaging.

The Cancer Immunology and Immunotherapy program studies how the immune system functions, how it can be manipulated to prevent and treat cancer, and the complications of cancer. The Cell Signaling and Developmental Pharmacology program studies cell signaling, cell cycle control and apoptosis to develop new pharmacologic approaches to cancer prevention and therapy. The Free Radical Cancer Biology program studies the role of oxidative events in the therapy of neoplastic disease, focusing on the use of in vitro, ex vivo, and small-animal systems to test oxidation-base therapeutic approaches to cancer therapy.

The purpose of the Tumor Imaging program is to integrate modern medical imaging techniques into basic, translation, and clinical cancer research. Specific areas of focus include metabolic assessment of response to therapy, iodine symporter as a reporter gene and as a novel therapy, cell trafficking, development of radiopharmaceuticals, and development of new analysis methodologies.

The Cancer Epidemiology program focuses on four areas: cancer etiology, cancer health services and outcomes, oral health and cancer, and cancer prevention and control. The program also administers the Iowa Cancer Registry, which is part of the NCI Surveillance, Epidemiology and End Results (SEER) program.

The Cancer Genetics and Computational Biology Program focuses on discovering genetic events involved in normal and malignant cell growth and investigating how these events affect cell behavior, with the ultimate goal of developing new cancer prevention and therapy strategies. Specific areas of focus include cancer genes and signaling pathways, genomic organization and gene expression, and papillomavirus carcinogenesis.

The Holden Center NCI Lymphoma Specialized Program of Research Excellence (SPORE) operates in conjunction with the Mayo Clinic Comprehensive Cancer Center. This project consists of five research projects, five core resources, and the Career Development and Developmental Research Program. The emphasis of the SPORE is on translational research, and a clinical trial or population study is included in each research project.

The Cancer and Aging Program is a joint project of the UI Center on Aging and the Holden Center. In 2003, the centers jointly received a five-year grant commitment from the NCI and the National Institute on Aging to study the relationship between aging and cancer.

SEE ALSO: Age; Education, Cancer; Genetics; Hospitals.

BIBLIOGRAPHY. Holden Comprehensive Cancer Center website, www.uihealthcare.com/depts/cancercenter (cited December 2006); The Iowa Consortium for Comprehensive Cancer Control website, www.canceriowa.org (cited December 2006).

SARAH BOSLAUGH
WASHINGTON UNIVERSITY SCHOOL OF MEDICINE

Honduras

THIS CENTRAL AMERICAN country was a Spanish colony until it achieved its independence on September 15, 1821. It has a population of 6,824,000 (2004) and has 83 doctors and 26 nurses per 100,000 people. Healthcare in Honduras remained underdeveloped until the late 20th century. Before then, many people did not live long enough to suffer from many cancers, although many people working in unhygienic mines and factories did develop tumors and occupational cancers. Cases of human T-cell leukemia–lymphoma virus have been found in some black former slave communities in Honduras.

There have been a number of studies of cervical cancer in Honduras with a mortality rate of 16.8 per 100,000, with an age-standardized incidence rate of 39.6 per 100,000 (compared with the United States, with rates of 2.8 and 1.2, respectively). One of the causes is believed to be smoke inhalation from wood kitchen fires. During the late 1990s, there was heavy promotion of increased screening procedures, Pap smears, and direct visual inspections.

Several people connected with Honduras died from cancer. Henri Louis Bischoffsheim, a financier connected with the 1867 Honduras Loan, succumbed to cancer. William Thornton Pryce, U.S. ambassador to Honduras from 1993 to 1996, died from pancreatic cancer. Gabriel Montalvo Higuera, papal nuncio to Honduras from 1974 to 1980, died from lung cancer.

There is a faculty of medicine at the Universidad Nacional Autonoma de Honduras. The Asociación Hondureña de Luchacontra el Cáncer, Honduras; and the Liga Contra el Cáncer, Honduras, are both members of the International Union Against Cancer.

SEE ALSO: Cervical Cancer; Developing Countries; Industry.

BIBLIOGRAPHY. "Cervical Cancer Prevention in Rural Honduras," www.med.unc.edu/hha/Cervical-Cancer-Prevention-Strategies.pdf (cited November 2006); A. Ferrera, et al., "Human Papillomavirus Infection, Cervical Dysplasia and Invasive Cervical Cancer in Honduras: A Case-Control Study," *International Journal of Cancer* (v.82, 1999); J. P. Velema, et al., "Burning Wood in the Kitchen Increases the Risk of Cervical Neoplasia in HPV-Infected Women in Honduras," *International Journal of Cancer* (v.97, 2002).

JUSTIN CORFIELD
GEELONG GRAMMAR SCHOOL, AUSTRALIA

Hong Kong Anti-Cancer Society

THE HONG KONG Anti-Cancer Society (HKACS), founded in 1963, has three principal aims: to promote, coordinate and undertake cancer research and cancer education; to promote, coordinate, and undertake relief work for cancer patients and survivors and their families; and to provide medical facilities for the diagnosis and treatment of cancer patients in Hong Kong.

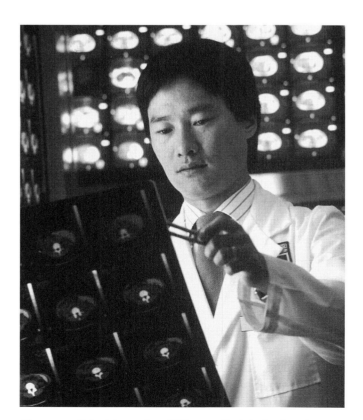

Above, a radiologist examines CAT scans. Such technology is promoted by the Hong Kong Anti-Cancer Society.

The society is funded by public donations and is a member agency of the Community Chest of Hong Kong, which provides funds to help meet HKACS operating expenses. The society is governed by an executive committee and has three subcommittees: Hospice Care Development, Cancer Education, and the Betterment Fund for Cancer Patients.

The HKACS provided the funding for construction of Nam Long Hospital, devoted entirely to the care of cancer patients, which opened in 1967. It was the only dedicated facility for cancer treatment and hospice care in Hong Kong at that time. Nam Long Hospital originally had 120 beds; this number was increased to 180 beds in 1978. In 1987, a hospice care program was established, and since 1989 more than 30 percent of the hospital beds have been devoted to hospice care. The hospital has been managed since 1991 by the Hospital Authority of Hong Kong, which manages all public hospitals in Hong Kong. Nam Long Hospital was converted to a cancer rehabilitation center in 2007.

The Hospice Care Development subcommittee advises the hospice-care team of Nam Long Hospital on hospice-care delivery services, organizes training courses and workshop for hospice-care professionals, and conducts public awareness campaigns to promote hospice care to the general public. The Cancer Education subcommittee organizes courses, lectures, and exhibitions for the medical profession and the general public, and publishes information pamphlets on cancer. The Betterment Fund for Cancer Patients manages a fund devoted to providing financial assistance to cancer patients and to supporting group activities for cancer patients. Most of the support for this fund is provided by the Hong Kong Jockey Club Charities Trust and the Brewin Trust Fund.

The HKACS provides funds for cancer research, concentrating on types of cancer common in Hong Kong, such as nasopharyngeal cancer and lung cancer. This in part reflects the research interests of the founder of HKACS, John H. C. Ho, a pioneer in cancer research and treatment. Ho established the first academic department of radiology and oncology at the Chinese University of Hong Kong. His greatest contributions may have been in the area of nasopharyngeal cancer; he discovered that feeding infants salted preserved fish, a common practice in southern China, was a primary risk factor.

SEE ALSO: Survivors of Cancer; Survivors of Cancer Families; Education; Hospice; Nasopharangeal Cancer.

BIBLIOGRAPHY. Jane Parry, "John H C Ho" [obituary], *British Medical Journal* (v.331, 2005); C.K. Li, et al., "Epidemiology of Paediatric Cancer in Hong Kong, 1982 to 1991: Hong Kong Cancer Registry," *Hong Kong Medical Journal* (v.5/2, 1999).

SARAH BOSLAUGH
WASHINGTON UNIVERSITY SCHOOL OF MEDICINE

Hong Kong Association of Blood Transfusion & Haematology Ltd.

THE HONG KONG Association of Blood Transfusion and Haematology Limited (HKABTH) was incorporated as a limited-liability company in January 1996. It was formerly known as the Hong Kong Blood Transfusion Society Ltd.

The primary objectives of the HKABTH are to advance knowledge in the fields of blood transfusion and hematology, promote high ethical and professional standards, facilitate the exchange of ideas and information in those fields, and develop connections with related organizations.

Membership in the HKABTH is open to persons with professional qualifications in fields such as medicine, nursing, technology, and research who are working in or have an interest in the fields of blood transfusion and hematology. As of 2006 the HKABTH had over 250 members. The association offices are located in Kowloon.

The HKABTH holds an annual general meeting and scientific symposium; it also organizes lectures and workshops for continuing professional education in blood transfusion and hematology throughout the year. Since 2001, the annual scientific meeting has been jointly organized with the Hong Kong Society of Haematology. The HKABTH is an accredited provider of Continuing Professional Development courses for Medical Laboratory Technologists in Hong Kong.

The HKABTH has issued guidelines on Preoperative Autologous Blood Deposit for Defined Use and Acute Normovolaemic Haemodilution; both are available on its website. The association published a newsletter distributed to its members, blood banks, hospitals, teaching institutes, and associated societies from 1995 to 2001; issues for 1999 and 2000 are available on the HKABTH website. Case histories and other articles intended for a professional audience are also available from the HKABTH website; presentation of these articles on the website serves as a partial replacement for the HKABTH newsletter. Links to professional resources in Chinese and English are also included on the website. PowerPoint presentations from some previous workshops and scientific meetings for 2002 and 2003 are available for download from the HKABTH website, as is *10th Anniversary Commemorative Album,* which contains essays and articles by the association's past and current presidents, as well as a comprehensive annotated bibliography of transfusion-medicine research conducted in Hong Kong or written by authors working in Hong Kong.

SEE ALSO: China; Education, Cancer.

BIBLIOGRAPHY. Hong Kong Association of Blood Transfusion and Haematology website, www.fmshk.com.hk/hkabth/home.htm; Edward Ma, "Hong Kong Association of Blood Transfusion and Haematology: History and Milestones," in *10th Anniversary Commemorative Album,* (Hong Kong Association of Blood Transfusion and Haematology, 2006).

SARAH BOSLAUGH
WASHINGTON UNIVERSITY SCHOOL OF MEDICINE

Hong Kong Cancer Fund

THE HONG KONG Cancer Fund (HKCF) was founded in 1987 as a small support group of cancer patients and their families, and has expanded to become a leading cancer organization in Hong Kong. The HKCF is an independent charity funded by donations and does not receive government funding.

The focus of the HKCF is on people-oriented care and on filling service gaps in cancer care; its motto is that no one should face cancer alone. Areas of cancer care targeted by the HKCF include the provision of psychological and social support services, helping survivors reintegrate themselves into society, improving nursing training, and making the hospital environment more pleasant for patients. The HKCF also educates the public on issues regarding cancer and funds cancer research.

Basic information about cancer is available in Chinese and English from the HKCF website, including incidence and mortality by type of cancer in Hong Kong, and information about cancer prevention and early detection.

The organization also produces 33 cancer information booklets in Chinese and English, covering two types of topics. The Understanding series offers information on various types of cancer, and the Coping series offers information and advice about topics such as pain, hair loss, and caring for someone with cancer. Both types of booklets can be downloaded from the HKCF website.

The HKCF publishes a newsletter in Chinese and English three times per year; the publication is available for download from the HKCF website or via e-mail subscription. The HKCF promotes professional education in cancer care by providing funds for medical professionals to attend overseas conferences; it also grants a scholarship in psycho-oncology for a doctoral student at the Centre for Psycho-Oncology Research and Teaching at the University of Hong Kong. The HKCF is also the main sponsor of the Psychosocial Symposium, which is held at the annual Hong Kong International Cancer Congress.

The organization has provided research funding for projects relating to the most common cancers in Hong Kong, including liver cancer, nasopharyngeal cancer, colorectal cancer, and breast cancer.

The HKCF has undertaken several projects to make cancer treatment less unpleasant, including renovation of the radiation-therapy rooms in Pamela Youde Nethersole Eastern Hospital and Tuen Mun Hospital to surround patients with soothing images and warm lighting. The oncology wards and waiting areas of Queen Elizabeth Hospital were renovated and outfitted with more comfortable furniture. A day-care center for cancer care, which allows patients to spend more time at home, was opened in Prince of Wales Hospital, funded jointly by the HKCF and the Hospital Authority. The HKCF also donated a van that Haven of Hope Hospice uses to provide care to terminally ill patients in their homes.

SEE ALSO: Education, Cancer; Survivors of Cancer; Survivors of Cancer Families.

BIBLIOGRAPHY. Hong Kong Cancer Fund website, www.cancer-fund.org/html/eng/index.asp (cite May 2007); C.K. Li, et al., "Epidemiology of Paediatric Cancer in Hong Kong, 1982 to 1991: Hong Kong Cancer Registry," *Hong Kong Medical Journal* (v.5/2, 1999).

SARAH BOSLAUGH
WASHINGTON UNIVERSITY SCHOOL OF MEDICINE

Hong Kong Paediatric Haematology & Oncology Study Group

THE HONG KONG Paediatric Haematology & Oncology Study Group is a member association of healthcare professionals working in the fields of pediatric hematology and oncology. Its purposes are to advance knowledge of pediatric hematology and oncology, to improve the standard of care for children suffering from cancer and blood diseases, and to promote child health relative to hematological and oncological conditions.

The Study Group is a member of the Federation of Medical Societies of Hong Kong, an organization of professional societies founded in 1965 to advance continuing education for health professionals and to facilitate cooperation among member professional organizations. The organization's offices are located in the Department of Paediatrics, Prince of Wales Hospital, Shatin, which is the teaching hospital of Chinese University of Hong Kong. Prince of Wales Hospital is a leader in research and treatment of pediatric cancers; it includes the Sir Yue Kong Pao Centre for Cancer and the Lady Pao Children's Cancer Centre, both opened in 1994.

Medical practitioners residing in Hong Kong with an interest in pediatric hematology and oncology are eligible to become full members of the organization, subject to approval by the Study Group Council. Persons who work with children suffering from oncological or hematological disorders but who do not reside in Hong Kong, or who are not qualified medical practitioners, may apply to become associate members, also subject to council approval.

Honorary members are people who have made major contributions to hematology or oncology and have been selected at the Study Group annual general meeting.

Study Group members have been influential in the study of childhood cancer in Hong Kong, including the epidemiological study of pediatric cancers in Hong Kong from 1982 to 1999, based on data collected in the Hong Kong Cancer Registry.

The Study Group website includes a bibliography of scientific publications and presentations by members; the text of the organization's constitution; and the names, affiliations, and contact information of officers and council members. Further information about Study Group activities, including courses offered and conferences, is available through the Federation of Medical Societies of Hong Kong website.

SEE ALSO: Childhood Cancers; China; Education, Cancer.

BIBLIOGRAPHY. Federation of Medical Societies of Hong Kong website, www.fmshk.org/fmshk.php?lang=eng (cited November 2006); Hong Kong Paediatric Haematology & Oncology Study Group website, www.fmshk.com.hk/hkphosg/home.htm (cited November 2006); C.K. Li, et al., "Epidemiology of Paediatric Cancer in Hong Kong, 1982 to 1991: Hong Kong Cancer Registry," *Hong Kong Medical Journal* (v.5/2, 1999).

SARAH BOSLAUGH
WASHINGTON UNIVERSITY SCHOOL OF MEDICINE

Hospice

THE TERM *HOSPICE* refers both to a facility that provides specialized services for persons with terminal illness and a philosophy of care that emphasizes maintaining the comfort, dignity, and quality of life of persons with serious or terminal illness. This care may be provided in a person's home, a hospital, a nursing home, or a specialized hospice facility.

Characteristics of hospice care include a focus on symptom management rather than cure of disease; a focus on maintaining the person's quality of life rather than using all possible means to extend its length; and application of a holistic philosophy that endeavors to meet the physical, social, psychological, and spiritual needs of patients and their families rather than simply providing medical care to the patients. Hospice care may include medical treatment but differs in its focus. Rather than attempting to cure a patient's disease, hospice care accepts that the disease is terminal and focuses on allowing the individual to live as fully as possible for whatever remaining amount of life he or she may have. Hospice care in the United States is available primarily to individuals who, in the judgment of their physician, would no longer benefit from curative treatment and are projected to be in their last six months of life.

The term *palliative care* is sometimes used in the same sense as hospice care, meaning care for a person with terminal illness that emphasizes pain control, symptom control, and quality of life rather than cure of disease. The term is also used in a much broader sense, however, to mean care that maintains a person's quality of life during treatment for any illness, including those from which the person is expected to recover. It is also sometimes applied to treatment for conditions that affect a person's quality of life without posing an immediate threat to survival. In fact, a large portion of hospice care consists of the application of palliative-care principles to persons with terminal illness, with the addition of elements that apply specifically to end-of-life care, such as financial planning and bereavement counseling to prepare the individual and family members for the anticipated death.

The World Health Organization (WHO) has stated that palliative care is an essential part of cancer control and can be provided simply and inexpensively in most cases. Because outside the industrialized world, persons with cancer typically do not see a doctor until their cancer is in an advanced stage, provision of palliative care is particularly important in developing countries. The WHO definition of palliative care includes statements that also apply to hospice care, including the provisions that palliative care regards dying as a normal process, neither hastens nor postpones death, provides relief from pain and other symptoms, includes the psychological and spiritual aspects of the patient's life, helps patients live as actively as possible, and offers support to the family during and after the illness.

The word *hospice* comes from the Latin word *hospitium* (guesthouse) and is also the root of the English word *hospitality*. Hospices were originally places

of shelter and rest for travelers or the indigent, often run by religious orders.

The term *hospice* was first used with reference to a facility providing medical care to the dying by the British physician Dame Cicely Saunders, who introduced the idea to the United States during a lecture delivered at Yale University in 1963. Saunders was instrumental in the creation of St. Christopher's Hospice, the first such facility in the world, in London in 1967. Saunders greatly influenced Florence Wald, then dean of the School of Nursing at Yale, who worked at St. Christopher's during a sabbatical year in 1968. The first hospice in the United States was The Connecticut Hospice, founded in Branford, Connecticut, in 1974, followed by a hospice established at the Yale Medical Center and a hospice program in Marin County, California.

Hospices now exist in over 90 countries, although terminology sometimes differs, and the services provided are partly dependent on the culture of each country and on how healthcare is provided and paid for in that country. In the United Kingdom and Ireland, for example, hospices are generally freestanding units on the grounds of a hospital. Services such as pain and symptom management provided elsewhere are referred to as palliative care rather than hospice care.

Acceptance of hospice care was greatly influenced by the publication in 1969 of *On Death and Dying* by the Swiss-American psychiatrist Elisabeth Kübler-Ross. In it, Kübler-Ross sharply criticized the treatment of dying patients in American hospitals, which she had observed as a physician and which she believed was based on the denial of death as a natural consequence of life. She believed that persons with terminal illness are often aware of their impending deaths and experience thoughts and emotions that can be characterized as a series of five stages. She also argued that terminally ill patients should be able to participate in decisions affecting their future, including the choice of dying at home rather than in an institution, which was a sharp contrast to the usual medical practice of the time.

PUBLIC FUNDING

The first legislation to provide federal funding for hospices was introduced in the United States in 1974 but was not enacted. In 1978 the Health Care Financing Administration (HCFA, which functioned in the same role as the Centers for Medicare and Medicaid Services

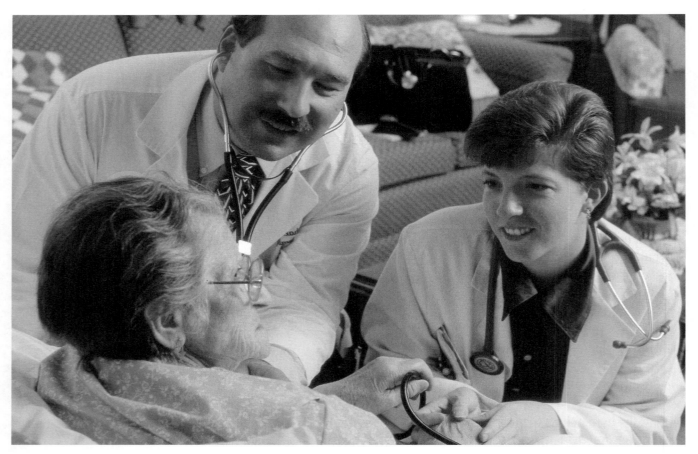

*The word **hospice** comes from the Latin word **hospitium** (guesthouse). Hospice care accepts that a patient is in a terminal stage of life and focuses on allowing the individual to live as fully as possible for whatever remaining amount of time that he or she may have.*

does today) issued a report citing hospice care as a humane and possibly cost-saving alternative to usual medical care for the dying. In 1979 HCFA initiated demonstration programs across the United States to determine decide what kind of care should be offered in a hospice and whether hospice care could be provided in a cost-effective manner. In 1982 Medicare initiated a hospice benefit, which became permanent in 1986. Also in 1986, states were given the option of including a hospice benefit in their Medicaid plans. Hospice care became an accepted part of a comprehensive healthcare package in the 1990s. It was recommended for inclusion in veterans' benefits packages in 1991 and was included as a guaranteed benefit in President Bill Clinton's healthcare reform proposal in 1993.

ASPECTS OF HOSPICE CARE

Hospice care is generally provided by a multidisciplinary healthcare team, which may include physi-
cians, nurses, dieticians, counselors, religious leaders, therapists, social workers, and home healthcare workers. Usually, members of the patient's family also are involved, and a family member may be designated as the primary caregiver. This person, who does not need special medical training, takes primary responsibility for assisting the patient with daily activities such as bathing and eating, and works closely with the professional staff in monitoring the patient's condition. Because of the importance placed on familial involvement in hospice care, even if care is provided within a hospital or nursing home, the patient's room will include accommodation for at least one member of his or her family.

Control of pain and other symptoms is the primary focus of hospice care. The goal is to provide the level of pain and symptom control that allows individuals to be comfortable and take part in any life activities that they are able to perform while remaining alert and able to make decisions.

Counseling for patients and their family members is an important aspect of hospice care and may be provided by many individuals, including clergy, psychologists, social workers, or trained volunteers.

A basic concept of hospice care is acknowledgment that death is a normal part of life and that the person receiving care is in the last stage of life. Counselors help the patient and his or her family prepare for the imminent death and support the family during the bereavement. They may also help the patient prepare in practical ways—to help get financial and legal affairs in order, for example.

Most hospice care is provided in the patient's home. When home hospice care is initiated, a medical caregiver typically visits the patient's home to assist in setting up the care situation, to train the family member who will be the primary caregiver, and to learn about the patient's needs. Return visits by the caregiver are scheduled regularly to monitor the patient's condition.

Hospital hospice care is an option for persons whose illness requires the regular services of the hospital. This type of care may be provided in a special unit of the hospital devoted to hospice care or may be provided by a hospice team that provides the care to eligible patients in any unit of the hospital.

Long-term-care facilities such as nursing homes may also have hospice units and may provide an intermediate solution for individuals who need more care than can be provided at home but do not need to be admitted to the hospital, or who do not have a family member who is able to serve as the primary caregiver.

Respite hospice care is provided in freestanding hospices, hospitals, and long-term-care facilities with a hospice unit. Respite care allows an individual who is usually cared for at home to be cared for in the hospice facility for a short period—often, five days—to provide a break for family members or to allow the family member serving as primary caregiver a few days to take care of personal business that he or she could not accomplish while serving as primary caregiver.

Medicare, a federal insurance program for persons who are over age 65 or who have certain medical conditions such as end-stage renal disease, has offered a hospice benefit since 1982. Because most people in hospice care in the United States are over age 65, willingness of Medicare to pay for hospice services has a major impact on the availability of hospice care.

Medicare pays for hospice care under the following conditions:

1. The individual is eligible for Medicare Part A.

2. The individual has less than six months to live, as certified by his or her doctor and the hospice director.

3. The individual signs a statement stating that he or she chooses hospice care.

4. The individual chooses a Medicare-approved hospice program.

Medicare pays for an initial consultation with a hospice medical director or physician to allow discussion of care options. It also pays for most hospice services related to the terminal illness, including nursing care, physician services, medical equipment and supplies, physical and occupational therapy, drugs for symptom control and pain relief, home healthcare, and short-term inpatient and respite care.

Medicare does not pay for treatment intended to cure the terminal illness (the choice of hospice care includes forgoing such treatment), prescription drugs intended to cure the illness, or room and board for those living in a residential hospice facility. Medicare payment for treatment of conditions other than the terminal illness is provided as it would have been before the individual elected hospice care.

Continuation of hospice benefits under Medicare requires regular evaluation of the individual's medical condition. Initially, coverage is provided for two 90-day periods of care, followed by an unlimited number of 60-day periods of care. At the start of each period of care, a hospice physician must recertify that the individual receiving benefits is terminally ill. Even if the individual lives longer than the originally anticipated six months, hospice benefits may continue as long as the hospice physician continues to certify that the individual is terminally ill.

An individual receiving hospice benefits has the right to end hospice care at any time and resume normal Medicare benefits, which would include curative treatment for the terminal disease. In addition, if the person's health improves (if cancer goes into remission, for example), he or she may resume normal Medicare benefits and return to hospice benefits when the disease is judged terminal.

Medicaid, a government insurance plan in the United States provided primarily for the impoverished, has offered a hospice benefit since 1986. Medicaid is funded jointly by the federal and state governments and administered by the states following guidelines set by the federal government. Benefits offered under Medicaid differ by state and may change frequently. Eligibility for benefits also differs by states, within guidelines set by the federal government.

The Medicaid hospice benefit is an option that individual states may choose to offer or not. In 2006, 47 states offered it. In general, the Medicaid hospice benefit covers similar services to the Medicare hospice benefit, although it may differ in specific details.

In addition, individual states may set more restrictive eligibility conditions or cover a different period of time from that provided under Medicare. For persons eligible for both Medicare and Medicaid (known as dual eligibles) who reside in a hospice facility, Medicare pays for the hospice program services, and Medicare pays the room-and-board charges.

Many private health insurance plans in the United States offer some hospice-care benefits, but the types of services covered and the amount of benefits available differ among individual policies and companies.

HOSPICE USE IN THE UNITED STATES

According to the National Center for Health Statistics, 106,000 patients in the United States were enrolled in hospice care in 2000. The average length of stay was 47 days, and the most common primary diagnosis (58 percent of the cases) was cancer. Of those patients, 621,100 were discharged in 2000, the most common reason (85.5 percent) being death. Other reasons for discharge included transfer to inpatient care (2.3 percent) and loss of eligibility due to recovery or loss of insurance coverage (7.9 percent); the reasons for discharge among the remaining cases were unknown.

Discharges were almost evenly split between males (49.8 percent) and females (50.2 percent). The population was primarily elderly, with most patients (79.6 percent) age 65 or older and 26.5 percent age 85 or older. Most patients (84.1 percent) were white, with the second-most-common ethnic group being African American (8.1 percent). Marital status was almost evenly split between married (47.2 percent) and unmarried (46.6 percent), with the marital status of 6.2 percent unknown.

The primary source of payment for hospice services was Medicare, which accounted for 78.6 percent of the total. Private insurance was the second-largest source of payment (13 percent), with Medicaid covering 5.1 percent of the cases and the remainder funded by other sources, including charity care.

Most persons discharged from hospice care (61.2 percent) in 2000 lived in a private or semiprivate residence, a category that includes private homes, boarding houses, and retirement homes. The second-most-common place of residence was a healthcare facility (34.9 percent), and the remainder lived in an assisted-living or residential-care facility (3.5 percent). Those not living in a healthcare facility were most likely to live with a family member (80.9 percent); 8.9 percent lived alone, and 7.9 percent lived with one or more nonfamily members. The primary caregiver was most often a relative (80.6 percent), and the relative was most often a spouse (41.9 percent) or child or child-in-law (29.5 percent).

In the 30 days before discharge, most hospice patients received skilled nursing services (91.8 percent), and 30.1 percent received physician services. Most patients received one or more type of psychosocial services, including referral or social services (71.9 percent), pastoral or spiritual counseling (59 percent), and counseling or psychological services (31.3 percent).

ETHICAL CONSIDERATIONS

The philosophy of hospice care is to provide a patient the highest possible quality of life in the last months of a terminal illness, which means admitting that the illness is indeed terminal and that further efforts will not be made to cure the patient. This philosophy has been termed a patient-centered rather than disease-centered approach to care because the focus is on treatment (such as pain control) relevant to the patient's quality of life rather than on treatment aimed at curing the disease.

Some people object to this philosophy, feeling that it is immoral to stop trying to cure a disease when means are still available to attempt to do so. Other people raise the question of whether hospice care would be recommended to individuals to save money that would otherwise be spent on their care—that is, to let them die sooner rather than later to avoid paying for further treatment. These objections have been largely met by the fact that hospice care is a choice made by the individual receiving the care and requires initial certification and regular recertification by one or more medical professionals that the patient is indeed terminal.

Hospitals   **445**

FINANCIAL CONSIDERATIONS

Independent of quality-of-life issues, the question of whether hospice care costs more or less relative to usual care is relevant because insurers have an obvious interest in controlling expenditures and are reluctant to offer additional benefits that will increase their costs. In addition, rising costs of healthcare must generally be reflected in rising insurance premiums for private insurance or in rising costs borne by taxpayers in the case of government-funded benefits such as Medicare and Medicaid. Adding benefits to insurance programs is counterproductive if it makes the policies too expensive for individuals or governments to afford.

Given such considerations, some states currently offering the Medicare hospice benefit have considered dropping it as a cost-saving measure. Therefore, there are legitimate reasons for examining the costs of hospice care versus usual medical care that would otherwise have been provided. This is a difficult question to examine, because individuals who choose hospice care are usually self selected: however, several studies have suggested that hospice care saves money in some circumstances and costs about the same or more in other circumstances.

D.E. Campbell and colleagues found that for persons receiving Medicare benefits, hospice care for persons with late-stage cancer saved money compared with usual care, particularly among persons with lung cancer and other very aggressive cancers who were diagnosed in the last year of life. For conditions other than cancer, hospice care costs were equal or higher than usual care costs, and costs increased relative to patient age. On average, costs for noncancer patients in hospices were 11 percent higher than usual-care costs, and the greatest increase in cost was for people hospitalized for dementia.

E.J. Emanuel surveyed a number of studies, including three that used randomization, and concluded that savings from hospice care and advance directives were greatest in the last month of life (25 percent to 40 percent) but decreased to 0 percent to 10 percent over the last year of life.

SEE ALSO: Age; Government; Insurance; Medicare and Medicaid; Pain and Pain Management; Psycho-Social Issues.

BIBLIOGRAPHY. *Access to Hospice Care: Expanding Boundaries, Overcoming Barriers: A Special Supplement to the Hastings Center Report* (Hastings Center, 2003), available for download from www.thehastingscenter.org/research/hchp05.asp (cited January 2007); D.E. Campbell, et al., "Medicare Program Expenditures Associated with Hospice Use," *Annals of Internal Medicine* (v.140, 2004); Centers for Medicare and Medicaid Services, *Medicare Hospice Benefits* (CMS, 2005), available for download from www.medicare.gov/Publications/Pubs/pdf/02154.pdf (cited January 2007); Ann Armstrong Dailey and Sarah Zarbock, eds., *Hospice Care for Children*, (Oxford, 2001); E.J. Emanuel, "Cost Savings at the End of Life: What Do the Data Show?" *Journal of the American Medical Association* (v.275, 1996); B.J. Haupt, *Characteristics of Hospice Care Discharges and their Length of Service: United States, 2000* (National Center for Health Statistics, Vital Health Statistics 13(154), 2003), available for download from www.cdc.gov/nchs/data/series/sr_13/sr13_154.pdf (cited January 2007); Hospice Foundation of America website, www.hospicefoundation/org (cited January 2007); Elisabeth Kübler-Ross, *On Death and Dying* (Macmillan, 1969); The National Hospice and Palliative Care Organization website, www.nhpco.org/templates/1/homepage.cfm (cited January 2006); Cicely Saunders, "A Personal Therapeutic Journey," *British Medical Journal* (v. 313, 1996); Denise Sheehan, *Hospice and Palliative Care: Concepts and Practice*, (Jones and Bartlett, 2003); World Health Organization, Palliative Care website, www.who.int/cancer/palliative/en (cited January 2007).

SARAH BOSLAUGH
WASHINGTON UNIVERSITY SCHOOL OF MEDICINE

Hospitals

HOSPITALS AND THEIR affiliated cancer centers are the primary sites for cancer treatment. Cancer treatment centers are divided into five categories and are specifically approved by government and medical organizations based on the services they provide. The types of cancer facilities vary dramatically, from centers that devote their time solely to cancer treatment and research to centers that comprise a small division of a hospital and that offer only basic diagnostic and treatment services.

Nationally recognized organizations such as the National Cancer Institute (NCI) evaluate and approve hospitals and cancer centers based on strict criteria. In addition to treatment, hospitals with advanced medical technology serve as foremost diagnostic facilities for cancer. The majority of the diagnosis is performed by the hospital's facilities and staff.

CHOOSING A TREATMENT CENTER

When a patient is searching for a cancer treatment center, he or she should consider various criteria. A patient can choose a comprehensive cancer center, clinical cancer center, community clinical oncology program, university-affiliated hospital or center, or community cancer center or local hospitals, based on the nature of the cancer and the location of residency. The NCI reassesses the comprehensive cancer centers, clinical cancer centers, and community clinical oncology programs every three to five years to ensure the highest standard of care. The periodic inspection elevates these three types of facilities above others in relation to the quality of cancer care provided.

Comprehensive cancer centers, so designated by NCI, offer the most recent developments in cancer detection and therapy. These centers are actively involved in community outreach and education programs about cancer, and participate in clinical trials. The benefits of these centers are advanced treatments, access to clinical trials, skilled healthcare specialists, and a unit or an affiliated center designated for stem-cell transplantation. NCI centers are usually found in larger cities.

Clinical cancer centers are NCI-approved centers that offer the same services as comprehensive cancer centers but may not emphasize community outreach and education about cancer prevention and control.

Community Clinical Oncology Programs are NCI-designated programs—not treatment facilities—combine the efforts of local and community oncologists, institutions, and researchers to use NCI-sponsored treatments in conducting clinical trials. A patient benefits from having access to NCI-funded treatments if an affiliation exists between a community center or local hospital and an NCI center.

University-affiliated hospitals or centers have an affiliation with a university hospital or a medical school. As a result of being a teaching hospital or center, the facility offers the most recent cancer treatment and care, as well as experienced staff, and has a unit that specializes in stem-cell transplantation. The abun-

dance of student physicians (medical students and residents) results in decreased privacy.

Community cancer centers at local hospitals located in rural communities appeal to local residents because of the nearby location and familiarity with the hospital staff. If the local facility lacks an affiliation with NCI or a university, it is advisable that the treating oncologist consult university oncologists or NCI researchers throughout the duration of treatment. Moreover, NCI-funded treatments may be available if the local facility or center is affiliated with a community clinical oncology program. The disadvantages of consulting a local cancer center or hospital are fewer treatment options, reduced access to NCI clinical trials, and lengthy distance to the nearest stem-cell transplantation center.

CERTIFYING ORGANIZATIONS

Several organizations provide a list of treatment facilities and assist in confirming a facility's credentials and qualifications. They include:

Joint Commission on Accreditation of Healthcare Organizations (JCAHO). JCAHO is an independent, not-for-profit organization that evaluates and accredits close to 20,000 healthcare organizations and programs in the United States. An online quality-check service is available to assist in determining whether a specific facility is accredited by the JCAHO and provides the institution's performance reports.

NCI. NCI appoints a variety of institutions as cancer centers by thoroughly evaluating the institutions' research programs. The title *comprehensive cancer center* is assigned to institutions that carry out broad research; the title *clinical cancer center* is assigned to institutions that have narrower research programs in conjunction with clinical care services. Institutions designated by NCI frequently offer effective clinical-care programs. A list of cancer centers and links is provided on the NCI website.

Commission on Cancer (CoC) of the American College of Surgeons. CoC includes 30 medical professional organizations that work together to set guidelines for cancer diagnosis and treatment. CoC-approved hospitals treat more than 70 percent of cancer patients, even though they comprise only 20 percent of U.S. hospitals.

The American Cancer Society offers a searchable database of over 1,400 Commission on Cancer approved programs in the United States.

CHARACTERISTICS OF TOP TREATMENT CENTERS

In addition to engaging in intensive cancer research, a cancer treatment facility is judged on the basis of having certain technical services. The top cancer centers should offer the following services:

A pathology lab and blood bank
Around-the-clock physician staffing
A tumor board
Social-services department
Medical, radiation, and surgical oncology
Respiratory therapies and rehabilitation services
Diagnostic imaging
Intensive-care unit

DIAGNOSIS

Upon suspicion of cancer, several crucial steps are taken to rule out other conditions and to identify and characterize the type of cancer. A physician who suspects that his or her patient has cancer will refer the patient to the nearest cancer treatment facility (preferably, a comprehensive cancer center, clinical cancer center, or a university-affiliated hospital or center) to undergo extensive diagnostic tests.

If a patient's history suggests the need for further testing, blood and urine tests are performed to rule out or diagnose the disease. Small amounts of blood and urine are collected and analyzed in the laboratory for abnormalities. If the tests reveal the presence of cancer cells, elevated or lowered cell counts, abnormal types of cells, or various other substances, a diagnosis of cancer is possible. Although blood and urine tests help diagnose the disease, other tests are usually required to make a successful diagnosis.

Diagnostic imaging is used to determine the location, size, and spread of cancer. Imagining tools include X-ray, magnetic resonance imaging (MRI), computerized tomography (CT), ultrasound, radionuclide scanning, and positron emission tomography (PET).

X-rays are usually used to check for cancers of the lungs, intestines, stomach, kidneys, and breasts. MRI is often employed to detect cancer of the brain, spinal cord, head and neck, liver, and soft tissues. CT scans are used to examine the brain, lungs, liver, pancreas, adrenal glands, and bones. Ultrasound technology helps diagnose cancers of soft tissues. Radionuclide scanning helps locate cancers of the bones or thyroid. Finally, PET scanning determines the location and the spread of the cancer. Unfortunately, not all cancers are detected by imaging technology; a tumor may be too small or in a location that is difficult to observe. In these instances, other tests may prove more successful.

A biopsy—always necessary to diagnose cancer—is the removal of a sample of tissue for careful examination by a pathologist. Several biopsy techniques are available.

Needle biopsy. A needle biopsy is the most common approach. A thin needle and a syringe are used to remove small pieces of tissue from a tumor. Two types of needle biopsies exist: fine-needle aspiration and core biopsy. Both procedures are fundamentally the same except that core biopsy requires the use of a larger needle to take out a small sample of tissue. This approach is used in any tissue, including the liver, lung, brain, and bone marrow.

Endoscopic biopsy. Endoscopic biopsy entails the insertion of a thin, flexible tube (endoscope) into a natural opening in the body, such as the mouth, throat, or rectum. The endoscope contains a fiber-optic light and a video camera at its tip to visualize the interior of the body on a screen. If abnormal tissue is observed on the external monitor, special instruments are inserted through the endoscope to excise a sample of the irregular tissue.

Surgical biopsy. As the name implies, a surgical biopsy involves an incision through the skin, and the entire tumor (excisional biopsy) or a portion of a tumor (incisional biopsy) is removed. Generally, local anesthesia is used; however, when the tumor is not easily accessible, such as inside the chest, general anesthesia is used.

Following the removal of a cancerous tissue, it is generally examined under a microscope by a pathologist to determine the nature of the cancer. With the information obtained from all the diagnostic tests, an oncologist determines the stage of the cancer. Cancer stages are assigned roman numerals from 0 to IV, with 0 being least advanced and IV being the most advanced. The stage of cancer determines the type of treatment(s).

SEE ALSO: American Cancer Society; American College of Surgeons; National Cancer Institute.

BIBLIOGRAPHY. Mayo Clinic, "You've Been Diagnosed with Cancer: What Happens Next," www.mayoclinic.com (cited January 2007); Memorial Sloan-Kettering Cancer Center, "Choosing a Hospital for Cancer Care," www.mskcc.org (cited

January 2007).American College of Surgeons, "What Is an Approved Cancer Program," www.facs.org/cancer/coc/whatis.html (cited January 2007); Leukemia & Lymphoma Society, "Choosing a Treatment Facility," www.leukemialymphoma.org/all_mat_toc.adp?item_id=9877 (cited January 2007); Mayo Clinic, "Diagnosing Cancer: Common Tests, Biopsies and Examinations," www.mayoclinic.com/health/cancer-diagnosis/CA00028 (cited January 2007);

BORIS ROZENFELD
INDEPENDENT SCHOLAR

HPV Vaccine

DURING THE SUMMER of 2006, the U.S. Food and Drug Administration (FDA) licensed the quadrivalent human papillomavirus (HPV) vaccine. Shortly afterward, the Advisory Committee on Immunization Practices issued recommendations for use of the first vaccine developed to prevent cervical cancer and genital warts in females.

Genital human papillomavirus (HPV) is the most common sexually transmitted infection in the United States; an estimated 6.2 million persons are newly infected every year. Although most infections cause no clinical symptoms and are self limited, persistent infection with oncogenic types of HPV can cause cervical cancer and other anogenital cancers in women. Nononcogenic HPV types can cause genital warts.

Cervical-cancer rates have decreased in the United States, largely because of the widespread use of Papanicolaou (Pap) testing, which can detect precancerous lesions of the cervix before they develop into invasive cancer. However, estimates were that in 2002 (the most recent data available), 12,000 new cases of cervical cancer were diagnosed, and approximately 4,000 women died from the disease. In many countries where cervical-cancer screening activities are limited, cervical cancer occurs more frequently.

The HPV vaccine licensed by the FDA protects against four HPV types: 6, 11, 16, and 18.

Two types together—HPV 16 and HPV 18—cause 70 percent of cervical cancers. The other two types together—HPV 6 and HPV 11—cause 90 percent of genital warts.

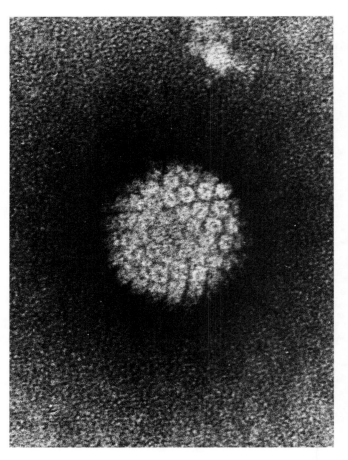

Electron micrograph of a negatively stained human papilloma virus (HPV) which may occur in warts. Cervical warts can be cancerous.

The licensed HPV vaccine is composed of proteins from the outer part of the virus that self-assemble into a viruslike particle (VLP). The VLP is similar in shape and size to a virus but does not contain infectious material.

This HPV vaccine was tested in more than 11,000 females (9 to 26 years of age) in many countries, including the United States. These clinical trials showed that the HPV vaccine was safe and caused no serious side effects. The main adverse event was pain at the injection site. This reaction was common but mild. The vaccine contains no thimerosal or mercury. Clinical trials of this vaccine showed positive results. Among females who had not been infected with HPV type 6, 11, 16, or 18, the vaccine had high efficacy in preventing persistent HPV infection, vaginal and vulvar cancer, precursor lesions to cervical cancer, and genital warts due to these HPV types. There was no evidence of protection against existing disease or infection.

The investigators concluded that females infected with one or more of these HPV types before vaccination would still be protected against disease caused by the other HPV types in the vaccine. There is no evidence that the vaccine protects against infection or disease due to HPV types not included in the vaccine.

The vaccine is administered by intramuscular injection. The recommended schedule is a series of three doses, with the second and third doses administered two and six months, respectively, after the first dose. The recommended age for vaccination of females is 11 to 12 years, but vaccine can be administered to girls as young as 9 years of age. Vaccination is recommended for females who are 13 to 26 years of age and have not been vaccinated. Vaccination is not a substitute for routine screening for cervical cancer, and vaccinated females should have cervical-cancer screening according to current recommendations. Vaccination of males with the quadrivalent vaccine may offer direct health benefits to males and indirect health benefits to females, but available data do not support use of HPV vaccine in males. Efficacy studies in males are ongoing, and information will be available in the future. Current studies indicate that the vaccine is effective for at least five years, with no waning of immunity.

Implementation of this vaccine faces several challenges. Administration of a three-dose vaccine to adolescents may be difficult because adolescents may not have regular or frequent health care. In addition, the cost of the vaccine is high. The catalog price of the vaccine is $120 per dose ($360 for the full series), and the price through the federal Vaccines for Children program is $96 per dose ($288 for the full series). The federal program will cover the cost of this vaccine for children who meet eligibility criteria; some insurance companies may cover the costs of the vaccine and administration. New public policies may help with implementation of this vaccine. Immunization of children is not required by federal law, but states can mandate immunizations for school attendance. Some states are considering legislation that will mandate school requirements for HPV immunization.

A bivalent HPV vaccine is in the final stages of clinical testing in females. This vaccine would protect against the two types of HPV (16 and 18) that cause 70 percent of cervical cancers.

HPV vaccines offer promising new approaches to the prevention of HPV and associated conditions.

SEE ALSO: Cervical Cancer; Clinical Trials; Vaccines.

BIBLIOGRAPHY. Centers for Disease Control and Prevention, *HPV and HPV Vaccine—Information for Healthcare Providers* (Centers for Disease Control and Prevention and National Cancer Institute, 2006); Centers for Disease Control and Prevention, *National Program for Cancer Registries* (Centers for Disease Control and Prevention and National Cancer Institute, 2006); Centers for Disease Control and Prevention, "Quadrivalent Human Papillomavirus Vaccine Recommendations of the Advisory Committee on Immunization Practices (ACIP)," *Morbidity and Mortality Weekly Report Recommendation and Reports* (in press, 2007); M. Schiffman, et al., "Cervical Cancer," in D. Schottenfeld and J. Fraumeni, eds., *Cancer Epidemiology and Prevention* (Oxford University Press, 1996); H. Weinstock, et al., "Sexually Transmitted Diseases among American Youth: Incidence and Prevalence Estimates, 2000," *Perspectives on Sexual and Reproductive Health* (v.36, 2004).

MONA SARAIYA
EILEEN DUNNE
LAURI MARKOWITZ
HERSCHEL LAWSON
CENTERS FOR DISEASE CONTROL AND PREVENTION

Hungary

THIS CENTRAL EUROPEAN country, as the kingdom of Hungary, was part of the Austro-Hungarian Empire until World War I. The largely ethnic Hungarian part of the former empire then became the kingdom of Hungary, ruled by a regent until World War II. After the war it was ruled by the communists until the fall of communism in 1989. It has a population of 10,032,000 and 357 doctors and 385 nurses per 100,000 people. An example of cancer incidence rates in Hungary includes 386.8 cases of cancer in males per 100,000, according to the International Agency for Research on Cancer.

When Hungary was part of the Austro-Hungarian Empire, many surgeons in Hungary trained in Vienna, which was a center of medical learning for much of central Europe. Systematic collection of information for a cancer database was established in Hungary in 1904, one of the earliest to be set up in Europe. It became more heavily systemized after World War II.

The most famous Hungarian cancer specialist was Móric Kaposi, after whom Kaposi's sarcoma is named. Born in Kaposvár in western Hungary, he was originally surnamed Kohn, changing his name when he converted from Judaism to Catholicism. He studied at the University of Vienna, becoming a world-famous dermatologist who discovered what was then a rare sarcoma; he first described the symptoms in 1872. Since the advent of human immunodeficiency virus (HIV) and acquired immune deficiency syndrome (AIDS), the sarcoma has become a common AIDS symptom attracting much new research. Josef Marek described the lymphoproliferative disease of chickens in 1907; it later became known as Marek's Disease. Another medical researcher who became a cancer researcher after leaving Hungary was Albert Szent-Györgyi. He was born in Budapest and gained his medical degree from the University of Budapest. Interested in biochemistry, he studied in Germany, the Netherlands, the United Kingdom, and the United States. His discoveries concerning the roles played by some organic compounds such as Vitamin C in the oxidation of nutrients by cells earned him the Nobel Prize for Physiology or Medicine in 1937. In 1947 he emigrated to the United States and there was appointed director of the Institute for Muscle Research, Woods Hole, Massachusetts, where he conducted research into cancer through his work on cell division.

RESEARCH PROGRAMS

In 1941 the State Oncological Institute of Hungary was established, but owing to World War II, it was not until 1947 that it became the major research and clinical cancer center in the country. With its head office in Budapest, it rapidly established branch offices throughout the country. During the 1960s and 1970s work was undertaken by I. Tóth, F. Gál, and S. Eckhardt from the National Cancer Institute at the Research Institute of Oncopathology, Budapest, into the Muramidase activity of transplantable myeloid rat leukemia induced by 7,12 dimethylbenzanthraceene. There was also work by E. T. Gláz on the preferential inhibition of DNA polymerase I deficient *E. coli* by dianhydrohexitols, tilorone, and metronidazole.

L. Nemeth and G. Elek of the State Oncological Institute in Budapest worked with C. Klausner and A. Furst of the Institute of Chemical Biology, University of San Francisco, on immunological experiments with the shay tumor. I. Nagy, M. Kossoru, M. Ats, and K. Majorossy from the Municipal Ambul. Laboratorium, Budapest, worked on the interrelation between the immune activity of tumor sera and their fraction distribution. B. Kellner of the Institute of Oncopathology in Budapest worked on a new method for the evaluation of chemotherapeutic drug effects as seen from combined treatment.

Laszlo Institoris of Chinoin Factory for Pharmaceutical and Chemical Products, Budapest, worked on transport parameters involved in the mechanism of action of cytostatric dibromohexitols. Karoly Lapis and Istvan Benedeczky from the Postgraduate Medical School of the Department of Pathology, Budapest, worked on the comparative studies of subcellular alterations caused by different chemotherapeutics in shay tumor of rats. Istvan Martos of the Hungarian Society of Radiology in Budapest worked on a new system for a movable radiation cobalt unit.

C. Sellei and F. Masszi of the National Cancer Institute, Budapest, worked on clinical trials with mannomustine-heparinate in connection with clinical chemotherapy. Among the Hungarians who have died from cancer, József Antall, prime minister from 1900 to 1993, died from lymphatic cancer.

SEE ALSO: HIV/AIDS-Related Cancers; Kaposi's Sarcoma.

BIBLIOGRAPHY. L. Madai, "Le premier enregistrement statistique des maladies cancereux dans l'année 1904, en Hongrie," *Genus* (v.37, 1981); Jakob Vikol, "Twenty-Five Years of Cancer Control in Hungary," in Jakob Vikol and C. R. Sellei, *Orszagos Onkologiai Ontezet: Twenty-Five Years in the Fight against Cancer* (State Oncological Institute, 1966).

JUSTIN CORFIELD
GEELONG GRAMMAR SCHOOL, AUSTRALIA

Huntsman Cancer Institute

AT THE UNIVERSITY of Utah, in Salt Lake City, the Huntsman Cancer Institute (HCI) focuses on understanding cancer at a molecular and genetic level. Its mission is to "find the causes of cancer, to develop new and better treatments, and to prevent people from ever developing cancer." It is an institution with extensive cooperation among scientists, physicians, and medical educators. The institute was named after the Huntsman family, which made a generous donation in 1995 to build the cancer-care center that was to become the HCI. It is led by executive directors, senior directors, and a clinical director emeritus. There is also a scientific advisory board that steers the HCI to promote innovative and promising research endeavors. Finally, a board of directors oversees the managerial aspects of the institute.

Researchers at HCI aim to understand cancer at its most basic levels: genetically and molecularly in the cell. To do so most effectively, they collaborate across disciplines. Investigators examine genetics of a specific cancer, effects of treatments, and nutritional relationships to cancer, among other fields.

The HCI is designated a cancer center by the National Cancer Institute (NCI). Several research programs at the HCI are Cancer Control and Population Sciences; Cell Response and Regulation; Gastrointestinal Cancers; Molecular Imaging, Diagnostics, and Therapeutics; and Nuclear Control of Cell Growth and Differentiation. Students can complete graduate studies in various programs, including Neurobiology, Cell and Molecular Biologies, Developmental Biology, and Biostatistics and Epidemiology.

Researchers at the HCI have access to shared core facilities and resources. These resources include those for biostatistics, cancer systems biology, DNA/peptides, DNA sequencing, flow cytometry, genomics, informatics, mass spectometry, microarrays, preclinical drug evaluation, and protein interactions, as well as a facility for tissue acquisition and distribution. Additionally, given the HCI's fortuitous position among the Mormon population in Utah, there is a pedigree and population resource using the Utah population database.

The unique demographics of the population of Salt Lake City allows for a high level of genetic analysis of cancer. The residents in and around Salt Lake City are typically in large, close families with detailed genealogical records. In collaboration with the Mormon church, The Church of Jesus Christ of Latter-Day Saints, the families have given to the HCI an enormous resource for research into the genetic etiology of cancer.

As a service to its patients, the HCI maintains a section of its website to disseminate information and provide important resources. The Huntsman Online Patient Education Guide offers books; relevant research and clinical articles from medical journals; frequently asked questions; and other information about cancer prevention, treatment, and research. There is also an explanation of the different cancers. Additionally, tips for coping, recognizing symptoms, and evaluation risk factors are offered.

Cancer clinics available at the HCI include those for brain, spine, and skull-base cancers; sarcoma; breast cancer; melanoma; thoracic cancer; gastrointestinal cancer; and urologic cancers. Additionally, the institute offers risk counseling for members of families with a history of cancer. A fitness program, social work, palliative care, children's care, and internal medicine acute care are also open to patients. The HCI also has a radiation oncology program.

The HCI follows a Cancer Awareness Calendar, as established by regional, national, and international organizations working with cancer. Each month has been recommended for increasing awareness and education about particular cancers. The HCI uses these recommendations to enhance its education efforts. In the appropriate month, the institute makes efforts to highlight the cancers in its initiatives. November, for example, is Lung Cancer Awareness Month.

To go along with this theme, the HCI highlights smoking-cessation programs. In December, rather than focusing on a particular cancer, the HCI stresses healthy nutrition. People are reminded to consume enough fruits and vegetables, and to avoid excess fats and sugars, which can be difficult in the holiday season. As an incentive to its patients to eat well, the HCI offers recipes and tips for eating well.

Additionally, the HCI encourages patients and other members of the public to undergo routine screening for cancers. This initiative is the Birthday Cancer Screening program. The HCI recommends that people have a relevant cancer screen on their birthdays and provides a simple flier to suggest which screens are important. People can follow the guide based on their age and gender.

Furthermore, monthly self-exams are advised, such as a testicular exam for men and a breast exam for women.

For patients who are interested in alternative and complementary care, the HCI offers information on Natural Standard, an independent program that educates users about these additional care options. The program, developed by clinicians and researchers, outlines evidence for uses of herbs and supplements. It also warns patients about combinations of drugs and herbs that could do more harm than good.

The HCI also offers clinical trials to its patients. Potential patients are thoroughly screened for their eligibility and are counseled so they can make the best decision regarding weighing the risks of treatments against the benefits.

In 2005 the HCI and Intermountain Healthcare (Intermountain) began a collaboration that will bring HCI's cancer care and research to all patients in the Intermountain network. Intermountain consolidates cancer knowledge and data from the Mountain States Region, which enables the HCI to have a broader base for its studies.

The joint program will establish multidisciplinary, tumor-specific cancer-care clinics throughout Utah so patients can address their cancer needs in one location, in one visit. Cancer centers will also be built across the state to expand outpatient care into broader regions.

Within these cancer centers will be cancer education centers to provide information resources to patients and public. An additional HCI center is the Huntsman Cancer Institute's Center for Children. Work here involves research on pediatric cancer, as well as a clinical pediatric oncology section of the Primary Children's Medical Center.

Researchers focus on diverse fields such as the childhood cancer retinoblastoma, embryonic development and how it relates to cancers resembling developmental defects, and individual-specific reactions to childhood leukemia treatments.

SEE ALSO: Alternative Therapy: Diet and Nutrition; Alternative Therapy: Herbs; Genetics; National Cancer Institute.

BIBLIOGRAPHY. John K. Cowell, *Molecular Genetics of Cancer (Human Molecular Genetics)* (Academic Press, 2001); G. Edward Griffin, *World without Cancer: The Story of Vitamin B17* (American Media, 1996); Shirley V. Hodgson, et al., *A Practical Guide to Human Cancer Genetics* (Cambridge University Press, 2006).

CLAUDIA WINOGRAD
UNIVERSITY OF ILLINOIS AT URBANA-CHAMPAIGN

Hypopharyngeal Cancer

HYPOPHARYNGEAL CANCER IS a disease affecting the hypopharynx, which is a tube linking the pharynx (throat) with the esophagus (muscular tube carrying food to the stomach). The cancer manifests itself in the form of thin, flat squamous cells that line the affected part of the hypopharynx.

Patients may present with the early stages of hypopharyngeal cancer, with symptoms such as persistent sore throat or ear pain. Physicians look for risk factors such as use of tobacco products (smoked or chewed), unbalanced and inappropriate diets, or excessive use of alcohol.

Approximately 2,500 new cases of the cancer are diagnosed annually in the United States, and the great majority of cases affect both men and women above the age of 50. Children are rarely affected by this form of cancer. It is possible that some geographical factors may lead to clusters of outbreaks in some parts of the world, but this is not clear, and if it is so, the causal factors are not well understood. Testing for the presence of the disease may be undertaken through physical examination or the use of X-rays, endoscopy, or magnetic resonance imaging. An alternative is taking tissue samples for subsequent bioscopy.

Treatment of the disease is usually possible, but it varies significantly based on the overall physical well being of the patient; the stage of the disease (i.e., to what extent it has spread throughout the length of the hypopharynx); and physical circumstances such as the extent to which a mass prevents or hinders a patient from speaking, eating, or breathing. Depending on the specific circumstances of the disease, it may be possible to tackle it through surgery, radiation treatment, or chemotherapy. The choice is complicated by the importance of the hypopharynx for normal procedures of life; treatment may require invasive modifications in the way that the patient breathes or eats, which generally reduce quality of life. Radiation treatment is often indicated but can be problematic because of the position of the mass or the effects it will have on the patient's quality of life.

The disease may pass through several distinct stages, depending on the size of the affected tissue mass, its location, and the extent to which it has spread to soft connective tissue. Symptoms are rarely identified at early stages of the disease, so physicians will generally be required to intervene when the disease has already reached a later stage, when intervention is more difficult.

Patients who have suffered from hypopharyngeal cancer are likely to be at an elevated risk of developing a secondary cancer elsewhere in the head or neck. Consequently, physicians will generally want to institute a strict and persistent follow-up and monitoring regime to investigate the possibility of future outbreaks.

SEE ALSO: Alcohol; Diet and Nutrition; Head and Neck Cancer; Tobacco Smoking.

BIBLIOGRAPHY. David J. Adelstein, ed., *Squamous Cell Head and Neck Cancer: Recent Clinical Progress and Prospects for the Future* (Humana Press, 2005); R. Pasha, *Otolaryngology: Head and Neck Surgery—A Clinical and Reference Guide* (Plural Publishing, 2005); National Cancer Institute website, www.cancer.gov/cancerinfo/pdq/treatment/hypopharyngeal/patient.

John Walsh
Shinawatra University

Hypothalamic and Visual Pathway Glioma, Childhood

VISUAL PATHWAY AND hypothalamic glioma, often called optic pathway glioma, is a type of brain tumor that predominantly afflicts children. It accounts for approximately 5 percent of childhood brain tumors, and most patients are diagnosed before 10 years of age in the United States. It can cause visual impairment as well as hormonal and developmental defects.

The visual pathway refers to the nerves that convey information from the eyes to the brain. It includes the optic nerves, optic chiasm, and optic radiations. Tumors can form anywhere along this path. Optic nerves radiate from each eyeball; converge near the center of the brain; and then split, forming an X called the optic chiasm. The optic radiations then relay this information to the visual cortex.

The hypothalamus is located directly above the optic chiasm; it controls metabolism and homeostasis.

Optic-chiasm gliomas usually involve the hypothalamus due to their proximity.

Gliomas are the most common types of brain tumors. They develop from glial cells, which are cells that support neurons. The unregulated growth and replication of star-shaped glial cells called astrocytes give rise to visual pathway gliomas. Fortunately, most of the tumors are benign and slow-growing. Optic-nerve gliomas typically have better survival rates compared with gliomas of the chiasm/hypothalamus and optic radiations.

A significant risk factor of developing visual pathway gliomas is if a child is diagnosed with neurofibromatosis type 1, also known as von Recklinghausen's disease. It is a hereditary neurocutaneous disorder in which approximately one out of three patients develops visual pathway gliomas. Rarely, adults can develop visual pathway gliomas, but unlike in children, the adult tumors are often fatal.

Visual loss is the most common sign of visual pathway gliomas. Other signs include—but are not limited to—protruding eyes, tilting head, and abnormal eye movements.

Hypothalamic involvement can cause developmental delay and hormonal dysfunction, such as early puberty and weight changes. Some tumors also increase

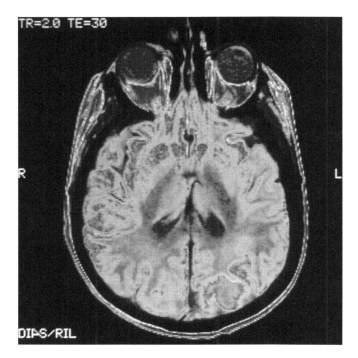

The use of magnetic resonance imaging (MRI) shows where cancer metastasizes in the occipital lobes.

intracranial pressure, causing nausea, vomiting, lethargy, irritability, and headaches.

Children affected by visual pathway gliomas are seen by a multidisciplinary team of physicians. The treatment options include chemotherapy, radiation therapy, and surgery. The treatments are effective, but their adverse side effects do not warrant their administration unless functionally debilitating symptoms arise. Asymptomatic tumors are typically observed, as they are often self limiting.

Chemotherapy is commonly administered as the initial treatment for symptomatic patients. Chemotherapy disrupts the tumor cells' ability to grow and replicate. This is an effective therapy, but side effects such as nausea, vomiting, and anemia can occur because the drugs do not differentiate between tumor and normal tissue. Radiation therapy uses high-energy rays to kill and shrink tumors.

Although it is also effective, serious long-term side effects such as cognitive, hormonal, and vascular complications may occur. Thus, radiation therapy is often avoided as the initial treatment and not recommended in young children. Surgery is also avoided if possible because the visual pathway can be damaged during resection of the tumor. Surgery is reserved to alleviate facial disfigurements and extended tumors, and to remove parts of tumors to relieve pressure on nerves.

Visual pathway gliomas are usually not life threatening. The primary goal of intervention and management is to preserve vision. Clinical trials and basic scientific research will enhance understanding of this childhood disease.

SEE ALSO: Brain Tumor; Cerebral Astrocytoma/Malignant Glioma, Childhood; Chemotherapy; Neurofibromatosis; Radiation Therapy.

BIBLIOGRAPHY. National Cancer Institute, "Childhood Visual Pathway and Hypothalamic Glioma (PDQ®): Treatment," www.cancer.gov (cited December 2006).

YOSHIHIRO YONEKAWA
WEILL MEDICAL COLLEGE OF CORNELL UNIVERSITY

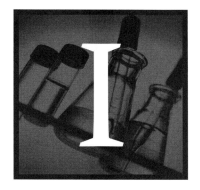

India

THIS NATION, WITH the second-largest population in the world, dominates southern Asia. It was ruled by the British, either directly or through a series of alliances and treaties, until independence in 1947. It has a population of 1,065,071,000 (2004) and has 48 doctors and 45 nurses per 100,000 people. An example of cancer incidence rates in India includes 99 cases of cancer in males per 100,000, according to the International Agency for Research on Cancer.

Indian medical practices have been recorded from ancient times. Balas, a fatal cancerous tumor that affects the throat, is mentioned in the Vedas, the oldest recorded story, dating from about 1000 B.C.E. There are other references from Aurvedic literature from 600 B.C.E., which are also believed to refer to cancers (which it diagnoses as Arbuda) and known to be fatal.

The Indian Cancer Research Centre was established in Bombay in 1922 as the Radium Service, and there was much interest in many parts of India in the work of Marie Curie. Indeed, in 1938, the postal authorities in French India issued a postage stamp to commemorate the fourth anniversary of the death of Marie Curie, and also to increase the awareness of cancer treatment and raise money for cancer research, as happened in many other French colonies.

A major advance in cancer treatment took place in early 1941, when Tata Memorial Hospital was opened for cancer patients. Studies of the people treated at Tata Memorial Hospital showed that between March 1941 and September 1943, more than 60 percent of patients were suffering from cancer at the base of the tongue and in the nostrils. Some 22.5 percent had cancer of the cheek, the floor of the mouth, and the alveolus, with cancer of the lip and anterior two-thirds of the tongue being rare. The studies were also able to highlight differences among the Gujaratis, Deccanis, other Hindus, Muslims, Indian Christians, Parsees, and non-Indians.

Plans were drawn up in the late 1960s by researchers at Tata Memorial Centre in Bombay to establish medical facilities in rural India for screening of the entire population by trained paramedical personnel, based on initial work at Tata Memorial Hospital that succeeded in covering 96,000 people in a smaller-scale project.

During the 1970s work was undertaken by S.V. Bhide and S.V. Khadapkar on the comparative study of the mechanism of urethan and thiocetamide carcinogenesis; by P. Raveendran, B.K. Batra, and Indira R. Menon on specific tumor regression with tumor cell extracts; by L.J. de Souza, D.J. Jussawalla, and P. Gangadharan, who studied cancer of the male breast; and G.G. Potdar, J.C. Paymaster, and P. Gangadharan, who worked on carcinoma of body uterus. J. N. Suraiya from Tata

Memorial Hospital was also prominent in his work on a history of cancer in India in ancient times.

The Indian Cancer Research Centre was formally opened in 1952, but by 1970 there were only five special cancer institutes in the whole of India.

Much work has taken place at the Cancer Research Institute in Parel, Bombay, including that by L. D. Sanghvi and Perin Notani, who studied the epidemiology of lung cancer in Bombay, concluding that although it is lower than in Western Europe, much of this is because of the smoking of Bibis as well as cigarettes.

Beatriz M. Braganca, A. Zaheer, and A.V. Hospattanakar of the Biochemistry Division worked on the cobra venom cytotoxin as a probe for the study of the surface properties of cells that cause Yoshida Sarcoma and tissue culture cell lines.

M.B. Sahasrabudhe, et al., studied the influence of host immune response on the incidence of cancer.

S.G. Gangal, et al., analyzed oncofetal cross-reactivity between human osteogenic sarcomas and fetal periostaeal fibroblasts grown in vitro. Most members of the team were also involved in research on the role of regional lymph nodes in immunity against osteosarcomas.

Devendra Patel from the Gujerat Cancer and Research Institute at Ahmedabad studied carcinoma of the esophagus, based on 650 cases in Gujerat State.

Saroj K. Gupta and Amiya P. Majumdar from the Department of Radiotherapy and Surgery at Chittaranjan Cancer Hospital, Calcutta, worked on malignant tumors in children, based on an analysis of 365 cases.

Cervical cancer is the most common gynecological cancer in India and has been the subject of much research. There have also been studies of oral cancer in India among people who chew betel nut and other substances.

British officials connected with India who suffered from cancer include Charles T. Metcalfe, who was forced to resign as governor of Jamaica because of his cancer; civil engineer William Moorsom; writer Grant Blairfindie Allen, who died from liver cancer; chemist Sir William Ramsay; and historian Shelford Bidwell.

Indians who died from cancer include cricket and tennis player Syed Mohammad Hadi; musician Vilayat Khan, who died from lung cancer; and philosopher Dimal Krishna Matilal.

Mention should be made of the canonization of the Roman Catholic nun Mother Teresa of Calcutta. Her healing of Monica Besra, who was suffering from a tumor, was one of the main elements in Mother Teresa's becoming a saint.

SEE ALSO: Breast Cancer; Esophageal Cancer; Nasopharyngeal Cancer; Women's Cancers.

BIBLIOGRAPHY. S.K. Acharya, et al., "Viral Hepatitis in India," *The National Medical Journal of India* (v.19.4, 2006); V.R. Khanolkar, "Oral Cancer in Bombay, India: A Review of 1,000 Consecutive Cases," *Cancer Research* (v.4, 1944); J.C. Paymaster and P. Gangadharan, "The Development of Cancer Treatment Facilities in India," *Oncology: Proceedings of the Tenth International Cancer Congress* (v.3, 1970); D.M. Parkin, et al., eds., *Cancer Incidence in Five Continents Vol VII* (International Agency for Research on Cancer and International Association of Cancer Registries, 1997); J.N. Suraiya, "Medicine in Ancient India with Special Reference to Cancer," *Indian Journal of Cancer* (v.10, 1973); E. Vallikad, "Cervical Cancer: The Indian Perspective," *International Journal of Gynaecology and Obstetrics* (v.95, 2006); Vishwanath and K. S. Grewal, "Cancer in India," *Indian Journal of Medical Research* (v.23, 24, 26, 1935–1939); "Indian Cancer Research Centre," *Cancer Bulletin* (v.12, 1960).

JUSTIN CORFIELD
GEELONG GRAMMAR SCHOOL, AUSTRALIA

Indiana University Cancer Center

THE ONLY CANCER care center designated as such by the National Cancer Institute (NCI) in Indiana is Indiana University Cancer Center (IUCC) in Indianapolis. IUCC is part of the Indiana University (IU) School of Medicine.

The center has faculty members from the IU schools of medicine, nursing, and allied health and dentistry. Faculty members also serve at the Purdue University School of Science. Additional members of the cancer-care team are scientists in basic and behavioral fields. The center is managed by a team of senior leaders, including a director, associate directors, administrator, and deputy director.

IUCC physicians and clinicians work with nurses and allied health professionals toward the center's mission: to "reduce the burden of cancer through innovation and dissemination." To achieve this mission, the IUCC has outlined four goals: to establish and develop research programs that promote interdisciplinary translational research; to use interdisciplinary clinical care to give optimal patient care; to develop interdisciplinary programs in graduate and postgraduate education and training; and to maintain its initiative in a cancer-control program for Indiana.

Although IUCC was established in 1992, its host institution, IU, has a long and comprehensive history in cancer research and care. This history began in 1921, when Long Hospital (which would become IU Hospital), installed its first radiation-therapy machine. In 1954 Riley Children's Hospital opened its cancer-research wing.

In 1974 Dr. Lawrence Einhorn developed cisplatin chemotherapy for testicular cancer and treated John Cleland, the first patient with this therapy. Since then, the cure rate of testicular cancer has increased from 10 percent to 95 percent. Legendary U.S. cyclist Lance Armstrong received treatment for his testicular cancer from the same doctor in 1996. Additionally, the first bone-marrow transplant in Indiana occurred in 1985 at IU's Riley Hospital for Children, performed by Dr. Jan Jansen.

Cancer patients at IUCC are treated by a team of caregivers, including experts on each aspect of cancer care. A patient might have on his or her team a dietician; a hematologist; a medical oncologist; a molecular geneticist; an oncology nurse; an oncology social worker; a pathologist; a psychologist or psychiatrist; a radiation oncologist; a surgical oncologist; and a physical, occupational, and/or speech therapist. With its team care strategy, IUCC offers comprehensive care so that a patient need not have multiple visits with multiple specialists. Teams are available for clinical care in adult hematology and hematologic malignancies, bone-marrow and stem-cell transplants, breast care and research, endocrine oncology, gastrointestinal cancer, genitourinary oncology, gynecologic oncology, head and neck oncology, melanoma, neuro-oncology, radiation oncology, sarcoma, testis cancer, thoracic oncology, and at Riley Hospital for Children.

IUCC provides patient care at its Indiana Cancer Pavilion. Additionally, patients may be seen at neighboring IU Hospital and its affiliated Riley Hospital for Children, the Richard L. Roudebush Veterans Administration Medical Center, or Wishard Health Services. Wishard Health Services specializes in community health, specifically related to the vulnerable populations of Indianapolis.

RESOURCES AND PATIENT SERVICES

Additionally, the center maintains a website designed to help patients and their caregivers navigate the process of cancer treatment, including prevention, diagnosis, treatment, and survival. The website provides resources for every aspect of cancer, as well as information to make a visit to IUCC as comfortable as possible.

IUCC recognizes that physical treatment of cancer is not the only part of the treatment process. To address the additional needs of its patients, the center created the CompleteLife initiative, which attends to the needs of cancer patients and family members beyond those treated chemically or with radiology. The services offered include counseling in nutrition, oncology pharmacy, psychology, psychiatric care, and spiritual care. Social-work services are also available. Art, music, and massage therapy help some patients through their cancer experiences as well. Financial counselors aid patients and their families in navigating the expenses of cancer treatment and care.

CLINICAL TRIALS AND RESEARCH

Clinical trials are an important method of testing the effectiveness and safety of novel cancer therapies. IUCC offers clinical trials to its patients. Eligible patients are given counseling to help them decide whether to participate by weighing the risks against the potential benefits.

Research is carried out primarily at the IU Cancer Research Institute, where investigators share the core facilities for flow cytometry, transplant and xenograft mouse, and vector production. Four other sites in Indianapolis house research laboratories and offices.

The Biotechnology Research and Training Center has a Transgenic and Knockout Mouse facility. The IU School of Nursing has the IUCC Cancer Prevention and Control Program's behavioral research office, as well as the Walther Oncology Institute's Mary Margaret Walther Program (MMWP). Research at the MMWP focuses on behaviors and their relations to cancer; for example, which behaviors can cause or prevent cancer, or increase the risk of developing cancer.

As of 2006, the construction of two more buildings was being planned. The first building was to be Research III, which would add much research space and would be completed in 2008. The other project was a renovation of the Van Nuys Medical Sciences Building to update and enlarge IUCC member research laboratories. Another building to be completed in 2008 was an expanded patient-care facility, a seven-story facility providing both outpatient and inpatient care, and connecting with IU Hospital.

PUBLIC INFORMATION AND EDUCATION

IUCC makes many efforts to increase education and awareness of cancer in the community. It is a NCI Cancer Information Services site, signifying that it disseminates information to the public on the latest developments in cancer research and care. Wishard Health Services, for example, has an IU Cancer Resource Center that opened in 2005. At the Resource Center, people can receive information on cancer and cancer-related issues. Additionally, the center participates in the Indiana Cancer Consortium, which works to reduce the negative impact of cancer by maintaining a state cancer-control plan.

The Summer Research Program at IUCC is an endeavor to increase the exposure of underrepresented minority high school and undergraduate students to the fields of biomedical and behavioral sciences. IUCC faculty members also participate in health fairs and community speaking engagements. Grand rounds, seminars, conferences, and meetings keep IUCC faculty and staff members educated in the fields of cancer research and care on a weekly basis.

SEE ALSO: Bone Marrow Transplants; Clinical Trials; National Cancer Institute; Testicular Cancer.

BIBLIOGRAPHY. Lance Armstrong and Sally Jenkins, *It's Not About the Bike: My Journey Back to Life* (Berkley Trade, 2001); Icon Health Publications, *The Official Patient's Sourcebook on Testicular Cancer: A Revised and Updated Directory for the Internet Age* (Icon Health Publications, 2002).

CLAUDIA WINOGRAD
UNIVERSITY OF ILLINOIS AT URBANA-CHAMPAIGN

Indonesia

THIS NATION, WHICH covers a large archipelago in Southeast Asia, was the Dutch colony known as the Netherlands East Indies until World War II. After the war, during which the colony was occupied by the Japanese, another conflict saw the Indonesian nationalists defeating the Dutch and achieving independence. Indonesia has a population of 238,453,000 (2004) and has 16 doctors and 50 nurses per 100,000 people. An example of cancer incidence rates in Indonesia includes 97.2 cases of cancer in males per 100,000, according to the International Agency for Research on Cancer.

Few of the Europeans connected with the Netherlands East Indies lived long enough to suffer from cancer. Many survived only two years in the region. Batavia, as Jakarta was then called, was one of the unhealthiest cities for Europeans in Asia. Gradually, as life expectancy increased for both Europeans and Asians, much more attention was given to the study of cancer.

During the 1920s, the Dutch colonial administration started research on cancer. In Bandung, in central Java, the Nederlands Indische Kanker Institute was formed in 1933; it became known in neighboring British colonies by its English-language name, the Institution for Cancer Control. It operated until 1942, when it was not funded by the Japanese, but it started up again in 1946, continuing after independence and being subsumed by the Cancer Control Foundation, which was established in 1962, with its headquarters in Jakarta.

Subsequently, several cancer foundations were established in the major cities of Java, including Bandung, Surabaya, Surakarta (Solo), and Yogyakarta. In 1974 the Ministry of Health established a Research Center for Cancer and Radiology, which was placed under the direction of the National Health Research Institute.

On April 17, 1977, the Indonesian Cancer Society was founded in Jakarta; it became the coordinating foundation for all these regional cancer foundations.

Although many hospitals throughout Indonesia, especially on the island of Java, treated cancer patients, the Cancer Center Hospital in Jakarta was opened in 1993 specifically for treating cancer patients, conducting oncology research, and training medical postgraduates in the field. It is affiliated with the Medical Faculty of the University of Indonesia and works closely with the official medical research center for the country, the Badan Penelitian dan Pengembangan Kesehatan (National Institute of Health Research and Development) in Jakarta. There are faculties of medicine in many universities throughout Indonesia.

In the 1960s Nugroho Kampono, et al., of the Cancer Sub-Division of the Department of Obstetrics and Gynecology at the School of Medicine, University of Indonesia, worked on an analytical epidemiology based on a study of 139 cases of malignant trophoblastic disease at Dr. Tjipto Mangunkusomo Hospital (now Dr. Cipto Mangunkusomo Hospital) in Jakarta. Recent research at the same hospital has been conducted by Didid Tjindarbumi and Rukmuni Mangunkusomo.

COMMON CANCERS

The major forms of cancer in Indonesia for women are cervical cancer and breast cancer, which constitute 28.66 percent and 17.77 percent of cancer cases in women, respectively (1991 figures).

For men, skin cancer (11.59 percent of cases) and nasopharyngeal cancer (11.27 percent of cases) are the two most common types. Despite high levels of smoking in cities, lung cancer causes only 3.99 percent of male cancers. The chewing of betel nut and similar substances is responsible for the higher rates of oral cancer.

In 1990 the Indonesian Ministry of Health established the National Cancer Control Action Plan to identify groups at high risk from particular cancers, to try to get screening of these groups, and to undertake a program of early treatment. Prominent Indonesians who suffered from cancer included Adam Malik, president of the United Nations General Assembly in 1970 and 1971, and vice president of the Republic of Indonesia from 1978 to 1983; he died from liver cancer. Ir. Soedarsono Hadisapoetro, minister for agriculture from 1978 to 1983, also died from cancer.

SEE ALSO: Nasopharyngeal Cancer; Netherlands; Skin Cancer (Melanoma); Skin Cancer (Non-Melanoma); Women's Cancers.

BIBLIOGRAPHY. M. N. Bustan, et al., "Oral Contraceptive Use and Breast Cancer in Indonesia," *Contraception* (v.47/3, 1993); R. D. Soebadi and S. Tejawinata, "Indonesia: Status of Cancer Pain and Palliative Care," *Journal of Pain and Symptom Management* (v.12/2, 1996); Didid Tjindarbumi and Rukmuni Mangunkusomo, "Cancer in Indonesia, Present and Future," *Japanese Journal of Clinical Oncology* (v.32/s1, 2002).

JUSTIN CORFIELD
GEELONG GRAMMAR SCHOOL, AUSTRALIA

Industry

INDUSTRY IS THE modern term for the large-scale production of a huge array of finished products from materials. Modern industry is a product of the Industrial Revolution, which began in England in the latter part of the 18th century. The 19th century saw advances in road surfacing, synthetic dyes, steamships, copper plating for the hulls of wooden ships, the making of tools, and a great many other technological developments.

The 20th century was an era in which petroleum fuels and petroleum products, steel, textiles, processed foods, steel battleships, horseless carriages, airplanes, and wires for telephones and electricity demanded an ever-growing and advancing set of inventions and technological developments. Supplies of raw materials, semi-finished goods, chemicals, and other materials meant that industry needed massive quantities of materials,

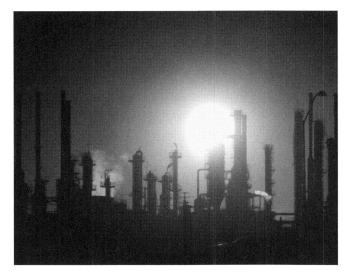

It has often been the byproducts of industrial processes that have come under scrutiny as possible carcinogens.

infrastructure, labor, and capital. The impact on the environment was tremendous. Forests were cleared. Vast mines and pits were dug for minerals and other raw materials. New lands were brought under cultivation. Some species went extinct under the onslaught of expanding industry. As inventions increased, however, education increased, and as commercial, financial, communications, and other infrastructures increased, so did health and quality of human life.

POLLUTION

The rise of modern industry has had tremendous benefits for billions of people. However, there has been a direct impact on the environment. The more severe forms of pollution have been those of radioactive materials and chemical wastes. Some chemical wastes are due directly to the activities of the chemical industry, while other chemical wastes are due to manufacturers and to activities of governments and to private citizens.

Solid wastes can be such things as used automobiles, newsprints, cans, glass bottles, vinyl materials, carpet, and old tires. These items were for years gathered into dumps. Recycling operations eventually turned some of them into other useful products. In some cases the wastes of industry are solids, but these wastes can become toxic if they are left to weather in the open.

Liquid wastes can enter the environment in many locations. For a time, phosphorous detergents were being used so heavily that streams were foaming with detergents that went either untreated or insufficiently treated into the watershed. Other liquid wastes included dyes and other chemicals that were simply dumped into rivers and creeks. In other instances metals such as mercury, lead, and arsenic in compounds that deteriorated into dangerous compounds were put into waste dumps or into rivers and streams. Unfortunately, it became apparent that these practices were poisoning not only the environment, but people as well.

HUMAN EFFECTS

Many people poisoned with mercury have been harmed by the neurological disease called Minamata, after the town of Minamata, Japan. Presenting symptoms resembling cerebral palsy, the people of Minamata were slowly poisoned by methyl mercury that had entered the food chain in fish. The local industry's wastewater had been laden with methyl mercury. Of great consequence is the carcinogenic poisoning that afflicts industrial workers. The list of carcinogenic chemicals in Group 1 (known to be carcinogenic to humans) and Group 2A (probably carcinogenic to humans) is not large, given the vast number of possible chemicals, but it includes some of the most widely used chemicals, many of which are chlorine compounds.

The dumping of chemical wastes in unapproved locations has led to people getting ill as well as developing cancer from the chemicals. Companies that illegally dumped toxic chemicals and operators who cut corners to dump them greatly increased the number of carcinogens in the environment. One particularly notorious case was at Love Canal in New York. Dow Chemical Co. had dumped chemicals for a long time in a location that the local government took over, using its power of eminent domain, despite Dow's vehement objections. Eventually, many people occupying the area developed cancer. This experience of chemical carcinogenic exposures has contributed to the increased rates of cancer.

With industrialization, there has been a steady migration to urban living. Industrial work processes have greatly decreased human energy expenditure in the workplace. Concurrent developments of mechanized transportation and changing urban plans have further reduced energy expenditure. These changes in lifestyle exacerbate cancer risk through reduced physial activity and increasing levels of obesity.

SEE ALSO: Chemical Industry; Pollution, Air; Pollution, Water.

BIBIOGRAPHY. Paul F. Deisler, Jr., *Reducing the Carcinogenic Risks in Industry* (Marcel Dekker, 1984); M. Sara Rosenthal, *Stopping Cancer at the Source* (Trafford Publishing, 2001); Richard J. Lewis, *Rapid Guide to Hazardous Chemicals in the Workplace* (Wylie and Son, 2000); William McDonough and Michael Braungart, *Cradle to Cradle: Remaking the Way We Make Things* (Farrar, Straus and Giroux, 2002); *Survey of Compounds Which Have Been Tested for Carcinogenic Activity* (National Cancer Institute, 2000); Richard P. Pohanish, ed., *Handbook of Toxic and Hazardous Chemicals and Carcinogens* (Noyes Data Corporation, 2002).

ANDREW J. WASKEY
DALTON STATE COLLEGE

Infection (Childhood, Sexually Transmitted Infections, Hepatitis)

NUMEROUS CARCINOGENS (or cancer-causing agents) have been implicated for their role in cancer causation; some biological organisms that cause infection are among these. *Infection* has been defined as the "invasion by and multiplication of pathogenic (capable of causing disease) microorganisms in a bodily part or tissue which may produce subsequent tissue injury and progress to overt disease through a variety of cellular or toxic mechanisms." Although numerous microorganisms have been implicated for their role in cancer causation, only those that have been classified as Group 1 carcinogens (carcinogenic to humans) by the International Agency for Research on Cancer (IARC) are examined in this article. The microorganisms discussed in this article can be categorized as bacteria, protozoa, and viruses.

BACTERIA

Bacteria are single-celled organisms that are capable of multiplying on their own. Not all bacteria are harmful; however, those that are (pathogenic bacteria) can cause illness and even disease.

Helicobacter pylori is a bacterium that has proved to have both protective and causative effects in relation to cancer. *H. pylori* infection has a protective effect against Barrett's esophagus, a precursor for adenocarcinoma of the esophagus. It has also been implicated for its role in the precancer process (i.e., chronic gastritis) associated with stomach cancer—more specifically, gastric adenocarcinoma and gastric MALT lymphoma. *H. pylori* has the ability to damage the mucous barrier, making it more vulnerable to carcinogens. Furthermore, it can increase the rate of proliferation of the gastric epithelium. Nevertheless, *H. pylori* is not the only risk factor for stomach cancer; factors such as diet and tobacco smoking (among others) also play important roles. *H. pylori* infection is known to be acquired in childhood; those who have been infected usually do not have any symptoms until later in life.

H. pylori is believed to be transmitted orally in two ways. The first is through the ingestion of food or water that has been contaminated with fecal matter. The second is through oral contact (i.e., kissing, drinking from the same cup/bottle, etc.). In light of this, it is not unusual that the risk of *H. pylori* transmission increases when other members of the family are infected.

The prevalence of *H. pylori* varies by geographical location, ethnic background, socioeconomic conditions, and age, with higher rates found in developing countries in comparison with developed countries. Among young children in developing countries, the risk factors for *H. pylori* include crowding, young age, and recurrent gastroenteritis.

Like bacteria, protozoa are single-celled organisms. Many forms of protozoa live in various environments (soil, water, etc.). They can also live within the body as parasites. Two well-known parasitic flatworm/fluke infestations have been associated with cancer causation: *Schistosoma haematobium* (*S. haematobium*) and *Opisorchis viverrini* (*O. viverrini*).

S. haematobium is a blood fluke that matures in the veins that drain the human bladder. Long-term infection with *S. haematobium* can lead to bladder cancer. Factors such as genetics, immune response, and other associated infections (such as hepatitis) play a role in the outcome of infection.

Humans are infected with *S. haematobium* after coming into contact (via skin or oral exposure) with water that has been contaminated with cercaria (parasitic larva). *S. haematobium* requires two hosts to complete its life cycle, the primary host being humans and the intermediary host being freshwater snails. The adult blood fluke can live in the human host for 30 years; during this time, it produces eggs, some of which leave the body via the urine or feces. These eggs hatch in water, infecting certain types of freshwater snails.

The infected snails then multiply asexually, producing cercaria larvae in the surrounding water. The eggs that remain in the human body can become trapped within the tissues, thereby leading to the development of bladder cancer.

Some ways in which people from high-risk areas may become infected include the use of contaminated water for domestic and/or hygiene reasons, recreational use, and occupational activities. *S. haematobium* is highly prevalent in regions of Africa and is widely distributed in the eastern Mediterranean and India.

O. viverrini is a liver fluke that matures under the surface of the human liver and can live in an infected host for more than 20 years. Chronic infection with

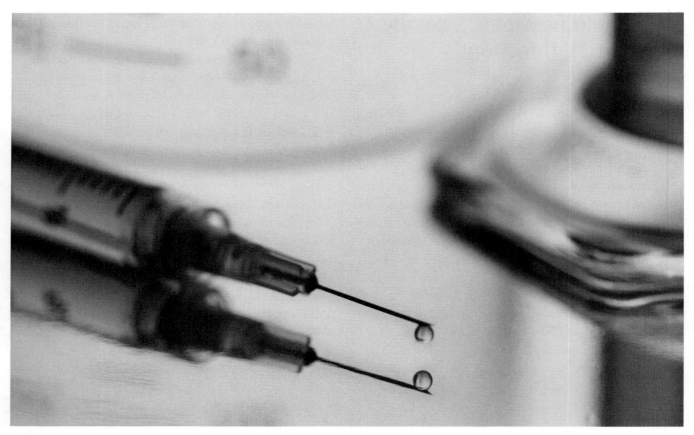

Scientists are developing vaccines that target some infection-related cancers in an attempt to minimize their potential future occurrence. Both risk factors and methods of transmission need to be addressed through educational measures.

O. viverrini has been implicated in cholangiocarcinomas (cancer that develops in the bile ducts inside the liver). *O. viverrini* requires two intermediary hosts to complete its life cycle. Similar to *S. haematobium*, it leaves the human host via urine or feces and uses the snail as the first intermediary. The second intermediary is freshwater fish, which are penetrated by the cercaria that have been produced by the snails. Humans are in turn infected with *O. viverrini* after consuming infected, raw, or undercooked freshwater fish. Infestations of liver-fluke parasites are most prevalent in Thailand and Southeast Asia.

VIRUSES

Unlike bacteria, viruses are not capable of multiplying on their own; they require a living host. A virus can be defined as "a small infectious agent consisting of a core of genetic material (DNA or RNA) surrounded by a shell of protein." Several viruses have been implicated for their role in cancer causation.

Chronic infections with hepatitis B and/or hepatitis C virus, human papillomavirus, Epstein-Barr virus, human T-cell leukemia virus-1, and human immunodeficiency virus-1 have been categorized as Group 1 carcinogens.

Chronic infection with hepatitis B (HBV), which is a DNA virus; hepatitis C (HCV), which is an RNA virus; or both has been associated with hepatocellular carcinoma (HCC). Infection with HBV often occurs at an early age, but usually does not appear until decades later. It is because of this lag time that researchers have implicated other factors as playing a role in the development of HCC; among these are exposures to aflatoxins, alcohol consumption, and coinfection with HCV. Naturally occurring aflatoxins, which are produced in dietary staples such as peanuts and maize, have also been classified as Group 1 carcinogens by the IARC (International Agency for Research on Cancer) and have been implicated for their role in the development of HCC.

HBV can be transmitted by exposure to infected blood (i.e., from infected mother to child during childbirth, or via infected needles, razors, or other sharp objects) or other bodily fluids (wound secretions, saliva, seminal and vaginal fluid, etc.). HCV is primarily transmitted by exposure to infected blood.

Risk factors for contracting HBV and/or HCV include unprotected sexual intercourse, sharing of infected needles (via drug use or improper hygiene practices at tattoo/piercing shops or other occupations that involve contact with infected blood, etc.), and blood transfusion that took place before hepatitis screening. Lengthy duration of infection with chronic hepatitis B and/or C is a risk factor for HCC. Further, chronic HCV and HBV have been associated with liver cirrhosis. Asia and Africa have been noted as highly prevalent areas for chronic HBV infection, whereas HCV infection is endemic in parts of Japan and Asia, the Middle East, and parts of Africa.

Human papillomavirus (HPV) is another virus that has been implicated for its role in the development of cancer. HPV are small, double-stranded DNA viruses. It has been documented that nearly all cervical cancers contain DNA from HPV. There are many types of HPV. HPV 16 and 18 are considered to be high-risk strains. Although some HPV infections resolve on their own, those that do not are usually high-risk strains that occasionally develop into a persistent infection, potentially leading to the development of cervical cancer if left untreated.

HPV is the most common sexually transmitted viral disease. Women who engage in sexual activity at a young age and who have several partners will most likely acquire HPV infection over their lifetimes. Furthermore, their partners' sexual histories also play a role. An increased number of sexual partners and smoking have been identified as relevant risk factors. Studies have shown that infection with genital HPV has also been associated with other cancers, such as those of the vagina, vulva, penis, and anus.

HPV is widely distributed in all human populations and is closely related to geographical patterns of cervical cancer. In an attempt to investigate HPV type by distribution, a study examining four regions of the world was carried out by G.M. Clifford, et al., in 2005. It reported that infection with HPV 16 was twice as frequent as any other high-risk type of HPV in regions of South America, Europe and Asia. Equally common rates of HPV 16 and HPV 35 infection were reported for Sub-Saharan Africa.

The risk of HPV 18 infection among HPV-positive women was found to be similar for all of these four aforementioned regions, with evidence of some heterogeneity within South America and Europe. Although not all regions of the world were included in this study, it did provide a comprehensive overview of the distribution of HPV types across some populations.

Epstein-Barr virus (EBV) is a member of the herpes virus family. EBV is found predominantly among adults; however, primary infection usually occurs in childhood. In nonindustrialized countries, virtually all children are infected with EBV by the age of 2, whereas in Western society, infection occurs later in life. EBV has been implicated for its role in Burkitt's lymphoma, Hodgkin's disease, non-Hodgkin's lymphoma, and nasopharyngeal carcinoma. Nevertheless, other risk factors also play a role in the development of these cancers. EBV has been detected in various lymphoepithelial carcinomas, particularly those found in the stomach, lung, and salivary gland, and in a small proportion of gastric adenocarcinomas. The role of EBV in these cancers has not been conclusively established, however.

EBV is transmitted through close contact via saliva (i.e., kissing). Recent studies suggest that transmission may also occur through sexual contact because EBV has been detected in both male and female genital secretions. Most people worldwide carry the virus; therefore, EBV is found throughout all human populations.

Human T-cell leukemia virus (HTLV-1) and human immunodeficiency virus 1 (HIV-1) are both retroviruses, and both have been implicated for their role in the development of various cancers. Some carriers of HTLV-1 have been found to develop adult T-cell leukemia-lymphoma after a long latent period. HIV-1 has been associated with Kaposi's sarcoma, non-Hodgkin's lymphoma, leiomyosarcoma in children, conjunctival squamous cell tumors in Africa, and Hodgkin's disease. Further, HIV-1 has been associated with the development of localized cervical cancer; however, this association may be attributed to the confounding role of HPV.

HTLV-1 and HIV-1 have similar routes of transmission, including mother-to-infant transmission (i.e., breastfeeding and childbirth), sexual transmission, and parenteral transmission (i.e., intravenous drug use and blood transfusions). Exposure to infected persons via these routes greatly increases the risk of contracting these viruses. Although HTLV-1 and HIV-1 have some similarities, they have differences in how they originated, their replication processes, and their associations with different cancers.

High-risk regions of HTLV-1 and HIV-1 are dissimilar, in that HIV-1 transmission patterns have been said to vary with time and geographical location, whereas infection with HTLV-1 is endemic in Japan, the Caribbean basin, Central and West Africa, and isolated areas elsewhere (i.e., parts of South America and Melanesia, Papua New Guinea, and the Solomon Islands), as well as among Australian aborigines.

PRECAUTIONARY MEASURES

Scientists are developing vaccines that target some infection-related cancers in an attempt to minimize their potential future occurrence. Nevertheless, a strong need still exists for greater awareness of the various precautionary measures that can be taken among high-risk populations. Both risk factors and methods of transmission need to be addressed through educational measures; changes in current high-risk practices, behaviors, attitudes, and perceptions; the adoption of safer alternatives; improved living and working conditions; and increased availability of and access to overall healthier environments. The implementation of strategies such as these are critical for decreasing the risks associated with the development of these infection-related cancers in the first place.

SEE ALSO: AIDS-Related Cancers; Anal Cancer; Bladder Cancer; Cervical Cancer; Esophageal Cancer; Gastric (Stomach) Cancer; Hepatitis B; Hepatitis C; Hepatocellular (Liver) Cancer, Adult (Primary); Hepatocellular (Liver) Cancer, Childhood (Primary); Liver Cancer, Adult (Primary); Liver Cancer, Childhood (Primary); Lymphoma, Burkitt's; Lymphoma, Hodgkin's, Adult; Lymphoma, Hodgkin's, Childhood; Lymphoma, Non-Hodgkin's, Adult; Lymphoma, Nasopharyngeal Cancer; Penile Cancer; Sarcoma, Kaposi's; Vaccines; Vaginal Cancer; Vulvar Cancer.

BIBLIOGRAPHY. G. Baseman Janet and Laura A. Koutsky, "The Epidemiology of Human Papillomavirus Infections," *Journal of Clinical Virology* (v.32/s1, 2005); F.X. Bosch, et al., "Prevalence of Human Papillomavirus in Cervical Cancer: A Worldwide Perspective," *Journal of the National Cancer Institute* (v.87/11, 1995); Ann N. Burchell, et al., "Epidemiology and Transmission Dynamics of Genital HPV Infection," *Vaccine* (v.24/s3, 2006); K. Celinski, et al., "*Helicobacter Pylori* Infection and the Risk of Adenocarcinoma of the Esophagus," *Annales Universitatis Mariae Curie Sklodowska Section D: Medicina* (v.59/1, 2004); G.M. Clifford, et al., "Worldwide Distribution of Human Papillomavirus Types in Cytologically Normal Women in the International Agency for Research on Cancer HPV Prevalence Surveys: A Pooled Analysis," *Lancet* (v.366/9490, 2005); Pelayo Correa, "Stomach," in Eduardo L. Franco and Thomas E. Rohan, eds., *Cancer Precursors: Epidemiology, Detection and Prevention* (Springer-Verlag, Inc., 2002); Dorothy H. Crawford, et al., "A Cohort Study among University Students: Identification of Risk Factors for Epstein-Barr Seroconversion and Infectious Mononucleosis," *Clinical Infectious Diseases* (v.43/3, 2006); Eduardo L. Franco and Alex Ferenczy, "Cervix," in Eduardo L. Franco and Thomas E. Rohan, eds., *Cancer Precursors: Epidemiology, Detection and Prevention* (Springer-Verlag, Inc., 2002); "Virus," in *Gale Encyclopedia of Neurological Disorders*, www.answers.com/topic/virus (cited October 2006); M. F. Go, "Natural History and Epidemiology of Helicobacter Pylori Infection," *Alimentary Pharmacology and Therapeutics* (v.16/s1, 2002); Luis A. Herrera, et al., "Role of Infectious Diseases in Human Carcinogenesis," *Environmental and Molecular Mutagenesis* (v.45/2–3, 2005); *IARC Monographs on the Evaluation of Carcinogenic Risks to Humans,* http://monographs.iarc.fr (cited October 2006).

ANN NOVOGRADEC
YORK UNIVERSITY

Insecticides

AN INSECTICIDE IS a pesticide developed to kill insects that are harmful to humans or food plants. Different types of pesticides have been developed to deal with different organisms that might reduce food production.

Insecticides are directed at insects; rodenticides are directed at rodents (such as mice and rats); fungicides, at fungi (such as blight and rust); and herbicides, at weeds (that is, any plants that grow where they are not wanted). During the 20th century the widespread use of insecticides greatly increased agricultural production throughout the world.

Insecticides used for agricultural purposes are classified according to the materials used to produce them and how they are applied to kill the insects. The first group of insecticides is applied directly to the plants. Insects feeding on the plants also eat the insecticide, resulting in their deaths. This group of insecticides is known as the systemic group.

Insecticides that are applied through aerosol distribution are known as contact insecticides, which kill the insects through contact.

Other insecticides come directly from nature itself and are known as natural insecticides. Over coevolution between plants and their pests, certain plants have developed a suit of chemicals that are injurious to their enemies. Citrus plants, for example, produce antifeedants, which are chemical agents that prevent certain insects from feeding by destroying their sense of taste. Some plants produce chemicals that destroy the hard protective outer cover of insects.

Other plants produce substances that are highly toxic to insects. One such potent natural pesticide is pyrethrum, which is extracted from the flowers of a daisylike plant.

The final group of insecticides is made inorganically in factories. These insecticides are manufactured from arsenates, copper, and fluorine compounds such as DDT that have been banned for their alleged harmful effects to humans and the ecosystem. Today, the most popular insecticides are organic insecticides, which are made from synthetic chemicals.

Different classes of insecticides have different modes of killing insects that may make them less or more toxic to other species such as fish, birds, and mammals.

Chlorine-based insecticides such as DDT do not kill the insect directly; they do so by opening the sodium channels in the nerve cells of the insect, resulting in the misfiring of neurons, uncontrolled spasms, and eventual death.

Organophosphate-based insecticides and chemical-warfare agents such as tabun, soman, VX, and sarin latch themselves to the neurotransmitter acetylcholinesterase and other cholinesterases, thereby disrupting the nervous impulses and in that way killing the insect.

ENVIRONMENTAL IMPACTS

Chlorine-based insecticides such as DDT and those based on organophosphates are very toxic and persistent in the environment, whereas those made from plants such as pyrethrum are nonpersistent and much less toxic. The pyrethroid insecticides are considered to be more environmentally friendly than synthetic or inorganic pesticides. Even though some insecticides have been banned, the number of insecticides on the market has skyrocketed. It is estimated that well over 1,000 different chemicals are used as insecticides and that they occur in more than 30,000 formulations.

Persistent and toxic insecticides have had deleterious effects, posing great danger to human health and the environment. Perhaps the most notorious case is that of DDT, which was initially introduced as a safer alternative to the lead and arsenic compounds that were used before the discovery of this chemical. DDT and similar insecticides do not distinguish between good and bad insects; they kill other nonpest species. This can result in the disruption of the natural pest-control mechanisms, such as parasitism and predation.

Joseph M. Moran, et al., reported the dangers of nondiscriminant killing of insects through the use of DDT in the Rio Grande Valley during efforts to control insect pests on cotton. DDT was widely used to control the three major pests: boll weevil, pink bollworm, and the cotton fleahopper. The widespread use of DDT resulted in the desired control of these three pests, increasing cotton yields. But the DDT also killed off the natural enemies of the tobacco budworm and the bollworm, which quickly proliferated and began to attack cotton, resulting in the reduction of cotton yields. Thus, although the farmers succeeded in controlling three major cotton pests, they accidentally got rid of insects that were the natural controls of two other pests, the budworm and the bollworm, thereby producing two additional pests.

One other environmental impact of the use of DDT in the Rio Grande Valley was increased resistance of the pests to the insecticide. By 1960 the bollworm and tobacco budworm had become increasingly resistant to DDT. The farmers then increased the dosage and frequency of applications, which resulted in further resistance to DDT so that by 1965 the pests could no longer be controlled by DDT. The farmers had to switch to a new organophosphate insecticide, methyl parathion. Unfortunately, within three years the tobacco budworm developed resistance to this insecticide as well.

With increased use of pesticides, the number of insects that are resistant has skyrocketed. It is estimated that over 450 species of insects have developed

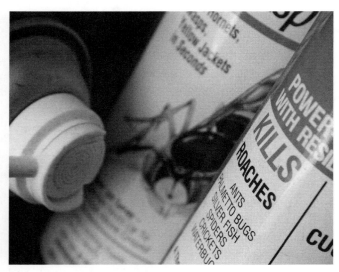

Many governments have opted to ban chlorinated hydrocarbons because of their alleged connection to cancer.

resistance to one or more pesticides. Thus, the use of pesticides can inadvertently contribute to the growth of a pest population that is composed primarily of resistant members.

PERSISTENT INSECTICIDES

Some insecticides are dangerous to the environment, as they remain in the environment as toxins for decades without breaking down. Often, such persistent insecticides pose great danger to both humans and animals.

The best example of such toxic insecticide is, once again, DDT. During the 1960s DDT was blamed for endangering certain species of birds, such as the bald eagle. DDT was blamed for reducing the thickness of the eggshells of predatory birds such as the bald eagle, the peregrine falcon, and the brown pelican. The shells became too thin for reproduction, resulting in dangerous reductions of bird populations.

As persistent pesticides remain in the environment, they are likely to be transported into aquatic ecosystems, easily contaminating them. Contamination of aquatic environments may affect the reproduction of some fish populations and may make such fish unfit for human consumption.

DDT and other chlorine-based insecticides have the tendency to bioaccumulate within the food chain. DDT, due to its stability and fat solubility, accumulates in the fat of animals and humans that ingest the chemical. In addition to bioaccumulating, DDT can

biomagnify, which causes progressively higher concentrations in the body fat of animals farther up the food chain. The result is that many countries have banned the agricultural use of DDT as an insecticide. There is great debate in the political and scholarly arenas as to the benefits of the use of this insecticide to control mosquitoes inside people's homes, particularly in the developing world, where malaria is endemic. Several other organochlorine-based pesticides have also been banned from most uses worldwide. These chemicals include aldrin, chlordane, DDT, dieldrin, endrin, heptachlor, mirex, and toxaphene. Their production is controlled by the Stockholm Convention on Persistent Organic Pollutants.

HUMAN HEALTH CONCERNS

Organochloride insecticides have been blamed as possible cancer-causing agents in humans. Beta-Benzene-hexachloride, an organochloride insecticide (also known under trade names such as HCH in Europe, hexachlor in Sweden, and hexachloran in the Soviet Union) has a number of health concerns, such as cancer and adverse impacts on the reproductive system, hormone system, stomach or intestines, brain, nervous system, cardiovascular system, blood, and immune system.

In the mid-1970s, the U.S. Environmental Protection Agency recommended a ban on further production of the insecticides aldrin and dieldrin on the grounds that they presented "a significant potential of an unreasonable risk of cancer in the American public." Although there was great debate concerning the evidence on which this decision was based, the EPA based its decision on the production in mice given diets containing aldrin or dieldrin of tumors in the livers, some of which moved into the lungs. It was argued in the scholarly community, however, that similar tumors occurred in mice on normal diets and could be produced by other compounds, including DDT. Because these insecticides were just as persistent as DDT, it was generally agreed that they should be phased out. It was emphasized, however, that the evidence that aldrin or dieldrin were carcinogenic to animals or to man was tenuous at best. To this day, the connection between certain insecticides and cancer or other health concerns in humans is hotly debated. Many governments have opted to ban chlorinated hydrocarbons and other persistent insecticides from general use because of their alleged connection to cancer and ecosystem contamination. In their place, other insecticides, especially those based on organophosphates, became more popular.

Organophosphates are less persistent than chlorinated hydrocarbons and, therefore, more environmentally friendly as they are less likely to accumulate in the food chain. Even organophosphates are hotly debated in terms of their health effects on humans, however. It is often argued that they are more toxic to humans than are chlorinated hydrocarbons and that they present a greater direct hazard to humans, especially to those persons who apply the pesticides. Humans have been fatally poisoned as a result of improper handling of organophosphates.

OTHER PEST-CONTROL METHODS

Those opposed to traditional environmentalism often cite the ban of DDT and other chlorine-based insecticides as an example of environmentalism going too far and interfering with the eradication of malaria, which has resulted in millions of deaths in the developing world.

Other pest-control methods have been advocated by those opposed to the use of persistent insecticides, such as DDT. Biological control, for example, has been suggested as an alternative method. In this case, a harmless bacteria or a predator or parasite to the pest is introduced in the ecosystem to reduce the pest to very low levels.

Bacillus thuringiensis, a bacterial disease of lepidopterans and some other insects, has been used to control insects. It is used as a larvicide against a wide variety of caterpillars. Because it has little effect on other organisms, it is considered more environmentally friendly than synthetic pesticides. The toxin from *Bacillus thuringiensis* has been incorporated directly into plants through the use of genetic engineering.

Genetic engineering is also being used to produce disease-resistant crops. The use of crop rotation to control pests is another method that is employed to control pests in an environmentally friendly manner.

Also, the concept of integrated pest management has been suggested as an effective way to deal with insect pests. This is defined as the coordination of all the suitable procedures and techniques that can be used in an environmentally compatible manner to maintain a pest population at levels low enough that no economic damage is incurred.

Moran, et al., noted that in the early 1970s, when cotton farmers no longer were able to control the insect pests with pesticides in the Rio Grande Valley, a new system of pest management was developed. That system included three basic components:

1. Cotton stalks were shredded and plowed under by mid-September, which reduced the number of weevils.

2. A rapid-fruiting, short-season cotton variety was cultivated, which could be harvested before the weevils would normally attack the cotton bolls.

3. A limited application of insecticides was carefully timed in the spring to kill overwintering adult weevils and to minimize the impact on the insect enemies of the bollworm and tobacco budworm.

Thus, when the farmers carefully adopted this method of controlling pests, cotton production increased again, and the pests declined significantly.

Learning from past mistakes, chemical companies are focusing their research efforts on developing new pesticides that are less persistent and more selective. Most of the newer insecticides are more specific in their actions and are designed to break down into nontoxic components within a few days of application. Nonetheless, misuse of insecticides remains an environmental, health, and economic issue.

SEE ALSO: Chemical Industry; Chlorine; Pesticide.

BIBLIOGRAPHY. Michael Crichton, *State of Fear: A Novel* (HarperCollinsPublishers, 2004); Ernest Hodgson and Ronald J. Kuhr, *Safer Insecticides: Development and Use* (M. Dekker, 1990); D. H. Hutson and T. R. Roberts, *Insecticides* (Wiley, 1985); International Agency for Research on Cancer, "Summaries and Evaluations: Occupational Exposures in Spraying and Application of Insecticides," (Group 2A), www.inchem.org/documents/iarc/vol53/01-insecticides. html (cited January 2007); Fumio Matsumura, *Toxicology of Insecticides* (Plenum Press, 1985); Joseph M. Moran, et al., *Introduction to Environmental Science* (W. H. Freeman, 1986); A. S. Perry, *Insecticides in Agriculture and Environment: Retrospects and Prospects* (Springer, 1998); Lester A. Swan, *Beneficial Insects—Nature's Alternatives to Chemical Insecticides: Animal Predation, Parasitism, Disease Organisms* (Harper & Row, 1964).

EZEKIEL KALIPENI
UNIVERSITY OF ILLINOIS AT URBANA-CHAMPAIGN

Insurance

LIFE IS FILLED with risk that harmful events may occur. These events may be accidents; illnesses; natural disasters such as floods, violent storms, or earthquakes; or other misadventures that disrupt the normal course of life with severe consequences. To minimize the financial damage that may result and that can be borne by a single individual, insurance was developed to distribute the risk of financial loss.

Historically, the rise of the insurance industry centered on the need to reduce the risk of loss to ship owners, shippers, and others. Storms, war, and pirates often caused significant losses to ships, crews, and cargoes. Spreading the risk among many investors made it possible to insure ships and cargoes against loss, so that a single loss did not wipe out an insurer's financial investments. Single losses on occasion were acceptable as part of the cost of doing business because the risk was distributed among many insurers. The profits from successful voyages made insurance profitable; if a loss occurred, the insurance money could be collected to cover the loss. Protecting against financial loss from all manner of risks has become a global industry. The most important types of insurance are life, health, and casualty (fire, floods, storms, thefts, or other forms of property losses).

Health insurance protects an individual against financial losses incurred from illness or accident. The insurer may be a private individual, a private company, a not-for-profit agency, or a government agency. In the United States, health insurance is generally market based and profit oriented. In other countries, the government is the insurer and also the medical provider that owns the hospitals and clinics, and that controls the delivery of medical services.

Health insurance began in the 19th century as a form of disability insurance. It was assumed that the working individual would return to work after his or her health was restored. Any expenses not covered by medical insurance were paid for by the patient on a fee-for-service basis. During World War II wage freezes prevented companies from increasing salaries or wages. To get around the freeze, many companies began to offer health insurance as a fringe benefit. By the 1970s the practice had become very widespread, with most people being insured by the companies or government agencies for which they worked.

CANCER INSURANCE

One of the greatest medical expenses is the cost associated with the treatment of cancer; therefore, cancer insurance has become popular in many quarters. Some people have even bought it with the superstitious hope that it would prevent them from getting cancer. This form of insurance, however, protects an individual in case cancer develops; it is not a substitute for comprehensive general health insurance. To be insured against any medical condition, including cancer, no previous existence of the disease can be known. If someone is insured for cancer, and it can be proved that the cancer was preexisting, the insurance may be nullified.

The cost of the insurance is an important consideration, because it is in addition to and not a substitute for a basic health insurance policy. People who are on Medicaid do not need cancer insurance, because they are already covered. People who are on Medicare can purchase a Medicare supplemental policy, which is usually much cheaper than private plans. Many expenses are not covered by a cancer policy. In addition, a policy may have a deductible clause, which means that the insured will pay a portion of the total cost of cancer treatment. Hospitalization for cancer treatment may also vary. Cancer patients often face large nonmedical expenses, such as home care, transportation, and rehabilitation costs. A cancer policy may not cover these expenses; if it does, the policy is very likely to cost much more.

The occurrence of cancer in the U.S. general population is relatively low. Overall, about 30 percent of the population ever gets cancer. If cancer occurs among many members of a person's family, however, the logic of purchasing cancer insurance increases. Only about 10 percent of total U.S. medical costs are due to cancer treatments.

Many kinds of cancer insurance policies are of limited value. Some policies charge premiums for hospital care, which is usually not needed because the average hospital stay for cancer is about two weeks. This means that a policy that promises to increase benefits after 90 continuous days of hospitalization is of little use for most people. In fact, most cancer treatments are given on an outpatient basis. It is not unusual for a cancer policy to have several fixed dollar limits. The limits may be for surgery, for radiation therapy, or fixed sums for each day in the hospital that are less than the hospital is likely to charge. In some cases, there are limits on the total medical costs that the policy will pay. Many cancer poli-

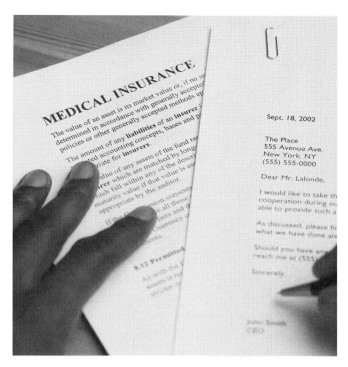

During World War II wage freezes prevented companies from giving raises and health insurance became a new fringe benefit.

cies set time limits. The insured must wait for a specified period for the insurance to become effective. Many policies stop paying benefits after two or three years.

SEE ALSO: Cost of Therapy; Government; Medicare and Medicaid.

BIBLIOGRAPHY. Jonathan Cohn, *Sick: The Untold Story of America's Health Care Crisis—and the People Who Pay the Price* (HarperCollins, 2007); David Edwards Marchinko and Hope Rachel Hetico, eds., *Dictionary of Health Insurance and Managed Care* (Springer Publishing Company, 2006); Dorothy E. Northrop, et al., *Health Insurance Resources: A Guide for People with Chronic Disease and Disability* (Demos Medical Publishing, 2006); Jo Ann C. Rowell and Michelle A. Green, *Understanding Health Insurance: A Guide to Billing and Reimbursement* (Thomson Delmar Learning, 2005); Harold D. Skipper, *Life and Health Insurance* (Prentice-Hall, 1999); Emmett J. Vaughn and Therese M. Vaughn, *Fundamentals of Risk and Insurance* (John Wiley & Sons, 2002).

ANDREW J. WASKEY
DALTON STATE COLLEGE

International Agency for Research on Cancer

THE INTERNATIONAL AGENCY for Research on Cancer/Centre International de Recherche sur le Cancer (IARC), founded in 1965, is an extension of the World Health Organization. IARC headquarters are in Lyon, France, where about 150 staff members are employed; about 600 scientists and trainees visit the headquarters each year.

The founding members of IARC are the Federal Republic of Germany (West Germany), France, Italy, the United Kingdom, and the United States. Today, IARC has 18 member countries: the original five plus Australia, Belgium, Canada, Denmark, Finland, India, Japan, Norway, the Netherlands, the Republic of Korea, Spain, Sweden, and Switzerland.

The primary mission of IARC is to conduct and coordinate research to identify the causes of cancer. It is not involved with issues of cancer treatment and care, and it is not involved in the implementation of control measures except when experimental intervention is necessary to assess the causes or mechanisms of cancer.

IARC places major emphasis on epidemiological research, environmental risk factors, and research training. This is based on the belief that 80 percent of cancers are linked to environmental factors and therefore are preventable—a belief supported by geographical variations in cancer incidence. Epidemiological studies conducted by IARC focus on descriptive studies of cancer incidence and mortality in different geographic locations and different populations, and on analytical studies of the relationships between risk factors and cancer incidence and mortality.

EDUCATION PROGRAMS AND PUBLICATIONS

IARC runs a summer school in cancer epidemiology that provides training for researchers and support workers involved in etiological research, cancer monitoring, and evaluation of interventions and care. The purpose of the summer school is to improve scientific knowledge and develop skills among research workers worldwide; for this reason, it emphasizes enrolling students from countries with limited resources to devote to cancer and other chronic diseases.

The organization recently inaugurated a Ph.D. training program in epidemiology and biostatistics.

Several types of research fellowships are available from IARC, including postdoctoral fellowships for junior scientists, a Visiting Scientist Award for an experienced investigator, and an Expertise Transfer Fellowship for an established investigator to work in a low- to medium-resource country to transfer knowledge and expertise to that country.

IARC produces several publications, including reports, handbooks, textbooks, and manuals, some of which are available for download from the organization's website. A bibliography of IARC scientific papers from 2003 to 2005 is available through the website as well. Recent press releases are available through the website. These press releases are primarily reports on current research by IARC staff on topics such as the health effects of passive smoke, dietary influence on cancer, and the cancer burden from the Chernobyl nuclear-plant accident.

SEE ALSO: Education, Cancer; France; World Health Organization.

BIBLIOGRAPHY. International Agency for Research on Cancer website, www.iarc.fr (cited November 2006).

SARAH BOSLAUGH
WASHINGTON UNIVERSITY SCHOOL OF MEDICINE

International Association for the Study of Lung Cancer

THE INTERNATIONAL ASSOCIATION for the Study of Lung Cancer (IASLC), founded in 1972, is an international organization dedicated to the study, treatment, and prevention of lung cancer and to the dissemination of information about lung cancer to the medical community and the general public. As of 2006 the association had about 2,000 members in 53 countries. The IASLC office is located in the University of Colorado Cancer Center in Aurora, Colorado.

The IASLC began with a group of researchers—including David T. Carr, Oleg S. Selawry, Lawrence Broder, and George Higgins—who had attended the First International Workshop for Therapy of Lung Cancer, held in Washington, D.C., in October 1972. These researchers wanted to establish a forum to continue the exchange of ideas from the workshop. The first organizational meeting of the IASLC was held in 1974, and the organization was incorporated as a not-for-profit corporation in that year. The IASLC organized the First World Congress on Lung Cancer in May 1978 at Hilton Head, South Carolina. Subsequent meetings were called World Conferences and were held first at two-year intervals and later at three-year intervals. World Conference locations have included Denmark, Japan, the Czech Republic, Poland, and Ireland.

The IASLC awards up to 17 fellowships annually. The Prevention/Translational Research Fellowship Award is awarded for two years for investigators working in lung-cancer prevention and translational research. The Lung Cancer Fellowship Award/Young Investigators Award is awarded for two years to provide training of fellows and young investigators who were recently awarded a Ph.D. or M.D. and are interested pursuing a career in lung-cancer diagnosis, treatment, or laboratory research. Further information about and applications for the fellowships are available from the IASLC website.

Journal of Thoracic Oncology (JTO), the official journal of the IASLC, is published by Lippincott Williams & Wilkins. It began publication in March 2006. All 2006 issues are available through the JTO website.

In 2005 the IASLC issued a much-cited Declaration on Tobacco, a copy of which is available from the IASLC website. This declaration states unequivocally that lung-cancer incidence is increasing in much of the world and that tobacco use is a primary cause.

The declaration also urged governments to ratify the Framework Convention on Tobacco Control, promote smoking-cessation and prevention programs, and increase taxes on tobacco; promoted the elimination of tobacco advertising; and encouraged all healthcare providers to receive training in antismoking counseling.

SEE ALSO: Lung Cancer, Non-Small Cell; Lung Cancer, Small Cell; Passive Smoking; Smoking Cessation; Tobacco Smoking.

BIBLIOGRAPHY. International Association for the Study of Lung Cancer, www.iaslc.org (cited November 2006); *Journal of Thoracic Oncology*, www.jto.org (cited November 2006).

SARAH BOSLAUGH
WASHINGTON UNIVERSITY SCHOOL OF MEDICINE

International Association of Cancer Registries

THE INTERNATIONAL ASSOCIATION of Cancer Registries (IACR) is a professional society whose members are cancer registries and individuals and organizations with an interest in cancer registration. It was founded in 1966 to facilitate the exchange of ideas among cancer registries and to improve data quality and comparability between registries. Two principal concerns of the IACR are establishing and promoting standards for cancer registries, and providing accurate information about worldwide cancer incidence.

There are four categories of membership: full members, which are established population-based cancer registries or associations of cancer registries that collect data on all cancer sites for an accurately enumerated population and can provide valid incidence rates; associate members, which are cancer registries that do not meet one or more of the standards for full membership; individual members, which are registries that have not yet begun operating and individuals interested in IACR activities; and corporate members, which are corporations involved in activities relevant to the IACR, such as pharmaceutical manufacturers and software companies.

Some IACR technical reports and guidelines are available from the IACR website; others are available from World Health Organization Press and Oxford University Press. IACR Press ceased operation in 2005. IACR also publishes two series of publications that are the leading source of information about adult and pediatric cancer incidence worldwide. Volumes in the series *Cancer Incidence in Five Continents* (C15) are published every five years and are the standard reference source on the international incidence of cancer. The first volume was published in 1966 and drew attention to the benefits to be derived from studying disease frequency in different areas and over a period of time. The most recent volume covers 1993 through 1997 and presents age-specific, standard, and cumulative incidence rates by sex for each type of cancer for each population.

A separate series, the *International Incidence of Childhood Cancer,* covers cancers in children. The first volume, which appeared in 1988, was the first comprehensive and systematic collection of data on worldwide pediatric cancer occurrence. A separate series for childhood cancers is needed because although they are theoretically included in the CI5 series, they are often missed because they are not well described by the International Classification of Disease categories used in that series. The IACR holds an annual scientific meeting in a different country each year to allow participation from the maximum number of members. Locations have included Brazil, Uganda, Cuba, Thailand, Portugal, and United States.

The Calum Muir Memorial Fellowship is awarded by the IACR to an individual working in cancer registries to broaden that person's experience through means such as attending workshops or training courses not available in his or her home country. Application forms are available from the IACR website.

SEE ALSO: Childhood Cancers; Survivors of Cancer.

BIBLIOGRAPHY. International Association of Cancer Registries website, www.iacr.com.fr (cited November 2006).

SARAH BOSLAUGH
WASHINGTON UNIVERSITY SCHOOL OF MEDICINE

International Cancer Alliance for Research and Education

WHEN A PATIENT goes through the long process of cancer care, the patient–physician relationship makes an impact on this process. The International Cancer Alliance for Research and Education (ICARE) is a not-for-profit organization dedicated to improving the patient–physician relationship, as well as to ameliorating the stresses and fears of patients and their families as they navigate diagnosis, treatment, and recovery. ICARE is based in Bethesda, Maryland.

A chief focus of the alliance is to bring researchers into the patient–physician dynamic, as well as to provide the latest knowledge and information available.

ICARE has a three-part mission statement:

1. It aims to organize the wealth of knowledge among researchers, clinicians, patients, and the media into a user-friendly format easily accessible by patients and their physicians.

2. It strives to hasten the transition of knowledge from the laboratory to the clinic.

3. It pledges to advocate for cancer research.

The alliance provides a Cancer Therapy Review (CTR) booklet to patients and their families. An individual booklet is published for each type of cancer. Patients are encouraged to register with ICARE to receive the booklet. CTR booklets are published for cancers of the bladder, brain, breast, cervix, colon, kidney, pancreas, prostate, and skin, as well as leukemia, lymphoma, and sarcoma. Patients with other cancers are asked to report these types, so that ICARE may address those cancers as well. Sections of the booklet cover descriptive aspects of the disease, procedures for detection, classification of the cancer stages, current treatments, and further information.

To spread information, ICARE posts news on its website. Each news story is summarized by a few sentences, free of jargon. The patient or physician can then choose to read the whole story. These full stories have enough detail to inform a physician, yet are carefully written so as to be understandable to a patient who may not have a scientific background.

Additionally, the website provides information on different types of cancer. Patients are guided through their cancer on the ICARE Highway to Health, a cartoon map of the stages of cancer and the treatment steps available at each stage. These treatments are explained by the acronym SCROCtA (Surgery, Chemotherapy, Radiation, Other, Clinical Trials, and Alternative). ICARE offers support for obtaining a second opinion. ICARE also guides patients through their cancers via a 12-part Patient Survival Guide. The Cancer Breakthrough Newsletter is an online newsletter updated with recent breakthroughs in cancer research.

ICARE Think Tanks are novel methods of addressing therapy. Five patients with a particular therapy concern are brought together with five leading cancer physicians for a one- or two-day meeting. At these meetings, the physicians gain an understanding of the therapy from the patients' perspectives, and improvements to these therapies are made.

Patients who want an electronic support group can request such a group from ICARE. These electronic chat rooms are private and available to patients with similar support-group needs.

The Clinical Trial Matching Program provides investigators in academia and the pharmaceutical industry information on patients eligible for clinical trials in breast, colon, and prostate cancers, as well as non-Hodgkin's lymphoma.

SEE ALSO: Clinical Trials; Pharmaceutical Industry; Survivors of Cancer; Survivors of Cancer Families.

BIBLIOGRAPHY. National Coalition for Cancer Survivorship, Barbara Hoffman, and Sam Donaldson, *A Cancer Survivor's Almanac: Charting Your Journey* (Wiley, 1996).

CLAUDIA WINOGRAD
UNIVERSITY OF ILLINOIS AT URBANA-CHAMPAIGN

International Committee of the Red Cross

THE INTERNATIONAL COMMITTEE of the Red Cross (ICRC) is a humanitarian organization headquartered in Geneva, Switzerland, that assists people throughout the world who are affected by international and internal armed conflicts. The ICRC maintains a permanent presence in over 60 countries and in 2003 had offices in 169 locations worldwide.

ICRC activities are funded through voluntary donations, primarily from National Red Cross and Red Crescent Societies and from national governments. As of 2006 the ICRC had about 800 staff members at its headquarters in Geneva, 1,400 staff members and delegates serving on field missions, and 11,000 local employees throughout the world.

The ICRC was founded in 1863 as the International Committee for the Relief of Military Wounded; in 1876 it was renamed the International Committee of the Red Cross. The first Geneva Convention was held in 1864, attended by representatives from 12 states and kingdoms; most notably, the delegates adopted 10 articles that established for the first time rules guaranteeing protection for injured soldiers, medical personnel, and humanitarian agencies during armed conflict. These rules have been revised several times but remain the international standard on the rights of soldiers and civilians during armed conflict.

The ICRC's specific concern is humanitarian law. It is part of the International Red Cross Movement, which includes the National Red Cross and Red Crescent Societies; it also is part of the International Federation of Red Cross and Red Crescent Societies, which coordinates activities among the national societies.

The *International Review of the Red Cross*, a specialized journal on humanitarian law, is published by the ICRC. It was first published in 1869 under the title *Bulletin international Sociétés des secours aux militaires blessés* and later as *Bulletin international des Sociétés de la Croix-Rouge.* The mission of the *International Review of the Red Cross* is to promote knowledge and reflection on humanitarian law; to product fundamental rights and values; and to provide a forum for discussion of contemporary humanitarian action and analysis of conflicts and the humanitarian problems they cause. Issues from 1995 to the present are available for free download from the ICRC website. The ICRC produces many other materials, including pamphlets, posters, books, DVDs, and films. Many of these materials are available for free download from the website or may be ordered from the ICRC.

SEE ALSO: Switzerland.

BIBLIOGRAPHY. David P. Forsythe, *The Humanitarians: The International Committee of the Red Cross* (Cambridge University Press, 2005); The International Committee of the Red Cross website, www.icrc.org/eng (cited November 2006).

Sarah Boslaugh
Washington University School of Medicine

International Myeloma Foundation

MULTIPLE MYELOMA IS the cancer of plasma cells (antibody-producing cells) in the bone marrow. It is currently incurable yet treatable. The International Myeloma Foundation (IMF) was established in 1990 with the mission of improving myeloma patients' quality of life while investigating the cure for and prevention of myeloma.

The IMF was conceived in 1989 in a coffee-shop conversation among myeloma patient Brian Novis, Susie Novis, and Dr. Brian Durie. The foundation became a reality in 1990. Although the IMF was es-

tablished in London, England, the international headquarters of the foundation are presently located in North Hollywood, California. The IMF is managed by a board of directors comprised of nearly 50 scientific advisers. Additionally, the IMF has a scientific advisory board that advises the foundation in its research and education funding endeavors.

Since 1993 IMG has provided an Info Pack to patients at no charge. The Info Pack includes information on living with myeloma. Additionally, a Concise Review of the Disease and Treatment Options and a Patient Handbook are available. Four times per year, the IMF publishes Myeloma Today, a newsletter for anyone affected by myeloma. Topics covered include the latest information on multiple myelomas and clinical breakthroughs. The foundation also produces the Myeloma Minute, an e-mail newsletter.

The foundation provides information on over 100 multiple-myeloma support groups to help patients find the support groups they most relate to. Furthermore, the IMF hosts Patients & Family Seminars across the nation, where guests can learn about current research and treatment options from a panel of myeloma experts. Information is offered in many languages, including English, Chinese, French, German, Greek, Hebrew, Italian, Japanese, Korean, Polish, Portuguese, Russian, Spanish, and Turkish.

Junior and senior investigators in the field of myeloma are supported by grants from the IMF. These grants are for one year. Applications are submitted in late summer; notification of acceptance is given by that fall, and funding begins the following January.

A special project of the IMF is Bank on a Cure, an international DNA bank of myeloma patients. Already, this project has discovered why thalidomide, a common treatment for multiple myeloma, causes blood clots in certain patients. Another offshoot of the foundation is the IMF Nursing Leadership Board, which holds meetings to share information and make recommendations for practices in myeloma nursing.

Every few years, the IMG hosts a gala benefit. Past benefits have been held in Philadelphia, Pennsylvania, and Universal City, California. To disseminate information on research and clinical advances, the IMF holds clinical conferences in cities around the world.

SEE ALSO: Genetics; Myeloma, Multiple.

BIBLIOGRAPHY. James R. Berenson, *Biology and Management of Multiple Myeloma (Current Clinical Oncology)* (Humana Press, 2004).

CLAUDIA WINOGRAD
UNIVERSITY OF ILLINOIS AT URBANA-CHAMPAIGN

International Psycho-Oncology Society

THE INTERNATIONAL PSYCHO-ONCOLOGY Society (IPOS) was founded in 1984 to facilitate multidisciplinary communication among people working in psychosocial and behavioral oncology, and to improve the care received by cancer patients and their families. The IPOS office is located in Charlottesville, Virginia.

The IPOS is concerned with two primary psychosocial dimensions of cancer: the response of patients, family, and staff to cancer and cancer treatment; and psychological, social, and behavioral factors that influence cancer progression and survival.

As of 2006 IPOS had over 200 members in 38 countries, from a variety of clinical and research fields including medicine, nursing, social work, psychology, social science, and education. Membership is available in three categories. Active members have a master's degree or doctoral-level qualification or the professional equivalent, and are actively involved in research or clinical work related to psycho-oncology. Associate members have an interest in psycho-oncology but do not have a professional qualification. Members-in-training are enrolled in training programs in fields such as medicine, psychology, and social work.

IPOS bestows three awards annually.

The Hiroomi Kawano New Investigator Award is given to a candidate who has completed graduate study or specialist training within the past five years; all candidates must be nominated by a member of IPOS or a national psycho-oncology society.

The Bernard Fox Memorial Award is given to honor an IPOS or community member who has made an outstanding contribution to psycho-oncology.

The Arnold M. Sutherland Award is given to an individual for lifetime achievement in psycho-oncology; the winner is invited to deliver a lecture at the World Congress of Psycho-Oncology.

Further information about and nomination forms for these awards are available from the IPOS website.

PUBLICATIONS AND RESOURCES

The journal *Psycho-Oncology* is published by Wiley on behalf of IPOS, the American Psychosocial Oncology Society, and the British Psycho-Oncology Society. It is published 12 times per year and includes articles from many disciplines related to the psychosocial aspects of cancer and AIDS-related tumors.

The IPOS website provides access to professional education materials, including a series of online lectures available in nine languages offering a core curriculum in psycho-oncology. Lecture topics in this series include psychosocial assessment in cancer patients, distress management in cancer, communication and interpersonal skills in cancer care, anxiety and adjustment disorders in cancer patients, and depression and depressive disorders in cancer patients.

MEETINGS AND EVENTS

IPOS holds regular scientific meetings that offer symposia, presentations, and training sessions in the field of psycho-oncology. The IPOS website provides a calendar of conferences, training courses, and similar events relevant to psycho-oncology.

SEE ALSO: American Psychosocial Oncology Society; Survivors of Cancer.

BIBLIOGRAPHY. International Psycho-Oncology Society website, www.ipos-society.org (cited November 2006).

SARAH BOSLAUGH
WASHINGTON UNIVERSITY SCHOOL OF MEDICINE

International Society for Cutaneous Lymphomas

THE INTERNATIONAL SOCIETY for Cutaneous Lymphomas (ISCL) is an international, not-for-profit association of medical and research professionals. ISCL offices are located in Zurich, Switzerland; Philadelphia, Pennsylvania; and New Haven, Connecticut.

The ISCL was founded in 1992 during the 18th World Congress of Dermatology, an annual scientific meeting sponsored by the International League of Dermatological Societies. Founding members of the ISCL came from many countries, including Austria, Italy, Spain, the United States, Canada, and Japan.

The society's primary aims are to increase knowledge of lymphoproliferative and related skin disorders, and to foster communication and stimulate interactions and collaborative efforts among regional, national, and international groups active in clinical, histomorphological, and research work related to cutaneous lymphoma. The ISCL sponsors an international registry of cutaneous lymphoma whose purpose is to collect clinical and epidemiological data about cutaneous lymphoma and to document rare cases that may aid in identifying the pathogenesis of this type of cancer. Cutaneous lymphomas are a type of cancer that begins in a lymphocyte (type of white blood cell) in the skin and belong to the class of non-Hodgkin's lymphoma.

The ISCL currently has about 220 members, primarily physicians and Ph.D.-level researchers: prospective new members must be approved by the ISCL executive committee on the basis of their professional interests in cutaneous lymphoma. The international focus of the ISCL is emphasized in its membership and organization. Not only are ISCL members located in many countries, but also, the ISCL bylaws specify that the executive committee must include representatives from the United States, Europe, and the other continents if those geographic regions are represented in ISCL membership.

MEETINGS AND EVENTS

The ISCL hosts a scientific session each year during the annual meeting of the American Academy of Dermatology, a worldwide organization of physicians working in dermatology, and holds a one- or two-day meeting every five years during the World Congress of Dermatology.

SEE ALSO: Lymphoma, Hodgkin's, Childhood; Lymphoma, Non-Hodgkin's, Childhood; Skin Cancer (Non-Melanoma).

BIBLIOGRAPHY. International Society for Cutaneous Lymphomas website, www-usz.unizh.ch/iscl/isclhome.htm (cited November 2006).

SARAH BOSLAUGH
WASHINGTON UNIVERSITY SCHOOL OF MEDICINE

International Society for Preventive Oncology

THE FIELDS OF predictive and preventive oncology focus on stopping cancer before it starts or immediately after it starts. The International Society for Preventive Oncology (ISPO) is a group based in Worcester, Massachusetts, whose members are dedicated to the studies of predictive and preventive oncology. The society is led by a board, for which biennial elections are held.

Predictive oncology is the identification and study of cancer causes and risk factors. It is involved in primary cancer prevention, which includes recognizing avoidable risk factors, genetic markers of cancer, and genetic predisposition to cancer, predicting a patient's response to anticancer treatment, among other areas.

Preventive oncology supports clinical screening and routine detection procedures involved in secondary cancer prevention. Secondary cancer prevention involves screening and detection methods as well as preliminary care for cancers.

The society studies the etiology of cancer and how certain factors can interact to enhance the risk of cancer development. With this knowledge, the ISPO hopes to determine how these etiologic factors have an effect on prevention, diagnosis, and treatment of cancer.

The ISPO's mission is to act as a "forum, committed to the study of interactive etiologic factors in cancer development and their impact on prevention, detection, and management of neoplastic diseases." To achieve its mission, the ISPO has outlined two priorities. It aims to identify and control cancer causes, specifically in high-risk individuals, and thereby support primary cancer prevention. Additionally, it works to detect and manage precancer lesions and cancer that is difficult to detect, thereby supporting secondary cancer prevention.

ISPO membership is open to all people actively involved in studying cancer prevention and detection. Members include physicians, epidemiologists, pathologists, hematologists, experimental oncologists, immunologists, social scientists, and educators. Membership is in five classes: active, associate, junior, life, and honorary. Active members can vote, hold office, and serve on standing committees. To be an active member, one must be a physician or other degreed doctor. Individuals working in preventive oncology at professional equivalence may also join the ISPO as active members.

EDUCATION AND PUBLICATIONS

The society makes many efforts to continue the education of its members through various activities. The ISPO holds regional workshops, symposia, and international meetings. Members of the ISPO agree to continue their educations in several fields, including the molecular biology of cancer and its agents, lifestyle impacts on cancer risks and socioeconomic factors, improved methods to diagnose and prevent cancers, and advances in understanding of risk factors and predictive markers, as well as new therapies.

Cancer Detection & Prevention is the official journal of the ISPO. It is published bimonthly and available free to society members.

SEE ALSO: Education; Psycho-Social Issues; Screening, Access to.

BIBLIOGRAPHY. Peter Greenwald, *Cancer Prevention and Control (Basic and Clinical Oncology, No 6)* (Informa Healthcare, 1994).

CLAUDIA WINOGRAD
UNIVERSITY OF ILLINOIS AT URBANA-CHAMPAIGN

International Society of Experimental Hematology

HEMATOLOGY IS THE study of blood cells. Several cancers involve blood cells, as well as the immune system, which is derived from white blood cells. The International Society of Experimental Hematology (ISEH) consolidates the latest information and knowledge from around the world to offer programs in education and training of hematology.

The society's mission is to "further basic translational and clinical research and to foster communication, education, collaboration in the field of experimental hematology and stem cell biology." Experimental hematology includes the study of cancer stem cells; cellular therapy; gene profiling and protein chips; gene therapy; hematopoeisis (the genesis of blood cells from precursors); the hematopoietic microenviron-

ment; hematologic malignancies (leukemia, lymphoma, myeloma); immunology; oncogenes; oncology; stem-cell niches; and stem-cell biology and transplantation, such as bone marrow, peripheral blood, and cord-blood transplantations and donations.

The ISEH is led by a board of officers consisting of a president, president-elect, vice president, treasurer, editor, and past president. Several counselors advise the board. Additionally, five committees steer the society: Scientific Program, Nominating, Emerging Leaders Task Force, Membership, and Publication.

An offshoot of the ISEH is the ISEH Society for Hematology & Stem Cells. This society holds an annual meeting to which all ISEH members are invited.

Members benefit from a free subscription to the ISEH's official journal *Experimental Hematology*, reduced registration fees to the ISEH meetings, eligibility to apply for society travel grants to support meeting attendance, eligibility to submit abstracts to the annual meeting (which will also be published in a special issue of *Experimental Hematology*), listing on and access to the membership directory, and the ability to serve on international committees acting in the field of experimental hematology.

The ISEH website has resources for experimental hematologists and a restricted site for members only. A calendar of events is updated to include global meetings and conventions regarding hematology and stem cells. The site also provides links to related societies, such as the American Association of Blood Banks; the International Society for Laboratory Hematology; the Leukemia and Lymphoma Society; the National Cancer Institute; and many national hematology societies, such as those of Germany, Denmark, Japan, Canada, and Belgium.

SEE ALSO: Bone Marrow Transplants; Leukemia Society of America; Lymphoma Research Foundation of America; National Cancer Institute.

BIBLIOGRAPHY. A. Victor Hoffbrand, et al., *Essential Haematology (Essential)* (Blackwell Professional Publishing, 2006); Ronald Hoffman, et al., *Hematology: Basic Principles and Practice* (Churchill Livingstone, 2004); G. J. L. Kaspers, et al., *Drug Resistance in Leukemia and Lymphoma III (Advances in Experimental Medicine and Biology)* (Springer, 1999).

CLAUDIA WINOGRAD
UNIVERSITY OF ILLINOIS AT URBANA-CHAMPAIGN

International Society of Nurses in Cancer Care

NURSES ARE IMPORTANT members of the cancer-care team. The International Society of Nurses in Cancer Care (ISNCC) is an international collaboration to provide education, training, and research knowledge to oncology nurses around the globe. Additionally, the society supports international networking of cancer nurses so that information can be shared across nations.

The ISNCC was founded in 1984, and 12 years later, 33 countries were represented in the society, as well as over 60 member groups within these countries.

To achieve its mission of fostering an international cooperation among cancer-care nurses and other health organizations, the ISNCC has outlined six objectives: to maintain a network for regional and international communication; to emphasize communication to nurses in countries without a national oncology nursing society; to aid nurses in establishing national and regional cancer-care nursing associations; to represent cancer-care nurses in the international arena and thus advise other organizations on nursing; to collaborate with other world health societies to achieve the ISNCC goals; and to disseminate knowledge and information about oncology nursing via the ISNCC publication International Cancer Nursing News.

The society has published three position statements in both English and Spanish. These mission statements cover the positions of the ISNCC on cancer pain, cervical screening, and tobacco use. The cancer-pain mission statement is also available in Portuguese, Turkish, and Xhosa (the language of the peoples of Bantu origins, presently living in southeastern South Africa).

The ISNCC offers research grants to support member nurses performing research on cancer-care nursing.

The society is a member of the World Health Organization with nongovernmental status and of the Pan American Health Organization (PAHO). It is affiliated with the International Council of Nurses and the International Union Against Cancer. The society is managed by a board of 18 trustees and one or two appointed members. The ISNCC has designated five global areas—Africa and the Middle East, Central

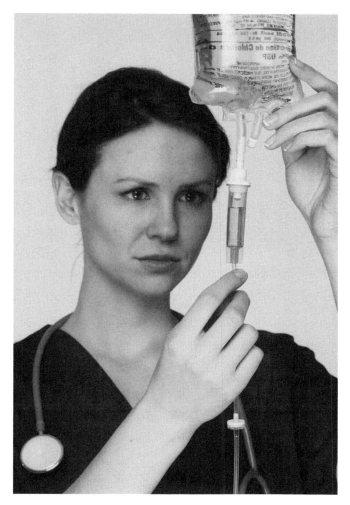

The mission of the International Society of Nurses in Cancer Care is to foster an international cooperation among cancer caregivers.

and South America, Europe, the Far East and Australia, and North America—and three board members must be from these areas.

Executive officers are the president, president-elect, and secretary/treasurer. These officers also serve as board members.

The society's website offers resources for oncology nurses, as well as links to related organizations such as the World Health Organization, the International Council of Nurses, the European Oncology Nursing Society, and several national societies of cancer-care nursing.

SEE ALSO: Canadian Association of Nurses in Oncology; European Oncology Nursing Society; Oncology Nursing Society; World Health Organization.

BIBLIOGRAPHY. Heather Porter, "International Affairs," *Cancer Nursing* (v.9, 1986); Connie Henke Yarbro, et al., eds., *Cancer Nursing: Principles and Practice (Jones and Bartlett Series in Oncology)* (Jones & Bartlett Publishers, 2005).

CLAUDIA WINOGRAD
UNIVERSITY OF ILLINOIS AT URBANA-CHAMPAIGN

International Society of Paediatric Oncology

THE INTERNATIONAL SOCIETY of Paediatric Oncology/Société International d'Oncologie Pédiatrique (SIOP) is an international organization focused on research and clinical care related to pediatric cancer.

SIOP's origins lie in the Club d'Oncologie Pédiatrique (Paediatric Oncology Club) founded in 1967 in the Paediatric Department of the Institut Gustave Roussy in Paris. The club held an assembly in 1969 in Madrid, Spain, and decided at that meeting to form the Société International d'Oncologie Pédiatrique, which remains the official name of the organization.

The central secretariat of SIOP is located in Eindhoven, The Netherlands.

SIOP has seven goals: to improvement knowledge of childhood malignant diseases and their management; to improvement the quality of life for children with these diseases and their families; to foster bonds among people working in pediatric oncology; to further scientific exchange in the field of pediatric oncology; to operate cooperative clinical trials; to foster collaboration with similar organizations; and to foster the training of healthcare professionals who work in the field of pediatric oncology. SIOP was clinically oriented in its early years, but this focus has expanded to include basic scientific research relating to pediatric oncology.

SIOP has established an alliance with the International Confederation of Childhood Cancer Parent Organizations to promote the interests of the families of children with cancer, including access to care regardless of financial status or national origin, and access to the best possible information to allow parents to decide on the optimal course of treatment for their children.

As of 2006 the society had over 1,150 members, primarily physicians, doctoral-level researchers, nurses, and other professionals working in pediatric oncology. Prospective members must be sponsored by a current member and approved by the annual general assembly.

PUBLICATIONS AND RESOURCES

Pediatric Blood and Cancer, previously known as *Medical Pediatric Oncology,* is the official journal of SIOP. This international journal is published by Wiley and carries articles concerning basic and clinical investigations of blood disorders and malignant diseases of childhood, as well as treatment options for those diseases. SIOP also publishes a newsletter that appears in July and December and that carries primarily news about SIOP. Newsletter issues from 2001 to the present are available from the society's website.

The society's website contains resources useful to people working in pediatric oncology, including notices of relevant courses, notices of meetings of related societies, a listing with contact information about clinical trials for pediatric cancers that have been endorsed by SIOP, and links to related organizations.

EDUCATION AND EVENTS

Scholarships are available to individuals under the age of 45 from economically less-developed countries. Details are available on the SIOP website.

SIOP sponsors an annual congress, including scientific sessions and a business meeting that alternates between European and non-European locations.

SEE ALSO: Childhood Cancers; Clinical Trials; Survivors of Cancer.

BIBLIOGRAPHY. International Society for Paediatric Oncology website, www.siop.nl (cited November 2006).

SARAH BOSLAUGH
WASHINGTON UNIVERSITY SCHOOL OF MEDICINE

International Society on Thrombosis and Haemostasis

THE INTERNATIONAL SOCIETY on Thrombosis and Haemostasis (ISTH) is a not-for-profit organization whose objectives are to advance research focused on medical problems relating to thrombosis, hemostasis, and vascular biology; to provide a forum for discussion of these topics; to foster the exchange of ideas and diffusion of research regarding these topics; and to encourage the standardization of nomenclature and methodology in thrombosis and hemostasis.

The origins of the ISTH lie in the first meeting of the International Committee for the Standardization of the Nomenclature of the Blood Clotting Factors in Basel, Switzerland, in 1954. This group was later re-named the International Committee on Thrombosis and Haemostasis and then the International Society on Thrombosis and Haemostasis. ISTH headquarters are located in Chapel Hill, North Carolina.

The effort to develop standard nomenclature in thrombosis and hemostasis remains a major concern of ISTH and is the focus of the ISTH Scientific and Standardization Committee. The committee pub-lishes a continually updated list of "Quantities and Units in Thrombosis and Haemostasis," first published in *Thrombosis and Haemostasis* in 1994, which aims to facilitate unequivocal communication in publica-tions and databases despite differences in terminology among medical specialties and differences in languag-es and alphabets. "Quantities and Units in Thrombosis and Haemostasis" is available on the ISTH website.

ISTH membership is open to researchers, edu-cators, clinicians, students, trainees, and postdoc-toral fellows with a continuing scientific education in thrombosis, hemostasis, and vascular biology. As of 2006 there were over 2,800 ISTH members from more than 70 countries.

Journal of Thrombosis and Haemostasis (JTH) has been the official publication of the ISTH since January 2003. JTH is a peer-reviewed journal published 12 times per year by Blackwell Publishing. Before 2003 the official journal of ISTH was *Thrombosis and Haemostasis,* pub-lished by F. K. Schattauer; this journal is still published but without the editorial supervision of the ISTH.

MEETINGS AND EVENTS
ISTH holds an biennial congress, which includes sci-entific presentations and symposia, guest lectures, and organizational meetings.

The Scientific and Standardization Committee of the ISTH and its scientific subcommittees meet an-nually; these committee meetings are held in con-junction with the congress in the years in which the congress is held.

Official communications of the Scientific and Stan-dardization Committee, as well as minutes and reports from the annual scientific subcommittee meetings for 1995 to 2006, are available from the ISTH website.

SEE ALSO: Childhood Cancers; Education, Cancer; Survi-vors of Cancer.

BIBLIOGRAPHY. International Society on Thrombosis and Haemostasis website, www.med.unc.edu/isth/welcome (cited November 2006).

Sarah Boslaugh
Washington University School of Medicine

International Union Against Cancer

THE INTERNATIONAL UNION Against Cancer/ Union Internationale Contre le Cancer (UICC) is a nongovernmental organization composed of more than 270 member organizations in over 80 countries. Members include voluntary cancer societies, tobac-co-control groups, patient support organizations, public health institutes, cancer research and treat-ment centers, and national ministries of health. The UICC was founded in 1933 and is headquartered in Geneva, Switzerland.

The UICC's objectives are to advance scientific and medical knowledge in cancer research, diagno-sis, treatment, and prevention, and to promote anti-cancer campaigns throughout the world. It has four strategic areas of focus: cancer prevention and early detection, tobacco control, knowledge transfer, and capacity building. The latter area includes promotion of national cancer-control planning efforts, fund rais-ing, and resource allocation.

International Journal of Cancer (IJC) is a peer-re-viewed scientific journal published by Wiley on be-half of the UICC. The IJC began publication in 1964 and currently publishes 30 issues per year, carrying scientific articles on a broad scope of topics relevant to experimental and clinical cancer research, includ-ing epidemiological studies.

Global Action Against Cancer, a frequently updat-ed booklet published jointly by UICC and the World

Health Organization, presents a global survey of the world's cancer burden and opportunities to improve prevention, early detection, care, and cure. The booklet is available in English, French, and Spanish for free download from the UICC website or may be ordered from the UICC.

The UICC selects about 150 fellows each year in the categories of beginning investigators, translational cancer research, bilateral research, transfer of cancer research and clinical technology, oncology nursing, and staff and volunteer training. Fellowships range from support for a full year of research funding to grants that allow a fellow to attend a single international conference or training. Upon completion of a UICC fellowship, fellows are invited to join the Association of UICC Fellows, which has over 1,000 members.

Further information and applications are available from the UICC website.

Accurate and consistent description of cancer staging (the extent or state of a cancer in an individual case) is necessary both for clinical care and for research, and the UICC has played a major role in developing and establishing international standards for cancer staging.

The global standard is the TNM (Primary Tumor, Regional Lymph Nodes, Distant Metastasis) system of classification, which was developed in the 1940s by Dr. Pierre Denoix. The UICC subsequently established a Committee on Clinical Stage Classification under Denoix's leadership; the committee is still in existence and working on refining the TNM system of cancer staging.

Principal TNM publications include the *TNM Classification of Malignant Tumors* (Wiley, 2002) and the *TNM Atlas* (Wiley, 2005). Tumor staging information is also available in a downloadable PDA version (*TNM Mobile Edition*) and online (*TNM Online*).

SEE ALSO: Education, Cancer; Government; Tobacco Smoking; World Health Organization.

BIBLIOGRAPHY. International Union Against Cancer website, www.uicc.org (cited November 2006).

SARAH BOSLAUGH
WASHINGTON UNIVERSITY SCHOOL OF MEDICINE

Investment, Wellness

CANCER IS PRESENT with few variations all around the globe and is responsible for 20 percent to 25 percent of all deaths, being the second-leading cause of death; thus, programs against cancer are implemented all over the world.

Partnerships are becoming more frequent between public and private sectors (connecting governments, health organizations, universities, private companies, and so on), and are aimed at projecting and implementing interventions to improve the population's general health and reduce the incidence of and mortality from cancer. Therefore, global investments that promote wellness and fight cancer encompass costs for initiatives in different areas of research (such as medicine, chemistry, computational biology, genetics, sociology, and nanotechnology) and prevention to reduce the risk of cancer and provide treatment and support for patients and their families.

In 2006 alone, the U.S. healthcare system spent about $210 billion for cancer-related medical costs. In the future, this amount is expected to be even higher, because life expectancy is rapidly increasing, and as people get older, they can be more easily subject to cancer. On the basis of current incidence rates, it is estimated that 33 percent of all people worldwide will develop a cancer during their lives.

It is widely believed, however, that four-fifths of all cancers are potentially avoidable and that if the rest could be diagnosed earlier, it would be possible to improve patients' chances of survival considerably. So it should be possible to reduce social costs and the economic burden at the same time.

A complete treatment—doctor's visit, hospital stays, surgery, chemotherapy, radiation care, etc—can cost up to $100,000 a year. Overall costs for cancer include not only direct medical costs, but also costs for lost productivity and mortality. Therefore, there is wide interest in strategies that can be effective in promoting general health and allowing a cost-effective use of resources.

PREVENTION STRATEGIES

Because bad lifestyles and environmental factors are considered to be responsible for almost two-thirds of all cancer deaths, millions of dollars are targeted at encouraging people to adopt healthy behaviors, such as changing to low-fat and low-alcohol diets; increasing physical activity; and avoiding smoking, excessive stress, and exposure to known cancer risk factors.

Primary prevention, a strategy that is not limited to people at high risk, has the potential for large reductions in the incidence of and mortality from cancer.

Other means that are considered to be effective in promoting wellness are early detection and diagnosis of tumors, quality treatments, and socio-psychophysical support for patients and their families.

The U.S. National Cancer Institute's budget for research projects, prevention, and care related to cancer for fiscal 2007 was almost $5 billion, 10 percent of which was for education and interventions in primary prevention. This kind of investment in wellness allows a cost-effective use of resources be-

cause, according to the Wellness Council of America, a $1 investment in wellness programs saves $3 in healthcare costs.

SEE ALSO: Cost of Therapy; Education, Cancer; Prevention, Health and Exercise; Tobacco Smoking; Western Diet.

BIBLIOGRAPHY. Atif B. Awad and Peter G. Bradford, eds., *Nutrition and Cancer Prevention* (Taylor and Francis, 2005); National Cancer Institute, "The Nation's Investment in Cancer Research," http://plan.cancer.gov (cited October 2006); Robert G. McKinnell, *Prevention of Cancer* (Chelsea House, 2006).

ALESSANDRA PADULA
UNIVERSITY OF L'AQUILA, ITALY

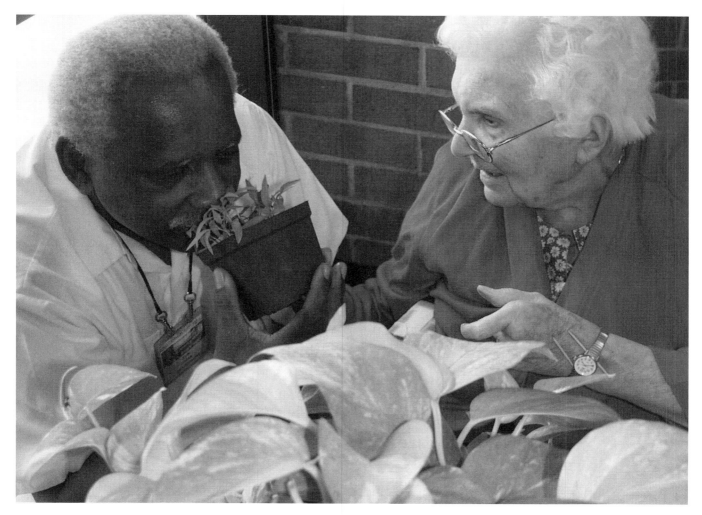

Global investments that promote wellness and fight cancer encompass costs for initiatives in different areas of research such as medicine, chemistry, computational biology, genetics, sociology, and nanotechnology, and prevention to reduce the risk of cancer.

Iran

THIS CENTRAL ASIAN country, known until March 21, 1935, as Persia, remains one of the most powerful countries in its region. It has a population of 69,019,000 (2004) and has 85 doctors and 259 nurses per 100,000 people. An example of cancer incidence rates in Iran includes 116.8 cases of cancer in males per 100,000, according to the International Agency for Research on Cancer.

There is a long history of medical research in Persia, with the university at Ahvaz being one where many doctors were trained.

The great Arab medical writer Avicenna was born in Baghdad but practiced in Persia; he was the first person to describe cancer of the esophagus and the first in Persia to conduct a mastectomy for breast cancer. He is also reported to have regularly performed surgery for the removal of carcinomas on the tongue. In his *Canon of Medicine*, he described how a cancer grows and can gradually take over the human body.

The medical scholar Jorjani lived in northeast Iran at present-day Gorgan, where he practiced cancer surgery and also described the symptoms of cancer of the esophagus, building on the work of Avicenna.

Cancer treatment in medieval and early modern, and indeed 19th-century Persia, continued to use the works of Avicenna and Jorjani. Cancer claimed the lives of many people during this period, including that of Jamal al-Din al-Afghani, a founding father of Islamic modernism.

EDUCATION AND RESEARCH FACILITIES

The Cancer Institute of Iran was established in 1955 by the Shire Khorshid Sorkh (now the National Red Cross Foundation). It was the 28th educational program of Tehran University, providing "a national point for diverse programs in prevention, early detection, patient care, education, cancer registry, community activities and international collaborations."

It is a matrix institution within the Tehran University of Medical Sciences & Health Services, with its headquarters at the Imam Khomeini Hospitals Complex in Tehran. The other major institutions connected with cancer in Iran are Imam Khomeini Medical Centre, the Research Centre of Gastroenterology and Liver Transplantation, and Shariati Hospital H.O.R.C.

Much research in Iran remains at the University of Tehran, with treatments of cancer involving nuclear medicine being conducted at the Nuclear Research Center, also in Tehran.

During the 1960s cancer statistics in Iran were collected by the different pathology laboratories in the Department of Pathology at Tehran Medical School, the Cancer Institute of Tehran, and the private pathology laboratories of Tehran.

This system resulted in the collection of much data showing that skin cancer was the most common cause of cancer in both sexes, with cervical cancer the most common cancer for women. The system of collecting data by different laboratories eventually proved unsuccessful. In 1968 a cancer registry was established in Iran as a collaboration among the International Agency for Research on Cancer and the School of Public Health, Tehran University. Its initial task was to study the high rates of esophageal cancer in Mazandran.

In 1976 a cancer registry was established at Fars, later expanding its work to cover Bakhtaran and Khozestan provinces. It initially restricted its work to histopathologically confirmed cases of cancer, later increasing its coverage. In 1980 the cancer registry was closed, but in 1984 the Iranian parliament, the Majlis, passed the Cancer Registration Bill, making it compulsory to register all cases of cancer with the Ministry of Health and Medical Education. The cancer registry was reopened in 1991, and three years later the Cancer Institute of Iran, with a grant from the Ministry of Health and Medical Education, set about merging the results collected from regional cancer registries throughout the country, with the plan of getting more accurate records for the entire country. The first major publication was a report of cancer incidence in Tehran between 1998 and 2001. In 1996 the Imam Khomeini Medical Center Hospital-Based Cancer Registry was established.

The major forms of cancer in Iran today for men are lung cancer, followed by stomach cancer, liver cancer, esophageal cancer, colorectal cancer, and prostate cancer. For women, breast cancer and cervical cancer remain the most important, with stomach cancer, colorectal cancer, lung cancer, and liver cancer also being important.

Mohammed Riza Pahlavi, the shah of Iran, sought treatment from the famous French doctor Dr. Georges

Flandrin when he began to suffer from cancer. When he was forced to leave Iran in February 1979, he went first to Egypt and then to Morocco, the Bahamas, and Mexico. He was suffering badly from non-Hodgkin's lymphoma and wanted to go to the United States to seek medical treatment. He was eventually allowed to go to New York for just over two months, from October to December 1979. From there, he left for Panama and then Egypt, where he died. One of the shah's younger brothers, Prince Ahmed Reza Pahlavi, died in Switzerland from lymphatic cancer in 1981. Sohrab Sepehri, a popular Iranian poet died from blood cancer. A bitter opponent of the shah, Zhoobin Razani, also died from cancer.

SEE ALSO: Skin Cancer (Melanoma); Skin Cancer (Non-Melanoma); Surgery.

BIBLIOGRAPHY. Cyril Elgood, *A Medical History of Persia and the Eastern Caliphate: From the Earliest Times Until the Year AD 1932* (Cambridge University Press, 1951); Cyril Elgood, *Safavid Medical Practice Between 1500 AD and 1750 AD* (B. Luzac, 1970); "Cancer Institute of Iran," http://194.225.51.19/CANCER/Default.htm (cited November 2006); Cyril Elgood, *Medicine in Persia* (P. B. Hoeber, 1934);

JUSTIN CORFIELD
GEELONG GRAMMAR SCHOOL, AUSTRALIA

Iraq

THIS MIDDLE EASTERN country, located astride the Tigris and Euphrates Rivers, was formed after World War I, officially gaining its independence from the Ottoman Empire on October 1, 1919, and from Britain on October 3, 1932. It has a population of 25,375,000 (2004) and has 55 doctors and 236 nurses per 100,000 people. An example of cancer incidence rates in Iraq includes 123.4 cases of cancer in males per 100,000, according to the International Agency for Research on Cancer.

The oldest reference to cancer in Iraq was made in Babylonian cuneiform from about 2000 B.C.E. There are also references to Mar-Samuel, director of a school of higher learning in Babylon, who de-

scribed his medical teachings in the Jewish Gemara, making mention of various forms of what are now known to be cancers.

In early medieval times, Avicenna, born in Baghdad, wrote his *Canon of Medicine,* in which he described how a cancer grows and gradually takes over the human body. He is said to be the first person to describe cancer of the esophagus.

During the early 20th century Baghdad underwent a partial revival, but the boom from the sale of oil after World War II resulted in more money being spent on medical health treatments, including cancer research. Khalid Qassab, professor of surgery at the College of Medicine in Baghdad, worked on the pattern of skin cancer in Iraq, and Tahseen Al-Saleem, Zuhair Bahrani, and Farhan Bakir worked on the pathology of malignant lymphomas of the small intestine.

In 1979 Saddam Hussein became president. Some biographies record that his older brother had died of leukemia when he was 13, just before Saddam Hussein's birth; others state that he did not have an older brother but lived with members of his extended family. During his first years as president, the health services in the country were improved, with more funds given to the cancer registry that had been established in 1976, one of the first in the region.

During the Iran-Iraq war, the war economy resulted in cutbacks of medical services in Iraq, and following international sanctions after Iraq's invasion of Kuwait in August 1990, medical services deteriorated badly. Western drugs for cancer treatment in Iraq became hard to import, and many people died prematurely.

EFFECTS OF WAR

A vast increase in cancer deaths was attributed by many commentators to the use of depleted uranium by the United States and its allies in Desert Storm in 1991. Certainly, Iraq pointed to this in government press releases. Following the U.S. invasion of Iraq, a large number of senior officials in the Saddam Hussein regime were detained by the Americans. On December 2, 2005, the U.S. authorities announced that one of them had died in their custody but did not name him.

Two days later in court, Barzan Ibrahim al-Tikriti named the man who had died as Mohammed Amza az-Zubeidi, prime minister of Iraq from 1991 to 1993. Barzan Ibrahim al-Tikriti stated that the former prime minister had died because of inadequate medical treatment.

Two women in Saddam Hussein's regime appeared in the world media during the invasion, both of whom were involved in cancer research. Dr. Rihab Rashid Taha al-Azawi, nicknamed "Doctor Germ" by the media, is a British-educated Iraqi scientist who was involved in work on, among other areas, aflatoxins that can cause liver cancer.

Huda Salih Mahdi Ammash, an Iraqi scientist dubbed "Miss Anthrax" by some U.S. newspapers, was the only woman featured in the Iraq "deck of cards." She completed her doctoral thesis on radiation at the University of Missouri-Columbia in 1983. She is now suffering from breast cancer, which may have been a result of her research on depleted uranium.

Sir Austen Layard, a British archaeologist who worked on the Assyrian capital at Nimrud, died from cancer. Other Britons with connections to Iraq who died of cancer were painter James Boswell; archaeological conservator Anna Plowden; and David Talbot Rice, a Byzantine scholar who worked initially as an archaeologist in Iraq.

There are close connections between Jordan and Iraq; the two royal houses are closely related. Prince Mi'red bin Ra'ad, second son of Prince Ra'ad, head of the royal house of Iraq, has been director of the King Hussein Cancer Foundation since 2003.

Elias Alsabti, an Iraqi medical researcher, posed as a member of the Jordanian royal family to gain a Jordanian government grant and wrote extensively on cancer research in the United States. It was later found that his articles, some with possibly bogus co-authors, had been reworked from other publications.

SEE ALSO: Breast Cancer; Chemotherapy; Radiation.

BIBLIOGRAPHY. A. M. Baruchin and H. Zirkin, "From the Times of Mar-Samuel to Those of Marjolin," *Burns Including Thermal Injuries* (v.12, 1985); William J. Broad, "*Would-Be Academician Pirates Papers: Five of his Published Papers Are Demonstrable Plagiarisms, and More Than 55 Others Are Suspect*," Science (v.208, 1980); Ronald W. Raven, *The Theory and Practice of Oncology* (Parthenon, 1990).

JUSTIN CORFIELD
GEELONG GRAMMAR SCHOOL, AUSTRALIA

Ireland

LOCATED ON THE island of Ireland, off the coast of Great Britain, the Republic of Ireland was occupied by the British until January 21, 1919, when the Irish Republic, or Eire, was proclaimed. It was recognized by the British on December 6, 1922. Eire had a population of 4,235,000 in 2006, with 219 doctors and 1593 nurses per 100,000. An example of cancer incidence rates in Ireland includes 273.6 cases of cancer in males per 100,000, according to the International Agency for Research on Cancer.

Until the foundation of the Dublin Society of Surgeons in March 1780, many barbers in Dublin continued the medieval practice of combining the cutting of hair with basic surgery, including the cutting out of tumors. Although this may have been preferable to some of the herbal concoctions, as well as those made from entrails of animals, said to cure cancer, the increasing number of scientific discoveries that occurred starting in the mid-18th century prompted the increased regulation of professions.

Over many years, large numbers of prominent Irish have been involved in medical research into cancer. Richard Thomas Tracy (1826–74), who later became a prominent surgeon in Australia, where he performed many operations for cancer of the ovary, was born in Limerick, Ireland. John Joly (1857–1933) was born in King's County and was a prominent geologist and physicist, who, in 1914, developed a method for extracting radium and was involved in pioneering its use in radiotherapy for cancer treatment.

Probably the most famous Irish cancer researcher was Denis Parsons Burkitt (1911–93), who was born in Enniskillen in Northern Ireland and who studied at the University of Dublin. He later moved to Africa where, in Uganda, he noticed a child with a large swelling, which led Burkitt to describe a new cancer that he called Burkitt's lymphoma.

During the 1960s and 1970s, many researchers worked in Ireland on anticancer treatments. R. Douglas Thornes of the Cancer Research Laboratories, Department of Medicine, Royal College of Surgeons in Ireland, studied antistromal therapy of human carcinomata. V.C. Barry, et al., from the Medical Research Council of Ireland, Trinity College, Dublin, worked on the relationship of chemical structure to anticancer activity in substituted thiosemicarbazide derivatives of dicarbonyl compounds. P.F. Fottrell and Carmel M. Spellman of the Department of Biochemistry, University College, Galway, worked on the similarities between pyruvate kinase from human placenta and tumors, and D. O'B. Hourihane, of the School of Pathology, Trinity College, worked on the links between asbestos and cancer.

In 1975, the Southern Tumour Registry was established—the first cancer registry in the Republic of Ireland. With staff drawn from the University College, Cork, it collected extensive data from 1977 until November 1991, when the Irish National Cancer Registry was established by the Department of Health, taking over the staff and the functions of its predecessor. By 1994, the registry covered the entire country, although still relying on staff from Cork, as well as the Department of Health and the Irish Cancer Society. Registration officers are based throughout the country to ensure that figures are accurate.

In Ireland, skin cancer and oral cancer rates are particularly high; historically, there have been 10 times the number of people in Ireland suffering from cancer of the lip than in England. In November 2006, the Cervical Screening Research Consortium was launched in Ireland with 1.25 million euros in funds from the Health Research Board.

SEE ALSO: Irish Cancer Society; Lymphoma, Burkitt's.

BIBLIOGRAPHY. Joan E. Cleary, *Breast Cancer: Experiences of Irish Women* (M.Phil. Thesis, Trinity College, 1994); Frank M.C. Forster, "Richard Thomas Tracy and His Part in the History of Ovariotomy," *Australian New Zealand Journal of Obstetrics and Gynecology* (v.4, 1964); B. Glemser, *Man Against Cancer: Research & Progress* (Bodley, 1969.

JUSTIN CORFIELD
GEELONG GRAMMAR SCHOOL

Ireland (Ohio) Cancer Center

THE IRELAND CANCER Center in Cleveland, Ohio, is part of the University Hospitals systems, which is affiliated with Case Western Reserve University. University Hospitals forms the largest center for biomedical research in Ohio and includes Rainbow Babies and Children's Hospital and MacDonald Women's Hospital. University Hospitals, formed in 1993, offers preventive care, screening, and primary care as well as tertiary medicine. Together, the University Hospitals have 947 beds and provide more than 3 million outpatient visits and 100,000 inpatient discharges annually.

TREATMENT FACILITIES

The Ireland Cancer Center has been designated as a Comprehensive Cancer Center by the National Cancer Institute (NCI) and provides care for over 200,000 patients annually. The center currently has 75 inpatient beds but is planning expansion to a freestanding building in 2009, which will increase the number of beds available to 200 and will bring all services and departments under one roof. Several community-based cancer centers in northern Ohio, known as Ireland Cancer Center Community Sites, are associated with Ireland Cancer Center and provide individualized, multidisciplinary treatment services in the same manner as the Ireland Cancer Center. Ireland Cancer Center Community Sites include the University Hospitals Chagrin Highlands Health Center, University Hospitals Landerbrook, University Suburban Health Center, University Hospitals Westlake Health Center, Community Health Partners Ireland Cancer Center, Lake/University Ireland Cancer Center, and Southwest General Hospital Ireland Cancer Center.

Patient care at the Ireland Cancer Center is provided through a multidisciplinary team, which may include experts in surgery, medical oncology, radiation therapy, diagnostic imaging, pathology, nursing, social work, behavioral medicine, genetic counseling, and psychology. Pediatric cancer care is offered through collaboration between the Ireland Cancer Center and Rainbow Babies and Children's Hospital. The Division of Pediatric Hematology/Oncology at Rainbow is a member of the Children's Cancer Group and a major referral center for children with leukemia, lymphoma, childhood solid tumors, and brain tumors. Special programs within pediatric cancer care include the Sickle Cell Anemia Center, the Pediatric Blood and Marrow Transplant Program, and the Hemophilia Treatment Center.

CLINICAL TRIALS AND RESEARCH PROGRAMS

Over 300 clinical trials are active at the Ireland Cancer Center, many featuring drugs developed at the center. The Ireland Cancer Center is one of only eight cancer centers in the United States to have access to a pipeline of new drugs for early-phase clinical trials through the NCI.

The Cancer Prevention, Control and Population Research Program at the Ireland Cancer Center aims to decrease cancer incidence, morbidity, mortality, and effect on quality of life by improving the delivery of cancer detection and prevention services in the primary-care setting, facilitating use of technology in genetic screening for cancer risk, identifying markers for cancer incidence, and increasing the utilization of cancer prevention and detection services among underserved populations.

The Cancer Genetics Program at University Hospitals includes personnel from the Ireland Cancer Center and the Center for Human Genetics. The Cancer Genetics Program provides families medical evaluations, genetic consultations, risk assessments, cancer screenings, and guidance. Testing is also offered for individuals who have a strong family history of cancer or who have already been diagnosed with cancer, to allow physicians to determine whether the patients are likely to develop other cancers and to plan prevention and screening programs. Diseases for which the Cancer Genetics Program offers testing include breast cancer, childhood overgrowth syndrome, colon cancer, Li-Fraumeni syndrome, multiple endocrine neoplasia types 1 and 2, neurofibromatosis type 2, ovarian cancer, osteosarcoma, prostate cancer, retinoblastoma, Von Hipple-Lindau syndrome, and Wilms' tumor.

SUPPORT SERVICES AND HOSPICE SERVICES

Support services at the Ireland Cancer Center are provided for cancer survivors and their families, including the services of specialized nurses, dieticians, social workers, psychologists, occupational and physical therapists, pharmacists, spiritual counselors, and music and art therapists.

In addition, the center provides a toll-free telephone line that offers advice, referrals, and information about clinical trials; cancer research and treatment; and cancer prevention, screening, and education. As of 2006 it logged nearly 4,000 calls annually.

The Center for Survivors of Breast Cancer allows survivors to meet with an interdisciplinary team—including nurse practitioners, social workers, dietitians, and other health professionals—to create an individualized plan to promote their health and lessen the health effects of cancer and cancer treatment. Resources are also available to address financial, employment, and insurance issues. Group classes and activities are available through the center to provide information and support to breast-cancer survivors and their families.

The Childhood Cancer Survivor Center at Rainbow Babies and Children's Hospital offers long-term follow-up and advocacy services for survivors and their families. Staff members at the center also conduct clinical and basic research that address issues central to childhood cancer survivors, including later risks of cancer or infertility due to radiation treatments, and psychological difficulties that may make it difficult for them to adjust to adult life.

SEE ALSO: Clinical Trials; Disparities, Issues in Cancer; National Cancer Institute; Survivors of Cancer; Survivors of Cancer Families.

BIBLIOGRAPHY. Ireland Cancer Center website, www.irelandcancercenter.org (cited December 2006).

SARAH BOSLAUGH
WASHINGTON UNIVERSITY SCHOOL OF MEDICINE

Irish Cancer Society

THE IRISH CANCER Society (ICS) is the national charity for cancer care in Ireland. Its chief priority is providing quality nursing care to Irish patients. The head office is in Dublin; there is another office in Cork.

The ICS mission statement declares the society as being dedicated to "eliminating cancer as a major health problem, and improving the lives of those living with cancer." To achieve this mission, the society has outlined six values: regard for the purpose, the role of leadership, teamwork, respect for the individual, responsibility and accountability, and stewardship.

Two subsections of the ICS are Action Breast Cancer (ABC) and Action Prostate Cancer (APC). ABC was started in 2001 to support breast-cancer research and provide support to patients and their loved ones. Services provided are free and confidential. APC was launched in 2006 to provide information on prostate cancer and support its patients and caregivers. Both programs have free telephone hotlines and numerous resources.

The ICS has a research division called Cancer Research Ireland (CRI), which was organized to evaluate cancer-research proposals in Ireland and to recommend projects to the society for funding. Cancer experts who sit on the CRI board are from Ireland as well as other nations.

Recently, the CRI opened funding to nursing research grants. Research may be carried out at hospitals and relevant institutions toward evidence-based nursing.

Additionally, nurses studying for a degree or a master's degree can receive financial support through Daffodil Bursaries. These funds are provided to defray the costs of education.

RESOURCES AND PUBLIC EDUCATION

The ICS website has resources for Irish cancer patients and their loved ones. A special resource is for patients who have recently been diagnosed with cancer. There are also a live chat/message board for anyone who wants to interact with others in the same position and resources for quitting smoking. The society manages many education and awareness initiatives to serve the public. One such initiative is the SunSmart program, which teaches communities how to prevent skin cancer, which is the most common cancer in Ireland.

The society maintains numerous support groups for patients and their families. These can be broadly categorized, such as Cancer Plus for parents of cancer patients and Can Teen for teenagers with cancer, or specialized, such as Men Against Cancer, a group for prostate- and testicular-cancer patients.

SEE ALSO: European Oncology Nursing Society; Oncology Nursing Society; World Health Organization.

BIBLIOGRAPHY. Irish Cancer Society, *One Day in Ireland* (Corgi, 1989); Heather Porter, "International Affairs," *Cancer Nursing* (v.9, 1986); Connie Henke Yarbro, et al., eds., *Cancer Nursing: Principles and Practice (Jones and Bartlett Series in Oncology)* (Jones & Bartlett Publishers, 2005).

Claudia Winograd
University of Illinois at Urbana-Champaign

Israel

THIS MIDDLE EASTERN country was founded in 1948 from what had been the British mandated territory of Palestine. As the only Jewish state in the world, it has a policy of encouraging Jewish people from all over the world to settle in the country, resulting in one of the most culturally diverse populations in the world. The Republic of Israel has a population of 7,047,000 (2006), with 385 doctors and 613 nurses per 100,000 people. An example of cancer incidence rates in Israel includes 295.6 cases of cancer in males per 100,000, according to the International Agency for Research on Cancer.

Cancer was known in ancient times, and a reference in the Tohoroth section of the Talmud appears to describe vaginal dermoid cyst. During much of the medieval and early modern periods there was extensive use of Arab surgical practices, but medical treatment was usually beyond the reaches of most people in the Holy Land.

In 1920 the Kupat Holim Clatit, the largest sickness fund, was founded by the General Federation of Labor in Palestine, with further sick funds established during the 1930s: the Amamit Sick Fund, the Leumit Sickness Fund, and the Mercazit Sick Fund. These and subsequent funds continue to provide health insurance for many people in the country, assisted significantly by Christian and other charitable organizations. In a small country with a highly developed medical insurance system, it was natural that mass screening of people should be introduced early. Nathan Trainin's evaluation for the Israel Cancer Association showed that mass screening of women for breast cancer has had positive results, with a fall in the number of women dying of breast cancer. Because the population of Israel has been drawn from all over the world, it has also been possible to study the incidence rates of cancer in these populations, often providing useful information for the health services in their countries of origin.

CANCER RESEARCH

In the 1960s much research on cancer took place in Israel. Michael Schlessinger from Hebrew University's Hadassah Medical School in Jerusalem worked on the isoantigens in thymic grafts in mice.

During the 1970s A. Adler, et al., from the Institute of Oncology, Hadassa Hospital, and Tel Aviv Medical

School worked on delayed-hypersensitivity skin reactions in 220 breast-cancer patients.

G. M. Goldberg from the Department of Anatomy and Anthropology at Tel Aviv University Medical School at Ramat Aviv worked on the incidence of malignant hepatoma in the Negev, discovering an incidence rate among the Bedouins in the Negev that was 6.6 times higher than that in the Jewish population.

J. Bar-Ziv and G. M. Goldberg of the Department of Radiology at the M. Soroka Negev Medical Center, Beer-Sheba, and the Department of Anatomy and Anthropology at Tel Aviv University Medical School worked on scar carcinoma of the lung. A. Yerushalmi of the Radiation Unit at the Weizmann Institute of Science at Rehevot researched a cure of a radioresistant tumor by simultaneous administration of heat and x-ray irradiation. E. Robinson, S. Sher, and T. Mekori from the Department of Oncology at Rambam University Hospital and the Aba Khoushy School of Medicine in Haifa worked on lymphocyte stimulation by phytohemagglutinin and tumor cells of malignant effusions H. J. Brenner, J. Medalie, and F. Ch. Izsack of Sheba Hospital, Tel Hashomer and Donolo Hospital, Jaffa, and Tel Aviv University Medical School studied multiphasic early detection screening systems.

Chloe Tal of the Laboratory of Experimental Neurology, Hadassah University Hospital, worked on the nature of the cell membrane receptor for the agglutination factor present in the sera of tumor patients and pregnant women.

G. M. Goldberg and Isidor L. Kozenitzki from the Institute of Pathology, Negev Central Hospital, Beer-Sheba, studied malignant lymphomas and leukemias.

Several senior Israeli politicians suffered from cancer, including Chaim Weizmann, president from 1948 to 1952, who lived with cancer for many years; his successor, Isaac Ben-Zvi, who died of cancer; Moshe Sharett, prime minister from 1953 to 1955, who succumbed to cancer; and Golda Meir, prime minister from 1969 to 1974, who died from leukemia. Mordechai Gur, chief of staff from 1974 to 1978, committed suicide after being diagnosed with terminal cancer.

The Israel National Cancer Registry, Jerusalem, was established in the early 1950s and joined the Middle East Cancer Consortium in 1996, sharing cancer information with Cyprus, Egypt, Jordan, the Palestinian Authority, and Turkey. The Israel Cancer Association is a member of the International Union Against Cancer, as is the Patient's Friends Society–Jerusalem (a nongovernmental Palestinian organization).

SEE ALSO: Breast Cancer; Insurance; Radiation Therapy.

BIBLIOGRAPHY. Solomon Robert Kagan, *Jewish Medicine* (Medio-Historical Press, Boston, 1952); D. M. Parkin, et al., eds., *Cancer Incidence in Five Continents,* vol. VII (International Agency for Research on Cancer and International Association of Cancer Registries, 1997); Alan D. Steinfeld and Henry C. McDuff, "An Ancient Report of a Dermoid Cyst of the Vagina," *Surgery, Gynecology & Obstetrics* (v.150, 1980); R. Steinitz, et al., *Cancer Incidence in Jewish Migrants to Israel 1961–1981* (International Agency for Research in Cancer, 1989); Andrew C. Twaddle, *Health Care Reform around the World* (Auburn House, 2002).

JUSTIN CORFIELD
GEELONG GRAMMAR SCHOOL, AUSTRALIA

Italy

THIS EUROPEAN COUNTRY, with a population of 58,000,000 (2004), has one of the best health services in Europe, with 554 doctors and 296 nurses per 100,000 people. An example of cancer incidence rates in Italy includes 321.3 cases of cancer in males per 100,000, according to the International Agency for Research on Cancer.

The history of cancer research in Italy dates back to ancient times, when Aulus Cornelius Celsus came up with the idea of the systematic teaching of medicine after being influenced by the ideas of Greek and Alexandrian doctors. Clarissimus Galen, born at Pergamon in Asia Minor, also studied at Alexandria and then became a physician in Rome. He described cancer with his humoral theory, which was accepted for nearly a thousand years.

Breast cancer was said to have afflicted Saint Agatha, who was tortured to death by Quintinian, a Roman consul whose advances she had spurned. The story of her life included having both her breasts cut off and then restored by Saint Peter just before her death. The patron saint of cancer patients, Peregrine Laziosi, was a friar from the Servite Order. He was said to have been cured of cancer and was canonized as Saint Peregrine in 1726. Some medical historians reading the surviving evidence, however, suggest it was more likely that he was suffering from an extremely bad case of varicose veins.

During the 16th century the centers for medical research were at Bologna, Padua, and Pisa, with many students from elsewhere in Italy, as well as France and other countries, studying there. Vasallius was professor of anatomy at Pisa and then Padua. One of his students, Gabriele Fallopis (or Fallopius), made some discoveries about uterine cancer. Mention should also be made of Marco Aurelio Severino, who wrote about cancers; his book contained pictures of surgical procedures and lesions. In these pictures he showed the differences between benign and malignant tumors, advising the excision of benign breast tumors because he felt that they could easily lead to malignant ones. In 1530 in Naples, Antonio Ferri was the first to describe prostate tumors, which caused bladder-outlet obstruction. In 1713 Bernardino Ramazzini, professor of medicine at the University of Padua, noticed that breast cancer was common among nuns and was one of the first to search for an environmental or occupational reason. He surmised that it was because of lack of sexual intercourse.

One advance in cancer treatment was made in 1835, when Zanobi Pecchioli, professor of surgery at the University of Siena, removed a meningioma. A wealthy Italian, Casare Mattei, developed a homeopathic cure that was alleged to have cured Lady Walburga Paget, wife of Sir August Paget, British ambassador to Vienna. Italian physician Tomasso De Amicis wrote a monograph about Kaposi's sarcoma in 1882. This cancer is particularly prevalent among African men and other men who live in the Mediterranean region. Marie Curie visited Italy in 1932, raising the profile of cancer research. After World War II, as Italy prospered, impetus was placed on health services and cancer research.

POST-WORLD WAR II RESEARCH

A. di Marco, et al., from the National Institute of Tumors, Milan, studied the metabolic degradation and antineoplastic activity of Daunomycin. Luciano Morasca and Chiara Rainisio of the Instituto di Ricerche Farmacologiche Mario Negri, Milan, worked on the perfusion of T.C. cells by the blood of animals treated with antineoplastic agents.

Augusto de Barbieri of the Instituto Sieroterapico Milanese, Milan, worked on the synthesis and screening of substances acting by alkylation and metabolic inhibition. A.M. Dogliotti and L. Caldarola of the Clinica Chirurgica dell'Università di Torino, Instituto di Oncologia di Torino, worked on endoarterial cancer therapy with radiating resin microspheres.

G.G. Cavallucci, et al., of the Institute of Cancer Research, Naples, worked on the effect of cortisone on the endothelial proliferation during the local growth of rat tumor Guerin T8. Natale Pennelli, et al., from the Division of Experimental Cancer at the Institute of Anatomy and Pathology at the University of Padua, worked on the presence and biological significance of the murane leukemia virus particles in megakaryicytes. Two Italians became prominent in cancer research in London. Renato Dulbecco was a virologist who spent five years as director of the Imperial Cancer Research Fund in London. He shared the 1975 Nobel Prize for Physiology or Medicine with Howard M. Temin and David Baltimore, both of whom had studied under him. Guido Pontecorvo was a geneticist who discovered the process of genetic recombination in the fungus *Aspergillus*. He moved to London in 1968 and worked at the Imperial Cancer Research Fund Laboratories until his retirement in 1975. Salvador Luria won the 1969 Nobel Prize for Physiology or Medicine for research on bacteriophages, viruses that infect bacteria. Five years later he became the director of the Center for Cancer Research at the Massachusetts Institute of Technology.

SEE ALSO: Breast Cancer; Education; Kaposi's Sarcoma.

BIBLIOGRAPHY. Arturo Castiglioni, *Italian Medicine* (P.B. Hoeber, 1932); Renato Giuffre, "Successful Radical Removal of an Intracranial Meningioma in 1835 by Professor Pecchioli of Siena," *Journal of Neurosurgery* (v.60, 1984); Robert Jackson, "St. Peregrine O.S.M.—Patron Saint of Cancer Patients," *Canadian Medical Association Journal* (v.111, 1971); D. G. Lytton, et al., "Galen on Abnormal Swellings," *Journal of the History of Medicine and the Allied Sciences* (v.33, 1978); James S. Olson, *Bathsheba's Breast: Women, Cancer and History* (Johns Hopkins University Press, 2002).

JUSTIN CORFIELD
GEELONG GRAMMAR SCHOOL, AUSTRALIA

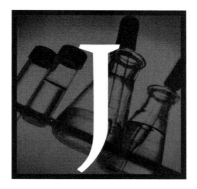

Jackson Laboratory

JACKSON LABORATORY (JAX-LAB) is a not-for-profit institution with a mission "to improve the quality of human life through discoveries arising from our own genetic research and by enabling the research and education of others." It maintains over 1,200 employees, nearly 500 of whom are dedicated researchers and nearly 200 of whom have a doctorate or similar qualification.

The laboratory has five major research areas: bioinformatics, development and aging related, immune system and blood disorders, metabolic diseases, and neurological and sensory disorders. It also conducts an extensive research program with respect to cancer.

MOUSE BREEDING

To facilitate research, JAX-Lab produces a wide range of mice for distribution to research laboratories internationally. Some 2.3 million such mice have been distributed to 12,000 laboratories.

The mice, which are supervised and protected by the Laboratory Animal Health Services program, are bred with 800 specified mutations, including cancer, heart disease, and Huntington's disease. Breeding these mice can be a complex process, as the various mutations induced in the animals can render them sterile or be otherwise problematic and hence require supplementary surgical techniques. The breeding

program takes place in an advanced-technology stable, where considerable information has been gathered and presented in the Mouse Genome Database. Sale of mice raised nearly $70 million in 2004, and this contributed greatly to the overall annual revenue of some $137 million.

The use of laboratory animals has been widespread throughout the history of experimental research, and many important discoveries have been attributed to their use. A significant element of people believe, however, that the use of laboratory animals in medical research is unacceptable on ethical grounds, irrespective of the care with which the animals are treated.

JAX-Lab was founded in 1922 by C.C. Little, who had served as president of the University of Maine and the University of Michigan, and who was active in mouse breeding for research purposes. The laboratory, then called Roscoe B. Jackson Memorial Laboratory, was established in Bar Harbor, Maine, with support from several Detroit-based industrialists. Mice were being sold to researchers elsewhere by 1933, and students had already begun to study at the laboratory under the supervision of a team of experienced researchers.

In 1940 William Russell successfully completed the first transfer of ovaries between mice, thereby greatly enhancing the ability of laboratory staff to breed mice with the required mutations and diseases. In the same decade, a major fire destroyed most of the laboratory and its mice; the importance of the laboratory to scientific understanding is apparent from the fact that donations of money and mice were received from around the world to assist in the reconstruction.

The facility is still vulnerable to fire. In 1989, a large fire at the Morrell Park headquarters in Maine led to the deaths of around 400,000 mice and, consequently, a lack of mice for research.

MOUSE GENOME DATABASE

The laboratory has continued to develop and to make new discoveries in support of its aims. It also took a leadership role in disseminating information and data to interested scientific parties, which resulted in the Mouse Genome Database and its availability online. Work by Joseph Nadeau and Ben Taylor published in 1983 demonstrated that the mouse genome represents a good approximation of the human genome, albeit with several known reversions.

New buildings and facilities were acquired as the research success of scientists led to new research grants, sponsorship, and support. By 1976, for example, the world's largest mammalian research program maintained some 700,000 mice with a total budget of $9 million.

The ability to transfer tissue between animals was significantly assisted by JAX-Lab researcher George D. Snell, who won the 1980 Nobel Prize for Physiology or Medicine. The laboratory is designated by the National Cancer Institute as a Cancer Center at which research is licensed; it is considered to be critical to the success of the national effort to combat cancer. It is the world's most important mammalian-management center for scientific and medicinal research.

JAX-Lab maintains an official website at www. jax.org. It also maintains a Mouse Genome Informatics website at www.informatics.jax.org; this site contains a great deal of data related to the Mouse Genome Database.

An autobiographical extract by George D. Snell is available at http://nobelprize.org/nobel_prizes/ medicine/laureates/1980/snell-autobio.html.

SEE ALSO: Genetics; Technology, New Therapies.

BIBLIOGRAPHY. Earl L. Green, ed., *Biology of the Laboratory Mouse*, 2d ed. (Dover Publications, 1966); Hedrich, Hans, ed., *The Laboratory Mouse* (Academic Press, 2004); J. H. Nadeau and B. A. Taylor, "Lengths of Chromosomal Segments Conserved Since Divergence of Man and Mouse," *Proceedings of the National Academy of the Sciences of the USA* (v.81, 1984).

JOHN WALSH
SHINAWATRA UNIVERSITY

Japan

THIS EAST ASIAN country, consisting of islands, has a recorded history going back to ancient times, with a royal family (previously the imperial family) that traces its ancestry back to 660 B.C.E. Japan has a population of 128,085,000 (2005), with 193 doctors and 745 nurses per 100,000 people. An example of cancer incidence rates in Japan includes 261.5 cases of cancer in males per 100,000, according to the International Agency for Research on Cancer.

Japan has one of the lowest rates of coronary heart disease in the world, and the incidence of lung cancer and of breast cancer in females is historically very low, although that of stomach cancer is high, possibly because of the Japanese diet. Breast and colon cancer incidence rates have recently caught up with rates observed in Western countries.

Cancer is one of the major causes of death in Japan, and it seems likely that this was the case for hundreds of years, before detailed records were kept. Archaeologists working on sites in Japan have unearthed skeletons from the medieval period that showed evidence of bone cancer. It is also believed that the militant Buddhist monk Nichiren died from cancer of the intestinal tract.

One recent study showed that the human T-cell leukemia–lymphoma virus was found in Japan but was limited to the coastal regions of Kyushu and Shikoku. When this extremely rare form of cancer also was found in Mozambique and South Africa, researchers concluded that the strain of cancer might be hereditary and could have been brought by Portuguese traders who lived in the Kyushu region during the 16th century. It is believed that the traders brought the disease from Africa.

During the late 19th century there was considerable improvement in Japan's medical services. The Japanese Foundation for Cancer Research was established in

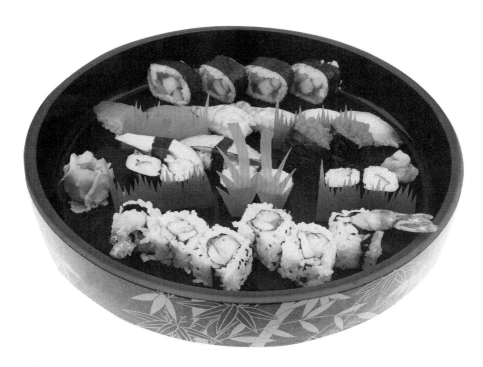

Japanese sushi delicacies: The incidence of stomach cancer in Japan is high compared to other developed countries, possibly a result of the traditional Japanese diet that includes raw fish but also rice and vegetables.

1908, and Japanese researchers have been prominent in cancer research since then. Beginning in the 1910s, Japanese contributions were published in *Journal of Cancer Research* and many other journals.

Japanese cancer researchers of that period included Katsusaburo Yamagiwa and Kokichi Ichikawa, who were involved in the first experimental production of tar cancer in rabbits by painting them with tar products. The work of Yamagiwa was so important that during the 1920s and 1930s Polish researchers were involved in following up his research in working out the causes of cancer in animals.

In the period after World War II, several studies of cancer rates among people in Hiroshima and Nagasaki who survived the nuclear bombing of their cities in 1945 showed much higher rates of many cancers. Continued follow up of survivors of the atomic bombs has contributed substantialy to the understanding of radiation and cancer risk.

In 1955 Hidao Umezawa developed phleomycin; 11 years later, he put together the compound drug bleomycin. The two most prominent Japanese medical specialists are Nobel laureates Susumu Tonegawa and Koichi Tanaka. In 1987 Tonegawa was awarded

the Nobel Prize for Physiology or Medicine for his discovery of the genetic mechanisms underlying the great diversity of antibodies produced by the vertebrate immune system. Tanaka won the 2002 Nobel Prize for Chemistry along with John B. Fenn and Kurt Wüthrich for developing techniques to identify and analyze proteins and other large biological molecules. Tanaka's soft laser desorption technique has since proved extremely useful in the early detection of certain types of cancer and other diseases.

Other Japanese cancer specialists include H. Baba, T. Harada, M. Ito, S. Morikawa, Y. Nakamura, and K. Yasuhira. Also, Tatsuhei Kongo, Hidehito Ichihashi, and Munehisa Imaizumi from the Department of Surgery at Nagoya University have contributed to medical understanding of the significance of host in the effectiveness of carcinostatic agents.

The many Japanese people and others connected with Japan who died of cancer include Emperor Hirohito, who died from complications from surgery for duodenal cancer; professional wrestler Shohei Baba; film director Shohei Imamura, who died from liver cancer; actor Kinji Fukasaku, who had prostate cancer; Tsuguharu Foujita, a prominent painter who died from cancer in Switzerland; and Sir Fred Warner, British ambassador to Japan from 1972 to 1975.

SEE ALSO: Gastric (Stomach) Cancer; Japanese Gastric Cancer Association; Radiation.

BIBLIOGRAPHY. R. Keith Cannan, "Contribution to the Work of the Atomic Bomb Casualty Commission," *Archives of Environmental Health* (v.21, 1970); Robert Gallo, et al., "Origin of Human T-Cell Leukemia-Lymphoma Virus," *Lancet* (v.2, 1983); F. Henschen, "Yamigawa's Tar Cancer and Its Historical Significance," *Gann* (v.59, 1968); Shigeo Hino, et al., "HTLV and the Propagation of Christianity in Nagasaki," *Lancet* (v.2, 1984); E. Murakami, et al., "Progress in Studies on Stomach Cancer in Japan," *Journal of Japanese Clinical Medicine* (v.25, 1965); Waro Nakahara, "A Pilgrim's Progress in Cancer Research 1918 to 1974: An Autobiographical Essay," *Cancer Research* (v.34, 1974); Toshio Oiso, "Incidence of Stomach Cancer and Its Relation to Dietary Habits and Nutrition in Japan between 1900 and 1975," *Cancer Research* (v.35, 1975); D. M. Parkin, et al., eds., *Cancer Incidence in Five Continents,* vol. VII (International Agency for Research on Cancer and International Association of Cancer Registries, 1997); T. Takahasi, "Historical Review of Cancer Research in Japan: Chemical Carcinogenesis and Biochemistry," *Protein Nucleic Acid Enzyme* (v.15, 1974).

JUSTIN CORFIELD
GEELONG GRAMMAR SCHOOL, AUSTRALIA

Japan Cancer Society

THE JAPAN CANCER Society (JCS) was established in 1958 for the purposes of furthering cancer control, promoting healthy diets and lifestyles, and minimizing cancer deaths through early detection and treatment. It is the oldest private anticancer society in Japan and was established as part of a program to commemorate the 80th anniversary of *The Asahi Shimbun* (*The Morning News*), a leading Japanese newspaper.

Funding for the JCS is partially supplied by the national and prefectural governments. Other sources of funding include the Japanese Keirin Association (which governs professional bicycle racing in Japan), the Postal Service, the Japan Lottery Association, and private donations. The main JCS office is located in Tokyo, and there are local chapters in 46 prefectures across Japan.

The JCS has three primary goals. The first is to reduce by half the number of Japanese who smoke. Activities focused on this goal include raising public awareness about the harmful effects of tobacco, targeting education to young Japanese with the intent of eliminating smoking among young people, and creating nonsmoking campaigns specifically aimed at women. The second goal is to lower the death rate from cancer by increasing the number of people who undergo cancer screening, including mammography for breast cancer and computed tomography (CT) scans for lung cancer. The third goal is to increase the survival rate for cancer patients and to improve the quality of life for both patients and cancer survivors. Efforts toward this goal include a campaign to educate the public that cancer is not necessarily a fatal disease, but one that may be cured or survived for many years.

The JCS provides over 10,000 free cancer consultations at its headquarters and local chapter offices annually, under the commission of the Ministry of Health, Labor and Welfare. Telephone consultations have also been available since 2002. JCS chapters offer mobile screening services (in specially equipped vans or buses) for the most common types of cancer, including stomach cancer; lung cancer; breast cancer; uterine cancer; and liver, gallbladder, and pancreatic cancers. The society also organizes lectures and seminars to inform the public about cancer-related topics.

PUBLICATIONS AND RESOURCES

The JCS produces and distributes pamphlets, flyers, brochures, and videos on topics such as the benefits of cancer screening, cancer prevention, and self-examination for breast cancer. The society also publishes *Cancer Society Journal,* a monthly journal.

Basic information about cancer in Japan, including trends in cancer mortality since the 1940s and mortality trends for different types of cancer since the 1970s, is available on the JCS website in English and Japanese.

SEE ALSO: Education, Cancer; Japan; Lung Cancer, Non-Small Cell; Lung Cancer, Small Cell; Screening, Access to; Smoking and Society; Tobacco Smoking.

BIBLIOGRAPHY. Japan Cancer Society website, www.jcancer.jp/en (cited November 2006).

SARAH BOSLAUGH
WASHINGTON UNIVERSITY SCHOOL OF MEDICINE

Japanese Gastric Cancer Association

THE JAPANESE GASTRIC Cancer Association (JGCA) is a scientific association that promotes basic and clinical research on gastric cancer. It was established in 1962 as the Japanese Research Society for Gastric Cancer; at that time it was a closed association whose membership consisted of 352 Japanese organizations.

In 1997 the JCGA changed its structure to that of an open association composed of individual members and adopted its current name.

Although the JGCA is primarily a Japanese organization and its official language is Japanese, the association accepts international members. In addition, the JCGA's official journal is published in English, and English-language presentations are included in some meetings and congresses. The JGCA office is located in Kyoto.

Gastric cancer is a topic of particular concern in Japan because incidence is very high. This form of cancer was the leading cause of cancer death in Japan until 1998, when it was overtaken by lung cancer. The JCGA is involved in several activities to promote the research and study of gastric cancer.

The JCGA Registration Committee oversees the nationwide registry of gastric cancer patients. The registry was founded in 1963. Currently, data on over 15,000 new patients are added each year.

The association also promotes cooperation in basic and clinical studies of gastric cancer with the International Gastric Cancer Association and the World Health Organization. A scientific congress is held each year.

PUBLICATIONS AND MEETINGS
Gastric Cancer is the official journal of the JGCA and the International Gastric Cancer Association. *Gastric Cancer* is a peer-reviewed journal published in English by Springer, including original articles, review articles, case reports, technical notes, meeting and conference reports, letters, and editorials related to stomach neoplasms.

The JCGS also publishes the *Japanese Manual of Gastric Carcinoma*, which was first published in English in 1995. A scientific congress is held each year.

SEE ALSO: Education, Cancer; Gastric (Stomach) Cancer.

BIBLIOGRAPHY. Japanese Gastric Cancer Association website, www.jgca.jp/gatkkai/foreigner.html (cited November 2006).

SARAH BOSLAUGH
WASHINGTON UNIVERSITY SCHOOL OF MEDICINE

Japan Lung Cancer Society

THE JAPAN LUNG Cancer Society (JLCS) was founded in 1960 as the Society for the Study of Lung Cancer; in 1966 the society assumed its current name. The JLCS has over 8,000 members. Its offices are located in Chiba.

The goals of the JLCS are to contribute to improvement in the study and treatment of lung cancer, to disseminate knowledge and understanding of lung cancer to the general public and medical practitioners, and to promote practical training in lung-cancer diagnosis and treatment.

Lung cancer is a particular focus of interest in Japan because it is the leading cause of cancer death. Paradoxically, although smoking rates (a prime risk factor for lung cancer) are high in Japan, lung-cancer rates are lower than in many other industrialized countries, such as the United States, and explanations have been sought in Japanese diet and lifestyle factors.

PUBLICATIONS AND MEETINGS
A particular emphasis of the society is the establishment of common rules for pathological and clinical description of lung cancer. In 1978 the JLCS published the first edition (in Japanese) of *General Rules for Clinical and Pathological Recording of Lung Cancer,* which sets forth practical and theoretical guidelines for uniform description of different types of lung cancer and aspects related to treatment and care, to allow comparison and study of clinical treatment results across

different hospitals and institutes. The first English edition was published in 2000 under the direction of Harubumi Kabo and the English Edition Subcommittee of the JLCS as *Classification of Lung Cancer*.

The JLCS publishes the *Japanese Journal of Lung Cancer* in Japanese and English. This journal publishes seven issues per year and includes original research articles, review articles, case reports, and short reports related to lung cancer. A searchable interface with links to electronic copies is available on the JLCS website. The JLCS holds annual scientific meetings.

SEE ALSO: Japan; Lung Cancer, Non-Small Cell; Lung Cancer, Small Cell; Smoking and Society; Tobacco Smoking.

BIBLIOGRAPHY. Japan Lung Cancer Society website, www.haigan.gr.jp/e (cited November 2006); The Japan Lung Cancer Society, *Classification of Lung Cancer* (Kanehara & Co. Ltd, 2000).

SARAH BOSLAUGH
WASHINGTON UNIVERSITY SCHOOL OF MEDICINE

Japanese Society for Therapeutic Radiology and Oncology

THE JAPANESE SOCIETY for Therapeutic Radiology and Oncology (JASTRO) was established in February 1988 as a membership organization of people working in healthcare or research in the fields of therapeutic radiology and oncology. The JASTRO office is located in Tokyo. The society's purpose is to promote communication and cooperation in clinical and basic research related to cancer diagnosis and treatment, particularly in radiotherapy and combined treatment modalities, including radiotherapy.

Prospective JASTRO members must be recommended by a current member and be approved by the board of directors. As of January 2005, JASTRO had over 2,600 members, primarily active members (researchers and individuals with medical or dental qualifications working in radiotherapy, diagnostic radiology, or nuclear medicine) and associate members (radiological technicians and nurses).

Three awards are bestowed at the annual meeting: the Abe Award (since 2004), the Umegaki Award for

the best paper of the year by a scientist under 40 years of age (since 1995), and the Excellent Educational Lecturer Award (since 2003). The society also provides funding for research projects of up to two years' length in radiation oncology.

JASTRO actively cooperates and exchanges information with other professional organizations, including the American Society for Therapeutic Radiation & Oncology, the European Society for Therapeutic Radiation and Oncology, and the Chinese Society of Radiation Oncology. Part of this cooperation is sending representatives from JASTRO to attend the conventions of the other radiation societies, welcoming representatives from those societies to JASTRO meetings, and including speakers from those societies at the JASTRO annual meetings.

PUBLICATIONS AND MEETINGS

Journal of the Japanese Society for Therapeutic Radiology and Oncology is the official journal of JASTRO. It is a peer-reviewed journal that has been published quarterly since 1989 and includes articles in either Japanese or English. Authors must be JASTRO members. All issues are available for free download from the society's website. JASTRO holds an annual scientific meeting. Notices of upcoming annual meetings are available on the society's website, as are informational materials from recent meetings.

SEE ALSO: American Society for Therapeutic Radiation & Oncology; European Society for Therapeutic Radiation and Oncology; Japan; Radiation; Radiation Therapy.

BIBLIOGRAPHY. Japanese Society for Therapeutic Radiology and Oncology website, www.jastro.jp/english (cited November 2006).

SARAH BOSLAUGH
WASHINGTON UNIVERSITY SCHOOL OF MEDICINE

Jensen, Elwood V.

AMERICAN ENDOCRINOLOGIST ELWOOD V. James was the winner of the Charles F. Kettering Prize of the General Motors Cancer Foundation in 1980 for "discovering the steroid receptor protein present in certain mammary cancers and for developing a method for determining which breast cancers were hormonally sensitive and thereby responsive to endocrine therapy."

Elwood Vernon Jensen was born January 13, 1920, in Fargo, North Dakota, the son of Eli A. and Vera Jensen (née Morris). His father, from Denmark, was the business manager of a college, and his mother was from North Dakota. He grew up in Springfield, Ohio, and attended Wittenberg College, graduating in 1940. He then went to the University of Chicago and gained his doctorate in organic chemistry in 1944. At that time, in the latter years of World War II, Jensen was involved in research on poison gas. From 1946 to 1947 he was a Guggenheim Fellow at the Swiss Federal Institute of Technology, his research being on synthetic rubber.

Jensen was an assistant professor in the department of surgery at the University of Chicago from 1947 to 1951 and an associate professor in the department of biochemistry from 1951 to 1960. He was a professor at the Ben May Laboratory for Cancer Research from 1951 to 1963; in 1969 he was promoted to director of the laboratory, holding that position until 1982. In 1958 he won a fellowship from the U.S. Public Health Service while he was visiting professor at the Max Planck Institute, Munich, Germany. He spent 1965 as a visiting professor at Kyoto University, Japan. Keeping up his contacts with Switzerland, he was research director of the Ludwig Institute for Cancer Research in Zurich from 1983 to 1987.

In 1990 Jensen, having reached the age of 70, had to retire. He became emeritus professor of biology at the University of Chicago and professor at the Institute of Hormone and Fertility Research at the University of Hamburg in 1992. Subsequently, he was appointed George and Elizabeth B. Wile Professor for Cancer Research at the University of Cincinnati and then John and Gladys Strauss Professor of Cancer Research at the Vontz Center for Molecular Studies at the University of Cincinnati's Medical Center.

RESEARCH

In 1947 Jensen started studying steroid hormones; he was involved in isolating estrogen receptors and discovering their importance in breast cancer. At that time much of the research was on the role of enzymes. He decided to work on whether there was a parallel between the inhibition of estrogen binding and the inhibition of cancer growth. In 1958 he used a radioactive marker to show that tissues that respond to estrogen must contain binding proteins.

In pioneering research in 1967, along with Jack Gorski of the University of Wisconsin, he showed that putative receptors were macromolecules that could be extracted from tissue.

This led to a breakthrough the following year, when Jensen was able to develop a reliable test for the presence of estrogen receptors in breast-cancer cells. During the 1970s Jensen identified an estrogen receptor in some breast cancers that made it possible to determine the effectiveness of using hormonal manipulation in some patients.

Jensen was awarded an honorary doctorate from Wittenberg College in 1963, from Acadia University in 1976, from the Medical College of Ohio in 1991, and from the University of Hamburg in 1994. He won the D. R. Edwards Medal in 1970, the La Madonnina Prize in 1973, the G. H. A. Clowes Award and the Papanicolaou Award in 1975, the Prix Roussel and the National Award from the American Cancer Society in 1976, the Amory Prize in 1977, the Gregory Pincus Memorial Award in 1978, the Gairdner Award in 1979, and the Charles F. Kettering Award in 1980, among many other awards.

In 2004 he won the Albert Lasker Award for basic medical research, for "his pioneering research on how steroid hormones, such as estrogen, exert their influence." He shared the award with Pierre Chambon of the Institute of Genetics and Molecular and Cellular Biology (Strasbourg, France), Ronald M. Evans of the Salk Institute for Biological Studies (La Jolla, California), and the Howard Hughes Medical Institute. In 2005 he was given an honorary doctorate from the University of Athens.

Jensen was made a member of the National Academy of Sciences in 1974. He is also a member of the American Academy of Arts and Science, the American Chemical Society, the American Society of Biological Chemists, the Endocrine Society (of which he was president in 1980 and 1981), the American Association for Cancer Research, and the American Association for the Advancement of Science.

SEE ALSO: Breast Cancer; Estrogens, Steroidal; United States; War Gases.

BIBLIOGRAPHY. *American Men and Women of Science* (R. R. Bowker/Gale Group, 1971–2003); Nathaniel I. Berlin, "The Conquest of Cancer," *Perspectives in Biology and Medicine* (v.22, 1979); Zachary Binney, "Elwood Jensen Discusses His Life at the University," *Chicago Maroon* (October 6, 2004); *International Who's Who* (Europe Publications, 1989–2003); *Who's Who in Technology* (Gale Research, 1989–1995).

JUSTIN CORFIELD
GEELONG GRAMMAR SCHOOL, AUSTRALIA

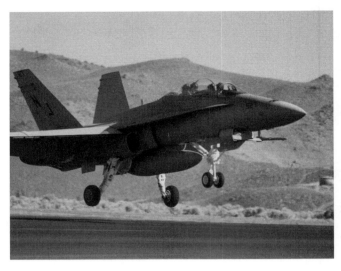

Some jet fuel additives are known carcinogens and exposure presents a risk of cancer to humans.

Jet and Rocket Fuels

JET ENGINES AND rockets burn different fuels to achieve jet propulsion. Jets and rockets are growing in numbers, and their fuels have become more sophisticated and carcinogenic in some cases.

Jets and rockets are similar in methods of propulsion. They differ in that jets take their oxidizer from the atmosphere, whereas rockets carry their oxidizer as part of their fuel package. Jets can reach near the top of the stratosphere at 40,000 to 50,000 feet. Rockets can fly in empty space because they do not need to draw oxygen from an atmosphere.

There are more than a dozen types of jet engines for jet aircraft. Most commercial and military jets use turbofan engines. Turboprop and turbojet engines are common as well. The many jet engines use fuels that vary in name and in formulation. Some are formulated for specific aircraft; others represent military designations. In practice, two main fuels are used: JET A-1 and JET B.

The most common jet fuel is JET A-1, which is produced according to an international set of specifications and is the only jet fuel used in the United States. It is an unleaded petroleum-based fuel that uses a type of paraffin.

It has a flash point above 38 degrees C (100 degrees F) and freezes at −47 degrees C. JET B fuel is a naptha–kerosene formulation that is good for cold-weather conditions. Because it has more volatile compounds, it is more flammable than JET A-1. It is dangerous to handle because of its flammability; however, in Arctic cold it is more likely to perform well.

JET FUEL ADDITIVES AND CARCINOGENS

To enhance their performance, both JET A-1 and JET B contain additives. Antioxidants are included to prevent gumming. These antioxidants are commonly alkylated phenols of some formula.

Antistatic agents are added to dissipate static electricity; otherwise, sparking might start a disastrous fire. A common antistatic formula contains the antistatic compound dinonylaphthylsulfonic acid (DINNSA).

To prevent corrosion, jet fuels contain corrosion inhibitors, which often vary in military and civilian planes. A mixture called DCI-4A is used in civilian planes, and DCI-6A is used in military planes. To prevent icing in the fuel system, icing inhibitors are added to jet fuel. These are generally called FSII agents. Di-EGME is one such mixture.

Studies of both civilian and military jet fuels have concluded that some of the additives are carcinogenic and that others are potentially carcinogenic. The jet fuel JP8, which is a special formula for military jets, contains ethylene dibromide (EDB), a known carcinogen. It has been an additive in leaded gasoline and has been used as a fumigant. Studies of laboratory animals showed that it can produce a variety of toxic effects. Rats exposed to JP8 developed tumors regardless of the routes by which they were exposed. Naphthalene is another component of jet fuel, formed from two benzene rings. Exposure for long periods presents the risk of cancer. Studies of laboratory mice showed that it produced carcinomas on the skins of mice and created bronchiolar adenomas. It is considered to be probably carcinogenic in humans. Workers exposed to it for long periods have developed laryngeal carcinomas, but these cases involved cigarette smokers. Toluene has been used in aviation gasoline and high-octane blending stock. In studies of laboratory rats, the results were inadequate to show that it was a carcinogen.

Rocket fuels may be liquid or solid. The giant space rockets used by the National Aeronautics and Space Administration (NASA) have generally used liquid, but most military rockets are solid-fuel rockets. Rockets use a fuel and an oxidizer. In the case of the rockets propelling the American space shuttles, the fuel is a mixture of liquid oxygen and liquid hydrogen. The hydrogen is the fuel, and the oxygen is the oxidizer. Other liquid fuels have been hydrogen peroxide and nitrogen tetroxide. Common skyrockets are propelled by gunpowder or some more stable mixture. Solid-fuel rockets used in the United States in the 1950 and 1960s were often made of ammonium perchlorate powder (oxidizer) and aluminum powder (fuel). In the 1970s intercontinental ballistic missiles were designed to use solid rocket fuel.

CARCINOGENS IN ROCKET FUEL

Hydrazine is a major component in solid rocket fuels, in the form of 1,1-Dimethylhydrazine. It has been classified as a Group 2B carcinogen (possibly carcinogenic to humans) by the International Agency for Research on Cancer. The U.S. Environmental Protection Agency also classifies it as a possible carcinogen. N-nitrosoamines are a class of chemicals including *N*-Nitrosodimethylamine (NDMA). These chemicals have been found in the areas around rocket-testing facilities in very high concentrations. They are suspected carcinogens with cancer potencies higher than those of the trihalomethanes.

SEE ALSO: Chemical Industry; Tobacco Smoking.

BIBLIOGRAPHY. James E. Conel, *Toxicity Caused by Benzene, Toluene, Ethelene/Propylene Glycol, Gasoline, Jet Fuel and Stoddard Solvent* (DIANE Publishing Co., 1993); Nicholas A. Cumpsty, *Jet Propulsion: A Simple Guide to the Aerodynamic and Thermodynamic Design and Performance of Jet Engines* (Cambridge University Press, 2003); Paul E. Damphousse, *Characterization and Performance of a Liquid Hydrocarbon-Fueled Pulse Detonation Rocket Engine* (Storming Media, 2001); Jeanne Jones, *Jet Fuel* (Random House, 1984); National Research Council, *Toxicologic Assessment of Jet-Propulsion Fuel 8* (National Academies Press, 2003); Jack D. Mattingly, *Elements of Propulsion: Gas Turbines and Rockets* (American Institute of Aeronautics & Astronautics, 2006); Gaberial Roy, *Chemical Propulsion Systems* (Elsevier Science & Technology Books, 2005); Gaberial Roy, ed., *Propulsion Combustion: Fuels to Emissions* (Taylor & Francis, 1998); Eckart Walter Schmidt, *Hydrazine and its Derivatives: Preparation, Properties, Applications* (John Wiley & Sons, 2001); Wolfgang Spyra and Kay Winkelmann, eds. *Conversion of Liquid Rocket Fuels Risk Assessment* (Springer-Verlag, 2004).

ANDREW J. WASKEY
DALTON STATE COLLEGE

Jimmy Fund (DFCI)

THE JIMMY FUND is one of the best-known organizations aimed at raising money for cancer research and care. Based at the Dana-Farber Cancer Institute (DFCI) in Boston, Massachusetts, the Jimmy Fund holds over 300 events annually to support the DFCI.

On May 22, 1948, a 12-year-old cancer patient identified as Jimmy was paid a visit by the Boston Braves baseball team. This visit was broadcast from Jimmy's hospital bedside at the Children's Cancer Research Foundation on Ralph Edwards' national radio program "Truth or Consequences." The Braves gave an honorary uniform to the boy, and listeners sent in donations to buy him a television set so that he could watch the Braves games.

The event was arranged by the Variety Club of New England (now the Variety Children's Charity of New England). The first donations far superseded the club's intent. Over $200,000 was donated that year; proceeds started the Jimmy Fund and have since been put toward research and care.

In 1953 the Braves moved to Milwaukee, but the new Boston Red Sox claimed the Jimmy Fund as the team's official charity. The Massachusetts Chiefs of Police Association followed suit.

In 1998, half a century after the initial 1948 radio broadcast, Jimmy was still anonymous. Nobody had imagined that he could still be alive. But Einar Gustafson stepped forward and revealed his identity as Jimmy. A false name had been used to protect his identity, per his doctor's demands.

When he was back in the public eye, Gustafson became an important spokesperson for the Jimmy Fund. He made many public appearances and frequently visited cancer patients at the DFCI. His presence was an inspiring story for research and care of juvenile cancer.

Gustafson passed away in 2001 from a stroke. He was 65 years old.

Sidney Farber, before becoming Jimmy's doctor, was a pathologist at Children's Hospital in Boston, working with leukemia patients. At that time, leukemia was treated in the same way as when it was first described in 1845; there wasn't any treatment.

Farber, inspired by recent advances in anemia treatments, was determined to find a treatment for leukemia. He knew that bone-marrow growth was stimulated by folic acid; therefore, he reasoned that a drug that blocked folic acid action might alleviate the aberrant growth in leukemia. At the same time, Aminopterin was a folic-acid-blocking drug under testing by the pharmaceutical company Lederle.

In November 1947, Farber treated 16 child leukemia patients with Aminopterin; 10 of these children showed remission of their leukemia. Unfortunately, when his results were published in June 1948, fellow physicians reacted with disbelief. Because nobody had ever shown a way to treat tumors that didn't involve surgical removal, people could not believe that a drug could cause remission of inoperable soft tumors. It didn't take long, however, for news to spread to patients and their families across New England and the rest of the nation. Soon, people began to accept this treatment for leukemia. By then, Farber had started the Children's Cancer Research Foundation, which was to become the Dana-Farber Cancer Institute.

The Jimmy Fund Clinic at the DFCI is designed around children and their families. Every detail is considered to make the stay as pleasant as possible for children. On Thursday mornings, outpatient children come to play in the Jimmy Fund Clinic. Toys, movies, videogames, coloring books, and more are provided so that the children can have a fun day amid their chemo schedules and other therapies.

The DFCI's mission is "to provide expert, compassionate care to children and adults with cancer while advancing the understanding, diagnosis, treatment, cure, and prevention of cancer and related diseases." Ultimately, the DFCI aims to end cancer, along with AIDS, related diseases, and their corresponding fears. The Jimmy Fund has a clear statement as well; it "funds research and care at Dana-Farber Cancer Institute."

Along with blood donations, the Jimmy Fund works with bone-marrow donations in collaboration with the National Marrow Donor Program. Through this program, the Jimmy Fund Clinic performs marrow and blood stem-cell transplants, as well as peripheral blood stem-cell donations. Because marrow and blood stem-cell donation is much more invasive than blood donation, the Jimmy Fund Clinic offers extensive information to potential donors before they become eligible. Jimmy Fund staff and volunteers work tirelessly to promote cancer awareness and raise money. The motivation for these efforts can be found in their slogan: "Because it takes more than courage to beat cancer."

FUND RAISING AND PUBLICATIONS

As of 2006, over 88 cents per dollar raised goes toward Jimmy Fund purposes. The Jimmy Fund often raises money by asking for spare change from the public. A major campaign was a brief ad during the previews at a cinema, followed by the passing around of a canister for collecting coins. Currently, a principal charity event is an annual bicycle ride across Massachusetts, called the Pan-Massachusetts Challenge. Started in 1980, it has grown to be the Jimmy Fund's largest event. Additionally, a Jimmy Fund walk covers the 26.2-mile route of the Boston Marathon.

Yet another annual fund-raising event is the holiday tree and wreath sale, led by Dan Murphy, Jr., and his family, and based in their backyard in Randolph, Massachusetts. This sale has continued since 1970, when Dan's son Dan III, now cancer free, was treated at DFCI for Hodgkin's disease.

The Jimmy Fund maintains an office in Palm Beach, Florida, for fund-raising purposes. The major event planned at this office is the Discovery Ball.

Newsletters published by the Jimmy Fund include the *Dana-Farber Report, Impact,* and *Paths of Progress.*

These newsletters can be accessed through the Jimmy Fund website. The website also provides information on seasonal fund-raising events and blood donation.

SEE ALSO: Clinical Trials; Dana-Farber Cancer Institute; Leukemia, Acute Lymphoblastic, Adult; Leukemia, Acute Lymphoblastic, Childhood; Leukemia, Acute Myeloid, Adult; Leukemia, Acute Myeloid, Childhood; Leukemia, Chronic Lymphocytic; Leukemia, Chronic Myelogenous; Leukemia, Hairy Cell; Leukemia Society of America.

BIBLIOGRAPHY. Cindy Anderson, "Thursday's Children," *Yankee Magazine* (September 1997); Archives Program of Children's Hospital, *Children's Hospital Boston (Images of America)* (Arcadia Publishing, 2005); James N. Parker and Philip M. Parker, *The Official Parent's Sourcebook on Childhood Acute Lymphoblastic Leukemia* (Icon Health Publications, 2002); Saul Wisnia, *The Jimmy Fund (Images of America)* (Arcadia Publishing, 2002).

CLAUDIA WINOGRAD
UNIVERSITY OF ILLINOIS AT URBANA-CHAMPAIGN

Johnson & Johnson (United States)

AS OF 2007, Johnson & Johnson had more than 200 companies under its umbrella in 57 countries. The company's products serve patients with such health problems as acne, arthritis, cancer, Crohn's disease, dandruff, epilepsy, fever, hair loss, hepatitis, joint replacement, hernia, lactose intolerance, and schizophrenia.

The mission of Johnson & Johnson is to "provide scientifically sound, high-quality products and services to help heal, cure disease and improve the quality of life."

R. W. Johnson wrote the company's credo in 1943. The credo directs the company philosophy in regard to its community, customers, employees, and shareholders. The document has been translated into 36 languages for international employees.

Johnson & Johnson was founded in 1886 in New Brunswick, New Jersey, by James Wood Johnson and Edward Mead Johnson. Initially, the company had 14 employees in a rented factory, producing antiseptic surgical dressings. The idea for sterile surgical dressings was that of the third Johnson brother, R. W. John-son, based on surgeon Sir Joseph Liston's lectures on germs. Before the surgical dressings offered by Johnson & Johnson, cotton sweepings from textile mill floors were used. R. W. Johnson joined the company later in 1886.

On October 28, 1887, the company was officially incorporated. In 1890 it became famous for its baby powder. In 1896 Johnson & Johnson marketed dental floss, originally made from silk.

In 1888 Johnson & Johnson published a book, *Modern Methods of Antiseptic Wound Treatment.* The company also published and circulated magazines to educate the public and medical society about healthful practices in life and medicine. These magazines served as excellent advertisements for Johnson & Johnson products.

SEE ALSO: Drugs; Surgery; United States.

BIBLIOGRAPHY. Ahmed F. Abdel-Magid and Stephane Caron, *Fundamentals of Early Clinical Drug Development: From Synthesis Design to Formulation* (Wiley-Interscience, 2006); Anne Clayton, *Insight into a Career in Pharmaceutical Sales* (Pharmaceuticalsales.com, Inc., 2005); Rick Ng, *Drugs—From Discovery to Approval* (Wiley-Liss, 2004); Adriana Petryna, et al., *Global Pharmaceuticals: Ethics, Markets, Practices* (Duke University Press, 2006).

CLAUDIA WINOGRAD
UNIVERSITY OF ILLINOIS AT URBANA-CHAMPAIGN

Jonsson Comprehensive Cancer Center at UCLA

THE JONSSON COMPREHENSIVE Cancer Center (JCCC) is affiliated with the University of California at Los Angeles (UCLA). The JCCC dates back to the 1960s, when a group of scientists and volunteers and UCLA began development of a cancer center that would combine excellence in research, education, and patient care; this goal was realized when the JCCC was designated a Comprehensive Cancer Center by the National Cancer Institute in 1976.

The JCCC is located principally within the Doris and Louis Factor Health Sciences Building in the Center for the Health Sciences on the Westwood campus of UCLA, along with UCLA's David Geffen School of Medicine, Dental School, College of Letters and Sciences, School of Public Health, School of Nursing, the Mattel Children's Hospital, and UCLA Medical Center; many faculty from these units are members of the JCCC.

The JCCC handles over 20,000 patient visits per year, conducts hundreds of clinical trials annually, and has a membership of over 230 physicians and scientists.

The JCCC has a team-oriented approach to patient care, drawing on experts from over 40 medical and scientific disciplines. Outpatient care is provided primarily in the UCLA Oncology Center and in clinics specializing in particular types of cancer. Inpatient care is provided primarily by the UCLA Medical Center and Mattel Children's Hospital. Psychosocial and supportive care for patients and their families is also provided within the JCCC and affiliated organizations.

The UCLA Oncology Center is located in the UCLA Medical Plaza and includes more than 50 physicians who treat cancer patients. It is affiliated with the UCLA Medical Center, a major teaching hospital, and offers comprehensive cancer services, including medical and surgical consultations, minor surgery, cancer detection and prevention, nutrition and dietary counseling, symptom management, chemotherapy, immunotherapy, transfusions, social services, and individual and family counseling. Related services—including laboratory testing, radiology, pathology, and nuclear medicine—are located in separate facilities in the UCLA Medical Plaza.

The Revlon/UCLA Breast Center, a component of the JCCC, offers a multidisciplinary approach to breast problems. Patient-care services include a diagnostic clinic for new and established patients; a follow-up clinic for women who are undergoing or have completed treatment for breast cancer; and a high-risk clinic for women with a family history of the disease or a personal history of risk factors, such as an abnormal breast biopsy. Research programs at the center include basic science research and clinical trials focusing on cancer treatment and quality of life.

The Ted Mann Family Resource Center at the JCCC provides a variety of support groups, counseling, and educational programs for cancer patients and survivors, as well as their families. Support groups include Living with Cancer (for newly diagnosed patients and their families); Couples Together; Friends and Family; Look Good, Feel Better (co-sponsored by the American Cancer Society, a group that helps women manage

physical-appearance changes brought about by cancer and cancer treatment); Among Friends (for women being treated for early-stage cancer); Looking Ahead (for women who have finished treatment and have no evidence of cancer); and the Grief Work Group (for men and women who recently lost an adult family member to cancer). Classes and seminars offered at the center include Qigong, journal writing, and meditation.

Research at the JCCC is organized into 12 programs in three divisions: Basic Research Programs, Clinical/Translational Research Programs, and Cancer Prevention and Control Programs.

Basic Research Programs is concerned with advancing the understanding of fundamental mechanism relating to cancer.

The Cancer Cell Biology Program focuses on clarifying the mechanisms that underlie fundamental biological processes in cells, and on highlighting and characterizing the differences between normal and cancer cells.

The Gene Regulation Program studies gene expression and the role played by misregulated gene expression in cancer.

The Signal Transduction and Therapeutics Program studies the role played by signaling pathways and signal transduction events in the development of cancer, and seeks to develop new methods to detect changes in signaling events and to develop inhibitors of signal transduction that could lead to new cancer therapies.

The Signal Transduction and Therapeutics Program is part of Clinical/Translational Research Programs.

The Tumor Immunology Program studies the basic biology of the immune system, its role as a tissue target of neoplasia, and its impact on the host response to malignancy.

Cancer Molecular Imaging studies cancer in living organisms by using molecular imaging, a process that allows noninvasive visualization of changes that occur when cancer develops.

The Clinical/Translational Research Programs are organized around disease areas reflecting interdisciplinary research strengths.

The Genitourinary Oncology Program investigates the molecular and immunologic mechanism responsible for genitourinary cancers and aims to translate those results into therapeutic trials.

The Hematopoietic Malignancies Program coordinates basic research in hematopoiesis, leukemia, lymphoma, and multiple myeloma at UCLA, and seeks to translate research findings into preclinical and clinical trials and to provide clinical research support and laboratory support for clinical trials.

The Thoracic Oncology Program seeks to understand the biology of lung cancer and develop more effective prevention, diagnosis, and treatment methods.

The Women's Cancers Program studies breast and reproductive cancers in women, and aims to create a more comprehensive approach to clinical and translational research.

The Cancer Prevention and Control Programs focus on research in particular study populations.

The Healthy and At-Rick Populations Program focuses on primary prevention, screening, and early detection in people who are healthy and/or are at increased risk for cancer; it includes an emphasis on cancer prevention and control among low-income, minority, and underserved populations.

The Patients and Survivors Program focuses on reducing morbidity and mortality among cancer patients and long-term survivors, as well as their family members and caregivers. Particular areas of focus include behavioral interventions, quality-of-life assessments, nutritional interventions, and symptom control.

The Molecular Epidemiology Program studies the interactions between environmental exposures, molecular genetic alterations, and the risk and progression of cancer.

The UCLA Family Cancer Registry, founded in 1998, combines expertise and resources from the JCCC and the UCLA Schools of Medicine and Public Health. The registry is a repository of information collected from people who have had cancer or who have a family history of cancer. The types of information collected includes pedigree data (the tracing of certain cancers through a family tree), survey data about health behaviors and lifestyles, biological specimens such as blood and tissue samples, and the results of genetic susceptibility testing.

The registry is open to people who have a type of cancer known to run in families, have a family history of cancer (defined as two or more blood relatives with the same type of cancer), have a family history of cancers known to be related (e.g., breast and ovarian cancer), or have been diagnosed as having a cancer-susceptibility gene. Data collected by the registry are confidential and may include family history, demographic and lifestyle characteristics, and personal medical and psychosocial history. Blood samples, and possibly tissue samples, are also collected.

The registry also provides counseling concerning genetic-susceptibility testing for individuals with a strong family history of cancer. Longitudinal information is gathered through regular collection of updated personal and familial medical history information from persons included in the registry.

Medical and health researchers may apply for access to the registry's resources for conducing research studies, both to analyze the data and biological samples collected by the registry, and to access contact information for people included in the registry who may want to participate in research studies.

SEE ALSO: Education, Cancer; Genetics; Survivors of Cancer; Survivors of Cancer Families.

BIBLIOGRAPHY. UCLA's Jonsson Comprehensive Cancer Center website, www.cancer.mednet.ucla.edu (cited December 2006).

SARAH BOSLAUGH
WASHINGTON UNIVERSITY SCHOOL OF MEDICINE

Jordan

THIS MIDDLE EASTERN country has borders with Israel to the west, Syria to the north, Iraq to the east, and Saudi Arabia to the south. It was created after the defeat of the Ottoman Empire in World War I. It then became the Hashemite Kingdom of Transjordan, occupying land on both sides of the River Jordan.

In 1967, during the Six-Day War, Jordan lost the lands to the west of the river—this area becoming known as the West Bank—to which it renounced claims in 1988, with certain conditions such as a continuing role in Muslim and Christian holy places in Jerusalem. The country has a population of 5,350,000 (2005), with 166 doctors and 296 nurses per 100,000 people. An example of cancer incidence rates in Jordan includes 117.9 cases of cancer in males per 100,000, according to the International Agency for Research on Cancer.

During the 1960s, A.S. Abu-Guora was involved in cancer support groups in Jordan, being a member of a panel on voluntary organizations held at the Ninth International Cancer Congress in Tokyo in October 1966. The Jordan Cancer Registry was established in 1996 and operates under the auspices of the Ministry of Health. It is a member of the Middle East Cancer Consortium, sharing information with Cyprus, Egypt, Israel, the Palestinian Authority, and Turkey.

King Hussein, who was always concerned with the welfare of the Jordanian people, established the King Hussein Cancer Center (KHCC) in Amman in 1997. It was originally called the Al-Amal Cancer Center but was renamed in November 2002 following the death of the king from cancer.

The KHCC is the only specialized cancer center in the Middle East that treats both adult and pediatric patients. A quarter of the 2,300 new patients treated each year come from neighboring countries.

Since 2003 the director of the King Hussein Cancer Foundation has been H. R. H. Prince Mir'ed bin Ra'ad. The senior researcher and oncologist is Mahmoud Sarhan. Some research is undertaken at the Faculty of Medicine at the University of Jordan, Amman. Fathi Arafat, brother of Yasser Arafat, practiced as a medical doctor in Jordan for many years and died of lung cancer in Cairo, Egypt.

King Hussein, who ruled Jordan from 1952 until 1999, died of complications from non-Hogkin's lymphoma after suffering from cancer for many years.

He had been treated at the Mayo Clinic in Rochester, Minnesota, for some time.

The Jordanian government was involved in a scandal surrounding Elias Alsabti, an Iraqi medical researcher who posed as a member of the Jordanian royal family to gain a Jordanian government grant to study cancer research in the United States in 1977. He was involved in reworking cancer articles from less well-known publications and submitting them to other journals. Overall, he is believed to have published 50 to 60 articles, some co-authored with people who are believed to be fictional.

SEE ALSO: Iraq; Lymphoma, Non-Hodgkin's, Adult.

BIBLIOGRAPHY. K. T. Ababneh, "Biopsied Gingival Lesions in Northern Jordanians: A Retrospective Analysis over 10 Years," *The International Journal of Periodontics & Restorative Dentistry* (v.26/4, 2006); William J. Broad, "Would-Be Academician Pirates Papers: Five of His Published Papers Are Demonstrable Plagiarisms, and More Than 55 Others Are Suspect," *Science (v.208, 1980)*; M. Al-Sheyyab, et al., "The Incidence of Childhood Cancer in Jordan: A Population-Based Study," *Annals of Saudi Medicine* (v.23/5, 2003).

JUSTIN CORFIELD
GEELONG GRAMMAR SCHOOL, AUSTRALIA

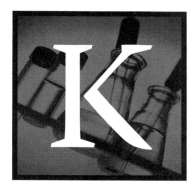

Kaplan, Henry S.

AMERICAN CANCER SPECIALIST Henry S. Kaplan was the winner of the Charles F. Kettering Prize of the General Motors Cancer Foundation in 1979 for "distinguished leadership in the development of a highly effective therapeutic regimen for Hodgkin's disease." His efforts ensured that radiotherapy became a new discipline in oncology. Kaplan also pioneered research in radiobiology and was involved in experimental work with the viral etiology of rat leukemia.

Henry Seymour Kaplan was born April 24, 1918, to Nathan M. and Sarah Kaplan (née Brilliant). He grew up in Chicago, and attended the University of Chicago (B.S., 1938), Rush Medical College (1940), and the University of Minnesota (M.S. in Radiology, 1940). He worked as an intern at Michael Reese Hospital in Chicago, becoming the resident in the radiation therapy and tumor clinic in 1941 and 1942. In 1943 and 1944 he had a fellowship at the National Cancer Institute (NCI). Later, he was an instructor in radiology at Yale Medical School (1944–45), assistant professor (1945–47), and radiologist at the NCI (1947–48).

Kaplan then moved to the School of Medicine at Stanford University, where he remained for the next 36 years, initially as professor of radiology and chairman of the department (1948–72); he was director of the biophysics laboratory from 1957 to 1964. During this period he used lymphangiographic mapping techniques to demonstrate that the spread of Hodgkin's disease was not unpredictable and random, but spread from one lymph node chain to the next. It therefore allowed possibilities for treatment that eventually earned him the Charles F. Kettering Prize.

In 1954 and 1955 he was a Commonwealth Fund fellow and visiting scientist at the National Institute of Health. In 1972 he became the Lyles D'Ambrogio professor of oncology and director of the cancer biological research laboratory, a post he held until his death in 1984. Beginning in 1977 he was also chairman of the science advisory committee at the Sharett Institute of Oncology, Hadassah Medical Center, Hebrew University, Jerusalem.

A member of many professional associations, Kaplan served on the committee for radiology of the National Research Council from 1950 to 1956, the gastrointestinal-cancer committee of the NCI, the pathology panel dealing with the effects of radiation at the National Academy of Science-NRC, and the advanced committee on biology at Oak Ridge National Laboratory from 1969 to 1975.

He was also a member of the subcommittee on radiation carcinogensis (chairman in 1957 and 1958) and the commission on research for the International Union Against Cancer. He was a member of the national advisory Cancer Council of California (1959–62), the board of division of scientific advisors for cancer treatment (1957–1979), the national consultative panel on cancer for the U.S. Senate (1970–71), and the council of analysis and projection of the American Cancer Society (1972–76).

He was a member of many professional medical bodies, and he received many honorary degrees and awards from the United States and overseas. Outside the United States, Kaplan was a member of the board of governors of the Weizmann Institute of Science, Rehovot, Israel (1974–84), and of Ben Gurion University, Beersheba, Israel (1979–84). He received the Légion d'Honneur from France, the Order of Merit from Italy, and the Shahbanou Award from Iran.

A prolific writer, Kaplan was co-author, with S. J. Robinson, of *Congenital Heart Disease: An Illustrated Diagnostic Approach* (McGraw-Hill, 1954; 2d ed., with H.L. Abrams and S.J. Robinson, McGraw-Hill, 1965); coauthor, with H.L. Abrams, of *Angiocardiographic Interpretation in Congenital Heart Disease* (C.C. Thomas, 1955); author of "Historical Aspects," in *Hodgkin's Disease* (Harvard University Press, 1972, 1980); editor, with P. J. Tsuchitani, of *Cancer in China* (A.R. Liss, 1978); coauthor, with R. Levy, of *Malignant Lymphomas* (Academic Press, 1978); and coauthor, with S. A. Rosenberg, of *Advances in Malignant Lymphomas* (1981).

Kaplan served on the editorial advisory boards of *Current Topics in Radiation Research Quarterly* from 1971 to 1977 and of *Cancer Proceedings of the National Academy of Science* from 1973 to 1978. He was advisory editor of the *International Journal of Radiation Oncology, Biology, Physics*. Interested in the history of cancer, he wrote several papers in this field.

Kaplan was recipient of the Lila Motley Cancer Foundation Award, the Modern Medicine Award for Distinguished Achievement in 1968, and the Atoms for Peace Award in 1969. In 1971 he received the Lucy W. James Award of the James Ewing Society, the R.R. de Villers Award of the Leukemia Society, and the Karnofsky Memorial Award of the American Society of Clinical Oncology. Many other awards followed, including the National Award of the American Cancer Society in 1972, Laureate of the Prix Griffuel for cancer research in France in 1975, and the G.H. A. Clowes Memorial Award of the American Association for Cancer Research in 1976.

In 1977 he was given the gold medal of the American Society for Therapeutic Radiologists; in 1978, he received the medal of honor of the Danish Cancer Society, the Ungerman-Lubin Award of the Taubman Foundation, and the Lila Gruber Memorial Award of the American Academy of Dermatology.

The award of the Kettering Prize in 1979 was followed by the Prentis Award of the Michigan Cancer Foundation in 1980 and the Walker Prize of the Royal College of Surgeons in 1981.

He died February 4, 1984. Stanford University School of Medicine honored him with the establishment of a new chair: Henry S. Kaplan and Harry Lebeson Professor in Cancer Biology.

SEE ALSO: National Cancer Institute; Radiation Therapy; United States.

BIBLIOGRAPHY. Z. Fuks and M. Feldman, "Henry S. Kaplan 1918–1984: A Physician, a Scientist, a Friend," *Cancer Survey* (v.4, 1985); Sherman B. Nuland, "The Lymphatic Contiguity of Hodgkin's Disease: A Historical Study," *Bulletin of the New York Academy of Medicine* (v.57, 1981); *Who Was Who in America 1982–1985* (Marquis Who's Who, 1985).

JUSTIN CORFIELD
GEELONG GRAMMAR SCHOOL, AUSTRALIA

Kazakhstan

THIS CENTRAL ASIAN republic was part of the Soviet Union as an autonomous republic in 1920 and as a Soviet republic from 1936. It gained its independence in 1991 as the Republic of Kazakhstan and has a population of 15,217,000 (2006), with 353 doctors and 649 nurses per 100,000 people. An example of cancer incidence rates in Kazakhstan includes 295.3 cases of cancer in males per 100,000, according to the International Agency for Research on Cancer.

During the Soviet Union period, cancer treatment became important as life expectancy rose; consequently, the number of people suffering from cancer also increased dramatically. As well as lung cancer and breast cancer, which continue to be major types of cancer prevalent in Kazakhstan, there was much occupational cancer from unhealthy work conditions and from use of asbestos and other carcinomas. In 1961 the number of cancer beds in Kazakhstan was

1,051, compared with 866 the previous year and only 180 in 1950. The government has established several cancer registries in the country to help provide researchers accurate records for all of Kazakhstan. In one study comparing the data from the Pavlodar, Semipalatinsk, and Ust-Kamenogorsk Regional Cancer Registries of Kazakhstan from 1996 to 1998, it was shown that the records were comprehensive and that they provided models for developing registries for different types of cancers. Many Soviet nuclear missiles were deployed in Kazakhstan, and many doctors and researchers have worked on connections between carcinomas in the Semipalatinsk part of Kazakhstan and rates in other parts of the country.

In one extensive study, conducted between 1960 and 1999, some 582,750 person-years of follow-up were conducted on 19,545 inhabitants of villages in the Semipalatinsk region, making the study one of the largest of its type in the world. It quickly became apparent that rates of mortality in general, as well as those from cancer in particular, greatly exceeded those in comparative populations in areas not affected by nuclear radiation.

As a result, to raise the level of cancer treatment in Kazakhstan, links have been established between Kazakh treatment centers and those overseas. One of the most successful was in Semipalatinsk, the site of the exposure to possible nuclear radiation. There, the local health network—involving the Regional Oncology Dispensary (200 beds, 22,000 outpatients annually), Regional Clinical Hospital (580 beds), Regional Children's Hospital (280 beds), Emergency First Aid Hospital, Semipalatinsk Gynaecological Hospital, and the Regional Diagnostic Treatment Center in Kurchatov. This led, in 1996, to the formation of the Semipalatinsk Medical Academy and also a nearby medical college for training nurses.

BREAST CANCER

There has also been a rise in breast cancer in Kazakhstan in recent years, partly because of the higher life expectancy. In November 2001, in an important study of women in Almaty, different rates were discovered in Kazakh Russian and Korean communities. Women in the Korean community, despite their higher-than-average educational levels, were less aware of the use of preventive methods, whereas Russian women were more active in regular breast screening.

RESEARCH

It had long been thought that exposure to oils also caused cancers, and during the 1960s M.A. Karymov and S.N. Nugmanov from the Kazakh Institute of Oncology and Radiology at Alma-Ata worked on applying oils from seven sources in Kazakhstan to rabbits, rats, Syrian hamsters, and mice. This experiment resulted in several tumors, some benign and others malignant. Rabbits were found to be the most sensitive. Furthermore, the researchers found that the curing soot used in the Guryev fish factory had marked carcinogenic properties.

At the same time, A.N. Sizganrov of the Kazakh Institute of Clinical and Experimental Surgery of the Academy of Medical Sciences of the USSR at Alma-Ata worked on the distribution and deposition of some carcinogenic compounds in the organism of animals. O.K. Kabyev and S.M. Vermenitchev, also from the institute, worked on leukoantocyanidines and catechines as a new class of anticancer compounds. S. B. Balmukhanov, et al., researched the acquired radioresistibility of tumor cells. K.I. Zholkiver, et al., worked on cancer radiotherapy using big dose fractions. V.A. Smirnov worked on the histogenesis of skin cancer as a study in cancer geography. N.I. Kolytcheva and M.K. Kayrakbayev worked on esophagus-cancer epidemiology in Kazakhstan. N.M. Alexandrova studied the etiology and pathology of oral cancer, and was able to show regional variations in the prevalence of different types of oral cancers. S.N. Nugmanov studied the climatic influences on cancer in Kazakhstan.

During the 1970s there was a campaign to reduce cancer of the esophagus, which came from the consumption of heavy meals including fatty foods late in the evening, and also from the heavy drinking of strong hot tea. With the recent large increase in the advertising budgets of cigarette manufacturers eager to sell their products in Kazakhstan, it is expected that lung-cancer rates among men will remain a major concern to the Kazakh government.

SEE ALSO: Breast Cancer; Esophageal Cancer; Lung Cancer, Non-Small Cell; Lung Cancer, Small Cell; Radiation; Russia; Tobacco Smoking.

BIBLIOGRAPHY. Susanne Bauer, et al., "Radiation Exposure Due to Local Fallout from Soviet Atmospheric Nuclear

Weapons Testing in Kazakhstan: Solid Cancer Mortality in the Semipalatinsk Historical Cohort, 1960–1999," *Radiation Research (v.164*, 2005); M. K. Kairakbaev, "Etapy razvitiia i stanovlenia onkologicheskoi sluzbhy v Kazakhskoi SSR za gody sovetskoi vlasti," *Voprosy Onkologii* (v.18, 1972); N. F. Kramchaninov, "Skin Cancer of the Extremities in Kazakhstan," *Voprosy Onkologii* (v.12, 1966); A. P. Pozdniakova, et al., "The Dynamics of Esophageal Cancer Morbidity in Kazakhstan" [in Russian], *Voprosy Onkologii* (v.38, 1992); S. N. Nugmanov, "Razvitie onkologii v Kazakhskoi SSR," *Voprosy Onkologii* (v.14, 1968); A. A. Suleimenov, et al., "Onkologicheskaia sluzhba Kazakhstana za 60 let SSR," *Voprosy Onkologii* (v.28, 1982); Irina V. Volguina, "Descriptive Epidemiology of Cancer in Three Regions of Kazakhstan" (M.S. thesis, University of Texas School of Public Health, 2001); T. Wan and P. S. Ho, "Factors Influencing Breast Cancer Preventive Practices of Older Women in Almaty, Kazakhstan," *Academy Health Meeting* (v.20, 2003); D. G. Zaridze, "Childhood Cancer Incidence in Relation to Distance from the Former Nuclear Testing Site in Semipalatinsk, Kazakhstan," *European Journal of Cancer* (v.31/s6, 1995).

JUSTIN CORFIELD
GEELONG GRAMMAR SCHOOL, AUSTRALIA

Kenya

THIS EAST AFRICAN country was briefly settled by the Portuguese, who established bases during the 16th century, and also by Arabs from Oman. In 1890 it became a British colony, remaining such until December 12, 1963, when it gained its independence, becoming a republic a year later. It has a population of 34,256,000 (2005), with 13 doctors and 90 nurses per 100,000 people. An example of cancer incidence rates in Kenya includes 155.2 cases of cancer in males per 100,000, according to the International Agency for Research on Cancer.

One type of cancer heavily associated with Kenya and nearby countries is Burkitt's lymphoma. During a 1932 dig in Kenya, the anthropologist Louis Leakey found an old skull dating from 500,000 B.C.E to 1,000,000 B.C.E. In Leakey's view, the skull showed that the person suffered from Burkitt's lymphoma, although later other doctors felt that the evidence of

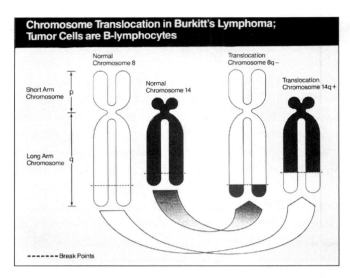

One type of cancer heavily associated with Kenya and nearby countries is Burkitt's lymphoma.

a tumor on the mandible came from a low-grade inflammation.

Certainly endemic, Burkitt's lymphoma has become the most common childhood cancer in Kenya, especially the western part of the country. Herman Autrup and Gerald P. Warwick of the Department of Pathology, the University of Nairobi, in Kenya's capital, were involved in research on the reductive cleavage of a potentially cytotoxic azo compound by human hepatocellular carcinoma. There have also been recent studies of cancer among Kenyans, including one by Jorgen Fogh, et al., focusing on a boy from the Msuba tribe of western Kenya. The Kenya Medical Research Institute was established in 1979 to improve the national healthcare delivery system. It includes areas for cancer treatment and has a research center specializing in medical technology.

SEE ALSO: Lymphoma, Burkitt's; Portugal, United Kingdom.

BIBLIOGRAPHY. Ann Beck, *A History of the British Medical Administration of East Africa 1900–1950* (Harvard University Press, 1970); Dennis Burkitt, "A Sarcoma Involving the Jaws in African Children," *British Journal of Surgery* (v.46, 1958–1959); Jorgen Fogh, et al., "Cultivation and Characterization of Cells from a Malignant Lymphoma in an African Child," *Cancer Research* (v.24, 1964); Ezekiel Kalipeni and Philip Thiuri, *Issues and Perspectives on Health Care in*

Contemporary Sub-Saharan Africa (Edwin Mellen Press, 1997).

JUSTIN CORFIELD
GEELONG GRAMMAR SCHOOL, AUSTRALIA

Kidney Cancer, Childhood

WILMS' TUMOR IS generally a solitary growth that may occur on any part of the kidney (either one). It accounts for almost all renal cancers in childhood and occurs in approximately equal frequency in both sexes and races, with an incidence of 7.8 million children under the age of 15 years. This type of tumor is seen with congenital anomalies such as genitourinary anomalies (4 percent), hemihypertrophy (3 percent), and sporadicaniridia (1 percent).

Wilms' tumor has developed in children of parents with hemihypertrophy and is seen in siblings of children with hemihypertrophy. Hemihypertrophy may not be obvious until the time of the adolescent growth spurt, however.

The child with asymmetric growth following treatment for Wilms' tumor may have hemihypertrophy rather than a complication of therapy.

The familial form of Wilms' tumor is more likely to be bilateral than the sporadic form. Patients with bilateral or familial disease have a higher incidence of congenital anomalies, which may make the tumor develop much earlier in life. It is estimated that a child of a patient with bilateral or familial Wilms' tumor has a 30 percent risk of developing the tumor. Renal cell carcinomas are very rare in the first decade of life, but they can occur within the teenage years.

SYMPTOMS AND DIAGNOSIS

The median age of diagnosis of Wilms' tumor is about 3 years old. At that time the most frequent finding is an abdominal mass, which is usually smooth and firm, and rarely crosses the midline of the abdomen. About 60 percent of patients have hypertension due to compression of the renal pedicle.

Patients usually have an abdominal ultrasound to determine whether the mass is cystic or solid and whether there is any involvement of the renal vein or the vena cava. An abdominal scan is needed to see the extent of the tumor and whether any regional lymph nodes are involved. Other types of renal cancers are nephroblastomatosis, mesoblastic nephromas, and renal cell carcinomas. Nephroblastomatosis is found in all patients with bilateral Wilms' tumor. They generally show manifestation of nephroblastomatosis. About one-third of patients show malformations or benign neoplasias, or both.

Patients on chemotherapy have a declining incidence of nephroblastomatosis tumors. It is important to follow patients with computed tomography (CT) scans, which are helpful in determining tumor growth and outcomes. The staging system used is the National Wilms Tumor Study. State I is limited to the kidney. State II extends beyond the kidney but can be surgically removed. State III has residual nonhematogenous extension of tumor and is confined to the abdomen following surgery. State IV has hematogenous metastases and most frequently involves the lungs.

TREATMENT AND PROGNOSIS

Mesoblastic nephromas account for the majority of congenital renal tumors. The tumor is generally benign, and surgical removal is best. If metastatic disease is present, patients require chemo and irradiation. Surgical resection is the best cure, but patients with postoperative residual disease have a grim prognosis.

Although the prognosis is made by favorable or unfavorable cell types, the unfavorable category has three histologic types: anaplasia, which occurs in older patients; rhabdoid, which occurs in younger patients; and clear cell sarcoma, which is more predominant among males. These three unfavorable types are found in 10 percent of Wilms' tumors but are responsible for 60 percent of the deaths.

SEE ALSO: Chemotherapy; Kidney (Renal Cell) Cancer; Surgery.

BIBLIOGRAPHY. Eric P. Cohen, ed., *Cancer and the Kidney* (Oxford University Press, 2005); Henry Ekert, *Childhood Cancer: Understanding and Coping* (Taylor & Francis, 1989); Robert A. Figlin, ed., *Kidney Cancer (Cancer Treatment and Research)* (Springer, 2003).

RICHARD WILLS
INDEPENDENT SCHOLAR

Kidney (Renal Cell) Cancer

THE MOST COMMON type of kidney cancer is renal cell carcinoma, followed by Wilms' tumor (also known as nephroblastoma) and tumors of the collecting duct system. Each year about 30,000 new cases of renal cell carcinoma are diagnosed in the United States. This accounts for about 12,000 cancer-related deaths annually. Overall, renal cell carcinomas represent around 85 percent of the primary tumors of the kidney, and about 2 percent to 3 percent of all adult cancers.

All renal cell carcinomas are derived from the surface layer of cells that line the urine-collecting tubes within the kidney. There are several subclassifications of renal cell carcinoma, the three most common of which are clear cell, papillary renal cell, and chromophobe renal carcinoma. Historically, renal cell carcinomas were classified based on their shape, size, and growth patterns. Advances in understanding of genetics have allowed researchers to classify these tumors based on the initiating cause of the disease on a molecular level.

Renal cell carcinoma can be both hereditary and spontaneous. Hereditary forms are usually discovered to involve both kidneys; the sporadic forms are more likely to involve just one. The most common subtype is clear cell carcinoma, which is caused by a defect in the VHL gene, a gene that normally suppresses growth. In the hereditary form, one defective copy of the gene is passed on to offspring. For a cancer to develop, there needs to be a spontaneous mutation of the other functional copy in any given cell of the kidney. In the spontaneous forms of clear cell carcinoma, one cell has to have two spontaneous mutations to eliminate the copy of the VHL gene on both chromosomes. Papillary and chromophobe renal carcinomas are not as common as clear cell carcinoma, and they involve different types of genes. As a result, each type has a slightly different appearance under the microscope. Risk factors for kidney cancer include smoking, obesity, sedentary lifestyle, and a number of workplace exposures, such as cadmium, herbicides, benzene, and organic solvents.

The presenting symptoms for renal cell carcinoma classically include blood in the urine, flank pain, and a palpable mass in the abdomen. The diagnosis of renal cell carcinoma is frequently challenging, however, because people rarely have the triad of symptoms mentioned. Of these symptoms, blood in the urine is the most common manifestation, occurring in about 50 percent of cases. Yet blood in the urine is a symptom for many other, more common urinary-tract problems, such as bladder infections, so the finding is rather nonspecific. Most frequently, renal cell carcinoma is found incidentally during an abdominal imaging study of the abdomen for another cause.

The outcome of renal cell carcinoma largely depends on the extent to which the disease has developed when treatment is initiated. The earlier the disease is diagnosed and treated, the better the long-term outcome. The life expectancy for people with advanced disease is around 13 months. The mainstay treatment is to remove the affected kidney in surgery, but treatments are frequently used in conjunction with surgery for patients with advanced disease.

SEE ALSO: Genetics; Kidney Cancer, Childhood; National Kidney Cancer Association.

BIBLIOGRAPHY. Herbert T. Cohen and Francis J. McGovern, "Renal Cell Carcinoma," *New England Journal of Medicine* (v.353/23, 2005); Vinay Kumar, et al., *Robbins Basic Pathology* (Saunders, 1971).

JARON SULLIVAN
TEXAS A & M COLLEGE OF MEDICINE

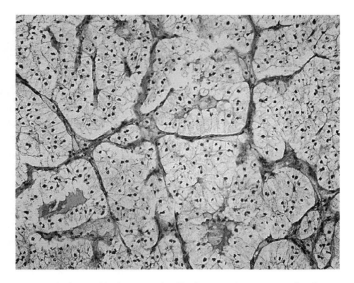

Histopathology of kidney renal cell adenocarcinoma. Renal cell carcinoma is the most common type of kidney cancer.

Kimmel Cancer Center

THE KIMMEL CANCER Center is in Philadelphia, Pennsylvania, and is part of Thomas Jefferson University, an independent medical school and medical research institution. It was established in 1991 through the philanthropy of Sidney Kimmel, who founded Jones Apparel Group, Inc., a designer, wholesaler, and marketer of branded apparel, footwear, and accessories. Kimmel remains chairman of the board of directors.

The center is a National Cancer Institute-designated Cancer Center. Initially, it had about 30 investigators in the basic sciences. Now the staff includes some 150 members. Physicians and scientists work in various fields and across fields to try to discover, develop, and record novel approaches for cancer treatment.

The mission of the Kimmel Cancer Center is "to increase the survival and quality of life of cancer patients by translating laboratory discoveries into new strategies to prevent, diagnose, monitor and cure human cancer." Toward this end, a major effort at the center is to translate the recent discoveries made in cancer research into specific ways of ensuring cancer prevention and treatment.

One of the major emphases of the center is dealing with cancer cells through a heavy focus on the advances made in human genetics. The center also focuses on cell biology biochemistry, structural biology pharmacology, and immunology of cancer. In 2005 the Kimmel Cancer Center achieved $70 million in sponsored research funding from U.S. federal and non-federal sources, including many private foundations and pharmaceutical companies. It is also involved in National Institutes of Health training programs for predoctoral and postdoctoral students, receiving $1 million annually for these training programs.

The center has a heavy training program, offering doctoral students the ability to research in the realms of biochemistry and molecular biology, genetics, immunology and microbial pathogenesis, and molecular pharmacology and structural biology. All these programs are undertaken through the College of Graduate Studies of Thomas Jefferson University.

Copies of many of the theses are held at the university's Scott Memorial Library, where they are consulted by staff members, other students, and researchers from around the world.

In addition to the library resources, the Kimmel Cancer Center has many shared resources, which include bioimaging, biostatistics, flow cytometry, microarray, nucleic acids, proteomics, transgenic/knockout mouse, and X-ray crystallography.

SEE ALSO: Education, Cancer; National Cancer Institute.

BIBLIOGRAPHY. Kimmel Cancer Center website, www.kimmelcancercenter.org (cited December 2006).

JUSTIN CORFIELD
GEELONG GRAMMAR SCHOOL, AUSTRALIA

Kuhl, David E.

AMERICAN RADIOLOGIST DAVID E. Kuhl was the joint winner, with Michael E. Phelps, of the Charles F. Kettering Prize of the General Motors Cancer Foundation in 2001 for "research in the development of positron emission tomography (P.E.T.) scanning and the use of this technology to study normal and abnormal cellular function."

David Edmund Kuhl was born October 27, 1929, in St. Louis, Missouri, and educated at Temple University (A.B., 1951) and the University of Pennsylvania (M.D., 1955). He was an assistant instructor in radiology at the School of Medicine of the University of Pennsylvania from 1958 until 1961 and was promoted from instructor to professor, remaining at the University of Pennsylvania until 1976.

He was also chief of the Nuclear Medical Division of the University of Pennsylvania Hospital from 1963 to 1976, professor of engineering at Moore School of Electrical Engineering from 1974 to 1976, and vice chairman of the Department of Radiology at the University of Pennsylvania Hospital from 1975 to 1976. After moving to California, Kuhl was chief of the Division of Nuclear Medicine at the Department of Radiology and Science at the School of Medicine at the University of California, Los Angeles; associate director of the Laboratory of Biomedical and Environmental Sciences; and chief of the Laboratory of Nuclear Medicine. He was professor of radiological sciences from 1976 to 1986 and vice chairman of the department from 1977 to 1986.

Concurrently with his other positions, Kuhl was a member of the advisory committee on the medical uses of isotopes, U.S. Atomic Energy Commission, National Research Council (1967–79), and a member of the Committee for Radiology at the National Academy of Sciences (1967–71). He was Radiation Study Secretariat at the National Institutes of Health from 1968 to 1973 and chairman of the Diagnosis Radiology Committee of the National Cancer Institute (NCI) from 1973 to 1977.

He was a fellow of the Council on Circulation of the American Heart Association in 1978, a member of the board of trustees of the James T. Case Radiological Foundation from 1982 to 1986, a consultant with the Outstanding Investigator Program of the NCI in 1984, and director of the Positron Emission Tomography Center at the University of Michigan in 1986.

Kuhl is a member of the Institute of Medicine at the National Academy of Sciences, a fellow of the American College of Radiology, a member of the Society of Nuclear Medicine, a fellow of the American Neurological Association, a fellow of the American College of Academic Sciences, and a member of the Association of American Physicians.

He is currently involved in work measuring altered cerebral neurochemistry using radiotracers and emission tomography in early degenerative brain disease.

AWARDS

Over his career Kuhl has received many awards, including honorary lecture awards and an honorary degree from Loyola University, Chicago, in 1993. He received the Nuclear Medicine Pioneer Citation from the Society for Nuclear Medicine in 1976; the Ernst Jung Prize Medal from the Ernst Jung Foundation, Germany, in 1981; the William C. Menniger Memorial Award from the American College of Physicians and the Javits Neurosi Investigator Award from the National Institute of Health in 1989; the Benedict Cassen Prize for Research from the Society for Nuclear Medicine; and the Outstanding Researcher Award from the Radiological Society of North America in 1996.

Kuhl is known to many Americans for his best-selling book on palliative care, *What Dying People Want: Practical Wisdom for the End of Life* (Public Affairs, 2002; Anchor, 2003). His research was funded by the Soros Foundation and drew on 15 years' involvement in palliative care, speaking to many dying people.

SEE ALSO: Radiation Therapy; Technology, Imaging.

BIBLIOGRAPHY. *American Men and Women of Science* (R. R. Bowker/Gale Group, 1982–2003); *Who's Who in America* (Marquis Who's Who, 1982–2003); *Who's Who in Medicine and Healthcare* (Marquis Who's Who, 1996–2000); *Who's Who in the Midwest* (Marquis Who's Who, 1992–2001); *Who's Who in the West* (Marquis Who's Who, 1982); *Who's Who in Science and Engineering* (Marquis Who's Who, 1994–2002).

JUSTIN CORFIELD
GEELONG GRAMMAR SCHOOL, AUSTRALIA

Kyrgyzstan

THIS CENTRAL ASIAN republic was part of the Soviet Union from the creation of the Kara-Kyrgyz Oblast (within the Russian Soviet Federated Socialist Republic), becoming the Kyrgyz Soviet Socialist Republic in 1936. It gained its independence in 1991 as the Kyrgyz Republic and has a population of 5,264,000 (2005), with 301 doctors and 750 nurses per 100,000 people. An example of cancer incidence rates in Kyrgyzstan includes 167.2 cases of cancer in males per 100,000, according to the International Agency for Research on Cancer.

The Soviet government introduced a free mass healthcare system after the Russian Civil War. Before the establishment of the Soviet Union there were only six hospitals (with 100 beds) in Kyrgyzstan, and this number had increased to 268 (with 33,500 beds) by 1973. Much of the healthcare system was concentrated in Frunze (now Bishkek), the largest city in the country, and Osh, the second-largest city, although there were doctors throughout the country.

In 1960 there were 197 beds for cancer patients in Kyrgyzstan, rising to 272 in the following year.

During the early 1960s several preliminary studies of cancer in the Kyrgyz Soviet Socialist Republic were conducted by A. I. Sayenko of the Oncology and Radiology Research Institute at Frunze. He found that the prevalence of skin cancer was 12.5 times less in people from the region, as opposed to Russians and

Ukrainians, and that there was a considerable difference in the incidence of cancer of the upper respiratory tract, the breast, and the uterus.

During the 1970s Sayenko worked on gastric cancer in Kyrgyzstan. He conducted a large study over successive years, using figures from 1958, when the precursor of the Kyrgyzstan Cancer Registry started collecting data. His study concluded that a massive improvement in diagnosis resulted in more patients seeking treatment earlier, which had a greater rate of success. In 1992 and 1993 the system of health-care provision changed; patients were still provided free hospital beds but had to pay for medication and treatment. Also, several hospitals were privatized. This resulted in the wealthy being able to afford bet-ter cancer treatment than they would have received before 1991, but the majority of the population was unable to pay for expensive cancer treatment.

SEE ALSO: Cost of Therapy; Gastric (Stomach) Cancer; Russia.

BIBLIOGRAPHY. Rafis Abazov, *Historical Dictionary of Kyrgyzstan* (Scarecrow Press, 2004); Jude Howell, "Poverty, Children and Transition in Kyrgyzstan: Some Reflections from the Field," *Journal of International Affairs* (v.52/1, 1998); World Bank, *A Survey of Health Reform in Central Asia* (World Bank, 1996).

JUSTIN CORFIELD
GEELONG GRAMMAR SCHOOL, AUSTRALIA

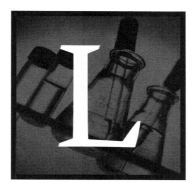

Laos

THIS LANDLOCKED SOUTHEAST Asian country, having borders with Thailand, Vietnam, China, Cambodia, and Myanmar (Burma), was dominated by Thailand during the late medieval and early modern periods. It was a French protectorate from its incorporation into French Indochina in 1893 until independence on July 19, 1949. In 1975 the Pathet Lao movement came to power, and the country was renamed the Lao People's Democratic Republic. Laos has a population of 5,924,000 (2006), with 24 doctors and 108 nurses per 100,000 people. An example of cancer incidence rates in Laos includes 108.9 cases of cancer in males per 100,000, according to the International Agency for Research on Cancer.

During the French period, small hospitals operated in Vientiane and Luang Prabang, the two major cities in the country, but these served only the Europeans and members of the small Lao elite. Cancer treatment tended to rely on surgery, with little knowledge or awareness of the disease in the wider community. Owing to the large number of men who chew betel nut, there is high prevalence of oral cancer; also, there are increasing levels of lung cancer from smoking. For women, breast cancer and cervical cancer are major causes of death in women of childbearing age. There are also increasing numbers of cases of nasopharyngeal cancer, which particularly affects the Chinese population of Laos. Australia has been involved in setting up projects in Laos to increase cancer awareness, and these projects have been fairly successful in encouraging cancer sufferers to seek earlier treatment.

Two people closely connected with recent Laotian history died from cancer: Dr. Thomas Dooley, an American Roman Catholic humanitarian in Laos and author of *The Night They Burned the Mountain*, who suffered from a malignant melanoma; and Sir Frederick Warner, British ambassador from 1965 to 1967.

SEE ALSO: Breast Cancer; Cervical Cancer; France; Nasopharyngeal Cancer; Tobacco Smoking.

BIBLIOGRAPHY. Steven Holland, *Impact of Economic and Institutional Reforms on the Health Sector in Laos: Implications for Health System Management* (Institute of Development Studies, 1995).

JUSTIN CORFIELD
GEELONG GRAMMAR SCHOOL, AUSTRALIA

Laryngeal Cancer

LARYNGEAL CANCER INVOLVES malignant cells occurring in the larynx. The larynx is composed of three parts: the supraglottis (an area above the vocal cords), the glottis (located in the middle of the larynx and containing the vocal cords), and the subglottis (which connects the vocal cords and the windpipe).

Symptoms of laryngeal cancer may include hoarseness, persistent sore throat, difficult or painful swallowing, and possibly pain in the ear or a lump in the neck. Approximately 95 percent of laryngeal cancer involves squamous cell carcinomas occurring in the lining of the throat, rather than in the muscle or cartilage cells. Roughly 5 percent of laryngeal cancer involves the less-aggressive, slower-moving, verrucous carcinoma.

Laryngeal cancer accounts for approximately 30 percent of all cancers of the throat, and between 2 percent and 5 percent of all cancers. Approximately 9,500 people in the United States were expected to develop laryngeal cancer in 2006, and it was estimated to cause around 3,700 deaths in that year.

Although it is the most common source of cancers in the larynx, accounting for approximately 60 percent of all larynx cancer, cancer in the glottis is slower to spread than cancer in the subglottis and the supraglottis. The supraglottis is the originating site of approximately 35 percent of laryngeal cancer; the remaining 5 percent originates in the subglottis.

Men are affected by laryngeal cancer far more than women, and people over the age of 50 are much more likely to develop it than younger people. African Americans have a much higher rate of laryngeal cancer than Caucasians. The primary behavioral risk factors for laryngeal cancer are smoking and alcohol. Secondary risk factors that may contribute include poor nutrition, human papillomavirus, chronic gastric reflux, a weakened immune system, and certain forms of chemical exposure. The single most effective way to prevent laryngeal cancer is to never smoke.

DIAGNOSIS, TREATMENT, AND PROGNOSIS

Tests and procedures that can be used in determining whether laryngeal cancer is present include biopsy; a head and neck exam involving fiber-optic laryngoscopes (narrow, flexible tubes inserted into the mouth or nose); examination of the larynx under general anesthesia; chest X-rays; a barium swallow; or an MRI, PET, or CT scan.

Such tests may show precancerous conditions called dysplasia, but although dysplasia may lead to cancer, in the vast majority of cases it does not.

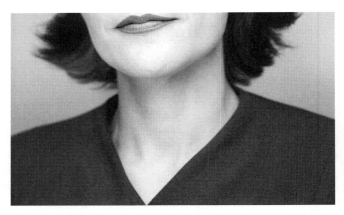

The larynx has three parts: above the vocal cords, the middle containing the vocal cords and from the vocal cords to the windpipe.

Treatment for laryngeal cancer depends on the specific location of the cancerous cells and the stage of the cancer. As with many other forms of cancer, the earlier laryngeal cancer is diagnosed, the more effective treatment becomes.

If laryngeal cancers are detected in Stage 0 (the earliest stage), they can almost always be cured by surgically removing them or vaporizing them. In Stage 1 and Stage 2, most laryngeal cancers can be treated successfully with radiation therapy, though surgery is sometimes another option. In Stage 3 and Stage 4, treatment can include total or partial removal of the larynx through surgery, chemotherapy, and radiation therapy, or any combination of those treatments. Surgery often includes neck dissection and the removal of lymph nodes.

One interesting (although small-scale) study conducted by Matthew C. Jepsen, et al., in 2003 found that poorer outcomes in terms of voice, speech, and swallowing were associated with adjuvant radiation therapy, compared with surgery.

Five-year survival rates for people diagnosed in the earliest stages of laryngeal cancer are estimated at above 80 percent.

SEE ALSO: Chemotherapy; Radiation Therapy; Surgery.

BIBLIOGRAPHY. Matthew C. *Jepsen, et al.,* "Voice, Speech, and Swallowing Outcomes in Laser-Treated Laryngeal Cancer," *Laryngoscope* (v.113/6, 2003).

MARK SHERRY
UNIVERSITY OF TOLEDO

Laryngeal Cancer, Childhood

CANCER OF THE larynx is rare; about 3.5 percent of all new malignancies diagnosed annually worldwide occur in the larynx. Most laryngeal cancers occur in adults, especially males in their 60s and 70s with a history of smoking and alcohol use. In children, laryngeal cancer is very rare. Since 1868 fewer than 100 cases of this cancer have been published in medical journals.

The larynx (or voice box) is a muscular tube in the neck that allows air to pass from the throat to the trachea (windpipe). It contains vocal cords that vibrate and make sound when air is directed against them. There are three main parts of the larynx: the glottis (where the vocal cords are located), the supraglottis (the tissue above the glottis), and the subglottis (the tissue below the glottis). The epiglottis is a flap at the top of the trachea that closes over the larynx to prevent food from entering the airways during the swallowing of food. Cancers of the larynx usually affect all its parts.

Different types of laryngeal cancer have been reported in children. In the past, the most common ones were squamous cell carcinomas, which start in squamous cells that form the outermost lining of the larynx. Currently, the most frequent pediatric laryngeal cancers are variants of rhabdomyosarcomas, which start in rhabdomyoblasts (primitive muscle cells).

Other laryngeal cancers in children are caused by the metastasis (spread) of other cancers, such as synovial sarcomas, non-Hodgkin's lymphoma, chondrosarcoma, Ewing's sarcoma, and primitive neuroectodermal tumor.

It is unclear why children and adolescents develop laryngeal cancers. The cancers are mainly attributed to genetic disease caused by damage to chromosomes. They are also attributed to exposure of children to radiation therapy, although many nonirradiated patients have this cancer.

In adults, factors that predispose one to laryngeal cancer include smoking or tobacco use, previous radiation therapy, and exposure to chemical carcinogens.

The early symptoms of laryngeal cancer are very unspecific and mimic those of many benign conditions that affect children. They include hoarseness, difficulty swallowing food, frequent choking on food, swelling in the neck, persistent sore throat, and breathing difficulty.

Laryngeal cancer in children is difficult to diagnose and is commonly detected after the cancer has progressed extensively. Reasons for its difficult diagnosis include the rarity of the cancer; the similarity of the cancer's early symptoms to those of benign, common childhood conditions; and the anatomic difficulties of examining children's larynxes. Therefore, the prognosis is poor in most cases of this cancer.

DIAGNOSIS AND TREATMENT

Diagnostic procedures include a complete medical history and physical examination in which the neck is carefully palpated for lumps, swellings, and other changes; laryngoscopies (insertion of a laryngoscope through the nose or mouth to visualize the larynx); biopsies (in which body samples are taken for examination under microscopes); and imaging procedures.

Laryngeal cancers in children are very aggressive and difficult to treat. Treatments usually include radiation therapy, surgery, and/or chemotherapy. In most cases the prognosis is poor.

To better manage children with this cancer, it would be helpful to have a pediatric and adolescent tumor registry to allow collection and sharing of information on the cancer.

SEE ALSO: Laryngeal Cancer; Lymphoma, Non-Hodgkin's, Childhood; Radiation Therapy; Rhabdomyosarcoma, Childhood.

BIBLIOGRAPHY. A. Rinaldo, et al., "Cancer of the Larynx in Children and Adolescents: A Neoplastic Lesion with a Different Etiology," *Acta Oto-laryngologica* (v.124/9, 2004); Health Publica Icon Health Publications, *Laryngeal Cancer—A Medical Dictionary, Bibliography, and Annotated Research Guide to Internet References* (Icon Health Publications, 2004).

KEMUNTO MOKAYA
YALE UNIVERSITY SCHOOL OF MEDICINE

Latitude

A LONG HISTORY of study has shown that cancer incidence varies according to latitude. A study in 1941

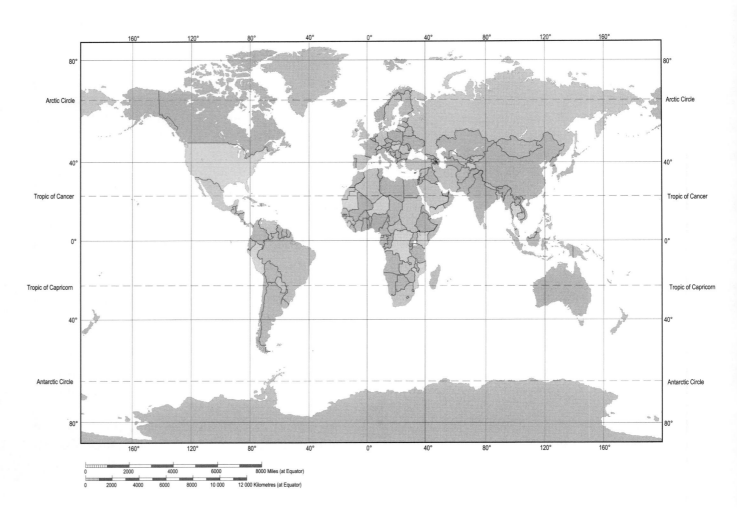

In general, the highest age-standardized cancer incidence rates are observed in latitudes distant from the equator. It was found that people living in northern latitudes had higher mortality from cancer than those living in southern states in the U.S.

reported that people living in northern latitudes including Vermont, Massachusetts, and New Hampshire had higher mortality from cancer than those living in Texas, South Carolina, and other southern states in the U.S. In general, the highest age-standardized cancer incidence rates are observed in latitudes distant from the equator. Such incidence patterns have been reported for cancers of the colon, breast, kidney, lung prostate, ovary, Hodgkin's disease, and pancreas. Morality from these cancers also follows the same latitude pattern as described for incidence.

VITAMIN D EXPOSURE

One mechanism or pathway for latitude to reduce cancer risk is through vitamin D status. Vitamin D is obtained by humans through exposure to the sun, from their diets, and from dietary supplements. Solar ultraviolet B radiation (wave length 290 to 315 nm) penetrates the skin and stimulates chemical reactions to produce vitamin D_3. This form of vitamin D is metabolized in the liver to 25-hydroxy vitamin D, which is then metabolized in the kidney to 1,25-dihydroxyvitamin D. This is the vitamin's active form and is tightly regulated in the blood. It is proposed that tissue in the colon, breast, prostate and other organs produces 1,25-dihydroxyvitamin D locally to control genes that help regulate cell functions and prevent cancer development or the survival of malignant cells.

Closer to the equator the solar irradiation is much stronger due to the angle of the sun, and higher levels of vitamin D are generated. On the other hand far from the equator (above a latitude of 37 degrees) the angle of the sun is lower, and in winter the sun is too weak to generate the production of any vitamin D. The impact of the sun on the generation of vitamin D can also be modified by clothing and by skin pigmentation—darker skin leads to lower levels of vitamin D. Over time our industrial evolution has led to a substantial shift away from outdoor work and an agriculture-based society to predominantly indoor work and urban living. A consequence of this evolution in the social structure of our population is a decrease in sun exposure. Thus the latitude cancer association is exacerbated by our societal evolution and can be explained in part by the sun and vitamin D pathways.

GEOGRAPHIC DISTRIBUTIONS OF UV RADIATION

In 1992 investigators examined the geographic distributions of UV radiation and prostate cancer mortality in 3,073 counties of the contiguous United States. The geographic distributions of UV radiation and prostate cancer mortality were significantly correlated inversely. Prostate cancer mortality exhibited a significant north-south trend, with lower rates in the South. These geographic patterns were not readily explicable by other known risk factors for prostate cancer. A growing body of epidemiologic evidence adds to the biologic plausibility of this vitamin D pathway as the explanation for the latitude association with cancer.

Prospective studies of blood levels of vitamin D and subsequent risk of cancer provide the strongest scientific evidence. For example, a prospective study of blood levels of 25-hydroxyvitamin D and risk of subsequent colon cancer showed an inverse relation between blood levels and colon cancer risk; a 50% reduction in risk was observed among women with the highest blood levels. Similar results based on prospective studies of men who have given blood samples showed an inverse relation with prostate cancer and among women an inverse association between blood levels and breast cancer risk.

PREVENTION

Future directions for cancer prevention that follow from the latitude association include strategies to increase sun exposure at a time when the angle of the sun is sufficient and vitamin D can be generated, and vitamin D_3 supplementation. One issue for supplementation that has not yet been resolved is the optimal blood level that should be obtained to achieve the highest cancer prevention. Furthermore as blood levels in the U.S. adult population currently vary by latitude and skin color, would we need different strengths of supplement pills to match our skin pigmentation and latitude of residence? These and other issues are being investigated to determine the optimal strategy to overcome the strong relationship between latitude and cancer.

SEE ALSO: Vitamin D.

BIBLIOGRAPHY. M. F. Hollick ,"Vitamin D Deficiency," *New England Journal of Medicine* (v.357, 2007); C. L. Hanchette and G. G. Schwartz, "Geographic patterns of prostate cancer mortality: evidence for a protective effect of ultraviolet radiation," *Cancer* (v.70, 1992); G. Melvyn Howe, (ed.), *Global Geocancerology: A World Geography of Human Cancers* (Churchill Livingstone, 1986); Rushton Gerard Staff, *Geocoding Health Data: The Use of Geographic Codes in Cancer Prevention and Control, Research and Practice* (CRC Press, Oct. 2007); Ric Skinner, Omar Khan (ed.), *Geographic Information Systems and Health Applications* (IGI Global, 2002).

GRAHAM COLDITZ
GENERAL EDITOR

Lauterbur, Paul C.

CHEMISTRY EDUCATOR PAUL C. Lauterbur was the winner of the Charles F. Kettering Prize of the General Motors Cancer Foundation in 1985 for "the discovery, development and subsequent refinement of the technique of magnetic resonance imaging." Eighteen years later he won the Nobel Prize in Physiology or Medicine jointly with Peter Mansfield for their discoveries concerning magnetic resonance imaging.

Paul Christian Lauterbur was born May 6, 1929, in Sidney, Ohio, to parents who had immigrated from Luxembourg and western Germany. His father was an engineer and part owner of Peerless Bread Machinery Co.

Lauterbur attended Holy Angels' School. As a boy he became interested in natural history from an aunt who taught at the demonstration school at Ball State Teachers' College (now Ball State University) in Indiana. He then attended Case Institute of Technology (Case Western Reserve University), Cleveland, specializing in chemistry and graduating in 1951. He became research assistant and associate at the Mellon Institute, Pittsburgh, from 1951 to 1953, and served as a corporal in the U.S. Army from 1953 to 1955. Returning to the Mellon Institute as a fellow in 1955, he remained there until 1963.

In 1961 Lauterbur completed his doctorate at the University of Pittsburgh, his topic being steric effects on C13 nuclear magnetic resonance spectra of substituted benzines. Two years later he was appointed associate professor of chemistry at State University of New York, Stony Brook, becoming professor in 1969, a post he held until 1984. In 1985 he moved to Urbana, Illinois, to become head of the department of medical information science and the department of chemistry at the University of Urbana-Champaign, and also director of the biomedical magnetic resonance laboratory. He was also distinguished university professor of the College of Medicine at the University of Illinois, Chicago.

PUBLICATIONS AND AWARDS

He has written extensively on many fields of cancer research and other areas, and was author or coauthor of 319 papers up to the time of his receiving the Nobel Prize in 2003.

Lauterbur has received numerous honorary degrees, including doctorates from the University of Liege, Belgium, in 1984; from Nicolaus Copernicus Medical Academy, Poland, in 1988; from Carnegie Mellon University in 1987; from Wesleyan University in 1989; from State University of New York in 1990; from Rensselaer Polytechnic Institute in 1991; and from the University of Mons, Hainaut, Belgium, in 1996.

His awards include the Gold Medal of the Society of Magnetic Resonance in Medicine in 1982; the Biological Physics Prize of the American Physics Society, the Howard N. Potts Medal of the Franklin Institute, and the Albert Lasker Clinical Research Award in 1984; the Kossar Memorial Award of the Society of Photograph-

ic Scientists and Engineers in 1985; and the Gairdner Foundation International Award in 1985, the year he was awarded the Charles F. Kettering Prize.

He was given the Distinguished Research in Biomedical Sciences Award of the Association of the American Medical College in 1986; the Roentgen Medal, the Medal of Honor from the Institute of Electrical and Electronics Engineers, and the National Science Medal in 1987; the National Medal for Technology in 1988; the Gold Medal Award of the Society for Computing of the Body Tomography and the Laufman-Greatbach Award of the Association for the Advancement of Medal Instrumentation in 1989; the International Society for Magnetic Resonance Award in 1992; and the Kyoto Prize from the Inamori Foundation, Japan, in 1994. In 2003 he won the Nobel Prize.

He was also the Jesse Beams Lecturer at the University of Virginia; the Smith Kline and French Lecturer at University College, London; and the H. H. Iddles Lecturer in Chemistry at the University of New Hampshire.

SEE ALSO: Technology, Imaging; United States.

BIBLIOGRAPHY. *American Men and Women of Science* (R. R. Bowker/Gale Group, 1971–2003); *Who's Who in America* (Marquis Who's Who, 19902004); *Who's Who in Medicine and Healthcare* (Marquis Who's Who, 1997–2000); *Who's Who in the Midwest* (Marquis Who's Who, 2000–2002); *Who's Who in Science and Engineering* (Marquis Who's Who, 1994–2000); *Who's Who in Technology* (Gale Research, 1989–1995).

JUSTIN CORFIELD
GEELONG GRAMMAR SCHOOL, AUSTRALIA

Lead

LEAD (PB) HAS been used since ancient times. It is commonly used in modern petroleum engineering, atomic reactors, and many organic (synthetic) compounds. Lead is a soft metal that has very little strength by itself. To add strength, it is usually combined with other metals to form alloys. Tin and antimony are often used to make lead alloys that have greater strength. Called plumbum by the Romans, pure lead is almost never found in nature; rather, it is found bonded with other compounds. Its most common form as an ore is galena, which is lead sulfide, a gray metallic ore.

Deposits of galena have been found all over the world. Numerous deposits have been mined in southwestern Wisconsin, Iowa, and Missouri, and in Cornwall, England. Joplin, Missouri, was a major galena-mining center for many years. Its galena deposits were worked as open-pit mines or deep shaft mines. Tailings of rock that contained the ore still cover large areas. Galena deposits frequently include copper, gold, and silver. Joplin's deposits also included zinc.

Galena ore is extracted from dirt, rocks, and other debris by crushing and by flotation. The process of flotation concentrates the ore in a tank containing a chemical such as copper sulfate or an oil of some type. The ore floats in the flotation bath, and the tailings sink to the bottom. Then the ore is skimmed from the flotation bath into a concentrated mass.

Concentrated galena is roasted to break the bonding with the lead. The roasting causes the sulfur to react with oxygen, forming sulfur dioxide (SO_2), which has many industrial uses, especially in the paper industry. Lead oxide (PbO_2) is also created in particulate form. Then the substance is sintered into pellets that can be reduced to pure lead by burning them with coke. The carbon in the coke reacts with the oxygen in the lead oxide to form carbon dioxide and a mass of metal. The resulting metal is rarely pure lead; instead, it is mixed with gold, silver, zinc, copper, and slag, which are separated in turn to produce pure lead.

PROPERTIES AND USES

Lead has a relatively low melting point of 327.5 degrees C (621.50 degrees F). It has numerous uses—as a covering to prevent leaks, for example. Its density makes it an excellent shield against X-rays in medical procedures. Lead is extensively used in atomic reactors to safeguard against radiation; it is also used as shielding on shipping containers for radioactive wastes and materials.

Chemical companies use lead for pipes because it resists corrosion. Lead is also used for shipping and storing many chemicals. Usually, the lead in these containers is an alloy of some type that adds strength to the lead's anticorrosive properties. Many electrical and electronic products use lead alloys to protect equipment from water corrosion. Power companies apply lead alloys to areas of power equipment that need protection. Lead is a component of solder, a tin–lead alloy that is used to join metal surfaces. The use of solder is common in the automotive and electronics industries.

The products that consume the greatest quantities of lead are lead–acid storage batteries, gasoline additives, and paints and dyes. In addition, large quantities are consumed in the manufacture of corrosion-resistant red and white lead paints, as well as explosives, insecticides, and some rubber products.

Lead–acid batteries, used in gasoline and electrical vehicles, consume most of all the lead currently produced. The dumping of these batteries has virtually ceased, and almost 100 percent of them are recycled globally, so lead–acid batteries are now insignificant sources of lead pollution.

Gasoline additives made with lead are used to reduce or prevent engine knocking. Tetraethyl lead was for a long time the second-largest consumer of lead. Leaded gasoline was standard for decades until its chemical-pollution drawbacks were identified. The use of tetraethyl lead as an antiknock chemical was discovered in 1922. DuPont Chemical Co. and General Motors created Ethyl Corp. in 1924 to manufacture and distribute tetraethyl lead. Almost immediately, the health risks were identified, and action to prevent its use was considered. The gasoline industry was able to block opposition and to use tetraethyl lead for decades, however. At the plants where tetraethyl lead was produced, some workers who handled it suffered illness or death from lead poisoning—one result of careless handling of tetraethyl lead or inadequate safety measures.

Beginning in the 1970s the U.S. Environmental Protection Agency took steps to ban lead as a gasoline additive. The sale of leaded gasoline in the United States has been illegal since 1995. Leaded gasoline is still manufactured, however, and is still used in farm machinery, race cars, and aviation.

Lead is used in paint to achieve many goals. It is used as a pigment; it is used to add durability, to keep the paint looking fresh for a longer period; and it is used to speed drying time and resist moisture that could cause corrosion. White and red lead paints are usually used to coat steel beams or steel plating. Lead paint is also used extensively on military

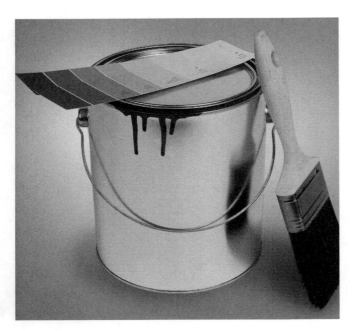

Since 1978 paint with lead content of more than .006 percent has been banned in residential housing (Code of Federal Regulations 1303).

equipment and to paint lines on roadways and parking lots. Since 1978 paint with lead content of more than .006 percent has been banned in residential housing (Code of Federal Regulations 1303), due to the danger that children will eat flaking lead paint. Lead is very harmful to children under the age of 6 because it can stunt growth, harm mental development, damage the nervous system, and destroy hearing. Some states seek to force paint companies to pay for the removal of lead paint from older housing. In 2006 several state cases involving issues related to lead paint reached the U.S. Supreme Court; decisions were expected in 2007.

HUMAN EFFECTS

Exposure to lead is usually through ingestion or inhalation. In addition, lead can be absorbed through the skin with long exposure. Inhaling lead particles or absorbing them through the skin poses is a danger to health, especially if exposure has been extensive and over a long period. The toxicity of lead arises from its similarity to other metals used by the human body, such as calcium, iron, and zinc. The proteins that combine with metals used by the body react with enzymes to perform necessary biological functions. Lead's reactivity displaces ions of calcium, iron, zinc,

and other metals to create a metabolic disorder. There is no known function for lead in the human body. Lead accumulates in the body, especially in the skeleton.

Lead poisoning is also called saturnism, plumbism, or painter's colic. It is a serious health condition that can, in severe cases, cause seizure, coma, and death. It disrupts the production of red blood cells and may damage the kidneys, liver, brain, and other organs.

Symptoms of chronic lead poisoning include neurological problems, nausea, stomach cramps, fatigue, insomnia, hyperactivity, headaches, and loss of mental capacities. Gastrointestinal symptoms include constipation, diarrhea, vomiting, and changes in appetite.

CARCINOGENIC PROPERTIES

To date, studies have found that lead is a carcinogenic agent in animals, but the evidence for human carcinogenetic reactions to lead is still inadequate. Studies strongly suggest that exposure to lead can be a secondary factor in the development of cancer.

The National Toxicology Program has reported through its Carcinogens Review Committee that lead and lead compounds should be considered to be possible human carcinogens. Four epidemiological studies have been made of workers in lead–acid battery plants and lead smelters. Those with obvious lead poisoning were examined, but only slightly higher rates of cancer were found.

The studies conducted to date did not report on smoking among the subjects of the study. The results were inconsistent in the events, locations, kinds of cancers, and other data points. The evidence is believed to be inadequate to determine whether lead is a human carcinogen.

Studies of laboratory animals produced tumors in rats and mice after exposure to soluble lead salts (phosphates and acetates). The studies found that lead affected gene expression. The studies examined different lead compounds but did not examine the carcinogenicity of lead in a systematic way. In the 10 studies of rats, for example, the strain of rats used was not reported. By contrast, hamsters given lead salts did not develop tumors.

Studies have indicated that lead compounds can create chromosomal changes. Lead has been shown to affect DNA structure and the molecular processes associated with gene expression. Lead exposure is a variable, but studies have not been able to demonstrate the effects of age, health, exposure duration, nutritional state, and other factors that may be connected with cancer events.

SEE ALSO: Battery Acid; Dyes and Pigments; Gasoline; Genetics; Insecticides; Paint.

BIBLIOGRAPHY. Jose Casas and Jose Sordo, eds. *Lead: Chemistry, Analytical Aspects, Environmental Impact and Health Effects* (Elsevier Science and Technology Books, 2006); H. Richard Casdorph and Morton Walker, *Toxic Metal Syndrome: How Metal Poisonings Can Affect Your Brain* (Penguin Group, 1994); Peter Kundig, ed., *Transition Metal Arene P-Complexes in Organic Synthesis and Catalysis* (Springer-Verlag, 2004); Michael J. Scoullos, et al., *Mercury—Cadium—Lead: Handbook for Sustainable Heavy Metals Policy and Regulation* (Kluwer Academic Publications, 2001); Helmut Sigel, et al., eds., *Neurodegenerative Diseases and Metal Ions: Metal Ions in Life Sciences* (John Wiley & Sons, Inc., 2006); ABBE Research Division Staff, *Lead (PB)(IARC-Rated as 2b Carcinogen) and Its Hostile Effects on Health in the U. S. A. Including Lead Poisoning in Adults and Children: Index and Medical Analysis of New Research Knowledge* (ABBE Publishers Association, 2004**);** ABBE Research Division Staff, *Lead (PB)(IARC-Rated as 2b Carcinogen) and Its Hostile Effects on Health in the U. S. A. Including Lead Poisoning in Adults and Children: Index and Medical Analysis of New Research Knowledge* (ABBE Publishing Association, 2004).

ANDREW J. WASKEY
DALTON STATE COLLEGE

Leukemia, Acute Lymphoblastic, Adult

ACUTE LYMPHOBLASTIC LEUKEMIA (ALL), less commonly referred to as acute lymphocytic leukemia, is a type of blood cancer caused by unregulated proliferation of white blood cells. These cells multiply excessively in the bone marrow, circulate in the bloodstream, and may infiltrate certain organs and tissues in the body. Adult ALL is less prevalent than childhood and adolescent ALL, encompassing 25 percent of ALL diagnoses. According to the National Cancer Institute, the annual incidence of adult ALL in the United States

is 0.4 to 0.6 cases per 100,000 people between 25 and 50 years of age. The incidence rises steadily during the older decades, however, and is twofold to threefold higher after the sixth decade of life.

Varying degrees of medical complications are common in ALL, depending on the pattern and extent of tumor-cell involvement. Adult ALL is generally more aggressive and less curable than childhood ALL. Although most patients are never cured, advances in current therapies are increasing patients' lifespan and the periods of disease-free remission.

Currently, the precise cause of ALL in adults is uncertain. Some evidence suggests that certain environmental exposures, such as chemotherapy or exposure to industrial chemicals, may increase the risk of developing ALL, but no definitive links have been proved.

Strong evidence indicates, however, that there is a genetic predisposition to ALL, including a higher incidence in both monozygotic and dizygotic twins of ALL patients. Interestingly, genetic abnormalities are very common in adults with ALL—much more so than in children with ALL. Genetic abnormalities have important clinical relevance for adult ALL, particularly relating to prognosis. ALL is slightly more frequent in men than women and maintains a higher incidence in Caucasians than in people of African origin.

The original cell that becomes malignant in ALL is believed to be a lymphoid stem cell that undergoes genetic alterations in the bone marrow. In becoming a malignant cell, it acquires attributes of white-blood-cell lymphoblasts (precursors to lymphocytes), and makes numerous identical copies of itself, a process known as clonal expansion. Such cells accumulate in the body because they lose the ability to mature and differentiate into other blood cells, and become unable to age and die like normal cells. In addition to residing in the bone marrow, replicated lymphoblasts circulate in the peripheral blood of ALL patients. The replicating cells in each ALL patient, otherwise known as the malignant clones, resemble either B or T lymphocytes (B- and T-cells) at various stages of development. Of total ALL cases, 75 percent involve B-cell ALL; the remainder are T-Cell ALL.

Significant heterogeneity exists among patients regarding the precise stage of cellular differentiation, however. Thus, ALL is more accurately understood as being a group of several disease subsets.

SYMPTOMS AND CLASSIFICATION

ALL patients have a variety of early disease signs and symptoms. Because of the acute onset, patients are often diagnosed following a recent development of symptoms. Typically, at least one of the normal blood-cell populations is suppressed due to malignant cells overcrowding the bone marrow, where blood cells are produced. As such, ALL patients may display fatigue; easy bruising or bleeding; or multiple infections due to loss of red blood cells, platelets, and normal white blood cells (such as neutrophils).

Constitutional symptoms—such as fevers, chills, and night sweats—frequently accompany other disease manifestations. In addition, the malignant cells have the potential to spread to the lymph nodes, spleen, liver, thymus, testes, and central nervous system, and may lead to liver, spleen, or lymph-node enlargement and a variety of associated pathologies.

The diagnosis and classification of ALL have evolved considerably since the end of the 20th century. Advances in understanding the immunological profiles of the malignant lymphoblasts have made it possible to subclassify ALL into extremely specific subtypes.

One of the first widely used classification schemas was the French-American-British (FAB) Co-operative Group subtyping. The FAB categorization of ALL depends on the morphological traits of the lymphoblastic clone and is subtyped L1 to L3, based on the size and intracellular staining of the lymphoblasts.

The World Health Organization subsequently devised a different classification system based on more specific immunological surface markers and genetic abnormalities, helping clarify ALL diagnosis for clinicians.

Currently, ALL is normally categorized in very specific immunological subtypes that can be considered to be different disease entities. Each unique subtype, such as pro B-Cell (i.e., pre-pre-B-cell) or mature T-Cell ALL, represents a clonal cell that became malignant at a different point in the continuum of lymphocyte development.

Increasingly, it is becoming clinically relevant to differentiate subtleties among subtypes, as both prognosis and response to therapy have been demonstrated to vary greatly among ALL subtypes.

TREATMENT AND PROGNOSIS

Therapy for ALL is usually aimed at reducing the burden of disease or achieving long-term disease remission. Therapy is highly dependent on particular ALL subtypes. Mature B-cell ALL is treated with short-term intensive chemotherapy, for example. All the other subtypes, however, usually involve prolonged treatment schedules, first employing induction therapy to attain remission, followed by long-term consolidation therapy with the aim of systematically eliminating all residual traces of disease.

Clinicians generally use combination chemotherapy regimens for induction therapy, including agents such as daunorubicin, vincristine, prednisone, and asparaginase. Currently, 60 percent to 80 percent of adults can be expected to attain complete remission after induction treatment, having no detectable cancer cells left in their bodies. After achieving remission, however, only about 30 percent to 40 percent of adult ALL patients achieve long-term disease-free survival. Patients at high risk for relapse or those with residual disease after induction treatment may be candidates for bone-marrow transplantation, which offers the chance of curing their disease.

Individualized and targeted therapies, including various small-molecule drugs and monoclonal antibodies, are being investigated for their efficacy in altering molecular pathways involved in the pathogenesis of ALL. The overall benefits, in terms of response rates and disease-free survival, of many of these new agents remain to be determined following randomized prospective clinical trials.

Overall, treatments for ALL are quite diverse, depending on the patient's age and other risk factors, and are constantly being retailored based on specific disease subtypes and genetic abnormalities.

SEE ALSO: Bone Marrow Transplants; Chemotherapy; Genetics; Leukemia, Acute Lymphoblastic, Childhood.

BIBLIOGRAPHY. American Cancer Society, *Cancer Facts and Figures 2006* (American Cancer Society, 2006); Nancy Lee Harris, et al., "World Health Organization Classification of Neoplastic Diseases of the Hematopoietic and Lymphoid Tissues: Report of the Clinical Advisory Committee Meeting-Airlie House, Virginia, 1997," *Journal of Clinical Oncology* (v.17, 1999); Ahmedin Jemal, et al., "Cancer Statistics, 2004," *CA: A Cancer Journal for Clinicians* (v.54, 2004); Ching-Hon Pui and William E. Evans, "Treatment of Acute Lymphoblastic Leukemia," *New England Journal of Medicine* (v.354, 2006); Lynne A. G. Ries, et al., eds., *SEER*

Cancer Statistics Review, 1975–2002 (National Cancer Institute, 2004).

ANDREW R. BRANAGAN
MEDICAL SCHOOL FOR INTERNATIONAL HEALTH
BEN-GURION UNIVERSITY OF THE NEGEV
COLUMBIA UNIVERSITY MEDICAL CENTER
ITAI LEVY
SOROKA UNIVERSITY MEDICAL CENTER
BEN-GURION UNIVERSITY OF THE NEGEV

Leukemia, Acute Lymphoblastic, Childhood

LEUKEMIA IS A cancer of the white blood cells. Lymphocytes are members of a specific group of white blood cells that function to help the body fight infections and are part of the immune system known as the lymphoid cells. Like other types of cells in the blood, lymphocytes originate in the bone marrow in immature forms. Before developing into fully mature lymphocytes, these cells are called lymphoblasts. A fast, unregulated overgrowth of lymphoblasts that neither develop nor function normally is defined as acute lymphoblastic leukemia, also known as acute lymphocystic leukemia, acute lymphoid leukemia, or simply ALL.

Although rare, ALL is the most common cancer in children in the United States, occurring in about 1 of every 29,000 children per year. Among those under 15 years of age, 23 percent of all cancers are due to ALL.

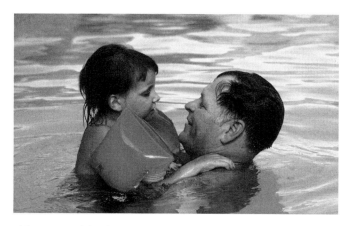

This 10 year-old girl was diagnosed at the age of 3 with a form of Acute Lymphoblastic Leukemia (ALL). She is in long-term remission.

The National Institutes of Health says that ALL is the cause of 80 percent of acute childhood leukemias. Most cases occur from ages 3 to 7. The Leukemia and Lymphoma Society reports that an average of 3,930 newly diagnosed cases of ALL in children occur each year in the United States. The frequency of this cancer in adults is lower than that of acute myeloid leukemia. There are approximately 1,000 new adult cases each year. Worldwide, the highest incidence occurs in Italy, the United States, Switzerland, and Costa Rica.

The cause of ALL has yet to be determined. Certain risk factors seem to be associated with this cancer, including having a sibling with leukemia; Down syndrome, radiation exposure; and exposure to chemicals such as benzene, alcohol, or immunosuppressant chemotherapy drugs. Chromosome abnormalities may also be involved. Being Hispanic or Caucasian, or living in the United States, may play a role as well.

There are many distinctive subtypes of ALL, based on the cell type that is affected, chromosomal changes, and the age at diagnosis. Among these, T-cell ALL, Philadelphia chromosome-positive ALL, and ALL diagnosed in infancy are approached differently from the other subtypes. Depending on the subtype, the patient is treated with different chemotherapeutic drugs. A patient's subtype may determine the survival rate. Infants with ALL have a very low survival rate, for example.

TREATMENT AND SURVIVAL RATE

In general, treating ALL requires using multiple chemotherapeutic drugs for two to three years, or bone-marrow transplantation when necessary. Currently, more than 85 percent of ALL children survive for over five years—a tremendous improvement in survival rate compared with less than 5 percent in the 1960s. St. Jude Children's Research Hospital promises a 90 percent cure rate of ALL in the coming years. Most important, allowing a child with ALL to receive care at an institution dedicated to treating patients with ALL provides the best prognosis for the child.

SEE ALSO: Bone Marrow Transplants; Chemotherapy; Genetics; Leukemia, Acute Lymphoblastic, Adult; Leukemia, Acute Myeloid, Childhood; St. Jude Children's Research Hospital.

BIBLIOGRAPHY. National Cancer Institute, "Acute Lymphoblastic Leukemia in Children: Fact Sheet," www.cancer.gov

(cited February 2007); St. Jude Children's Research Hospital, "St. Jude Announces 90% Survival Rate for Leukemia," www.stjude.org (cited February 2007); The Leukemia and Lymphoma Society, "Acute Lymphoblastic Leukemia," www.leukemia-lymphoma.org (cited February 2007); U.S. National Library of Medicine, "Acute Lymphoblastic Leukemia (ALL)," www.nlm.nih.gov (cited February 2007).

Susanna N. Chen
Western University of Health Sciences

Leukemia, Acute Myeloid, Adult

ACUTE LEUKEMIA IS a disease belonging to the group of hemoblastoses (malignant cancers of the blood related to genetic mutation in bone-marrow cells). In acute leukemia, the malignant cells do not attain maturity, and the blastic forms prevail in peripheral blood. Acute leukemia occurs in two forms: acute myeloid leukemia (AML) and acute lymphoid leukemia (ALL). In AML, the myeloid series—granulocytes, monocytes, erythrocytes, and platelets—is affected.

Factors that increase the risk for AML include exposure to radiation (including previous radiotherapeutic treatment and nuclear disasters), contact with chemicals (benzene), contact with chemotherapeutic agents (including previous treatment for cancer and some antibiotics), and old age. Men are at greater risk for developing AML than women.

Impaired differentiation in tumor cells results in a discrepancy between proliferation and differentiation. Rapid, unchecked proliferation of malignant cells suppresses normal hematopoiesis—that is, normal erythrocytes, platelets, granulocytes, and monocytes are no longer produced.

In later stages, malignant cells spread to peripheral blood, lymph nodes, the central nervous system, the skin, and the spleen. In some patients, the brain cov-

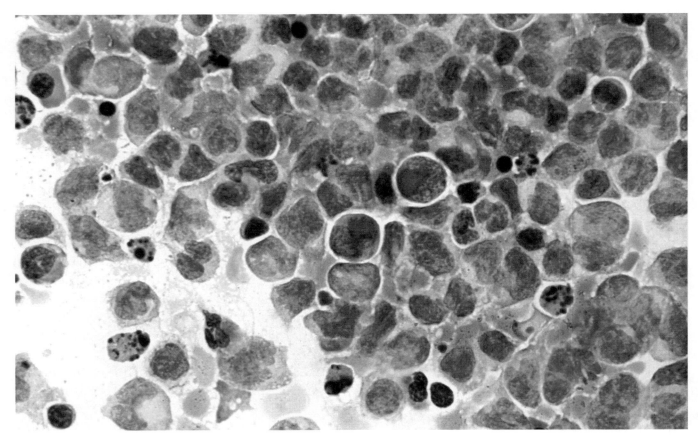

Human cells with acute myelocytic leukemia (AML) in the pericardial fluid, shown with an esterase stain at 400x. Acute leukemia occurs in two forms: acute lymphoid leukemia (ALL) and acute myeloid leukemia (AML).

erings (meninges) become involved, in a form of the disease called meningeal leukemia.

The clinical signs of AML vary. Some patients experience only symptoms such as tiredness, loss of appetite, and fever. Other patients show signs of anemia and hemorrhages (petechiae, bruises) due to the decrease of erythrocytes and platelets in blood. Anemia is a common presentation and can be marked by fatigue, dizziness, chest pain, tachycardia, and pale mucosa and nail beds. Pain in the bones and lymph nodes and spleen enlargement are usually late signs of the disease. Secondary infections occur frequently in patients with acute leukemia. Fever, tonsillitis, and swollen gums are common.

Diagnostic tests to identify AML include a complete blood count (to calculate the amount of erythrocytes, leucocytes, and platelets) and a peripheral blood smear (to determine the presence of blast cells and any abnormalities in blood cells). Additional tests include bone-marrow aspiration and biopsy (the bone-marrow sample is reviewed by a pathologist for signs of cancer) and cytogenetic analysis (to look for chromosomal abnormalities). Immune phenotyping (to identify the subtype of AML on the basis of specific antigenic markers) and polymerase chain reaction are usually done. When a diagnosis of AML has been confirmed, additional tests are used to determine whether the disease has spread outside the blood and bone marrow. A lumbar puncture or spinal tap, x-ray of the chest, and ultrasound investigation of the abdomen are essential.

There is no standard staging system for diagnosis of AML, but the World Health Organization and French-American-British classifications are widely used.

TREATMENT AND PROGNOSIS

Treatment of AML aims to achieve three goals: suppress the proliferation of the abnormal cells, recover normal hematopoiesis, and control symptoms. The modalities of treatment depend on the subtype of the AML; typically, the patient receives combination therapy consisting of two or more drugs. Allogenic stem-cell transplantation may be done in a patient experiencing a period of remission if a compatible donor is available.

The prognosis depends on the subtype of the AML, the stage of disease at the time of diagnosis, and the presence of concomitant diseases.

SEE ALSO: Genetics; Leukemia, Acute Lymphoblastic, Adult; Leukemia, Acute Lymphoblastic, Childhood; Leukemia, Acute Myeloid, Childhood.

BIBLIOGRAPHY. Robert C. Bast, Jr., et al., eds., *Cancer Medicine*, 5th ed., www.ncbi.nlm.nih.gov/books/bv.fcgi?call=bv.View..ShowTOC&rid=cmed.TOC&depth=2 (cited August 2006); Cancer Research Foundation website, www.cancer-researchfoundation.com (cited August 2006); Leukemia and Lymphoma Society website, www.leukemia-lymphoma.org (cited August 2006); Wikipedia website, www.wikipedia.org (cited August 2006).

RAHUL PANDIT
ST. PETERSBURG STATE MEDICAL ACADEMY, RUSSIA

Leukemia, Acute Myeloid, Childhood

ACUTE MYELOID LEUKEMIA (AML)—also called acute myelogenous leukemia, acute myeloblastic leukemia, acute granulocytic leukemia, or acute non-lymphocytic leukemia—is a cancer in which the bone marrow overproduces immature, abnormal white blood cells inside the bone marrow; these cells then circulate into the blood. A reduction in the growth of normal blood cells is present, resulting in deficiencies of the red blood cells, platelets, and other important white blood cells.

Those afflicted with AML experience numerous infections, anemia, and bleeding dysfunctions, and are at risk of bone-marrow failure. They may even have bone pain and difficulty walking.

About 15 percent to 20 percent of leukemia cases in childhood are acute myeloid leukemias; the risk of AML increases significantly with age. About 500 new cases of AML in children are diagnosed in the United States each year. AML is the second-most-common cancer in children who have been treated for a previous malignancy.

Normally in the bone marrow, precursor blood cells develop into various types of mature blood cells that are involved in the immune response and blood clotting. These stem cells are termed myeloblasts and differentiate into granulocytes, monocytes (cells with immune function), and platelets (cells for coagulating blood). Granulocytes include neutrophils, eosinophils, and basophils. (AML does not, however, involve lymphocytes, as in acute lymphoblastic leukemia.) The cancerous cells in AML may eventually replace the normal cells in the bone marrow and spread to other areas of the body, such as the central nervous system, spleen, liver, kidneys, gonads, skin, and gums.

Many risk factors may contribute to the risk of AML. Having a sibling with leukemia; having a history of myelodysplastic syndrome or aplastic anemia; exposure to radiation or certain chemicals; exposure to cigarette smoke or alcohol before birth; having genetic disorders including Down syndrome, Fanconi anemia, neurofibromatosis type 1, or Noonan Syndrome; or being of Hispanic background may all increase the risk of AML. AML may be differentiated into various subtypes based on the types of blood cells affected. The subtypes reflect the stages of development of the myeloblasts.

TREATMENT AND PROGNOSIS

Treatment is through various chemotherapeutic agents and possibly antibiotics, depending on the AML subtype. Stem-cell transplantation is a less commonly used treatment option. For patients with Down syndrome or acute promyelocytic leukemia, the therapies vary from those of other AML subtypes. In particular, promyelocytic leukemia is treated with all-trans retinoic acid (ATRA), which induces the immature promyelocytes to mature into neutrophils while reducing the number of leukemic myeloblasts. Chemotherapy is given simultaneously to achieve remission. Arsenic trioxide may be given if the patient is not treatable with ATRA.

Prognosis is better when certain chromosomal changes are present in the cells. Currently, 80 percent to 90 percent of children with AML may experience remission after treatment, but only 40 percent to 50 percent of those children have long-term remission.

Novel methods of therapy are under study, including clinical trials studying AML gene-expression profiles currently in progress at St. Jude's Children's Research Hospital.

SEE ALSO: Chemotherapy; Genetics; Leukemia, Acute Lymphoblastic, Childhood; Leukemia, Acute Myeloid, Adult; Myelodysplastic Syndromes; Myelodysplastic/Myeloproliferative Diseases; St. Jude Children's Research Hospital.

BIBLIOGRAPHY. National Cancer Institute, "General Information about Childhood Acute Myeloid Leukemia and Other Myeloid Malignancies," www.cancer.gov (cited February 2007); St. Jude Children's Research Hospital, "Leukemias/Lymphomas: Acute Myeloid Leukemia (AML)," www.stjude.org; The Leukemia and Lymphoma Society, "Acute Myelogenous Leukemia (AML)," www.leukemia-lymphoma.org (cited February 2007).

SUSANNA N. CHEN
WESTERN UNIVERSITY OF HEALTH SCIENCES

Leukemia and Lymphoma Society of America

IN THE 1940S, leukemia was a fatal disease. Thus, a prominent New York family established the foundation of the Leukemia Society of America to raise funds for research and to educate the public about leukemia. The orannization is based in White Plains, New York, and has regional offices in Virginia, Ohio, and California.

The society's mission is to "cure leukemia, lymphoma, Hodgkin's disease and myeloma, and improve the quality of life of patients and their families." To achieve its mission, the society has established a set of strategic goals: research, patient services, advocacy, revenue generation, public awareness, and human resources. In addition to funding research for leukemia and lymphoma, the society funds research on myeloma.

The society grew out of the Robert Roesler de Villiers Foundation, which Rudolph and Antoinette de Villiers started in 1949 in memory of their son, who had passed away from leukemia in 1944. They formed the foundation in the hope of preventing further suffering from this disease. The name The Leukemia Society of America was adopted in the 1960s to express the organization's national concerns. Lymphoma was added to the name in 2000 to reflect the society's focus on all blood cancers. The society collaborates with several other organizations—including Community Health Charities, the National Health Council, the Cancer Leadership Council, and the Cancer Appropriations Working Group—to bring the best service to leukemia and lymphoma patients. Additionally, many corporations and organizations have contributed to the cause and are acknowledged as sponsor partners.

The society supports three new research initiatives: the Specialized Center of Research, which fosters collaboration among research institutions; the Translational Research Program, which funds promising translational research projects; and the Career Development Program, which supports young investigators in the fields of blood cancer. The Leukemia and Lymphoma Society of America's website is available in English, French, Portuguese, and Spanish.

SEE ALSO: Myeloma, Multiple.

BIBLIOGRAPHY. Tariq Mughal, et al., *Understanding Leukemias, Lymphomas and Myelomas* (Taylor and Francis, 2005).

CLAUDIA WINOGRAD
UNIVERSITY OF ILLINOIS AT URBANA-CHAMPAIGN

Leukemia, Chronic Lymphocytic

CHRONIC LYMPHOCYTIC LEUKEMIA (CLL), the most frequent form of leukemia in the Western countries, is characterized by clonal proliferation and accumulation of neoplastic B lymphocytes in the blood, bone marrow, lymph nodes, and spleen. The annual incidence is 2 to 3 per 100,000; the male-to-female ratio is 2:1; and the median age at diagnosis is 65 to 70 years. CLL is suspected whenever an absolute lymphocytosis in the peripheral blood occurs in an adult. Minimum requirements for the diagnosis of CLL include an absolute lymphocyte count in the peripheral blood of more than 10,000 per microliter, and a normocellular to hypercellular bone marrow with lymphocytes accounting for more than 30 percent of all nucleated cells.

The most consistently abnormal finding on physical exam of the patient with CLL is lymphadenopathy. Other commonly encountered physical findings are splenomegaly and hepatomegaly.

Rai and Binet devised staging systems that remain the cornerstones on which decisions regarding medical follow-up and treatment are built. The Rai system has been the most widely used staging system in North America. The Rai system uses the presence or absence of lymphadenopathy, organomegaly (spleen and liver), and cytopenias to separate patients into groups with widely different anticipated survival times.

The definitive cause of CLL remains unknown. CLL might result from a multistep process, beginning with an antigen-driven polyclonal expansion of CD5+ B lymphocytes that, under the influence of mutational agents, would eventually be transformed into monoclonal proliferation. In recent years, it has been suggested that B lymphocytes in CLL either avoid death through the intercession of external signals or die by apoptosis, only to be replenished by proliferating precursor cells.

Recent studies have provided important biological markers that can be further used to predict the course of CLL. Cases can be divided into two subgroups on the basis of the presence or absence of somatic mutations in the specific immunoglobulin heavy-chain variable-region (IgVH) genes used by the leukemic cells. Mutations in these genes are somehow closely linked to the clinical course, because patients whose leukemic B cells express IgVH genes with somatic mutations fare much better than those without such mutations.

The disparity in life span is very striking, with a median survival of more than 24 years and 6 to 8 years, respectively. Studies are currently under way to identify more prognostic markers and their surrogates, which will soon allow physicians to offer individual patients with CLL a much more definitive projection of their clinical course than is currently possible.

TREATMENT AND PROGNOSIS

During the past few years, important advances have been made in the understanding of the biology, natural history, and treatment of CLL. Chlorambucil was the standard first-line treatment for CLL. Clinical trials have now established the effectiveness of various other agents, such as fludarabine, a purine nucleoside analogue, and rituximab, an anti-CD20 monoclonal antibody. Because of this potential benefit and the modest side effects of rituximab, the addition of rituximab to purine nucleoside analogue-based therapy has been widely adopted as the first line of treatment.

The course of the disease is variable. Whereas some patients with CLL have a normal life span, others die within five years after diagnosis. Some patients with CLL survive for many years without therapy and eventually succumb to unrelated diseases, whereas others have a rapidly fatal disease despite aggressive therapy.

SEE ALSO: Clinical Trials; Leukemia, Chronic Myelogenous.

BIBLIOGRAPHY. T. Shanafelt, "Narrative Review: Initial Management of Newly Diagnosed, Early-Stage Chronic Lymphocytic Leukemia," *Annals of Internal Medicine* (v.145, 2006).

NAKUL GUPTA
ROSS UNIVERSITY SCHOOL OF MEDICINE

Leukemia, Chronic Myelogenous

CHRONIC MYELOGENOUS LEUKEMIA (CML) is a malignant clonal disorder of hematopoietic stem cells that results in increases in myeloid cells, erythroid cells, and platelets in the peripheral blood. Philadelphia (Ph) chromosome, formed via translocation t (9; 22), is the cytogenetic hallmark of CML. The translocation forms a chimeric gene, bcr-abl, that generates BCR-ABL, a fusion protein that constitutively activates ABL tyrosine kinase and causes CML.

CML has an incidence of 1 to 2 cases per 100,000 people per year and accounts for 15 percent of leukemias in adults. The median age at presentation is about 55 years. Of all patients, 20 percent to 50 percent are asymptomatic, with the disease first being suspected from routine blood tests, which characteristically show uncontrolled production of maturing granulocytes, predominantly neutrophils. Among symptomatic patients, systemic symptoms (fatigue, malaise, weight loss), abdominal fullness, and bleeding episodes are common. The most common abnormality on physical examination is splenomegaly, which is present in up to half of patients.

The Ph chromosome causes a BCR-ABL-positive myeloproliferative disease, which can be diagnosed by cytogenetics, reverse transcription-polymerase chain reaction (RT-PCR), and fluorescence in situ hybridization (FISH). CML has a triphasic clinical course: a chronic phase, which is present at the time of diagnosis in most patients; an accelerated phase, in which neutrophil differentiation becomes progressively impaired and leukocyte counts are more difficult to control with medications; and blast crisis, a condition resembling acute leukemia in which myeloid and lymphoid blasts fail to differentiate.

The cause of CML is the translocation of regions of the *BCR* and *ABL* genes to form a *BCR-ABL* fusion gene. In at least 90 percent of cases, this event is a reciprocal translocation termed t (9; 22), which forms the Ph chromosome. The product of the *BCR-ABL* gene, the BCR-ABL protein, is a constitutively active oncoprotein tyrosine kinase that phosphorylates substrates of remarkable diversity, including RAS, that activate multiple signaling pathways.

Because RAS serves as a critical control point for signal transduction from cell membrane to nucleus, the BCR-ABL–mediated over expression of RAS appears to alter signal transduction in a target stem cell, leading to abnormal mitosis and neoplastic expansion. In addition, BCR-ABL reduces cellular adhesion to stromal matrix, which allows myeloid progenitor cells to remain longer in the proliferative phase before undergoing differentiation. BCR-ABL also diminishes cellular responsiveness to apoptotic stimuli, providing a survival advantage to the leukemic clones.

TREATMENT AND ALTERNATIVE TREATMENT

Although allogeneic hematopoietic-cell transplantation is the only proven curative treatment for CML, the procedure is an option in only about 25 percent of patients and carries substantial risks. Novel target therapies such as imatinib mesylate have dramatically diminished the use of allogeneic stem-cell transplantation for CML. Imatinib mesylate, an ABL tyrosine kinase inhibitor, is a novel drug that binds to and stabilizes the inactive form of BCR-ABL. Imatinib voids the effects of BCR-ABL oncoprotein through inhibition of BCR-ABL autophosphorylation, inhibition of proliferation, and induction of apoptosis. With the introduction of imatinib, major advances in the treatment of CML have been achieved.

As with many other anticancer drugs, clinical resistance to imatinib monotherapy has emerged. The need for alternative treatments has led to a second generation of target therapies, such as AMN107, which are still in their early phases.

SEE ALSO: Alternative Therapy: Pharmacological and Biological Treatment; Genetics; Leukemia, Chronic Lymphocytic.

BIBLIOGRAPHY. C. Sawyers, "Chronic Myeloid Leukemia," *New England Journal of Medicine* (v.340/17, 1999). The Leukemia and Lymphoma Society, "Acute Myelogenous

Leukemia (AML)," www.leukemia-lymphoma.org (cited January 2007).

NAKUL GUPTA
ROSS UNIVERSITY SCHOOL OF MEDICINE

Leukemia, Hairy Cell

HAIRY CELL LEUKEMIA (HCL) is a B-cell lymphoproliferative disorder that, though uncommon, has received much attention due to the disease's unknown pathogenesis, unique characteristics, and varying clinical presentations.

HCL is characterized by abnormal B cells that express abnormal surface antigens, causing the cell to be recognized by the body as atypical and ultimately sequestered in the spleen. HCL is rare, with only about 700 new cases of the disease per year in the United States. The disease is not distributed equally between the genders, being four times more common in men than in women.

Both environmental and genetic conditions are implicated in possible causes for the disease. Suspected environmental causes include radiation exposure, Epstein-Barr virus (the virus that causes mononucleosis), farming, and organic chemicals such as pesticides. Genetic conditions that predispose an individual to HCL involve the human leukocyte antigen (HLA), a group of genes in the cell that codes for a particular type of tissue or group of cells. In this case, the HLA codes for white blood cells.

The physician must be careful and astute when examining a patient with splenomegaly and, though rare, to keep HCL in the differential diagnosis. Splenomegaly may be massive; thus, patients may present with abdominal distension or fullness. Patients may also feel weak and tired, and may bleed extensively because platelets are sequestered in the spleen and may not be able to contribute to clotting. Many patients with HCL show pancytopenia (low white-blood-cell count, low red-blood-cell count, and low platelet count).

Diagnosis of HCL includes microscopic analysis of white blood cells. Almost all patients with HCL show a characteristic hairy cell in peripheral blood smears with Romanovsky stain. The hairy-cell appearance

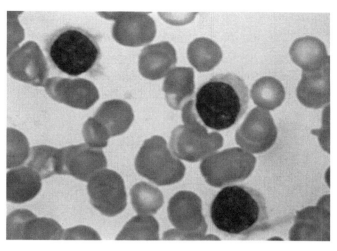

A histological slide of hairy cell leukemia. HCL is characterized by abnormal B cells that express abnormal surface antigens.

is due to cytoplasmic projections from the cell, giving the cell an abnormal and irregular border. Other methods of detecting HCL in a patient include bone-marrow trephine biopsy, reticulin staining of the bone-marrow trephine biopsy, and tartrate-resistant acid phosphatase activity on peripheral blood smear.

TREATMENT AND PROGNOSIS

Recent advances have replaced splenectomies as a treatment of choice, with highly successful pharmaceutical approaches proving to be successful in increasing complete remission rates. Purine analogs like Cladribine and Pentostatin effectively kill both resting and dividing lymphoid cells (the cells that are prone to becoming hairy cells). Pentostatin inhibits adenosine deaminase, an enzyme that enables lymphoid cells to work. Cladribine accumulates in lymphoid cells and causes a reaction whereby lymphoid cells kill themselves.

HCL, though a rare disease, has recently become a type of leukemia that has shown great promise to the medical profession. Pharmaceutical advances and extensive research have allowed patients a very high rate of complete remission. The treatment for HCL is a perfect example of how the cure for cancer can, in many cases, not necessarily target the mechanism of cell proliferation but kill malignant cells and those cells that are prone to becoming malignant.

SEE ALSO: Drugs; Genetics; Pesticides; Radiation.

BIBLIOGRAPHY. National Institutes of Health, "Leukemia, Adult Chronic," www.nlm.nih.gov/medlineplus (cited January 2007); National Cancer Institute, "Hairy Cell Leukemia," www.cancer.gov/cancertopics/pdq/treatment/hairy-cell-leukemia.

BRADLEY E. GOLDSTEIN
LAKE ERIE COLLEGE OF OSTEOPATHIC MEDICINE

Levy, Ronald

AMERICAN CANCER SPECIALIST Ronald Levy was the winner of the Charles F. Kettering Prize of the General Motors Cancer Foundation in 1999 for "demonstrating that the administration of monoclonal antibodies can produce objective clinical responses in patients with B cell lymphomas."

Ronald Levy was born in Carmel, California, and educated at Harvard University (B.S., 1963) and Stanford University (M.D., 1968). He also has a diploma from the American Board of International Medicine. Levy worked as an intern at Massachusetts General Hospital in Boston from 1968 to 1969 and as a researcher from 1969 to 1970. Levy was a Helen Hay Whitney Foundation fellow in the Department of Chemistry and Immunology at the Weizmann Institute of Science, Rehovot, Israel, from 1973 to 1975.

From 1975 to 1981 he was assistant professor in medicine at the division of oncology at Stanford University, becoming associate professor in 1981 and professor of medicine in 1987. Also in 1987 he was appointed Robert K. Summy Professor, as well as Frank and Else Schilling American Cancer Society Clinical Research Professor. Six years later Levy became chief of the division of oncology at Stanford. He was also concurrently investigator at the Howard Hughes Medical Institute (1977–82), chairman of the board of scientific counselors at the division of cancer treatment of the National Institutes of Health (1989–93), and member of the scientific advisory board of the Fred Hutchinson Cancer Research Center.

His early research on cancer was at the National Cancer Institute. His wife, Shoshana, was a cancer biologist. The main emphasis of his work was looking for answers to cancer in the human immune system. Specifically, he focused on components of the immune response called B-cells, each of which had a unique protein on its surface. When one of those cells reproduces uncontrollably, a tumor—and cancer—results. Thus, Levy was keen on finding a solution to the B-cells from within the body, which would remove the need for drastic surgery or chemotherapy, with the obvious side effects. Much of his research during the 1980s was on developing antibodies that were sufficient to treat cancer but not so much as to lead to major side effects. According to former colleagues, he often tested drugs and then treated patients. Many people tried his treatment methods. In 2004 Philip Karr testified that when he was 67, before he was treated by Levy, he was unable to swim the width of a pool. Interviewed at the age of 90, he said that after Levy's treatment, he could easily swim the length of a pool and was soon declared cancer free.

AWARDS AND PUBLICATIONS

Levy has won many awards, including the Armand Hammer Award for Cancer Research in 1982, the Ciba-Geigy/Drew Award in Biomedical Research in 1983, the Dr. Josef Steiner Prize for Cancer Research in 1989, and the Karnofsky Award of the American Society of Clinical Oncology in 1999 (the year he also won the Charles F. Kettering Prize). He won the Centeon Award from the 6th International Conference on Bispecific Antibodies later in 1999. He won the C. Chester Stock Award of the Memorial Sloan-Kettering Cancer Center, the Medal of Honor of the American Cancer Society, and the Key to the Cure Award of the Cure for Lymphoma Foundation in 2000. He won the Evelyn Hoffman Memorial Prize if the Lymphoma Research Foundation of America in 2001, the Jeffrey A. Gottleib Memorial Award of the M.D. Anderson Cancer Center in 2003, and the Discovery Health Channel Medal of Honor in 2004.

Levy has published extensively in many scientific journals, and has served on the editorial and advisory boards of many prestigious bodies.

SEE ALSO: Chemotherapy; National Cancer Institute; Surgery.

BIBLIOGRAPHY. *American Men and Women of Science* (R. R. Bowker/Gale Group, 1994–2003); *Who's Who in America* (Marquis Who's Who, 1984–1995); *Who's Who in Medicine and Healthcare* (Marquis Who's Who, 1996–1998);

Who's Who in Science and Engineering (Marquis Who's Who, 1994).

JUSTIN CORFIELD
GEELONG GRAMMAR SCHOOL, AUSTRALIA

Libya

THIS NORTH AFRICAN country was occupied by the Ottoman Turks from the 16th century until 1911, when it was captured by Italy. The Italians called it Libya (or Libia) in 1934 and held it until World War II. After the war, it was under British control (with the French holding Fezzan). It became independent on December 24, 1951, as the Kingdom of Libya. After a revolution in 1969 it was renamed the Libyan People's Socialist Arab Jamahiriya. Libya has a population of 5,673,000 (2006), with 128 doctors and 360 nurses per 100,000 people. An example of cancer incidence rates in Libya includes 99.3 cases of cancer in males per 100,000, according to the International Agency for Research on Cancer.

Before Italian colonial rule, healthcare in much of the country was extremely limited, although some Arab surgeons using the works of Avicenna and others were involved in successful surgical procedures for treating tumors. During Italian rule, healthcare improved dramatically for the European population and the local elite. It was not until after the discovery of oil that Libya became extremely wealthy, which resulted in a massive increase in health services in the country.

RESEARCH

During the 1960s, Elie N. Arida, director of laboratories at Benghazi University Hospital, researched the clinical purposes for the differentiation of leukemoid reactions from true leukemia.

In 2003 the first figures were collected by the Benghazi Cancer Registry, and these figures started to provide researchers in Libya detailed data on the prevalence of cancer throughout the eastern part of the country, although some figures are available for the early 1990s. There has also been recent interest in whether beta-glucan from dates grown in Libya have antitumor properties, with some evidence that glucans can help treat some particular cancers. The Faculty of Medicine at Alfateh Medical University in Tripoli is the main medical research center in the country, with much research work undertaken at Benghazi Hospital.

SEE ALSO: Diet and Nutrition; Italy; United Kingdom.

BIBLIOGRAPHY. A. S. Bakka, et al., "Frequency of Helicobacter Pylori Infection in Dyspeptic Patients in Libya," *Saudi Medical Journal* (v.23/10, 2002); M. El Mistiri, et al., "Cancer Incidence in Eastern Libya: Preliminary Result of the Year 2003," *Le Tunisie Medicale* (v.83/s12, 2005); O. Ishurd, et al., "Antitumor Activity of Beta-D-glucan from Libyan Dates," *Journal of Medicinal Food* (v.7/2, 2004); M. A. Jaber, "Intraoral Minor Salivary Gland Tumors: A Review of 75 Cases in a Libyan Population," *International Journal of Oral and Maxillofacial Surgery* (v.35/2, 2006).

JUSTIN CORFIELD
GEELONG GRAMMAR SCHOOL, AUSTRALIA

Ling, Victor

CHINESE-BORN CANADIAN SCIENTIST Victor Ling was the winner of the Charles F. Kettering Prize of the General Motors Cancer Foundation in 1991 for "the elucidation of the biochemical basis of multidrug resistance in tumor cells." In the same year he also received the Steiner Award.

His work has helped with the understanding of the existence and mechanisms of drug-resistant chemotherapy, which has provided help for patients suffering from leukemia, breast and ovarian cancers, and cystic fibrosis.

Victor Ling was born March 16, 1943, in China, and emigrated to Canada as a child. He was educated at the University of Toronto (B.Sc. in biochemistry, 1966) and the University of British Columbia (B.C., Ph.D. in biochemistry, 1971); his thesis was titled "Biosynthesis of Protamine in Trout Salmo Gairdnerii Testis." He undertook postdoctoral training with Nobel Prize laureate Fred Sanger at Cambridge University. He then became staff scientist at the Ontario Cancer Institute from 1971 to 1996; concurrently, he was professor of medical biophysics at the University of Toronto from 1983 to 1996 and head of the Division of Molecular and Structural Biology from 1989 to 1996.

In 1996 he was appointed vice president of research at the British Columbia Cancer Research Center and professor in the Department of Pathology and Biochemistry at the University of British Columbia. He was subsequently appointed assistant dean of the faculty of medicine at the University of British Columbia and vice president of discovery at the British Columbia Cancer Agency in Vancouver.

Ling's main area of research is the development of cancer, in particular the role played in genes that help malignant cells survive, thus limiting the effects of many anticancer drugs.

His research team was the first to discover the protein P-glycoprotein, which was found on the surface of cancer cells that were capable of resisting multiple cancer drugs. This protein protects the cancer cells by pumping out drugs before they can inflict lethal damage on the cancer cells.

Using recent research in genome science, the team has located more than 50 genes in the human genome in which this protein is present. This research has led to work by Ling and others in analyzing the human genome in the Cancer Genomics Program.

AWARDS AND PUBLICATIONS

He was awarded the Cancer Research Award of the Milken Family Medical Foundation in 1988, the Charles F. Kettering Prize of the General Motors Cancer Foundation in 1991, the International Award of the Gairdner Foundation in 1992, the Bruce F. Cain Memorial Award of the American Association for Cancer Research in 1993, and the Order of British Columbia from the government of British Columbia in 2000.

Also in 2000, he was appointed a member of the governing council of the Canadian Institutes of Health Research. In 2006 he was awarded an honorary doctorate from Trinity Western University.

His recent publications include articles written (and cowritten) for journals including *Nature Genetics, Journal of Biological Chemistry, Genomics, F.E.B.S. Letters,* and *Journal of Cell Physiology.*

SEE ALSO: Breast Cancer; Canada; Chemotherapy; China; Genetics.

BIBLIOGRAPHY. *American Men and Women of Science* (R. R. Bowker/Gale Group, 1994–2003); *Who's Who in America* (Marquis Who's Who, 2005); *Who's Who in Science and Engineering* (Marquis Who's Who, 1994–1996).

JUSTIN CORFIELD
GEELONG GRAMMAR SCHOOL, AUSTRALIA

Liver Cancer, Adult (Primary)

PRIMARY LIVER CANCER, or hepatocellular carcinoma (HCC), usually occurs in the setting of chronic liver disease or viral hepatitis.

Patients are often asymptomatic initially but often present with an abdominal mass, jaundice, and early satiety. Patients may also have fevers, weight loss, and bone pain due to bony metastasis, as well as acute stomach pain and distention due to tumor rupture and bleeding. Other systemic symptoms may develop due to the paraneoplastic syndrome, wherein the malignant tissue secretes hormonelike molecules that can cause watery diarrhea (vasoactive intestinal peptide), hypoglycemia (insulin), bleeding abnormalities (polycythemia), and hypercalcemia (parathyroid hormone).

Because the liver is involved in producing many essential proteins, laboratory examination may reveal low levels of platelets, albumin, and bilirubin. Furthermore, patients may have electrolyte disturbances, such as low levels of sodium or potassium.

There is no definitive way to diagnose HCC, but modalities used include imaging, the use of serum markers, and biopsies. The biologic marker alpha fetoprotein (AFP) is especially helpful in the diagnosis of liver cancer. Although the majority of patients with liver cancer have elevated levels of AFP in their blood, AFP can also be elevated in other types of cancer and disease states. Furthermore, a very high level of AFP and a rebound of AFP levels after treatment can indicate recurrence and poor prognosis.

The exact cause of primary liver cancer is unknown, but risk factors include viral hepatitis B and hepatitis C, cirrhosis, alcohol use, exposure to certain toxins, and intake of anabolic steroids. Although these risk factors seem to be synergistic, hepatitis B and hepatitis C infection seem to be the most significant causes of HCC worldwide. Aflatoxin, a substance produced by mold and found in certain foods, is a significant risk factor

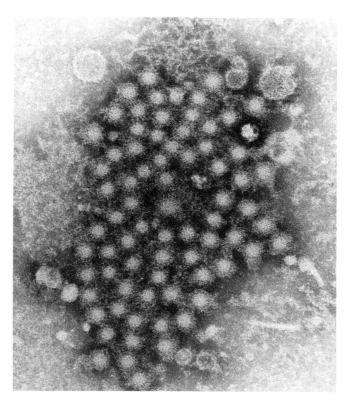

An electron micrograph (TEM) of numerous hepatitis virions. Hepatitis B and C are risk factors for primary liver cancer.

in certain parts of the world. Industrial exposures to chemicals such as vinyl chloride have also been associated with liver cancer. In the patient with liver cancer in the setting of viral hepatitis, care must be taken to avoid reactivating latent viral infection with the administration of immunosuppressive chemotherapies and pretransplant conditioning regimes.

TREATMENT AND PROGNOSIS
Treatment of HCC usually involves partial hepatectomy, a surgical procedure whereby a portion of the liver is resected. Many patients are not able to undergo surgery, however, due to diagnosis at a very late stage. Such patients have very little hepatic reserve, meaning that if the cancerous portion of the liver is removed, the remaining potion will not be able to function adequately due to disease. For this reason, the median survival at diagnosis is 6 to 20 months. Other treatment modalities include liver transplantation, radio frequency ablation (thermal energy administered through a radio frequency charged probe essentially cooks the diseased tissue), percutaneous ethanol or acetic acid ablation, transarterial chemo-

embolization (chemotherapy is injected directly into the hepatic artery to achieve higher localized concentrations), cryoablation (freezing diseased tissue), radiation therapy (HCC is not particularly radiosensitive, but healthy liver tissue is), and systemic chemotherapy (HCC is generally unresponsive to chemotherapy).

Prognosis in HCC depends on the size of the tumor, degree of spread, and hepatic reserve. Large tumor size with invasion into blood vessels and metastasis is also associated with a poor prognosis. Hepatic reserve is a measure of how well the unaffected liver tissue is functioning. If the patient has ample hepatic reserve, he or she is more likely to be able to tolerate a surgical procedure to remove the diseased tissue.

CHILDS-PUGH CRITERIA
Generally speaking, the treatment plan is determined by first assessing tumor size and resectability. If the tumor is deemed unresectable, and surgery is not an option, the patient's condition is assessed according to the Childs-Pugh criteria, which include presence or absence of ascites, bilirubin and albumin levels, encephalopathy, and the ability of the blood to clot properly. If the patient is considered to be Child Pugh class C, the patient is recommended for transplant. If the patient is not an appropriate transplant candidate or falls into class A or B, he or she usually is recommended for one of the aforementioned alternative treatments.

SEE ALSO: Chemotherapy; Hepatitis B; Hepatitis C; Liver Cancer, Childhood (Primary); Surgery.

BIBLIOGRAPHY. Eric K. Nakakura and Michael A. Choti, "Management of Hepatocellular Carcinoma," *Oncology* (v.14/7, 2000); Keith E. Stuart, "Hepatic Carcinoma, Primary," www.emedicine.com/med/topic2664.htm (cited June 2006).

JENNIFER HELLAWELL
CORNELL UNIVERSITY SCHOOL OF MEDICINE

Liver Cancer, Childhood (Primary)

LIVER CANCER IS very rare in the pediatric population, accounting for between 0.5 percent and 2 percent of all pediatric neoplasms. In children, liver cancer can be divided into two major groups based on histology: hepatoblastoma and hepatocellular carcinoma (HCC).

Hepatoblastomas account for 1 percent of all pediatric malignancies and 79 percent of all liver cancers in children under the age of 15. HCC accounts for about 0.5 percent of all pediatric malignancies and usually presents later in life, and hepatoblastomas usually present before the age of 3. Although the incidence of hepatoblastoma has doubled in the past two decades, the incidence of HCC in children appears to have remained stable.

Patients usually present with a painless abdominal mass and may also experience obstructive jaundice, diarrhea, vomiting, and weight loss. In more advanced cases, patients may also develop abdominal pain due to tumor rupture or effects on nearby structures. Laboratory examination often reveals high levels of bilirubin in the blood, altered liver-function tests, and abnormalities in blood clotting.

Risk factors for hepatoblastoma include premature birth and genetic disorders including Beckwith-Wiedemann syndrome, Simpson-Golabi-Behmel syndrome, and other variants of hemihypertrophy syndromes. Children with the genetic disorder familial adenomatous polyposis (FAP) are also at increased risk of developing hepatoblastoma, as are children with mutations in the β-catenin gene. HCC is most often associated with hepatitis B and hepatitis C infection, especially if children become infected right around the time of birth.

It is hoped that that widespread hepatitis B immunization may decrease the incidence of hepatocellular carcinoma. The time course to development of HCC in children infected with viral hepatitis is much shorter than in adults. Other risk factors for HCC in children include mutations in the met/hepatocyte growth factor receptor gene; other liver conditions, including tyrosinemia or biliary cirrhosis; and alpha-1-antitrypsin deficiency.

Diagnosis for HCC or hepatoblastoma involves imaging of the mass through ultrasound, computed tomography (CT), or magnetic resonance imaging (MRI). Definitive diagnosis can be made only based on histology of a tumor biopsy. Staging of the disease also involves visualizing extent of the tumor through imaging. As in adult liver cancer, most pediatric patients with either hepatoblastoma or hepatocellular carcinoma have a serum tumor marker—alpha-feto-protein—that reflects disease activity. Elevated levels of AFP in the setting of HCC may indicate poor response to therapy and recurrence. Unlike in HCC, however, the absence of AFP in hepatoblastoma is associated with a poor prognosis. Another serum marker, beta-human chorionic gonadotropin (β-hCG), may also be elevated in pediatric liver cancer. This serum marker is not as sensitive or as specific a marker of liver cancer in children, so it is usually followed in addition to AFP levels.

TREATMENT AND PROGNOSIS

The mainstay treatment for both forms of primary liver cancer in children involves surgical resection. Although the prognosis after complete surgical resection is favorable, a minority of patients are able to undergo adequate surgical resection. In such cases, chemotherapy may be administered in advance of surgery (neoadjuvant) in an effort to reduce the size and extent of the tumor. As in adults, other treatment options include chemoembolization, ethanol injection, radio frequency ablation, and orthotopic liver transplantation. In the latter process, liver tissue from a donor is transplanted into another part of the abdomen, thus allowing more complete resection of the recipient's disease.

Because hepatoblastoma usually presents as one lesion, whereas HCC presents multifocally, HCC can be more difficult to cure with surgery. The overall survival rate for children with hepatoblastoma is 70 percent, but it is only 25 percent for those with HCC.

SEE ALSO: Chemotherapy; Genetics; Hepatitis B; Hepatitis C; Liver Cancer, Adult (Primary); Surgery.

BIBLIOGRAPHY. Anil Darbari, et al., "Epidemiology of Primary Hepatic Malignancies in U.S. Children," *Hepatology* (v.38/3, 2003); Sukru Emre and Greg J. McKenna, "Liver Tumors in Children," *Pediatric Transplantation* (v.8/6, 2004); Paul R. Exelby, et al., "Liver Tumors in Children in the Particular Reference to Hepatoblastoma and Hepatocellular Carcinoma: American Academy of Pediatrics Surgical Section Survey—1974," *Journal of Pediatric Surgery* (v.10/3, 1975).

JENNIFER HELLAWELL
CORNELL UNIVERSITY SCHOOL OF MEDICINE

Lombardi Comprehensive Cancer Center

THE LOMBARDI COMPREHENSIVE Cancer Center (LCCC) was established in 1970 at Georgetown University Medical Center in Washington, D.C., with funds from the university, the federal government, and private sources. Georgetown is a private university, founded in 1789, affiliated with the Roman Catholic Church and the Jesuit order.

The LCCC was designated a National Cancer Institute Comprehensive Cancer Center in 1990, a designation that was renewed in 2003. The LCCC is named after Vince Lombardi, legendary football coach of the Green Bay Packers, who was treated for cancer at Georgetown University Hospital. The primary objectives of the LCCC are to provide the best and most advanced cancer care available and to find a cure for cancer. The LCCC treats almost every type of cancer, with a particular emphasis on adult and pediatric hematological cancers and solid tumors. The LCCC is affiliated with Georgetown University Hospital, which in 2000 became part of MedStar Health, a not-for-profit network of seven hospitals in the Washington, D.C., and Baltimore, Maryland, areas. The LCCC and MedStar are working together to create a multisite research network, expand access to clinical trials, expedite the clinical research process, and increase minority accrual.

The Betty Lou Ourisman Breast Health Center opened at LCCC in 1998. It combines comprehensive breast-health services in a single location, including breast examinations; imaging; second opinions; genetic testing and counseling; and diagnostic procedures, including ductal lavage and core breast biopsies.

The Jess and Mildred Fisher Center for Familial Cancer Research offers genetic counseling and testing to patients who have been diagnosed with cancer or who have a family history of hereditary cancers. Every new patient is automatically enrolled and completes a familial risk profile during the registration process, which allows doctors to identify and counsel individual who are at high risk. The Fisher Center was established in 2006 as one of several programs funded through a $6.5 million gift from the Robert M. Fisher Memorial Foundation.

Several support services are offered to cancer patients and survivors, as well as to their families. Active support groups include the Amputee Support Group, the Breast Cancer Support Group for Young Women under 40, the Head and Neck Cancer Support Group, the Hemophilia and Other Complications Support Group, the Look Good ... Feel Better program, the Lung Cancer Support Group, and the Women and Cancer Support Group (for women over 40).

The Nina Hyde Resource Room provides patients and families access to pamphlets, books, audiotapes, and videotapes on cancer-related topics.

The Palliative Care and Symptom Management program, established in 1996, helps patients control their pain and symptoms while undergoing cancer treatment, and improve their quality of life.

Pastoral-care, social-work services, and ethnics consultations are also available through the LCCC.

The Lombardi Institute for the Quality of Life, a joint initiative between the Palliative Care program, Psychosocial Oncology, and the Lombardi Arts and Humanities program, was established in 2005 with the assistance of a grant from the Prince Foundation. It focuses on the quality of care and quality of life of cancer patients, and promotes the emotional, physical and spiritual well being of patients, their families, and their caregivers.

The LCCC has nearly 200 full-time faculty members and 220 ongoing clinical trials as of 2006, and receives more than $100 million in research grants. Research is organized in seven programs: breast cancer, cancer control, cancer genetics and epidemiology, growth regulation of cancer, molecular targets and developmental therapeutics, angiogenesis, invasion and metastasis, and radiation biology and DNA repair. Three specialized research programs study tobacco use, molecular genetics, and the relationship between alcohol consumption and breast cancer. In addition, programs are being developed in prostate cancer, neuro-oncology and childhood cancers, nano-oncology and integrative cancer biology, and drug discovery and development.

The breast-cancer research program is centered at the Nina Hyde Center for Breast Cancer Research, which was founded in 1989 by Ralph Lauren and Katharine Graham in honor of Nina Hyde, who served as fashion editor of the *Washington Post* from 1972 until her death from breast cancer in 1990. The program focuses on translational research, with the mission of improving diagnosis, therapy, and prevention of the disease. The specific aims of the program are to identify new mechanisms in the onset and progression of breast cancer, to explore the effects of environmental and genetic risk factors in breast cancer, to establish new methods of screening and early detection, and to test new methods of prevention and treatment in the clinical setting.

The Cancer Control program studies populations across the human life span and includes research projects from the cellular level up through the societal and policy levels. The goal of the program is to reduce the incidence and mortality of cancer among high-risk populations through the development, evaluation, and dissemination of innovative cancer control interventions.

The Cancer Genetics and Epidemiologyprogram aims to understand the genetic and environmental bases of host response and carcinogenesis.

The Molecular Targets and Developmental Therapeutics program is a translational research program whose aims are to identify candidate molecular targets and compounds for cancer treatment, to test hypotheses in preclinical and clinical settings, to develop technologies to enhance the progress of candidate therapies, and to design and execute cancer clinical trials.

The Growth Regulation of Cancer program studies the fundamental aspects of the regulation of cell growth and cell death and their impact on cancer, with a major focus on steroid hormones and nuclear receptors. The specific research aims of the program are to determine the role of signal transduction in the growth and survival of human cancer cells and in DNA repair and cell death, and to determine the role of steroid hormones and nuclear receptors in the cancer process and how they interact with other signal transduction pathways.

The Angiogenesis, Invasion, Metastasis program studies the interaction between cancerous cells and surrounding tissues, focusing on the mechanisms that induce and drive angiogenesis, invasion, and tumor metastasis, as well as on translational research that will lead to novel therapeutic approaches and improved understanding of the underlying biology.

The Radiation Biology program aims to develop a research that integrates basic radiation biology and molecular biology. Specific aims include defining mechanisms of tumor response to radiation, understanding the mechanisms of radiation injury that lead to carcinogenesis, and identifying targets for therapeutic gain.

The Tobacco Research Center takes a transdisciplinary approach to smoking behavior, including behavioral science, genetics, epidemiology, basic research, and public policy, with particular emphasis on harm reduction.

The Institute for Molecular and Human Genetics (IMHG) was established in 1996 to strengthen biomedical research at the Georgetown University Medical Center. It links and expands Georgetown's resources in genetic technology, molecular and cell biology, and clinical practice. A major emphasis of the IMHG is research, which translates basic science advances into improved genetic diagnostics.

The Breast Cancer Center of Excellence, funded by the U.S. Department of Defense, studies the relationship between alcohol consumption and breast cancer. The center includes researchers from Georgetown, the University of Buffalo, the National Institutes of Health, and Catholic University of America, as well as experts in epidemiology, basic science, imaging, and biomarkers.

SEE ALSO: Alcohol; Breast Cancer; Education, Cancer; Genetics; Smoking and Society; Tobacco Smoking.

BIBLIOGRAPHY. Lombardi Comprehensive Cancer Center at Georgetown University website, www.lombardi.georgetown.edu (cited December 2006).

SARAH BOSLAUGH
WASHINGTON UNIVERSITY SCHOOL OF MEDICINE

Lung Cancer, Non-Small Cell

LUNG CANCER IS a significant public health problem in the United States. Tobacco smoke is the leading cause of lung cancer, but family history and other environmental exposures are risk factors as well. It is the second-most-common malignancy next to breast cancer in women and prostate cancer in men. In 2005 there were approximately 172,570 new cases of the disease. Lung cancer is the leading cause of cancer-related mortality in both men and women, with over 73,020 deaths in 2005. Survival rates are low, and there are no established screening methods for early detection. As a result, the majority of cases are found in later, less treatable stages.

Small cell and non-small cell types are the two major forms of lung cancer. Non-small cell lung cancer (NSCLC) is the most common, representing approximately 87 percent of all lung cancers.

NSCLC is comprised of three cell types: adenocarcinoma, squamous cell carcinoma, and large cell undifferentiated carcinoma. Less common forms include pleomorhic and carcinoid tumors.

Adenocarcinoma is the most prevalent cell type, comprising about 35 percent to 40 percent of NSCLC cases. It begins in the cells that line the alveoli and make substances such as mucus. It is typically found toward the peripheral portions of the lung and tends to be the type of NSCLC found in nonsmokers. Adenocarcinoma appears to be increasing in incidence and affecting women at a disproportionate rate.

Squamous cell carcinoma accounts for 20 percent to 25 percent of NSCLC cases and begins in the squamous cells of the lungs. These masses tend to be centrally located and are slow growing, taking longer to move from solitary tumors to invasive malignancies. Squamous cell is often linked with smoking history.

Large cell undifferentiated carcinoma represents the remaining 10 percent to 15 percent of the non-small cell group and, like adenocarcinoma, is located on the outer portions of the lung. It is strongly associated with smoking history and tends to be more aggressive by metastasizing more quickly than the other types of NSCLC. Although there are no standard screening mechanisms for NSCLC, chest x-ray, sputum cytology, computed tomography (CT) scan, or positron emission tomography (PET) scan are used to detect malignancy. More invasive procedures such as bronchoscopy, thorascopy, mediastinoscopy, and fine-needle aspiration are used to confirm the presence of NSCLC.

Staging is done on a Stage I to IV basis, using the common TNM (Tumor, Node, Metastasis) system. Five-year survival rates are based on the extent to which the cancer has metastasized.

Stage I disease, the most amenable to surgical resection, has a 47 percent five-year survival rate. Stage IV disease indicates a distant metastatic spread and has a five-year survival of only 2 percent.

Treatment options include surgery, chemotherapy, and radiation therapy. Complete surgical removal of the cancer offers the highest long-term survival. Surgical resection is an option only about 30 percent to 35 percent of the time, however, due to late detection.

Surgery, chemotherapy, radiation, or biologic therapies are used alone or as part of a multimodality treatment, depending on the severity of the disease.

Research on NSCLC focuses on identifying genomic targets, developing effective screening mechanisms, and developing novel drugs.

SEE ALSO: Chemotherapy; Lung Cancer, Small Cell; Tobacco Related Exposures.

BIBLIOGRAPHY. Jack A. Roth, *Thoracic Oncology* (W. B. Saunders, 1988); Howard A. Gitman, *Lung Cancer and Mesothelioma* (Xlibris Corp., 2005); Arthur Skarin, *Multimodality Treatment of Lung Cancer* (Dekker, 2000).

LAURA HOFFMEISTER
HARVARD UNIVERSITY

Lung Cancer, Small Cell

LUNG CANCER IS a significant public health problem in the United States. Tobacco smoke is the leading cause of lung cancer, but family history and other environmental exposures are risk factors as well.

It is the second-most-common malignancy next to breast cancer in women and prostate cancer in men. In 2005 there were approximately 172,570 new cases of the disease. All forms of lung cancer are the leading cause of cancer-related mortality in both men and women, with over 73,020 deaths in 2005.

Survival rates for all forms are low, and there are no established screening methods for early detection. As a result, the majority of cases are found in later, less treatable stages. Small cell and non-small cell types are the two most common forms of lung cancer. Small cell lung cancer (SCLC) is the less common of the two, compromising only 15 percent of all types of lung cancers. This type of cancer arises in the bronchi and in the center of the chest, and is characterized by cells that divide more rapidly than their non-small cell counterparts. SCLC is comprised of three major types: oat cell carcinoma, mixed small cell carcinoma, and combined small cell carcinoma. Oat cell is the most common of the three.

SCLC is rarely found in nonsmokers and occurs slightly more frequently in men than in women.

Although there is no standard screening method to detect SCLC, symptomatic patients may be given a chest X-ray, sputum cytology, computed tomography (CT) scan, or positron emission tomography (PET) scan. Less common invasive diagnostic procedures include bronchoscopy, fine-needle aspiration, and mediastinoscopy. One third of patients have limited disease at the time of diagnosis; however, microscopic spread that is not clinically visible has probably already occurred.

Staging is less valuable for treatment purposes because of the limited resectability of SCLC. It is largely based on diagnostic imaging and results in the disease's being categorized as limited or extensive.

Limited disease involves tumors that are confined to one side of the chest or central lymph nodes. Extensive disease is characterized by the spread of tumors to both sides of the chest or distant metastasis—typically, to the brain, bones, liver, and adrenal glands.

Patients with limited-stage SCLC are typically treated with chemotherapy and radiation therapy, whereas those with extensive disease are often treated with chemotherapy alone. SCLC responds rapidly to chemotherapy and radiation. Some patients with limited disease may experience response rates as high as 80 percent to 100 percent. In the extensive stage, 60 percent to 80

percent of patients respond to treatment. In most cases, however, SCLC relapses within two years, and median survival rates with recurrent disease are around two to three months. The median survival rate from the time of diagnosis is approximately 15 to 20 months for limited disease and 8 to 13 months for extensive disease. Five-year survival rates range from 1 percent to 10 percent, depending on the extent of the disease.

Research on SCLC focuses on novel drug development, detection tools, and biologic therapy.

SEE ALSO: Chemotherapy; Lung Cancer, Non-Small Cell; Tobacco Related Exposures.

BIBLIOGRAPHY. Jack A. Roth, *Thoracic Oncology* (W. B. Saunders, 1988); Howard A. Gitman, *Lung Cancer and Mesothelioma* (Xlibris Corp., 2005); Arthur Skarin, *Multimodality Treatment of Lung Cancer* (Dekker, 2000).

LAURA HOFFMEISTER
HARVARD UNIVERSITY

Lydon, Nicholas B.

CANCER SPECIALIST NICHOLAS B. Lydon was the joint winner, with Brian J. Druker, of the Charles F. Kettering Prize of the General Motors Cancer Foundation in 2002 for "contributions to the identification and clinical development of the tyrosine kinase inhibitor STI-571 (Gleevec™), a prototype 'targeted therapeutic' with efficacy in the treatment of patients with chronic myelogenous leukemia (CML), gastrointestinal stromal tumors (GIST), and possibly other malignancies."

Nicholas Lydon completed his B.S. from the University of Leeds in England and his doctorate in biochemistry from the Medical Sciences Institute of the University of Dundee, Scotland. His doctoral thesis, which was completed in 1982, was titled *Studies on the Hormone-Sensitive Adenylate Cyclase from Bovine Corpus Luteum*. He then began working on kinase inhibitors, becoming famous in cancer circles for his discovery and preclinical development of Gleevec as a kinase inhibitor for CML and GIST.

In business, Lydon initially worked as program team leader for tyrosine protein kinase inhibitors at CIBA-

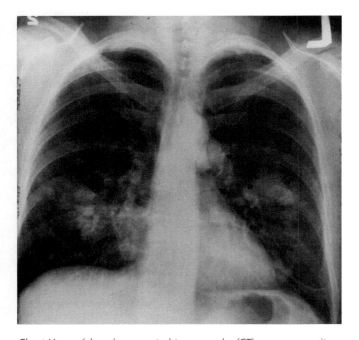

Chest X-rays (above), computed tomography (CT) scans, or positron emission tomography (PET) scans are used for detection.

GEIGY/Novartis AG, where his team discovered and developed Gleevec. He was vice president of small-molecule drug discovery and research informatics at Amgen, Inc., and also president and CEO of Kinetix Pharmaceuticals. The latter company focused on accelerating the discovery and optimization of selective kinase inhibitors. He managed the acquisition, by Amgen, of Kinetix after only three years of operations. He founded the company Granite Biopharma, LLC.

SEE ALSO: Carcinoid Tumor, Gastrointestinal; Leukemia, Chronic Myelogenous; Pharmaceutical Industry.

BIBLIOGRAPHY. Theresa Mikalsen, et al., "Inhibitors of Signal Transduction Protein Kinases As Targets for Cancer Therapy," www.sigtrans.org/publications/pkiRev (cited November 2006); Daniel Vasella and Robert Slater, *Magic Cancer Bullet: How a Tiny Orange Pill May Rewrite Medical History* (Collins, 2003).

JUSTIN CORFIELD
GEELONG GRAMMAR SCHOOL, AUSTRALIA

Lymphoedema Association of Australia

THE LYMPHOEDEMA ASSOCIATION of Australia (LAA) was founded in 1982 to encourage research on lymphoedema and its treatment, and to educate patients, medical professionals, and therapists.

Lymphoedema (also known as lymphedema) is a medical condition characterized by long-term swelling of parts of the body and is caused by lymphatic-system failure. Lymphoedema may be primary or secondary. Primary lymphoedema is caused by a lack of lymphatic vessels in the body or their failure to work properly. Secondary lymphoedema is caused by a disturbance of the lymphatic system due to surgery, radiotherapy, parasitic infection, or other reasons. Removal of the lymph nodes during cancer surgery is a common cause of secondary lymphoedema.

One of the drugs commonly used to treat lymphoedema, benzo-pyrone, was developed and first tested in Australia. Also, the LAA conducted and published the first large-scale study of complex physical therapy, which has become a common treatment for lymphoedema.

The LAA website provides a great deal of information about lymphoedema and available treatments for patients and medical professionals. The website includes a layperson's explanation of lymphoedema, discussions of available treatments, summaries of research on the efficacy of different therapies, an outline of the Training Course in Complex Lymphatic Therapy offered by the LAA, a list of LAA-trained therapists, and a list of support groups in Australia and abroad. The site also provides an extended section on the selection and use of compression bandages and compression garments, as well as a list of suppliers.

The LAA produces informational materials—including books, music tapes, and CDs—to accompany exercises, videos, charts, and computer software, all of which may be purchased through the LAA website.

SEE ALSO: Radiation; Radiation Therapy; Surgery; Survivors of Cancer.

BIBLIOGRAPHY. Judith R. Casley-Smith and John R. Casley-Smith, "Treatment of Lymphedema by Complex Physical Therapy, with and without Oral and Topical Benzopyrones: What Should Therapists and Patients Expect," *Lymphology* (v.29/2, 1996); Lymphoedema Association of Australia website, www.lymphoedema.org.au (cited November 2006).

SARAH BOSLAUGH
WASHINGTON UNIVERSITY SCHOOL OF MEDICINE

Lymphoma, AIDS-Related

ACQUIRED IMMUNODEFICIENCY SYNDROME (AIDS) is caused by the human immunodeficiency virus (HIV) and is characterized by a progressive destruction of the immune system.

Over 40 million individuals are infected with HIV worldwide, and these people have an increased risk of acquiring opportunistic infections and developing several malignancies, including Kaposi's sarcoma, invasive cervical cancer, and AIDS-related lymphoma. The initial presenting illness for 2 percent to 3 percent of those with AIDS is an AIDS-related lymphoma.

The lymphatic system is a network of tubes and nodes that carries lymph throughout the body. Lymph is a clear, watery fluid containing white blood cells (lymphocytes) that are part of the human immune system. In addition, organs such as the spleen, thymus, and tonsils are part of the immune system.

Lymphoma is a cancer of lymphocytes and can be divided into two general categories: Hodgkin's and non-Hodgkin's lymphoma. The tumor types are differentiated by looking at the tumor cells under a microscope. Both types can occur in a person living with HIV, but non-Hodgkin's lymphomas are considered to be AIDS-related because their incidence and severity are increased in those living with HIV.

Possible symptoms of AIDS-related lymphoma include weight loss; fever; night sweats; painless, swollen lymph nodes in the neck, chest, underarm, or groin; and a feeling of fullness in the abdomen. In patients with AIDS, lymphomas are more aggressive, and patients often present with tumors in sites other than lymph nodes, such as the bone marrow, liver, meninges (lining of brain), gastrointestinal tract, anus, heart, bile duct, and muscles. AIDS-related lymphoma can also begin in the brain or spinal cord and is then termed primary central nervous system lymphoma, as opposed to systemic/peripheral lymphoma. Because lymphomas occur within the lymph network, they frequently spread to many parts of the body before they are diagnosed.

The diagnosis of AIDS-related lymphoma involves a physical examination, blood tests showing HIV infection, and a biopsy of a lymph node for examination under a microscope. In addition, a bone-marrow biopsy, chest X-ray, or laparotomy (surgical examination of the abdominal organs for signs of cancer) may be needed to determine the extent of spread of the lymphoma.

After the AIDS-related lymphoma is found, treatment relies on an accurate staging of the tumor and on grading the tumor as indolent (slow growing) or aggressive. Stage I means that the cancer is found in one set of lymph nodes or one area/organ other than the lymph nodes. Stage II involves a tumor in two or more lymph groups on the same side of the diaphragm. Stage III tumors are found in lymph groups on both sides of the diaphragm. In Stage IV the tumor is in multiple organs and possibly in lymph groups distant from the organ site.

Treatment of AIDS-related lymphoma is difficult because patients with AIDS already have weakened immune systems, and the chemotherapy drugs used to kill tumor cells often further damage the immune system. In some cases patients are treated with lower doses of chemotherapy. Under other circumstances, patients are treated with antiretroviral (anti-HIV) medicines along with the chemotherapy. Radiation therapy—the use of high-energy x-rays to kill cancer cells—is used either alone or in combination with chemotherapy.

Treatment is expensive and not accessible to those living in the developing world. Without treatment, the median survival is often less than six months; with treatment, median survival is still less than one year.

SEE ALSO: Cervical Cancer; Chemotherapy; Radiation Therapy; Sarcoma, Kaposi's.

BIBLIOGRAPHY. *The Official Patient's Sourcebook on AIDS-Related Lymphoma: A Revised and Updated Directory for the Internet Age* (Icon Health Publications, 2002).

CHRISTINE CURRY
INDEPENDENT SCHOLAR

Lymphoma, Burkitt's

BURKITT'S LYMPHOMA (BL) is a monoclonal non-Hodgkin's lymphoma of B-cell origin and high-grade malignancy. The tumor consists of high-grade, diffuse, small-noncleaved B-cell lymphocytes.

A defining feature of BL is the presence of a translocation between the c-*myc* gene on chromosome 8 and the *IgH* gene on chromosome 14. Although Epstein-Barr virus (EBV) is associated with BL, its precise role in the pathogenesis of BL is still unclear.

Burkitt's lymphoma occurs in children and young adults throughout the world.

Three clinical variants of BL have been described: endemic, sporadic, and immunodeficiency BL.

The endemic form is most commonly observed in equatorial Africa, in children age 4 to 7 years, with frequent involvement of the jaw and kidneys. The particularly high incidence of BL in equatorial Africa (50-fold higher than in the United States) and the geographic distribution of this tumor, corresponding to the distribution of endemic malaria, have led to its designation as endemic BL. EBV is found in almost all cases of endemic BL.

The sporadic form of BL most commonly presents with abdominal tumors and is not specific to any geographic location. This clinical variant accounts for 1 percent to 2 percent of all adult lymphomas in Western Europe and the United States.

The immunodeficiency subtype is frequently observed in the setting of human immunodeficiency virus (HIV) infection. In a study performed before widespread use of highly active antiretroviral therapy, BL was estimated to be 1,000 times more common in HIV+ individuals than in the general population. The diagnosis of BL in an HIV+ individual often represents the first AIDS-defining criterion and involves lymph nodes; bone marrow; and extranodal sites, most often in the abdomen.

In addition to the clinical variants of BL, two morphologic variants have been identified: classic BL and atypical or Burkitt-like lymphoma (BLL).

Classic BL is found in cases of endemic BL and most cases of sporadic BL affecting children. In classic BL, the neoplastic cells are uniform and medium-size, with round nuclei and several or multiple small basophilic nucleoli. A "starry sky" appearance has been described in this type of BL because of its abundant proliferative rate, frequent apoptosis, and numerous macrophages containing ingested apoptotic tumor cells. The BLL variant has greater pleomorphism in nuclear size and shape, with fewer nucleoli than classic BL.

Eighty percent of BL cases harbor t(8;14), resulting in the juxtaposition of the *c-myc* gene on chromosome 8 with *IgH* enhancer elements on chromosome 14, which drive c-Myc mRNA and protein production. This translocation leads to an enhanced production of the *c-myc* gene, which has wide-ranging effects on progression through the cell cycle, cellular differentiation, apoptosis, and cell adhesion. c-*myc* rearrangement is a pivotal event in lymphomagenesis; it results in a perpetually proliferative state.

Complex chemotherapy regimens containing cytotoxic agents can successfully cure or control most patients with BL.

Short-duration, intensive regimens that minimize treatment delays and maintain serum drug concentrations over at least 48 to 72 hours have the greatest efficacy in treating BL. Such therapy—which includes agents such as cyclophosphamide, vincristine, methotrexate, doxorubicin, and cytarabine—has improved the outcome in patients with BL.

SEE ALSO: AIDS-Related Lymphoma; Chemotherapy; Genetics; Lymphoma, Non-Hodgkin's, Adult; Lymphoma, Non-Hodgkin's, Childhood.

BIBLIOGRAPHY. J. Shapira, "Burkitt's Lymphoma," *Oral Oncology* (v.34, 1998); A. Aisenberg, "Coherent View of Non-Hodgkin's Lymphoma," *Journal of Clinical Oncology* (v.13, 1995).

NAKUL GUPTA
ROSS UNIVERSITY SCHOOL OF MEDICINE

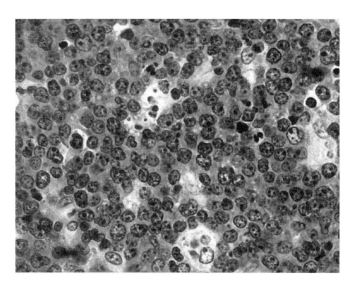

Malignant B-cell lymphocytes seen in Burkitt's lymphoma, stained with hematoxylin and eosin (H&E) stain.

Lymphoma, Hodgkin's, Adult

HODGKIN'S LYMPHOMA IS a lymphoproliferative malignancy involving lymph-node tissue, spleen, liver, and bone marrow. This malignancy is also called Hodgkin's disease. It was first described by Thomas Hodgkin in 1832. It has continued to be commomly called Hodgkin's disease because patients are often cured.

Hodgkin's lymphoma results from the monoclonal outgrowths of germinal center B cells that escape apoptosis through mechanisms such as viruses (such as the Epstein-Barr virus) or regulator genes and eventually give rise to Reed-Sternberg cells.

Hodgkin's lymphoma differs from non-Hodgkin's lymphoma in its histology. Involved lymph nodes contain Reed-Sternberg cells and more normal reactive, inflammatory cells than neoplastic cells. Reed-Sternberg cells have abundant cytoplasm and two (mostly) or three nuclei, each with a single nucleolus. The cancer cells spread through lymphatic channels and blood. Many risk factors have been identified, such as immune deficiency, genetic susceptibility, infections with microorganisms such as Epstein-Barr virus, treatment with immunosuppressive drugs, chemotherapy, and radiotherapy. Patients with immune supression are at higher risk.

In advanced disease, Hodgkin's lymphoma itself causes immune deficiency; patients are infected with microorganisms easily. Slightly more men than women develop this malignancy. There is an age-related bimodal incidence for Hodgkin's lymphoma. The first peak occurs in early adulthood, with a second rise in old age. Symptoms would include the following. Painless cervical adenopathy is the most common presentation. If the patient feels pain in the adenopathy region after drinking alcohol, it is a positive diagnostic sign suggesting Hodgkin's lymphoma. Fever, night sweats, and unintentional weight loss exceeding 10 percent of baseline body weight over six months are B symptoms.

Clinical signs differ according to distant metastasis and tumor masses. These signs include edema secondary to lymphatic obstruction; vertabral lesions, pain, and compression fracture secondary to bone involvement; superior vena cava syndrome (facial swelling, dyspnea, dilatation of the veins in the chest wall and neck) secondary to a huge mass; severe dyspnea secondary to tracheobronchial compression; pain in abdomen secondary to enlargement of organs, such as the liver or spleen; jaundice secondary to obstructions; and neurological pain secondary to invasion or compression of spinal cord.

Fatigue, pallor, dizziness, chest pain, tachycardia secondary to anemia, bleeding secondary to thrombocytopenia, and infections secondary to neutropenia signify bone-marrow involvement. Diagnosis is based on histopathology. Biopsies of the suspicious adenopathy (preferably excisional biopsies) should be reviewed by a competent hematopathologist. The World Health Organization classification is used for stating histopathologic subtypes. Each subtype has different epidemiologic characteristics, treatment options, and prognosis.

After diagnosis, staging should be made to choose treatment options. The Ann Arbor classification is used for clinical stagement referring to physical examination, imaging tests, and laboratory examinations such as bone-marrow biopsy.

TREATMENT AND PROGNOSIS

Treatment consists of chemoradiotherapy (mostly in earlier stages) and chemotherapy alone (mostly in advanced disease). Autolog transplantation increases the chance of cure. In an autologous stem-cell transplant, stem cells from the patient's own marrow are removed, stored, and then returned to the body (engrafted) after the patient receives high doses of chemotherapy and/or radiotherapy. Sometimes cancer cells are eliminated from the marrow before it is returned to the patient. Autolog transplantation is used to increase the dose of chemotherapy, which plays a huge role in treatment success. It should be considered for elective patients.

The prognosis depends on the histopathological subtype and clinical stage. Systemic symptoms such as B symptoms (fever, night sweats, and unintentional weight loss exceeding 10 percent of baseline body weight over six months) confer a poor prognosis, and they usually occur in advanced disease. If no systemic symptoms are involved, the prognosis is good.

SEE ALSO: Chemotherapy; Lymphoma, Hodgkin's, Childhood; Lymphoma, Non-Hodgkin's, Adult; Radiation Therapy.

BIBLIOGRAPHY. Lillian M. Fuller, Margaret P. Sullivan, Fredrick B. Hagemeister, and William S. Velasquez, eds., *Hodgkin's Disease and Non-Hodgkin's Lymphomas in Adults and Children* (Lippincott Williams & Wilkins, 1988).

GÜLNIHAN EREN
EGE UNIVERSITY FACULTY OF MEDICINE, TURKEY

Lymphoma, Hodgkin's, Childhood

CHILDHOOD HODGKIN'S LYMPHOMA is a disease in which malignant cancer cells form in the lymph system. It is one of the few pediatric cancers that share many of its attributes with adult cancer. Because lymph—a colorless fluid that travels through the lymph system and carries white blood cells—travels through the entire body, lymphoma can start nearly anywhere and metastasize throughout the body.

There are two types of childhood Hodgkin's lymphoma: classical Hodgkin's lymphoma and nodular lymphocyte predominant Hodgkin's lymphoma.

Age, gender, and Epstein-Barr virus infection have all been linked to childhood Hodgkin's lymphoma. Children between the ages of 5 and 14 are more susceptible to the disease, and lymphoma is more common among boys than girls. The Epstein-Barr virus is a common virus that usually remains dormant in most people and is linked to a few cancers. Having a sibling with Hodgkin's lymphoma can also put a person at higher risk.

Hodgkin's lymphoma is defined as having a number of multinucleated giant cells known as Reed-Sternberg cells or large mononuclear cells, Hodgkin's cells, in an inflammatory environment. This inflammatory environment contains lymphocytes, histiocytes, epithelioid histiocytes, neutrophils, eosinophils, plasma cells, and fibroblasts in varying portions. Nearly all cases of Hodgkin's lymphoma arise from germinal center B-cells, a type of white blood cells unable to synthesize proteins that make antibodies or receptors.

Approximately 80 percent to 85 percent of cases of childhood Hodgkin's lymphoma involve the lymph nodes and/or spleen. This involvement is classified as stages I, II, and III. The other 15 percent to 20 percent of patients typically have involvement of extranodal sites, including the lung, liver, bones, or bone marrow.

The most common symptom is adenopathy, or swelling of the glands, usually above the clavical or near the cervical area but also at the chest, underarms, or groin. Approximately 25 percent of patients experience systemic symptoms such as fever, night sweats, weight loss, or itchy skin.

A physical exam can be done to screen for any signs of disease. Blood-chemistry studies can be performed to monitor the components of the blood and detect any abnormal proportions. A lymph-node biopsy may have to be performed to test the area for cancer. This procedure can be an excisional biopsy (removal of the entire lymph node), an incisional biopsy (removal of part of the lymph node), or a needle biopsy (removal of part of the lymph node using a needle). Immunophenotyping is a test in which the blood or bone marrow is examined under a microscope to determine the types of malignant lymphocytes that are contributing to the lymphoma.

TREATMENT AND PROGNOSIS

When treatment began for childhood Hodgkin's lymphoma, it was modeled after adult treatments, which caused complications due to the high radiation doses involved. Therefore, chemotherapy and low-dose radiation began to be used, resulting in a 90 percent to 95 percent cure rate among children with Hodgkin's lymphoma. Complications can arise post-treatment, however. Some patients have experienced second cancers, severe organ damage, and other life-threatening disabilities or impairments later in life. Pediatric oncologists work to minimize these side effects to improve patients' overall quality of life.

Several factors can contribute to recovery among patients. The stage of the cancer, size of the tumor, response to treatment, the patient's symptoms upon diagnosis, and the features of the cancer cells can all contribute to the prognosis.

SEE ALSO: Chemotherapy; Lymphoma, Hodgkin's, Adult; Radiation.

BIBLIOGRAPHY. "Childhood Hodgkin's Lymphoma (PDQ): Treatment," www.cancer.gov (cited November 2006); W. Balwierz and A. Moryl-Bujakowska, "Late Complications of Treatment for Hodgkin's Disease in Childhood and Adolescents," www.pubmed.gov (cited December 2006).

LAUREN RIEDMUELLER
ST. EDWARD'S UNIVERSITY

Lymphoma, Hodgkin's, During Pregnancy

HODGKIN'S LYMPHOMA, NAMED for the English physician who first described it in 1832, is a distinct lymphatic cancer (cancer of the immune system). According to the National Cancer Institute, over 8,000 new cases of Hodgkin's lymphoma were confirmed in the United States in 2007, and over 1,000 deaths occurred the same year. The cause of Hodgkin's lymphoma is unknown, but it is a potentially curable illness. Hodgkin's lymphoma is characterized by the presence of unique cells in lymph tissues called Reed-Sternberg cells and occurs more frequently in men than in women. Hodgkin's lymphoma during pregnancy is not common, affecting approximately 1 in 1,000 to 1 in 6,000 pregnancies. It is considered to be a disease of young adulthood; those typically affected are between 15 and 34 years of age.

Hodgkin's lymphoma causes symptoms of fever, night sweats, weight loss, itchiness, and swelling in the lymph nodes. Although pregnancy itself is not a risk factor for development of Hodgkin's lymphoma, being infected with the Epstein-Barr virus is.

The majority of women who are diagnosed in the early stages of Hodgkin's lymphoma can be successfully treated with single-agent chemotherapy. Though research indicates that women with Hodgkin's lymphoma have similar outcomes, treatment of Hodgkin's lymphoma during pregnancy must be approached with caution, as many treatments are unsafe for the developing fetus.

Hodgkin's lymphoma during pregnancy can also pose a threat to maternal health. Previous cancer treatment can render the mother more susceptible to pulmonary and cardiac problems exacerbated by the stress of pregnancy. Additionally, the risk of breast cancer incurred through radiation therapy increases further with the onset of pregnancy.

The majority of women diagnosed with Hodgkin's lymphoma are of childbearing age. Thus, retaining the ability to bear children is a priority for both female adolescent cancer patients and their providers. The choice of treatment depends largely on several conditions, including the stage of the lymphoma, the overall health of the patient, her wishes, and how far along she is in pregnancy (i.e., the age of the fetus).

The National Cancer Institute describes four types of therapy used in treating Hodgkin's lymphoma during pregnancy: radiation therapy, chemotherapy, steroid therapy, and simply watching and waiting.

Radiation therapy involves introducing X-rays and other forms of radiation to the cancer site. Because of its potentially harmful effects on the fetus, radiation therapy is recommended postdelivery.

Chemotherapy uses a combination of drugs to halt the proliferation of cancer cells. ABVD (adriamycin, bleomycin, vinblastine, dacarbazine), developed in the 1970s, has become the standard chemotherapy treatment for Hodgkin's lymphoma because of its superior disease-free survival outcomes in patients compared with other regimens. A recent comparison of pregnancy outcomes demonstrated that female survivors of Hodgkin's lymphoma who had received ABVD did not experience significant changes in fertility compared with controls that did not have the disease.

In general, research supports the conclusion that pregnancy outcomes are similar for women with Hodgkin's lymphoma and women who do not have the disease. Termination of pregnancy is considered when radiation therapy is recommended, as the risk of disturbance to the fetus is high in these cases. Those women who are diagnosed with Hodgkin's lymphoma while pregnant are likely to achieve full recovery.

SEE ALSO: Breast Cancer; Chemotherapy; Childhood Cancers; Lymphoma, Hodgkin's, Adult; Lymphoma, Hodgkin's, Childhood; Lymphoma, Non-Hodgkin's During Pregnancy; Radiation Therapy.

BIBLIOGRAPHY. D. C. Hodgson, et al., "Fertility among Female Hodgkin Lymphoma Survivors Attempting Pregnancy Following ABVD Chemotherapy," *Hematological Oncology* (v.25, 2006); F.T. Ward and R.B. Weiss, "Lymphoma and Pregnancy," *Seminars and Oncology* (v.16, 1989); National Cancer Institute, "Hodgkin's Lymphoma," www.cancer.gov/cancertopics/types/hodgkinslymphoma (cited May 2007); L.R. Schover, "After the Deluge: The Emerging Landscape of Childbearing Potential in Pediatric Cancer Survivors," *Journal of the National Cancer Institute* (v.98, 2006).

LAREINA NADINE LA FLAIR
HARVARD MEDICAL SCHOOL

Lymphoma, Non-Hodgkin's, Adult

NON-HODGKIN'S LYMPHOMAS (NHLS) are strikingly heterogeneous and accounted for 4 percent of cancer diagnoses and 4.2 percent of cancer deaths in the United States in 2003. With approximately 53,400 cases diagnosed and 23,400 deaths from NHL each year, this group of malignancies constitutes a serious public health problem in the United States, as it does in most developed countries.

In general, men are more likely than women to develop NHL, but in both men and women, NHL occur-

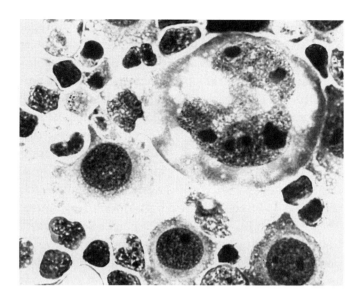

Human lymphoma tumor cells in the pleural fluid stained with a Defquick stain and magnified to 400x.

rence has risen steadily and dramatically in most parts of the world for several decades. Worldwide, rates are lowest in Asia and highest in Western Europe and North America.

In many populations, an epidemic of NHL caused by human immunodeficiency virus (HIV) infections contributed to the long-term rise in occurrence. The causes of most NHLs remain unexplained, however. The two predominant NHL subtypes—diffuse large B-cell lymphoma and follicular lymphoma—account for approximately 31 percent and 22 percent of all cases of NHL, respectively. Worldwide, it is estimated that 90 percent of all cases of NHL are B-cell NHL. T-cell NHL is relatively uncommon and accounts for roughly 12 percent of all cases of NHL.

NHL originates in lymphatic organs during lymphoid development. B and T lymphocytes develop and mature in the bone marrow and thymus, respectively. The mature lymphocytes migrate to peripheral lymphoid organs, including the lymph nodes, spleen, blood, tonsils, and other lymphoid tissues located in the gastrointestinal and respiratory tract.

It is estimated that 55 percent to 75 percent of NHLs worldwide present in the lymph nodes. Initial symptoms include swollen lymph nodes, itching, night sweats, fatigue, unexplained weight loss, and intermittent fever. There is no screening program for detecting NHL early.

Although the causes of most NHLs remain unexplained, known risk factors include advancing age, a family history (e.g., parent, sibling) of NHL, and factors that affect the immune system. In addition to HIV infection, other known infectious causes of NHL include human T-cell lymphotrophic virus type I (HTLV-I), an endemic infection in the Caribbean and Japan that causes a specific type of NHL called adult T-cell leukemia–lymphoma.

Two herpesviruses—Epstein-Barr virus (EBV) and human herpesvirus 8 (HHV-8)—cause Burkitt's lymphoma and primary effusion lymphoma, respectively. *H. pylori* infection causes gastric B-cell lymphoma, and infection with the hepatitis C virus has recently been linked to NHL.

Individuals with immune suppression are particularly prone to NHL, such as organ-transplant recipients who receive immunosuppressive therapy. Although incidence is rare, patients with primary or inherited immune deficiencies have greatly increased risk for NHL. Some common immune deficiencies have also been linked to NHL, including rheumatoid arthritis, Sjogren's syndrome, systemic lupus erythematosus, and celiac disease. Other causes of NHL include exposure to high doses of ionizing radiation and some pesticides.

Current NHL research includes refined classification of NHL subtypes that confer different survival characteristics. Identifying genetic variations that confer differential NHL risk and survival is also under way. It is hoped that the multipronged approach to understanding NHL etiology and survival will reveal the causes of NHL and lead to early NHL detection and to improved treatments and survival.

TREATMENT AND PROGNOSIS

Treatment regimens and survival after NHL diagnosis vary widely by NHL subtype. In general, treatment for NHL comprises radiation and/or chemotherapy.

Overall five-year relative survival among patients diagnosed with NHL is 56 percent, ranging from a high of 61 percent among white women to a low of 42 percent among black men. Survival rates are higher among patients diagnosed at younger compared with older ages and exceeded 72 percent among white women diagnosed under age 65 years.

SEE ALSO: Chemotherapy; Genetics; Hepatitis C; Pesticides; Radiation.

BIBLIOGRAPHY. P. Hartge, et al., "Non-Hodgkin Lymphoma," in D. Schottenfeld and J. F. Fraumeni, Jr., *Cancer Epidemiology and Prevention*, 3rd ed. (Oxford University Press, 2006).

Sophia S. Wang
Patricia Hartge
National Institutes of Health

Lymphoma, Non-Hodgkin's, Childhood

NON-HODGKIN'S LYMPHOMA (NHL) is a cancerous growth of cells in the lymphatic system. It is estimated that there are over 63,190 cases each year, with 5 percent of those cases occurring in children.

In children, NHLs typically present as four different types. (By contrast, there are 29 types of adult-onset NHL.) The type of NHL is determined by which lymphocytes are affected and how they present. The most common NHL in children is Burkitt's lymphoma, which accounts for 40 percent of all childhood NHL. There are two types of Burkitt's NHL: endemic and sporadic. Endemic Burkitt's lymphoma affects children between the ages of 5 and 10, and is localized to regions in Africa that are close to the equator. This type of Burkitt's lymphoma is associated with Epstein-Barr virus (EBV) infection and the presence of the c-myc gene. The disease is more common in male children.

The second type, known as sporadic Burkitt's lymphoma, is found throughout the world and is associated with c-myc gene mutations and less commonly with EBV. This type of Burkitt's lymphoma also involves male children, although they tend to be older than those affected by the endemic form.

The second-most-common NHL in children is lymphoblastic lymphoma, which affects children and adolescents. Most patients have tumors that occur above the diaphragm. This type of lymphoma accounts for 30 percent of all cases of childhood NHL but is highly curable when treated with chemotherapy. The long-term survival rate and complete remission rate is 96 percent with aggressive treatment.

Diffuse large B cell lymphoma accounts for 20 percent of all childhood cancers. This cancer does not differ by geographic area and is thought to be caused by a genetic component. There are various subtypes and variants of this type of lymphoma. This cancer is typically treated with chemotherapy. Some clients may go on to have radiation therapy. The least common form of childhood NHL is anaplastic large cell lymphoma (ALCL), which accounts for just 10 percent of NHL cancers.

There are two types of ALCL. One type is limited to the skin and presents as a slow-growing nodule. The cancer is typically staged, and lymph nodes are examined to assess for lymph-node involvement. The lymph nodes are affected 25 percent of the time. Remission and relapses are common. If a spontaneous remission does not occur, radiation and excision are the treatments of choice. Chemotherapy can be used for individuals with generalized lesions. If the skin over the lymph nodes is involved, the prognosis is typically not as favorable. The systemic form of ALCL is more common in children than in adults and is linked to a chromosomal abnormality. This type is typically treated with chemotherapy.

Children may also be affected by lymphoproliferative disease, which is associated with a weakened immune system. In rare cases, children may develop adult non-Hodgkin's lymphoma. As with adult NHL, the cancer is staged, and treatment regimens vary according to the type, stage, and the child's overall health status.

SYMPTOMS AND PROGNOSIS

The most common symptoms associated with childhood lymphomas include shortness of breath, difficulty breathing, wheezing, high-pitched breathing sounds, swollen lymph nodes, difficulty swallowing, nontender swelling in the lymph nodes, night sweats, unexplained weight loss, and fever. Children with these symptoms should have complete workups to determine whether they have lymphoma.

The five-year survival rate for children with cancer has risen to just over 75 percent. Many children are now treated in specialized children's treatment centers that focus on childhood cancers.

SEE ALSO: Chemotherapy; Genetics; Lymphoma, Burkitt's; Lymphoma, Non-Hodgkin's, Adult; Radiation Therapy; Surgery.

BIBLIOGRAPHY. John Graham-Pole, editor. *Non-Hodgkin's Lymphomas in Children* (Masson Publishing, 1980); Edward

C. Halperin, Louis S. Constine, and Nancy J. Tarbell. *Pediatric Radiation Oncology* (Lippincott Williams & Wilkins, 2004); Lillian M. Fuller, Margaret P. Sullivan, Fredrick B. Hagemeister and William S. Velasquez, eds., *Hodgkin's Disease and Non-Hodgkin's Lymphomas in Adults and Children* (Lippincott Williams & Wilkins, 1988); J.J. Sotto, C. Vrousos, Florence Vinvent, and Marie-France Sotto, eds., *Non-Hodgkin's Lymphomas: New Techniques and Treatments* (Karger, S. Inc., 1985).

MICHELE R. DAVIDSON, PH.D.
GEORGE MASON UNIVERSITY

Lymphoma, Non-Hodgkin's, During Pregnancy

LYMPHOMAS ARE CANCERS that form in the lymphatic system and are generally classified as either Hodgkin's or non-Hodgkin's lymphoma. Hodgkin's lymphoma is characterized under the microscope by the presence of unique cells in lymph tissues called Reed-Sternberg cells. Non-Hodgkin's lymphoma is classified as either B- cell or T-cell lymphoma. Though lymphomas are the third-most-common childhood cancer, 95 percent of non-Hodgkin's lymphoma cases occur in adults. Most cases occur in individuals over 60 years old. According to the American Cancer Society, the lifetime risk of non-Hodgkin's lymphoma is 1 in 50, with men two to three times more affected than women. The National Cancer Institute predicted over 63,000 new cases of non-Hodgkin's lymphoma in the United States in 2007, with over 18,000 of those cases being fatal.

Non-Hodgkin's lymphoma may cause symptoms of fever, night sweats, unexplained weight loss, abdominal pain or swelling, coughing, chest pain, and swelling in the lymph nodes. The cause of non-Hodgkin's lymphoma is unknown, but there are several associated risk factors: a weakened immune system; certain infections, such as the Epstein-Barr virus, human immunodeficiency virus (HIV), and hepatitis C; and older age.

It is highly uncommon for non-Hodgkin's lymphoma to present during pregnancy, but when it does, it presents at a higher disease stage and is more disseminated compared with Hodgkin's disease, thus necessitating difficult treatment decisions sooner. Aggressive and immediate chemotherapy may be needed.

Rituximab, a monoclonal antibody, used alone or with chemotherapy, has been shown to be effective in the treatment of aggressive lymphomas during pregnancy with positive birth outcomes. Remission of non-Hodgkin's lymphoma during pregnancy may occur in 40 percent to 80 percent of cases, though the disease may continue postpartum. Several factors influencing prognosis of the lymphoma are the type of non-Hodgkin's lymphoma, the stage the cancer has reached, and the levels of the enzyme lactate dehydrogenase in the blood. Other factors for consideration before making a decision about the type of treatment administered include the stage of the lymphoma, the age and overall health of the patient, the patient's wishes, and how far along she is in pregnancy (i.e., the age of the fetus).

SEE ALSO: Chemotherapy; Childhood Cancers; Hepatitis C; Infection (Childhood, Sexually Transmitted Infections, Hepatitis, Etc.); Lymphoma, Hodgkin's, Adult; Lymphoma, Hodgkin's, Childhood; Lymphoma, Hodgkin's During Pregnancy.

BIBLIOGRAPHY. American Cancer Society, "Overview: Lymphoma, Non-Hodgkin Type," www.cancer.org (cited May 2007); G. Constantinos, et al., "Non-Hodgkin's Lymphoma During Pregnancy: Case Report," *European Journal of Obstetrics & Gynecology and Reproductive Biology* (v.79, 1998); A. B. Gelb, et al., "Pregnancy-Associated Lymphomas: A Clinicopathologic Study," *Cancer* (v.78, 1996); F.T. Ward and R. B. Weiss, "Lymphoma and Pregnancy," *Seminars and Oncology* (v.16, 1989); National Cancer Institute, "Non-Hodgkin's Lymphoma During Pregnancy," www.nci.nih.gov/cancertopics/pdq/treatment/non-hodgkins-during-pregnancy (cited May 2007); L.R. Schover, "After the Deluge: The Emerging Landscape of Childbearing Potential in Pediatric Cancer Survivors," *Journal of the National Cancer Institute* (v.98, 2006).

LAREINA NADINE LA FLAIR
HARVARD MEDICAL SCHOOL

Lymphoma, Primary Central Nervous System

PRIMARY CENTRAL NERVOUS system lymphoma (PCNSL) is a malignancy of the lymphatic system (non-Hodgkin's lymphoma) that occurs primarily in the brain, eye, spinal cord, and meninges. It is unique because the brain, unlike other parts of the body, lacks lymph nodes or lymph channels.

Previously a rare disease, the incidence of PCNSL has increased by sevenfold to tenfold in the past decade. It occurs more frequently in individuals with depressed immunity, especially among transplant recipients and people with acquired immune deficiency syndrome (AIDS) or other forms of immune deficiency. PCNSL is seen in about 6 percent to 20 percent of patients who test positive for human immunodeficiency virus (HIV).

Although a direct causal relationship has not been proved, human herpesvirus (HHV-8) and Epstein-Barr virus (EBV), which also causes mononucleosis, have been implicated in the development of the disease. Virtually all patients with AIDS have exposure to EBV.

The average age of onset of PCNSL is about 58 years, with a slightly higher incidence in males. The tumor tends to grow rapidly. As with other brain tumors, the patients may initially complain of no symptoms. Symptoms arise due to pressure or destruction of the surrounding brain. PCNSL most commonly involves the frontal lobes, deep structures around the ventricles, and the corpus callosum (a large white-matter structure that joins the right and left lobes of the brain). A third of patients may have multiple tumors. Symptoms occur due to pressure on structures of the brain and include changes in behavior and cognitive function, memory, irritability, paralysis, and disturbances in speech. Seizures occur in about 15 percent of patients. Headaches and vomiting result from increase in spinal-fluid pressure or spread to the meninges that surround the brain.

All patients with suspected brain tumors should undergo imaging. A magnetic resonance imaging (MRI) scan administered with contrast dye is the test of choice. The tumor appears as an irregular mass in the deep white matter of the brain, with surrounding swelling. Toxoplasmosis (a parasitic disease caused by *Toxoplasma,* an organism found in cats) in patients with depressed immunity, and other primary brain tumors or metastasis (spread) from other cancers, should be considered in the differential diagnosis. As with other malignancies, a brain biopsy is required to make a definitive diagnosis. When the diagnosis is made, the extent of disease is assessed by performing a lumbar puncture for analysis of spinal fluid for the presence of malignant cells, as well as eye examina-tion to exclude involvement of the eye. An HIV test is part of the diagnostic workup, given the strong association with AIDS.

TREATMENT AND PROGNOSIS

PCNSL is a very aggressive tumor, the optimal treatment of which has yet to be established. There are two modalities of treatment: radiation and chemotherapy. In immunocompetent patients, total brain radiation therapy increases survival to about 18 months. Current studies and protocols are ongoing; in some studies, the addition of chemotherapy increases survival to 44 months. The side effects, including dementia, are significantly higher among patients who receive combination therapy, however.

Patients with AIDS have worse outcomes; the median survival is marginally increased to 4.4 months with radiation therapy. Treatment options are based on the patient's disease, immune status, and age. Several ongoing clinical trials may change therapy in the future.

SEE ALSO: Chemotherapy; Clinical Trials; Lymphoma, Non-Hodgkin's, Adult; Lymphoma, Non-Hodgkin's, Childhood; Radiation Therapy.

BIBLIOGRAPHY. "Primary Brain Tumours in Adults" (review), *Lancet* (v.361/9354, 2003).

PRIYA RADHAKRISHNAN
CATHOLIC HEALTHCARE WEST

Lymphoma Research Foundation of America

IN 2001 TWO leading organizations for the support of lymphoma research joined forces to form the Lymphoma Research Foundation (LRF). The two original groups were the Lymphoma Research Foundation of America, Los Angeles, California, and the Cure for Lymphoma Organization, based in New York City. The new foundation holds offices in both parent cities. It is managed by a volunteer board consisting of a president, vice presidents, chairmen, treasurer, founders, and additional members.

The mission of the new volunteer-run foundation is to "eradicate lymphoma and serve those touched by this disease." Lymphoma is a cancer of the blood, specifically of a subset of white blood cells. A chief function of the foundation is to fund promising new research in the field of lymphoma treatments and cures.

For assistance in choosing applications to fund, the LRF created the Scientific Advisory Board (SAB), a panel of volunteers who are experts in lymphoma research and oncology. Members of the SAB review proposed research projects and make final recommendations to the LRF on funding. The SAB meets annually to discuss areas of research that the LRF should enter and then advises the foundation so that it can address these areas. An offshoot of the LRF is the Blood Cancer Coalition, an advocacy group that asks the U.S. Congress to make efforts to improve treatments for blood-cancer patients. Its aim is to provide rapid access to cancer care for these patients.

To support its endeavors, the LRF hosts an annual fund-raising gala. As of 2006 more than 85 cents per dollar raised are put toward the funding goals of the foundation. As a service to lymphoma patients and their families, the LRF maintains a website of information and links to further resources. The website offers Lymphoma Awareness for Multicultural Populations in English, Spanish, and Chinese. *Lymphoma Today*, the newsletter of the LRF, is published four times per year. It highlights research funded by the foundation, as well as advances in research and treatment.

SEE ALSO: Leukemia Society of America.

BIBLIOGRAPHY. Elizabeth M. Adler, *Living with Lymphoma: A Patient's Guide* (The Johns Hopkins University Press, 2005); David A. Scheinberg and Joseph G. Jurcic, *Treatment of Leukemia and Lymphoma, Volume 51 (Advances in Pharmacology)* (Academic Press, 2004).

CLAUDIA WINOGRAD
UNIVERSITY OF ILLINOIS AT URBANA-CHAMPAIGN

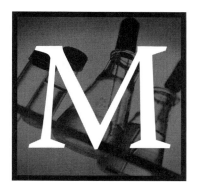

Madagascar

THIS ISLAND, OFF the east coast of Africa, was independent until 1883, when it became a French protectorate. It gained its independence June 26, 1960, as the Malagasy Republic. It has a population of 18,606,000 (2005), with 11 doctors and 22 nurses per 100,000 people. An example of cancer incidence rates in Madagascar includes 142.7 cases of cancer in males per 100,000, according to the International Agency for Research on Cancer.

During the French colonial period, knowledge of cancer in Madagascar was extremely limited. Formal healthcare, including access to hospitals, was usually restricted to the European population, wealthy Asians, and the small local elite.

Since independence, there has been some research in Madagascar, much of it centered on the native flora of the island. One project studied the properties of the leaves of Phellolophium madagascariense Baker (Apiaceae), an herb endemic to Madagascar that was believed to have caused antiproliferative effects in isopentenylated coumarins. Another project studied whether the root and bark of Podocarpus madagascariensis could help women suffering from a particular type of ovarian cancer.

Cancer and other medical research in the country is coordinated by the Institut Pasteur de Madagascar in Antananarivo. People connected with Madagascar who have died from cancer include James Louis Moulton, who was involved in the Allied occupation of Madagascar in 1942.

SEE ALSO: France; Women's Cancers.

BIBLIOGRAPHY. Ezekiel Kalipeni and Philip Thiuri, *Issues and Perspectives on Health Care In Contemporary Sub-Saharan Africa* (Edwin Mellen Press, 1997); C. Riviere, et al., "Antiproliferative Effects of Isopentenylated Coumarins Isolated from Phellolophium Madagascariense Baker," *Natural Product Research* (v.20/10, 2006); M. Reynolds, et al., "Cytotoxic Diterpenoids from Podocarpus Madagascariensis from the Madagascar Rainforest," *Natural Product Research* (v.20/6, 2006).

JUSTIN CORFIELD
GEELONG GRAMMAR SCHOOL, AUSTRALIA

Malawi

THIS LANDLOCKED SOUTH-CENTRAL African country was formed into the British Central Africa Protectorate in 1891 and the Nyasaland Protectorate in 1907. The British started growing tobacco in large amounts in Malawi; it remains the second-largest producer in Africa, after Zimbabwe.

Malawi was part of the Federation of Rhodesia and Nyasaland from 1953 to 1963, gaining its independence July 6, 1964, and becoming a republic two years later. It has a population of 12,884,000 (2005), with 8.8 doctors and 32 nurses per 100,000 people. An example of cancer incidence rates in Malawi includes 115.9 cases of cancer in males per 100,000, according to the International Agency for Research on Cancer.

During the British colonial period, medical treatment, including access to hospitals, was largely restricted to Europeans, wealthy Asians, and the local elite. Before independence, two well-known locals were trained as doctors: Daniel Sharpe Malekebu and Hastings Banda (prime minister of Malawi 1963–66 and president 1966–94). Neither practised in Malawi, and medical care remained rather limited during the initial period after independence.

Recent research in Malawi includes a study of pediatric malignancies in Blantyre from 1998 to 2003 by R.L. Sinfield, et al., of the Department of Paediatrics, College of Medicine, Blantyre, and a study by P. Hesseling, et al., of the Faculty of Health Sciences, University of Stellenbosch, South Africa, on Burkitt's lymphoma. There have also been studies of the prevalence of Kaposi's Sarcoma, increasingly common with the increase in human immunodeficiency virus (HIV) infections.

The Medical Association of Malawi publishes the *Malawi Medical Quarterly* and is the official medical research organization for the country.

Paul Fentener van Vlissingen, a Dutch philanthropist who developed game reserves in Malawi and other countries, died from pancreatic cancer.

SEE ALSO: Lymphoma, Burkitt's; Sarcome, Kaposi's; Tobacco in History; United Kingdom.

BIBLIOGRAPHY. M. M. Beyari, et al., "Inter- and Intra-person Cytomegalovirus Infection in Malawian Families," *Journal of Medical Virology* (v.75/4, 2005); P. Hesseling, et al., "The 2000 Burkitt Lymphoma Trial in Malawi," *Pediatric Blood & Cancer* (v.44/3, 2005); Ezekiel Kalipeni and Philip Thiuri, *Issues and Perspectives on Health Care in Contemporary Sub-Saharan Africa* (Edwin Mellen Press, 1997); Michael and Elspeth King, *The Story of Medicine and Disease in Malawi: The 130 Years Since Livingstone* (Montfort Press, 1991).

JUSTIN CORFIELD
GEELONG GRAMMAR SCHOOL, AUSTRALIA

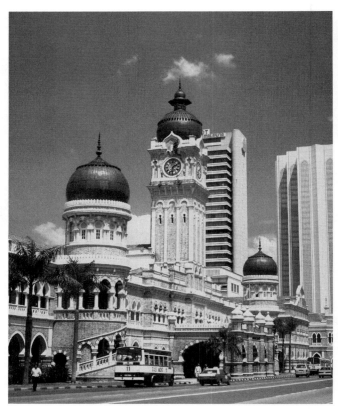

The modern capital city of Kuala Lumpur: During 1990s the medical system in Malaysia became one of the best in the region.

Malaysia

THIS SOUTHEAST ASIAN country was ruled by the British for many years, beginning in 1786, when the British East India Company took control of Penang Island. Province Wellesley was added in 1798, followed by Malacca (now Melaka), previously a Dutch possession, and then the rest of West Malaysia, which was divided into the Federated Malay States (Negri Sembilan, Pahang, Perak, and Selangor), the Unfederated Malay States (Kedah, Kelantan, Perlis, and Trengganu, now Terengganu), and the state of Johore (now Johor).

In northern Borneo, the Brooke family established themselves as hereditary rajahs of Sarawak in 1842, and the British North Borneo Company occupied North Borneo (now Sabah). The entire region was captured by the Japanese in 1941 and 1942. At the end of World War II, British rule was changed dramatically with the eventual creation of Malaya (West Malaysia), which became independent in 1957, gaining Sarawak and

Sabah in 1963 and becoming the Federation of Malaysia (which included Singapore from 1963 to 1965). Malaysia has a population of 26,849,000 (2006), with 66 doctors and 113 nurses per 100,000 people. An example of cancer incidence rates in Malaysia includes 106.3 cases of cancer in males per 100,000, according to the International Agency for Research on Cancer.

During the British colonial period, cancer treatment was largely restricted to Europeans, wealthy Chinese, and members of the Malay elite, with many people in Malaya and northern Borneo not living long enough to suffer from cancer.

Health services were considerably improved after independence, and during the 1980s and 1990s, the medical system became one of the best in the region. The National Cancer Registry of Malaysia, supported by the Ministry of Health, collects cancer data for the entire country. It has shown how cancers vary among people of different races. This has been easier to follow with the merging of the regional cancer registries in Penang, Sabah, and Sarawak. The highest incidence of breast cancer is among the Chinese population, with 59.7 cases per 100,000 in 2004. Among the Indian community there are 55.8 cases per 100,000; there are 33.9 cases per 100,000 for the Malays. Lung-cancer rates are also high, with large numbers of all races being smokers.

Many important Malaysians have died from cancer, including Tun Abdul Razak, prime minister from 1970 to 1976, who died from leukemia while seeking medical treatment in London. There are faculties of medicine at Universiti Kebangsaan Malaysia (National University of Malaysia), Bangi, and at Universitu Malaya (University of Malaya), Kuala Lumpur. There is also a school of medical sciences at Universiti Sains Malaysia (University of Science, Malaysia), Penang.

SEE ALSO: Breast Cancer; Tobacco Smoking; United Kingdom.

BIBLIOGRAPHY. E. L. Ho, et al., "Quality Assurance in Mammography: College of Radiology Survey in Malaysia," *Medical Journal of Malaysia* (v.61/2, 2006); C. H. Yip, et al., "Epidemiology of Breast Cancer in Malaysia," *Asian Pacific Journal of Cancer Prevention* (v.7/3, 2006); National Cancer Registry website, www.acrm.org.my/ncr (cited November 2006).

JUSTIN CORFIELD
GEELONG GRAMMAR SCHOOL, AUSTRALIA

Mali

LOCATED IN WEST Africa, Mali was the center of a large empire until it became a French colony in 1880, being administered as part of French West Africa. It gained its independence from France September 22, 1960. It has a population of 11,957,000 (2004), with 4.7 doctors and 13 nurses to every 100,000 people. An example of cancer incidence rates in Mali includes 52.8 cases of cancer in males per 100,000, according to the International Agency for Research on Cancer.

During the French colonial period hospitals were established in Mali's capital, Bamako. Medical care for cancer and other medical conditions has improved markedly in Bamako, but in remote areas healthcare is often lacking.

Liver cancer, stomach cancer, and cancer of the bladder are the main causes of death from cancer among men, with skin cancer, prostate cancer, lung cancer, and cancers of the colon and rectum also present at much smaller levels. For women, the main cancers are uterine and cervical cancers, liver cancer, breast cancer, and stomach cancer.

In January 1986 the Cancer Registry of Mali was created as part of the pathology service of the National Institute of Public Health Research. Initially, it recorded only data from Bamako, but now it also covers mortality rates from nearby areas. Data are supplemented by details drawn from the death registers of each town, as the cause of each death is registered, and burials are not allowed without death certificates. All information from regional cancer registries is now collated every three months and then computerized to eliminate problems coming from multiple registrations of deaths. Cancer research in the country is coordinated by the Institut Marchoux (Marchoux Institute) in Bamako. It has a section dealing with epidemiology, although its main focus is leprosy.

One of the most famous people from Mali, musician Ali Farka Touré, died in Bamako in 2006 after a long battle with bone cancer.

SEE ALSO: Breast Cancer; France; Prostate Cancer; Tobacco Smoking.

BIBLIOGRAPHY. Robin Denselow, "Ali Farka Touré," *The Guardian* (March 8, 2006); Jon Parales, "Ali Farka Touré, Malian Celebrated for His Music," *International Herald*

Tribune (March 8, 2006); D. M. Parkin, et al., eds., *Cancer Incidence in Five Continents,* vol. VII (International Agency for Research on Cancer and International Association of Cancer Registries, 1997).

JUSTIN CORFIELD
GEELONG GRAMMAR SCHOOL, AUSTRALIA

Marketing, Drugs

MARKETING IS A broad term that is used to describe many activities associated with the manufacturing and distribution of goods and services. Among these activities are the locating of manufacturing plants, distribution centers, and sales offices; sales; and advertising. The sale of a product, including pharmaceutical drugs, may involve educating the consumer. In the case of prescription drugs, pharmaceutical companies have specialists who visits physicians and medical centers to provide information about newly released drugs. This activity is an important and legitimate marketing activity that provides information to physicians who then may prescribe the drug. There have been unethical and illegal activities associated with the practice, however.

Because there has been a history of the sale of quack remedies, the sale of prescription drugs in the United States is regulated by the federal government. Over-the-counter remedies are scrutinized as well. The U.S. Food and Drug Administration (FDA) supervises the manufacture and sale of pharmaceuticals. In addition, the Federal Trade Commission examines the claims of many products, including nonprescription compounds or drugs.

The Prescription Drug Marketing Act of 1987 was enacted to ensure the safety and effectiveness of prescription-drug products purchased by consumers. Because the sale of counterfeit drugs is a lucrative crime, the FDA seeks to protect consumers from fraudulent sales. It also seeks to protect consumers from medicines that can be harmful. Some states, such as California, have also adopted codes that forbid physicians to accept gifts or incentives from drug companies.

The marketing of drugs involves such huge sums of money that the temptation to deliver drugs of little value is significant. Drug companies have been accused of ethical violations such as hiding negative data from clinical trials of a specific drug, such as harmful side effects. In some cases, there have been allegations of bribery and kickbacks. Another complication is the interest of financial promoters in small pharmaceutical companies. If a biotech company can bring a new cancer treatment to the marketplace, the product could be worth billions of dollars. Companies that specialize in bringing initial public offerings of a new stock can also make huge profits. This business is legitimate but very competitive; in the process, information that may be vital to consumers' health may not be presented.

The American advertising industry has joined with television networks to flood the airwaves with commercials proclaiming the benefits of all manner of drugs. Many of these drugs involve intimate bodily activities. The justification for the presentation of immodest commercials is the claim that it educates consumers. However, many patients now engage in researching drugs on their own and attempt to order their physicians to prescribe specific drugs.

SEE ALSO: Clinical Trials; Drugs; Food and Drug Administration; Pharmaceutical Industry.

BIBLIOGRAPHY. Adriana Petryna, *Global Pharmaceuticals: Ethics, Markets, Practices* (Duke University Press, 2006); Bonnie Highsmith Taylor, et al., *Pharmaceutical Marketing* (Hayworth Press, 2002).

ANDREW J. WASKEY
DALTON STATE COLLEGE

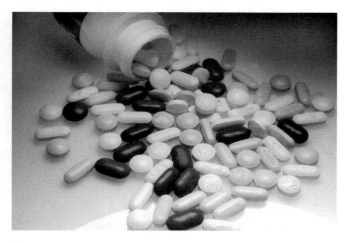

The marketing of drugs involves such huge sums of money that the temptation to deliver drugs of little value is significant.

Marketing, Hospitals and Clinics

HOSPITALS IN THE Western world for centuries were owned and operated by religious bodies. Today, there are still hospitals owned and operated by Roman Catholics, Baptists, and others. Since the end of World War II, however, there has been an increase in the commercialization of medicine practiced in hospitals and clinics. The costs of getting a medical degree and the costs of operating a physician's office, a clinic, or a hospital have forced the medical system to focus on the business side of medicine. Medical services and products cost significant sums of money no matter where medicine is practiced. The costs are real even in charity hospitals. To reduce costs, medicine has increasingly been subjected to competition, so that patients are customers who are sold medical services and products.

Some hospitals use call centers to identify the kinds of patients they may get and to justify the cost of marketing efforts designed to capture medical dollars. Call centers may record the requests of callers for a particular type of physician, service, or health information, as well as calls to register for health-education classes. In this marketing system, advertising appeals to the public to use this or that hospital or clinic for a medical service. Some hospitals focus on pediatrics, for example, seeking to encourage women to have their babies in those hospitals. The long-term goal is to secure the family's repeat medical business during the 18 or so years of childhood. In some cities, hospitals and clinics spend millions of dollars on radio, television, billboards, and other media to deliver their messages. Critics claim that such advertising can lead to a false view of the realities of disease and the medical community's ability to heal. Also, studies have shown that marketing affects physicians' behaviors in ways that may compromise patient care.

SEE ALSO: Hospitals; Marketing, Drugs.

BIBLIOGRAPHY. Steven G. G. Hillestad and Eric N. Berkowitz, *Health Care Market Strategy: From Planning to Action* (Jones & Bartlett Publishers, 2003); Lawrence F. Wolper, ed., *Health Care Administration: Planning, Implementing, and Managing Organized Delivery Systems* (Jones & Bartlett Publishers, 2003).

ANDREW J. WASKEY
DALTON STATE COLLEGE

Massachusetts Medical Society

THE MASSACHUSETTS MEDICAL Society (MMS) is the oldest continuously operating medical society in the United States. It was established in 1781 by the Commonwealth of Massachusetts as a professional organization of physicians. The MMS can license physicians in the state of Massachusetts. It actively advocates for physicians and their patients, including those working with and affected by cancer.

The mission statement of the MMS is as follows: "The purposes of the Massachusetts Medical Society shall be to do all things as may be necessary and appropriate to advance medical knowledge, to develop and maintain the highest professional and ethical standards of medical practice and health care, and to promote medical institutions formed on liberal principles for the health, benefit and welfare of the citizens of the Commonwealth."

The MMS outlines strategic priorities to achieve its mission. These priorities are updated every few years. Recent priorities included the viability of physician practices, involving equitable reimbursement, professional liability/patient safety/quality improvement; health-system reform, involving universal affordable coverage and disaster preparedness; and membership, involving the provision and development of benefits of value and focusing education and publications. An additional priority is the strategic direction of information technology.

The MMS represents 20 district medical societies in Massachusetts, coordinated by regional offices in Waltham, Lakeville, and Wilbraham. The society also communicates with the American Medical Association and other state, national, and international health organizations.

The MMS is led by a house of delegates and a board of trustees. The house of delegates is the legislative and policymaking body; the board of trustees implements those policies. The house of delegates meets twice annually at locations throughout Massachusetts; the board of directors meets six to seven times per year. Board meetings are held at the MMS headquarters in Waltham. Each of the 20 district medical societies has a representative on the board.

The MMS also has committees; member-interest networks; and member sections, which work with issues related to organized medicine and MMS programs and activities.

The society encourages its members to participate in Continuing Medical Education (CME), a nationwide initiative whereby degreed physicians attend seminars and courses to stay abreast of recent advances in medical research and practices. CME credit can be obtained at a CME event, through an online course, or via home study.

In 1812 the society established the *New England Journal of Medicine and Surgery and the Collateral Branches of Science.* This journal merged with *Medical Intelligencer* (established in 1823) to form the weekly *Boston Medical and Surgical Journal* in 1828. In 1928 the journal's name changed to the *New England Journal of Medicine.*

The MMS website includes resources for physicians and patients, as well as a members-only section titled My MMS. Patients can access the website for information on finding a physician, including physician profiles, a physician-referral service, and tips on choosing a doctor. Further patient resources include safety resources, medication information, and an outline of patient-medical-records rights in Massachusetts.

SEE ALSO: Education, Cancer; Insurance.

BIBLIOGRAPHY. Walter L. Burrage, *A History of the Massachusetts Medical Society: With Brief Biographies of the Founders and Chief Officers, 1781–1922* (Plimpton Press, 1923); Myrna Chandler Goldstein, *The Massachusetts Medical Society at 20th Century's Close: An Oral History of One Organization's Struggles in Support of Patient Care* (Massachusetts Medical Society, 2001); Everett R. Spencer, *A Society of Physicians: An Account of the Activities of the Members of the Massachusetts Medical Society, 1923–1981* (Massachusetts Medical Society, 1981).

CLAUDIA WINOGRAD
UNIVERSITY OF ILLINOIS AT URBANA-CHAMPAIGN

Massey Cancer Center

THE MASSEY CANCER Center is located on the campus of the Medical College of Virginia, which is also home to the Health Sciences Division of Virginia Commonwealth University (VCU), a public university located in Richmond. Physicians, scientists, and researchers of the Massey Center are affiliated with over 25 academic departments at VCU. The Massey Center's primary location (the Flagship Center) is in downtown Richmond; there are also several satellite locations in the Richmond area, and outreach services are provided to people living in rural areas in Virginia. The Massey Center was named a National Cancer Institute Cancer Center in 1974.

Research at the Massey Center is organized into five programs: Cancer Cell Biology, Cancer Prevention and Control, Immune Mechanisms, Radiation Biology and Oncology, and Structural Biology and Drug Design. Shared resource facilities, which offer services to all Massey clinicians and researchers, include facilities dedicated to biostatistics, flow cytometry, histopathology, mydridoma and cell culture, nucleic acids, molecular biology, structural biology, and transgenic mice.

The Cancer Cell Biology program is an interdisciplinary group that conducts basic, translational, and clinical research, and includes members from the School of Medicine, the College of Humanities and Sciences, and the Life Science Initiative at VCU. Its primary focus is cellular and molecular events important for the development and progression of cancer. The program's objectives include enhancing and strengthening research in molecular signaling of cancer; identifying new signal-transduction inhibitors and translating those results into new cancer therapies; promoting interdisciplinary research and training programs that bridge basic and clinical science; promoting the translation of scientific research into clinical practice; and applying modern methods of molecular, cellular, and structural biology to cancer-cell signaling research problems.

The Cancer Prevention and Control program focuses on developing a multidisciplinary, integrated research program in cancer control and risk reduction, with the ultimate goal of reducing the cancer burden. The program has four principal areas of interest: genetic epidemiology, including research on tobacco and marijuana use; palliative care and symptom management, including research on pain, dyspnea, and the outcomes of palliative care; health services, including labor-market outcomes, cost-effectiveness analysis, and health disparities; and behavioral studies in cancer prevention, including behavioral-change interventions focused on diet, exercise, smoking, cancer screening, as well as studies of addiction and craving, development of risk-tailored messages, and the psychoneuroimmunology of cancer treatment. The program also focuses on determining and meeting the needs of rural, minority, and underserved populations in Virginia.

The Immune Mechanisms program includes investigators from a number of basic and clinical departments of the VCU School of Medicine, the College of Humanities, and the School of Nursing. The program has two principal aims: to understand the cellular and molecular mechanisms of the regulation of cell growth, differentiation, and modulation; and to characterize antitumor immune effector mechanisms and develop immunologic approaches to cancer treatment.

The Radiation Biology and Oncology program includes basic scientists and clinicians from the Radiation Oncology, Radiology, Neurosurgery, Biochemistry, and Pharmacology and Toxicology departments of the VCU School of Medicine. The principal objectives of the program are to conduct research on molecular radiobiology and medical physics, leading to clinical trials in radiation oncology; to provide a research environment conducive to scientific collaboration; and to develop novel approaches to improving radiation therapy.

The Structural Biology and Drug Design program includes members from the VCU departments of Biochemistry, Chemistry, Medicinal Chemistry, and Pharmacology and Toxicology; it also includes faculty members from the Institute for Structural Biology and Drug Design. The goals of the program are to stimulate collaborative research aimed at identifying and understanding the functions of proteins fundamental to cancer research; to identify gene products of interest to therapeutics or that are involved in angiogenesis, tumor development, and progression; to study protein–protein interactions involved in processes central to cancer; and to employ structure-based drug design to study target proteins and to develop potential therapeutic compounds.

The Massey Center offers a number of predoctoral and postdoctoral programs that emphasize preparation for successful research careers in the context of interdisciplinary programs. Fields in which postdoctoral training is available include Developmental Therapeutics, Cancer Cell Biology, Cancer Genetics and Epigenetics, Immune Mechanism, Radiation Biology, and Cancer Prevention and Control.

Patient care at the Massey Center is provided through a multidisciplinary team approach. Most patient care is provided at the Flagship Center, where facilities include the Dalton Oncology Clinic, Radiation Oncology, the Bone Marrow Transplant Unit, the Thomas Palliative Care Unit, and the Medical/Surgical Oncology Units. Other locations where the Massey Center provides services include the Massey Cancer at Stony Point (Richmond), the Massey Cancer Center at Hanover Medical Park (Mechanicsville), and the McGuire Veterans Administration Medical Center (Richmond).

The Rural Cancer Outreach program was founded after it was determined in 1988 that oncology care was not available to many people living in rural areas of Virginia and that death rates from cancer were much higher than the national average in those areas. To correct those disparities, the Massey Center created partnerships with community hospitals and established clinics in Emporia, Kilmarnock, and Grundy. Each location serves a population of approximately 50,000 people. Oncologists and nurses from the Massey Center travel once per week to each clinic and provide diagnoses, follow-up visits, referrals to radiation therapy, and consultation with local physicians. The rural centers provide chemotherapy, transfusion, and pain-control services supervised by their own staff. The program is funded by a combination of private donations and public funds granted by the Virginia General Assembly.

Palliative care is a particular focus of the Massey Center. The Thomas Palliative Care program offers hospitalwide consultative services from a team of physicians and advanced-practice nurses who assist with pain and symptom management, consult on referrals, and help define the goals of care. The Virginia Initiative for Palliative Care, codeveloped by the Massey Center and Capital Hospice of Falls Church, and funded by the state of Virginia, provides free training to doctors, nurses, chaplains, social workers, and other professionals involved in patient care. The Palliative Care Leadership Center at the Massey Center is one of six sites nationally selected to participate in the Palliative Care Leadership Center Initiative. This program provides two-day training sessions to palliative-care teams from other hospitals and a mentoring services for a year following. The two-day training program assists care teams in designing a program structure and implementation plan for palliative-care service, developing business plans, and conducting financial analyses.

SEE ALSO: Disparities, Issues in Cancer; Pain and Pain Management; Radiation Therapy; Tobacco Smoking.

BIBLIOGRAPHY. VCU Massey Cancer Center website, www.massey.vcu.edu (cited December 2006).

SARAH BOSLAUGH
WASHINGTON UNIVERSITY SCHOOL OF MEDICINE

Mayo Clinic Cancer Center

THE MAYO CLINIC Cancer Center (MCCC) is part of the Mayo Clinic, the first and largest integrated, not-for-profit group medical practice in the world. The Mayo Clinic Cancer Center has been a National Cancer Institute (NCI) Cancer Center since that designation was created in 1971. In addition, it is designated as an NCI Comprehensive Cancer Center, one of only 38 in the United States as of 2006. This designation requires that the center conduct integrated research activities in laboratory, clinical, and population-based research.

The Mayo Clinic Cancer Center was originally located in the Mayo Clinic in Rochester, Minnesota, but in 2002 the NCI granted permission to incorporate the other two Mayo Clinic locations—in Jacksonville, Florida, and Phoenix/Scottsdale, Arizona—into the center. This incorporation made the Mayo Clinic Cancer Center one of the largest cancer centers in the nation, treating over 16,000 patients per year as of 2006. Although most Mayo Clinic Cancer Center patients are currently treated at the Rochester clinic, it is anticipated that one-third will be diagnosed at the Jacksonville and Scottsdale/Phoenix clinics.

The goals of the Mayo Clinic Cancer Center are to understand the biology of cancer; to discover new ways to prevent, diagnose, and treat cancer; and to transform the quality of life for cancer patients. The Mayo Clinic Cancer Center is guided by the philosophy that medicine is a cooperative science; for this reason it emphasizes collaboration among clinicians, researchers, and laboratory workers, and

is a leader in translating knowledge gained from research into improved patient care.

RESEARCH PROGRAMS

The Mayo Clinic Cancer Center has 12 major research programs.

Cancer Imaging focuses on four aspects: technology development, cancer detection, cancer therapy, and imaging informatics.

Cancer Prevention and Control evaluates and identifies innovative approaches to prevent cancer and to prevent or treat symptoms associated with cancer or side effects of cancer treatment. This program includes researchers and clinicians from 10 departments within the Mayo Clinic and includes interventions aimed at improving the psychological, social, and spiritual aspects of life for cancer patients.

The Cell Biology program focuses on increasing basic understanding of normal and abnormal cell processes, with the goals of understanding the transformation of normal cells into malignant cancer cells, the growth of tumor cells, and the metastasis of cancer cells; providing insight into normal and aberrant functions of genetic alterations in cancer cells; and providing a foundation of molecular cell biology to support the Mayo Clinic Cancer Center's organ-based cancer programs.

The Developmental Therapeutics program focuses on developing more effective cancer treatments and treatments with fewer side effects than standard therapies. This program has four major areas of concentration: pathways that contribute to cancer-cell survival and proliferation, laboratory studies examining mechanisms that make cancer cells resistant to currently available treatments, clinical trials of new anticancer drugs, and the relationship between an individual patient's genetic makeup and the side effects he or she suffers during chemotherapy.

The Gastrointestinal Cancer group focuses on topics ranging from the biology of gastrointestinal cancer to novel therapies for treating it. The group was one of three in the United States granted a Specialized Program of Research Excellence (SPORE) grant from the National Institutes of Health for research on pancreatic cancer.

The Gene and Virus Therapy group targets cancer on the molecular level by changing the genetic makeup of cancer cells. Research pursued by this group includes using an engineered measles virus to kill cancer cells through controlled cell fusion, engineering vectors and viruses targeted for gene expression to change the genetic makeup of a cancer cell and kill it, determining which cell types are most effective at delivering virus and vector cells, and introducing marker genes that allow researchers to track gene expression through blood tests or imaging rather than repeated biopsies.

The Genetic Epidemiology and Risk Assessment program performs observational studies with large numbers of patients or community members to determine cancer patterns, risk factors, and genes that predispose some people to develop cancer. One major study conducted by this program was analysis of more than 9,000 Minnesota women at risk for breast cancer through the Minnesota Breast Cancer Family Study. This large-scale study allowed the group to draw a number of conclusions about the relationship between individual risk factors such as smoking and oral-contraceptive use, and family history of the disease, in a woman's risk of developing breast cancer.

The Hematologic Malignancies program studies cancers of the blood and includes the oldest and largest myeloma program in the United States. It was granted a SPORE grant in 2003 to study multiple myeloma.

The Cancer Immunology and Immunotherapy program focuses on identifying substances that stimulate the immune system and providing effective therapies to target specific tumors.

The Neuro-Oncology program includes clinicians and basic, clinical, and population-science researchers whose primary focus is brain cancer. Its goals are to identify factors that lead to the development of primary brain tumors, to identify the mechanism of primary brain-tumor initiation and progression, to identify biomarkers to diagnose brain tumors and determine prognosis and response to therapy, and to develop new therapeutic approaches and interventions.

The Prostate Cancer program is one of 11 recipients of SPORE grants to study prostate cancer. Research focuses on identifying genetic susceptibility to prostate cancer to develop new prevention strategies and identify men at increased risk of developing the disease.

The Women's Cancer group focuses on breast and gynecological cancers, with the goals of identifying genetic alterations underlying these cancers, defin-

ing key cellular systems and pathways in the biology of these cancers, improving identification of women at high risk for these cancers, and developing and testing innovative management strategies for these strategies. The program also looks at personal issues important to women with cancer, including the impact of cancer on the patient's husband and the effect of spirituality on quality of life for ovarian-cancer patients. The group received a SPORE grant in 2005 to study breast cancer.

The conduct of clinical trials is an important aspect of research at the Mayo Clinic Cancer Center. The clinical-trials website includes search facilities by keyword, condition, or disease, and locations of open clinical trials conducted by the Mayo Clinic Cancer Center.

The Mayo Clinic Cancer Center has undertaken several initiatives to reduce health disparities in cancer. Taking advantage of the ethnic and racial diversity of the patient population at its three locations, the center has developed targeted interventions, including a breast-cancer screening program for African American women in Jacksonville, and cancer-screening and education programs for American Indians in Arizona. The Mayo Clinic Cancer Center also developed the American Indian/Alaska Native Cancer Information Resource Center and Learning Exchange to provide cancer-related materials and training for healthcare professionals and community members involved in the education and healthcare of Native Americans and Alaska Natives.

SEE ALSO: Clinical Trials; Disparities, Issues in Cancer; Mayo Clinic Cancer Center—Jacksonville; Mayo Clinic Cancer Center—Scottsdale; National Cancer Institute.

BIBLIOGRAPHY. Yvonne Hubmayr, "One Mayo Clinic Cancer Center," *Mayo Alumni* (v.39/3, 2003), available for download from www.mayo.edu/alumni/publications.html (cited November 2006); Mayo Clinic Clinical Trials website, http://clinicaltrials.mayo.edu (cited November 2006); Mayo Clinic Cancer Center website, www.mayoresearch.mayo.edu/mayo/research/cancercenter (cited November 2006); John Thompson Shepherd, *Inside the Mayo Clinic: A Memoir* (Afton Historical Society Press, 2003).

SARAH BOSLAUGH
WASHINGTON UNIVERSITY SCHOOL OF MEDICINE

Mayo Clinic Cancer Center—Jacksonville

THE MAYO CLINIC Cancer Center—Jacksonville (MCCCJ), which opened in 1986, is one of three branches of the Mayo Clinic Cancer Center (MCCC), which in turn is part of the Mayo Clinic; the other two branches are located in Rochester, Minnesota, and Scottsdale/Phoenix, Arizona.

The Mayo Clinic Cancer Center was established in 2002 with approval from the National Cancer Institute (NCI) to become the first multicenter healthcare institution to establish a cancer center across all its major locations. Although most MCCC patients are currently treated in Rochester, it is anticipated that one-third will be diagnosed at the Jacksonville and Scottsdale/Phoenix locations.

Ultimately, the Mayo Clinic intends to use the MCCC model to create seamless, comprehensive services across all three locations for other specialties.

The Mayo Clinic Cancer Center received over $46 million in funding from the NCI in 2002 and is an NCI-designated Comprehensive Cancer Center. This designation requires it to participate in basic, clinical, and population-based research; research in cancer prevention and control; research that bridges the previously named areas; and outreach and education directed to both healthcare professionals and the general public.

One of the advantages to the Mayo Clinic Cancer Center of having three widely separated geographic locations is the greater racial and ethnic diversity of patients who visit the clinics. Reduction in health-care disparities is a priority of the MCCC, which has developed prevention programs for specific ethnic groups, including a breast-cancer screening program for African American women in Jacksonville, and cancer-screening and education programs for American Indians in Arizona.

The Mayo Clinic Cancer Center Jacksonville provides primary and tertiary care in over 50 specialties, medical education, and laboratory research that focuses on cancer and the neurosciences. In 2005 almost 5,000 staff members were employed and more than 91,000 patients were treated and diagnosed in Jacksonville. About 80 percent of the patients came from Florida.

Cancer treatment is a particular focus of the Jacksonville clinic, and patients with more than 200 types of cancer seek treatment there annually. Areas of emphasis within the Mayo Clinic Cancer Center Jacksonville include breast cancer, gynecologic oncology, hematology and oncology, neuro-oncology, and radiation oncology.

The Griffin Cancer Research Building in Jacksonville, a $22 million facility completed in 2002, is devoted to cancer laboratory research; it is named for C. V. and Elsie Griffin, longtime Mayo Clinic patients and benefactors.

Clinical trials are conducted at each location of the MCCC, and a searchable interface for open trials is available through the Mayo Clinic website. Open clinical trials at the Jacksonville location in 2006 included a study devoted to different types of cancer, including anal and rectal cancer, anaplastic astrocytoma, biliary-tract cancer, breast cancer, colon cancer, endometrial cancer, fallopian-tube cancer, leukemia, lymphoma, melanoma, and prostate cancer.

The Melanoma Study Group, founded in 1999, was one of the first Mayo Clinic study groups to integrate across all three sites. It includes 90 clinicians and scientists from 15 disciplines; its core members meet four times per year by videoconference. The Melanoma Study Group conducted 15 clinical trials in 2006 and has developed unified practice guidelines for melanoma, which are revised annually and posted on the Mayo Clinic website. Hundreds of patients are treated for melanoma each year at the Mayo Clinic Cancer Center Jacksonville, and three clinical trials for melanoma were open to patients in Jacksonville in 2006.

SEE ALSO: Clinical Trials; Disparities, Issues in Cancer; Mayo Clinic Cancer Center; Mayo Clinic Cancer Center—Scottsdale; National Cancer Institute.

BIBLIOGRAPHY. Yvonne Hubmayr, "One Mayo Clinic Cancer Center," *Mayo Alumni* (v.39/3, 2003), 2-7), available for download from www.mayo.edu/alumni/publications.html (cited November 2006); Mayo Clinic in Jacksonville, Florida, website, www.mayoclinic.org/jacksonville (cited November 2006).

SARAH BOSLAUGH
WASHINGTON UNIVERSITY SCHOOL OF MEDICINE

Mayo Clinic Cancer Center— Scottsdale

THE MAYO CLINIC Cancer Center (MCCC) is a not-for-profit organization dedicated to the diagnosis and treatment of complex illnesses, including cancer. The three locations are Rochester, Minnesota; Jacksonville, Florida; and Scottsdale/Phoenix, Arizona. The Mayo Clinic logo is three seals, for patient care, medical research, and academic education, the chief priorities of the clinic. The clinic in Scottsdale, the Mayo Clinic Cancer Center—Scottsdale, (MCCCS) offers international services in English, Spanish, Arabic, and Turkish.

At the Mayo Clinic Cancer Center Scottsdale, patients receive a team approach to cancer treatment, whereby a team of experts is assembled and tailored to the individual patient. A patient can therefore make one appointment to see each specialist, rather than multiple visits over multiple days. In fact, doctors are called consultants, because each physician on a patient's cancer-care team is encouraged to discuss the treatment options and to debate these methods. This open communication among doctors leads to optimal patient care. Care is offered for adrenal, anal, bile-duct, bladder, bone, brain, breast, carcinoid, cervical, colon, small-bowel, esophageal, kidney, liver, lung, nasal-cavity (esthesioneuroblastoma), ovarian, pancreatic, prostate, rectal, skin, gastric, testicular, thyroid, tongue-base, uterine, vaginal, and vulvar cancers.

The Mayo Clinic Cancer Center Scottsdale offers clinical trials in a number of areas, including specific cancer types, side effects of the cancer or its treatment, and related diseases. Patients are thoroughly screened for eligibility before being advised of the available clinical trials; they are also counseled on weighing the risks of participating in a clinical trial against potential benefits, to assist their decision-making.

Clinical trials under way in late 2006 included a molecular staging study of endometrial cancer and a randomized study of combination chemotherapy drugs with and without calcium/magnesium in patients with metastatic colorectal cancer.

The Mayo Clinic Cancer Center Scottsdale maintains a Breast Clinic that offers research, high-quality services, and education in breast cancer. Healthcare providers use these resources to personalize the evaluation and treatment plan of each patient. Diagnosis, imaging, and treatment are offered to patients. Patients also come to the Breast Clinic following abnormal mammograms, breast lumps, breast pains, fibrocystic pains, or breast-cancer diagnosis. They receive screening, genetic counseling, biopsies guided by magnetic resonance imaging (MRI), treatment strategy options, second opinions, educational programs, possible access to clinical trials, and social services.

Teams at the Breast Clinic may be comprised of clinical social workers, diagnostic and interventional radiologists, genetic counselors, internists specializing in women's health, oncologists, oncology-certified nurses, pathologists, physical therapists, and surgeons. The Breast Clinic also specializes in male breast cancer (gynecomastia) and other breast-associated disorders, such as nipple discharge and changes in breast skin.

Physicians at the Mayo Clinic Cancer Center Scottsdale are affiliated with the North Cancer Central Treatment Group, which addresses cancer in the United States, Canada, and Mexico; and with the Eastern Cooperative Oncology Group, which conducts clinical trials on many adult cancers. Both initiatives are funded by the National Cancer Institute.

SEE ALSO: Breast Cancer; Breast Cancer, Male; Mayo Clinic Cancer Center; Mayo Clinic Cancer Center—Jacksonville; National Cancer Institute.

BIBLIOGRAPHY. Mayo Clinic, *Mayo Clinic Fitness for Everybody* (Mayo Clinic Trade Paper, 2005); Mayo Clinic, *Mayo Clinic Guide to Women's Cancers* (Mayo Clinic Trade Paper, 2005); Donald Hensrud and Mayo Clinic, *Mayo Clinic Healthy Weight for Everybody* (Mayo Clinic Trade Paper, 2005); Donald Hensrud and Mayo Clinic, *The New Mayo Clinic Cookbook: Eating Well for Better Health* (Oxmoor House, 2004).

CLAUDIA WINOGRAD
UNIVERSITY OF ILLINOIS AT URBANA-CHAMPAIGN

Meat, Cooking

ONE OF THE most notable findings by those who study cancer and longevity was the association of meat consumption and the likelihood of developing cancer. Meat intake—specifically, intake of red meat—has been consistently reported in numerous studies to have a strong correlation to cancer. Studies have shown that individuals who are sustained on the Asian diet or the Mediterranean diet generally have lower incidence of cancer than those on the typical Western-style diet, which is high in proteins and fat derived from animal products.

RISK FACTORS

A number of hypotheses have tried to explain the relationship between meat consumption and cancer risk. Meat is devoid of fiber and other nutrients that have a protective effect, and the process of cooking and the content of the meat itself can cause damage. Steady dietary consumption of meat influences carcinogenesis by two methods: (1) the cooking of meat, which induces the production of heterocyclic amines and polycyclic aromatic hydrocarbons, which are potent carcinogenic compounds; and (2) the induction of excessive steroidal hormones, which affect tissues and organs (such as the breast and prostate gland) that are sensitive to these hormones. The presence of carcinogenic compounds and excessive steroidal hormones that induce abnormal cellular growth is a major factor in carcinogenesis.

A report published by the World Health Organization has determined that at least 30 percent of all cancers in the Western Hemisphere are due to dietary factors. The key fact that consistently emerges from studies of cancer is that a diet based on vegetables and fruits helps reduce risk, whereas a diet that derives most nutrients from animal products is frequently found to increase risk.

In large studies conducted in Western Europe, individuals who consume meat regularly are 40 percent more likely than vegetarians to develop cancer.

The Physicians' Health Study, which followed close to 15,000 male physicians in the United States, showed a positive association between prostate-cancer incidence and meat consumption in individuals who consumed red meat at least five times a week. In these individuals, the relative risk of developing prostate cancer was close to three times higher than in those who rarely ate meat.

In another study conducted in the late 1980s that followed more than 52,000 male health professionals, the data demonstrated a statistically strong positive correlation between red-meat consumption and cancer. In the study, those individuals with advanced stages of prostate cancer were found to have high intakes of red meat. Individuals who ate red meat more than five times a week also had four times the risk of developing colon cancer than those who consumed red meat less than once a month.

For women, a comparable study—the Nurses' Health Study, which followed 122,000 married registered nurses from 30 to 55 years old in the 11 most populous states—showed that those who ate the largest amount of fat derived from animal products were twice as likely to develop colon cancer as nurses who consumed the least.

Why is the consumption of red meat risky? The fat contained in the meat and the carcinogens formed during the cooking process play major roles. Another factor may be the exclusion of vegetables, fibers, and grains from a diet dominated by meat.

HOW COOKING MEAT CAUSES CANCER

The consumption of raw or inadequately cooked meat can cause certain diseases. Pork may contain parasites that cause trichinosis or cysticercosis, for example. Outbreaks of *Salmonella* sometimes can be traced to undercooked chicken, and Creutzfeldt-Jakob disease in humans can be caused by prions contained in beef derived from cows infected with "mad-cow disease."

Although meat that is thoroughly cooked offers an obvious safety advantage, chemical reactions involving the natural components of meat—such as amino acids, creatine, fatty acids, and sugar compounds—during the cooking process can generate a number of carcinogenic molecules that are then ingested and absorbed into the body.

Two classes of carcinogenic compounds can be produced during the cooking process: heterocyclic amines and polycyclic aromatic hydrocarbons.

Heterocyclic amines are formed during the cooking process. The major classes of heterocyclic amines are IQ-type compounds (such as amino-imidazo-quinolines and amino-imidazo-quinoxalines) and PhIP-type compounds (such as amino-imidazo-pyridines). The optimal conditions for generation of heterocyclic amines are high cooking temperature (between 150 degrees C and 200 degrees C), long cooking times, and charring. Meat juices contain the highest concentration of heterocyclic amines.

A case-control study of 620 colon-cancer patients conducted in North Carolina examined meal intake by cooking method and found that high levels of heterocyclic amines are formed when meat is fried. Studies have showed that high frying temperatures increased colon-cancer risk twofold and increased rectal-cancer risk by more than 50 percent.

Numerous experimental studies have demonstrated a dose-dependent association of certain classes of heterocyclic amines and tumor formation in animals and cell lines. These heterocyclic amines induce numerous enzymatic and transcriptional changes to promote abnormal cellular growth or repair. Heterocyclic amines can also induce the formation of deoxyribose nucleic acid (DNA) adducts, which interfere with normal gene replication and transcription, leading to uncontrolled cell growth, which in turns leads to neoplasm.

Finally, studies have demonstrated that heterocyclic amines, once ingested, can be distributed to mammary glands in the breast and activated by the body to exert carcinogenic effects.

Polycyclic aromatic hydrocarbons are generated when meat is grilled and barbecued. When fat drips down to the heat source, fat pyrolyzes and generates polycyclic aromatic hydrocarbons. These compounds arise with the smoke, adhere to the food, and are then ingested and absorbed.

Studies of certain types of stomach cancer have implicated dietary exposure to polycyclic aromatic hydrocarbons. Studies have also demonstrated in animals and during in vitro studies that the application of polycyclic

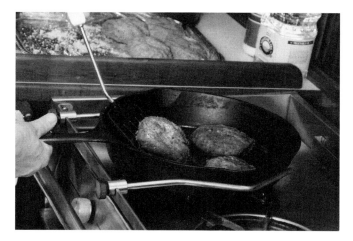

During the cooking process amino acids, creatine, fatty acids, and sugar compounds can generate carcinogenic molecules.

aromatic hydrocarbons resulted in cancer growth and numerous abnormal cellular-growth processes.

In one study of 82 patients diagnosed with colorectal adenoma, a precursor of colorectal cancer, the consumption of charbroiled red meat and meat-derived polycyclic aromatic hydrocarbons was associated with the risk of developing colorectal adenoma. In the study, the investigators demonstrated the formation of polycyclic aromatic hydrocarbons-DNA adducts and found a positive association between adduct levels and adenoma prevalence. The risk of developing colorectal adenomas was about three times higher for those with polycyclic aromatic hydrocarbons-DNA adduct than those with low or no adduct.

An additional risk for cancer from meat is the production of so-called secondary bile acids. Normally, bile acids are produced by the liver and stored in the gallbladder. When an individual consumes a meal, the bile acids are released from the gallbladder into the intestine. The bile acids are necessary for the chemical modifications of ingested fat so that the fat can be absorbed into the body. However, the presence of naturally occurring bacteria that reside in the intestine can form carcinogenic substances from the secreted bile acids. These cancer-promoting substances are called secondary bile acids.

Therefore, the process of cooking meat can form carcinogenic compounds, and the consumption of meat itself can also promote the release of bile acids and the growth of bacteria that cause the formation of carcinogenic secondary bile acids.

Consumption of dietary fat derived from animal products drives the production of steroidal hormones, inducing the growth of cancer cells in hormone-sensitive organs such as the breast and the prostate gland. The relationship between breast cancer and estrogen was demonstrated more than a century ago, when bilateral oophorectomy (the removal of the ovaries) resulted in the remission of breast cancer in premenopausal women.

In countries with a high intake of animal fat found in meat and dairy products, the incidence of breast cancer is proportionally higher than that in countries with low intake of animal-derived products.

The traditional Japanese diet, for example, is much lower in fat than the typical Western diet, and as such, breast-cancer rates are low. Right after World War II, less than 10 percent of the calories in the Japanese diet were derived from fat, and breast-cancer incidence was rare.

Studies have showed that when Japanese girls are reared on Westernized diets, in which up to 35 percent of calories are derived from fat, the rate of breast cancer increases dramatically. A 2003 National Cancer Institute study found that by increasing vegetables, fruits, and grains, and by lowering the amount of animal-derived fat in the diet, the girls (ages 8 to 10) were able to reduce the amount of estrogen by 30 percent to a lower and safer level for the next several years.

Experimental studies have showed that estradiol, the active compound of estrogen, can induce angiogenesis, the growth of vasculature in solid tumors and in breast tissues. Estrogens promote the differentiation and proliferation of mammary tissues. The excessive hormonal stimulation of mammary tissues may result in a progression from normal growth to hyperplasia to neoplasia.

SEE ALSO: Asian Diet; Breast Cancer; Breast Cancer and Pregnancy; Estrogens, Steroidal; Prostate Cancer.

BIBLIOGRAPHY. Peter A. Baghurst, "Polycyclic Aromatic Hydrocarbons and Heterocyclic Amines in the Diet: The Role of Red Meat," *European Journal of Cancer Prevention* (v.8, 1999); Vincent T. Devita, et al., *Cancer: Principles and Practice of Oncology* (Lippincott Williams & Wilkins, 2004); Ellen L. Goode, et al., "Inherited Variation in Carcinogen-Metabolizing Enzymes and Risk of Colorectal Polyps," *Carcinogenesis* (v.28, 2007); David W. Layton, et al., "Cancer Risk of Heterocyclic Amines in Cooked Foods: An Analysis and Implications for Research," *Carcinogenesis* (v.16, 1995); Minako Nagao and Takashi Sugimura, "Carcinogenic Factors in Food with Relevance to Colon Cancer Development," *Mutation Research* (v.290, 1993); The Nurses Health Study, www.channing.harvard.edu/nhs/index.html (cited February 2007); Manjinder S. Sandhu, et al., "Systematic Review of the Prospective Cohort Studies on Meat Consumption and Colorectal Cancer Risk: A Meta-Analytical Approach," *Cancer Epidemiology Biomarkers and Prevention* (v.10, 2001); World Health Organization Global Report, "Preventing Chronic Diseases: A Vital Investment," www.who.int/chp/chronic_disease_report/contents/en/index.html (cited February 2007).

JAMES S. YEH
BOSTON UNIVERSITY

Meat Processing

EATING PROCESSED MEAT—SUCH as sausages, frankfurters, bacon, liver pâté, cooked sliced ham, and other cold cuts—appears to increase the risk of colorectal cancer. Research conducted in the United States and Europe in the past decade has shown this over and over, but there are indications that the risk has been decreasing recently. It is speculated that nitrosamines, formed by a chemical reaction between the preservative nitrite and other substances in the meat, contribute to the risk. Besides colorectal cancer, processed meat is suspected to increase the risk of stomach cancer.

RECENT COHORT STUDIES

During the past 15 years, a substantial number of ongoing cohort studies that investigated the role of diet as a possible cause of cancer in various parts of the world have published their results. Cohort studies typically investigate large groups of people, ranging between 10,000 and 500,000. At the start of a cohort study an extensive dietary questionnaire is administered, after which the cohort is followed up for cancer for many years. Cancer incidence is subsequently compared among cohort subgroups with contrasting eating habits. Fourteen such studies have reported on the association between consumption of processed meat and the risk of colorectal cancer. With the exception of one study, all found that cohort members who were used to eating processed meat regularly had a higher risk of colorectal cancer than those who did not. This effect was not unique for processed meat; fresh red meat also increased the risk of colorectal cancer in many, but not all, studies.

According to a meta-analysis summarizing all the data extracted from the cohort studies, the association was stronger for processed meat when expressed as risk per quantity of meat consumed daily. Eating 30 g of processed meat per day over a long period appeared to increase the risk of getting colorectal cancer by, on average, 9 percent. The meta-analysis also showed evidence that the risk of colorectal cancer from processed meat has been decreasing in recent years. The five studies published before 2000 found higher risks than those published in and after 2001. The same trend was seen within specific cohorts. One study, a Dutch cohort of 120,000 men and women initiated in 1986, found a substantially increased risk of colon cancer (72 percent) during the follow-up period up to 1989 for persons eating more than 20 g of processed meat per day. This increased risk was reduced to 40 percent in the follow-up period up to 1992 and decreased further after longer follow-up.

It is thought that colon cancer and rectal cancer—taken together as colorectal cancer—do not have exactly the same etiology, although they share many risk factors. For processed meat, it is not yet clear whether the risk for colon cancer is different from that of rectal cancer. By the same token, it has not been possible to distinguish the effects of specific types of processed meat on the risk of colorectal cancer. It has been hypothesized that the increased risk of colorectal cancer for consumers of processed meat is due to the nitrosamines present in processed meat, as was detected in the 1970s. Nitrosamines, or N-nitroso compounds (NOCs), are established carcinogens in animals. Some of them are classified as probable or possible human carcinogens by the International Agency for Research on Cancer. Nitrosamines are formed by a chemical reaction between nitrite (added as a preservative) and precursor compounds (mostly amino acids) in the food.

CURING OF MEAT

Most processed meat has undergone some form of preservation. Besides smoking, fermenting, and drying, the most common preservation method is salting. Most of the meat is salted with nitrite salt, a small amount of sodium nitrite combined with sodium chloride. This process is called curing. Nitrite is particularly useful in preventing growth of Clostridium botulinum spores, which can produce a deadly toxin. Nitrite is also responsible for the pink color of cured-meat products, caused by the formation of nitrosomyochromogen. After processing and during storage, the nitrite content decreases. In the ready-to-eat product, nitrite content is below 50 mg/kg. Ascorbate (vitamin C) and tocopherol (vitamin E) are usually added to serve as antioxidants and to achieve color stability; they are also helpful in blocking nitrosating reactions, thus reducing the potential for formation of nitrosamines. Although research on alternatives to nitrite for preserving processed meat has been done for decades, it has not yet resulted in satisfactory solutions.

The addition of nitrite is subject to regulation. In Europe, the amount permitted to be added was reduced

from a maximum of approximately 500 mg/kg in the 1960s and 250 in 1986 to a maximum level of 150 mg/kg in 2005. Other countries, such as the United States and Canada, took similar regulatory measures.

Data on nitrosamine content of foods including processed meat are mostly derived from the 1980s. Typical NDMA (an important nitrosamine) concentrations in processed meat ranged from 0.5 µg to 3 µg per kg of meat, with occasional extreme outliers. Due to the more restrictive use of nitrite salt and application of antioxidants, concentrations are probably lower in processed meat today.

Although definite proof that nitrosamines in cured meat cause colorectal cancer is lacking, circumstantial evidence is in agreement with this mechanism. The temporal trend in risk seems to follow the decrease over time in nitrosamine content. The relatively strong and consistent association with processed meat compared with that of fresh red meat also supports the hypothesis. Furthermore, several studies have shown that total dietary nitrosamine intake increase the risk of colorectal cancer. Finally, a marker of nitrosamine exposure has been found in tissue from the large intestine. This marker, O6-carboxymethylguanine, attaches to DNA in cells lining the intestine. Nevertheless, the situation is likely to be more complex. It has been shown that nitrosamines can also be formed within the body, particularly in the large intestine. Endogenously produced nitric oxide may react with precursors present in meat—in particular, red meat (beef, pork, and lamb)—as has been found in a series of studies from the United Kingdom among human volunteers residing in a metabolic suite, where diet was carefully controlled and excreta were collected. As the formation of nitrosamines in the gastrointestinal tract depends on the presence of both a nitrogen source and precursor compounds, it is clear that a variety of foods and food combinations may cause an increased risk of colorectal cancer. A study in The Netherlands showed that patients with Inflammatory Bowel Disease who have a high endogenous production of nitric oxide have much more NDMA in their stools than healthy persons. When these patients receive only a liquid formula diet, however, NDMA levels are more comparable to those of healthy persons.

Although the most abundant data are available on processed meat and colorectal cancer, other sites in the gastrointestinal tract have been investigated.

Stomach cancer appears to be consistently associated with consumption of processed meat. For esophageal cancer, the data are limited and so far negative; the picture is inconsistent for pancreatic cancer.

SEE ALSO: Colon Cancer; Gastric (Stomach) Cancer; Meat, Cooking; Rectal Cancer; Western Diet.

BIBLIOGRAPHY. Susanna Larsson and Alicja Wolk, "Meat Consumption and Risk of Colorectal Cancer: A Meta-Analysis of Prospective Studies," *International Journal of Cancer* (v.119, 2006); A. R. Tricker, "N-nitroso Compounds and Man: Sources of Exposure, Endogenous Formation and Occurrence in Body Fluids," *European Journal of Cancer Prevention* (v.6, 1997).

SANDRA GOLDBOHM, PH.D.
TNO QUALITY OF LIFE, THE NETHERLANDS
PIET VAN DEN BRANDT, PH.D.
MAASTRICHT UNIVERSITY, THE NETHERLANDS

Media

IT IS ESSENTIAL to understand how issues related to cancer are represented culturally, because these media depictions can influence how patients perceive medical professionals, causes of cancer, and effective treatments. Through cultural assumptions presented in media messages, issues related to cancer are defined in society, which can lead to public support for specific medical policies and treatments of cancer.

Cultural messages can also reinforce perceptions and norms about potential causes and treatments for cancer. Within our culture, the media messages we watch, hear, and read shape our opinions about groups of people, societal structures, and our cultural institutions, including the medical institution. This process is part of the socialization of individuals in a culture.

In his historical analysis of depictions of doctors on television, for example, Joseph Turow points out that programs in that genre have historically focused on the physicians, not the patients. These messages, he suggests, contribute to the construction of the institution of medicine in society, reinforcing the perception of doctors as authorities.

By analyzing the discourse about cancer presented in news, television, and film media, we can identify shared media messages and determine the connotation, or social construction, of cancer in society.

News reports have been shown to educate the public effectively about the need for cancer screenings. Perhaps the best-known news report related to cancer screenings in recent years aired on the NBC morning program *Today* in March 2000, when Katie Couric—whose husband, Jay Monahan, died of colon cancer in 1998—was shown on live television having a colonoscopy. Following that airing, doctors reported a surge in the number of people seeking colonoscopies, and this became known in medical circles as the "Katie Couric Effect." *USA Today* reported that colonoscopy rates increased more than 20 percent following the original airing, and the higher rate continued for a year after.

Lance Armstrong, seven-time Tour de France winner, has also effectively used media messages to garner support for The Lance Armstrong Foundation, a not-for-profit organization he founded in 1977 after he battled testicular cancer, which also spread to his lungs and brain. Armstrong's foundation sells yellow rubber bracelets with the motto "Livestrong" embossed on them (www.livestrong.org). The bracelets are a way to raise money for cancer research and are a visible symbol of support for people who struggle with the effects of the disease.

Several not-for-profit organizations have created public service announcements to raise awareness of cancer-related causes. Following the efforts of AIDS activists in the 1980s who used red ribbons to enable people to display their support for people who have AIDS, they have created their own symbols to be identified with cancer-related issues.

These organizations have used new forms of media technology, particularly the Internet, to convey messages about cancer research and survival.

For more than 20 years, The Susan G. Komen Breast Cancer Foundation (www.komen.org), founded in 1982 by Susan's sister, Nancy Goodman Brinker, has offered research funding and educated the public about breast cancer. Each year, the foundation hosts the Komen Race for the Cure.

Corporations have also supported breast-cancer awareness. Ford Motor Co. (www.fordcares.org) has partnered with the Komen Foundation for its Warriors in Pink campaign, selling products such as scarves

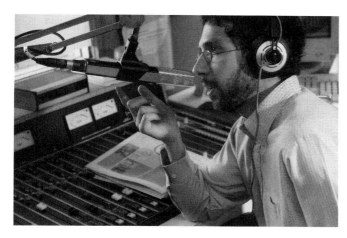

News reports, public service announcements, and talk shows raise the public awareness of cancer and cancer-related causes.

and T-shirts to raise funds for breast-cancer research and to encourage people to show support publicly for breast-cancer research. These products were advertised on ABC's talk show *The View*, an official partner with Ford in promoting the issue and supporting the Komen Foundation. Two hosts of *The View*, Rosie O'Donnell and Elisabeth Hasselbeck, repeatedly discussed their mothers' battles with breast cancer.

Since 1996 Lee, the jeans manufacturer, has sponsored Lee National Denim Day, held the first Friday in October, which is Breast Cancer Awareness Month. Each year a spokesperson is named to appear on morning talk shows to encourage people to make a $5 donation to Lee's foundation and also to wear jeans on that day to demonstrate support for breast-cancer survivors. In 2006 actor Pierce Brosnan served in this role.

Magazines have discussed issues related to cancer, including the women's magazine *Glamour*. In 2001 an employee of the magazine, Erin Zammett Ruddy, now 29, wrote several articles about her treatment for chronic myelogenous leukemia (CML), which she cited as a cancer that is often fatal.

Ruddy is currently in remission but has continued to write about issues related to cancer for the magazine, including her 2006 interview of Diem Brown, a star of MTV's reality show *Real World/Road Rules Challenge*, who discovered at age 24 that she had Stage 2 ovarian cancer. Brown was depicted in the MTV television programs as dealing with sociological and psychological issues, such as losing her hair following the cancer treatments.

In addition to nonfiction news reports and public service announcements related to cancer, fictional media messages have focused on the disease.

The 1971 made-for-television movie *Brian's Song*, starring James Caan and Billy Dee Williams, depicts the real-life story of NFL football player Brian Piccolo, who died of lung cancer in 1970.

The 1991 film *Dying Young*, starring Julia Roberts and Campbell Scott, portrays a young man suffering from a form of blood cancer.

My Life, a 1993 film starring Michael Keaton and Nicole Kidman, tells the story of a man who is diagnosed with kidney cancer as the couple is preparing for the birth of their child. Keaton's character videotapes messages to his unborn child.

In 1998 the film *Stepmom*, starring Susan Sarandon and Julia Roberts, illustrates the challenges of a divorced mother who struggles with her ex-husband's girlfriend to form a relationship with her children. Later, the mother relies on the girlfriend to strengthen that relationship when the mother discovers that she has cancer and will die soon because no treatments are available.

In each of these films, cancer is shown to be incurable, and the disease is a catalyst for dramatic reactions among the characters. One exception is the 1991 film *The Doctor*, starring William Hurt, which depicts a surgeon who discovers that he has throat cancer. The beginning of the film shows Hurt's character as an insensitive doctor, but that situation changes when he becomes a patient himself and understands the importance of developing a proper bedside manner.

That theme is echoed in the 1998 film *Patch Adams*, based on a true story. The film stars Robin Williams as an unconventional doctor who entertains his patients and advocates the need to treat the whole patient: body, mind, and spirit.

Medical dramas have been a popular genre on television for decades. Two programs airing in 2007, *ER* and *Grey's Anatomy*, portrayed patients dealing with cancer diagnoses and treatments.

A 2005 episode of *ER* showed an unmarried woman in her early 30s who tested positive for a breast cancer gene mutation, which researchers say increases the likelihood of developing breast cancer and ovarian cancer. A female doctor informed the patient that she could elect to have a preventive mastectomy involving the removal of her breasts to reduce the risk of developing breast cancer. A 2005 episode of *Grey's Anatomy* depicted a similar scenario.

In October 2006 *Grey's Anatomy* also portrayed a young mother in her 20s who was diagnosed with breast cancer, countering the public perception— supported by recommendations that mammogram screenings begin at age 40—that breast cancer generally affects women over 40. According to www.cbsnews.com, the episode was part of Ford's Warriors in Pink campaign and was specifically aired during Breast Cancer Awareness Month to educate the public on the issue.

Other types of cancer have been represented in *Grey's Anatomy* episodes. A 2005 episode depicted an elderly woman experiencing pain in her abdomen. While removing her gallbladder, doctors discovered that she had gallbladder cancer and that there were no options for treatment. In a 2006 episode, one of the main characters learned that his father had stomach cancer.

With so many fictionalized media depictions of cancer diagnoses and treatments, viewers may wonder what is based on real statistics and information, and what is included by producers to create the most dramatic moments.

To answer some of these questions, the website www.cancer.gov, operated by the National Cancer Institute, posts articles that include factual information about the types of cancer discussed in the fictional depictions. These reports explain symptoms, treatments, and other information related to the fictionalized depictions, and provide links for those who seek additional information.

SEE ALSO: Advertising (Drugs and Treatment Centers); Breast Cancer; Marketing, Drugs; Marketing, Hospitals and Clinics.

BIBLIOGRAPHY. Todd Gitlin, *Inside Primetime* (Pantheon, 1985); Michelle Healy, *USA Today*, "'Katie Couric Effect' Boosts Colonoscopy Rates" (July 14, 2003); Richard Kilborn, "Framing the Real: Taking Stock of Developments in Documentary," *Journal of Media Practice* (v.5/1, 2004); Joseph Turow, *Playing Doctor* (Oxford University Press, 1989).

MARIA SIANO, PH.D.
RAMAPO COLLEGE OF NEW JERSEY

Medicare and Medicaid

MEDICARE AND MEDICAID are U.S. government health insurance programs administered by the Centers for Medicare and Medicaid Services (CMS), formerly known as the Health Care Financing Administration. Both programs were created as part of the Social Security Act signed into law by President Lyndon Johnson July 30, 1965. Because the two programs have similar names, and because they were created by the same legislative act, the two programs are often equated in the public mind, but they are in fact quite different programs with different purposes. Among the most important differences are the facts that Medicare is an entitlement plan for which eligibility is based on age and disability status, and is funded by the federal government; Medicare is a social-welfare program for which eligibility is based largely on impoverishment and is supported by a combination of federal and state funding, with different eligibility rules and benefits applicable in different states.

MEDICARE
Medicare is primarily for people age 65 and older; other people who may receive Medicare benefits include people with end-stage renal disease and people with certain disabilities. Medicare is the second-largest social insurance program in the United States. In 2005 over 42.5 million Americans received benefits through Medicare, and total expenditures were over $330 billion. Medicare is partially financed by payroll taxes paid by employees and employers; these taxes were imposed by the Federal Insurance Contributions Act (FICA) and Self-Employment Contributions Act of 1954.

Medicare has four principal parts.

Medicare Part A covers hospital visits and, under certain conditions, nursing-home stays. Most Americans automatically become eligible for Part A when they turn age 65, assuming that they or their spouses worked at least 40 quarters in which they paid FICA taxes. Coverage under Part A does not require the payment of premiums, although there are deductibles and co-insurance payments.

Medicare Part B is optional medical insurance that covers primarily outpatient care and physician services, including laboratory and diagnostic testing. It also covers, in part or in whole, durable medical equipment such as prosthetic devices, wheelchairs, and home oxygen equipment. Coverage under Medicare Part B is voluntary and requires payment of monthly premiums; however, 95 percent of those eligible for Part B choose to participate.

Medicare Part C is Medicare Advantage (MA), an option offered to Medicare recipients since 1997. In Part C, Medicare benefits are provided through private health insurance plans.

Medicare Part D is a prescription-drug benefits plan established by the Medicare Prescription Drug, Improvement, and Modernization Act of 2003, which took effect January 1, 2006.

Two surveys are conducted regularly to collect data about Medicare beneficiaries.

Longitudinal information about Medicare beneficiaries is collected through the Medicare Current Beneficiary Survey (MCBS). The MCBS has been conducted continuously since 1991, using a rotating panel design that collects data from each single respondent for up to four years. Data collected by the MCBS include health status and functioning; demographic and socioeconomic characteristics; and healthcare utilization, expenditures, and insurance coverage.

Data about quality of care—defined as the changes in physical and mental functioning of covered individuals, delivered by Medicare-managed healthcare plans (currently known as MA plans)—are collected through the Medicare Health Outcomes Survey (HOS). The HOS was first administered in 1998 as part of the Health Plan Employer Data and Information Set. The HOS collects data longitudinally (at baseline and two years later) on a sample of individuals covered by each MA plan and is the largest survey undertaken by CMS. It was developed jointly by CMS and the National Committee for Quality Assurance, and is administered by approved private survey vendors.

Medicare is extremely popular and is generally considered to be successful in meeting its original goals. When Medicare was enacted in 1965, for example, fewer than half the elderly individuals in the United States had any kind of health insurance; today, virtually all elderly are insured.

The Medicare program is also valued because it allows recipients to choose their own doctors and hospitals, and because Medicare has outperformed private insurers in containing administrative costs.

The program has also been criticized on a number of points. The first is financial: The rising costs of medical care and the aging of the U.S. population have increased the burden of paying for Medicare. Current Medicare benefits are paid by current employees, and the ratio of working people paying Medicare taxes to persons receiving Medicare benefits is projected to drop as low as 2:4 by 2030.

In addition, the prescription-drug benefit (Part D) has been severely criticized for being confusing and for barring the federal government from negotiating drug prices with pharmaceutical companies on behalf of Medicare.

MEDICAID

Medicaid is primarily for low-income and disabled persons. The program is funded by the federal and state governments, and administered by the states. State participation in Medicaid is voluntary, but all states have participated since 1982.

Medicaid is the largest joint federal/state entitlement program in the United States and is governed by a combination of federal and state laws. The federal government sets guidelines within which each state may determine who is eligible for Medicaid benefits and what services are covered.

Medicaid coverage is not necessarily available to all impoverished individuals. It is estimated that in 1996 only 46 percent of poor Americans were covered by Medicaid. Because coverage and services offered differ widely by state and may change frequently within each state, specific and current information about Medicaid within any particular state should be sought from the relevant state government.

States that participate in Medicaid are required by the federal government to cover certain types of individuals and eligibility groups.

People eligible because they are considered to be categorically needy include recipients of Supplemental Security Income (SSI), pregnant women and children under age 6 whose family income is at or below 133 percent of the federal poverty level, caretakers of children under age 18, and individuals and couples living in medical institutions who have monthly incomes at or below 300 percent of the SSI income standard.

Some states (35 in 2005) also cover persons who are considered medically needy although they may have income or savings that make them ineligible for coverage based on poverty. People covered in this category include pregnant women (including a 60-day postpartum period), children under age 18, certain newborns, and certain blind persons. Some states extend the medically needy category to include children up to age 21, caretaker relatives, persons age 65 and older, and blind and/or disabled persons.

For persons judged categorically needy for Medicaid, the categories of care that the states are required to cover include inpatient and outpatient hospital care, laboratory and X-ray services, physician services, nursing-facility services, family-planning services and supplies, pregnancy and postpartum services, and home health services for beneficiaries entitled to nursing-facility services under the state's Medicaid plan.

For persons judged to be medically needy, services that must be covered include home health services for individuals eligible for nursing-facility services under the state's Medicaid plan, prenatal and delivery services, and postpartum services for beneficiaries under age 18.

Medicaid extends health services to many Americans who otherwise might not receive them and provides an important source of insurance for many who otherwise would not be covered due to poverty, disability, or lack of employer-sponsored coverage.

Medicaid has also been criticized on many scores. One is that Medicaid costs continue to increase, due to the increased costs of medical care and (in some cases) expanded enrollment.

Ironically, Medicaid has also been criticized for failing to cover many impoverished Americans. Because rules about who is eligible and what benefits are included vary from state to state, the provision of benefits or lack thereof may seem arbitrary and capricious. Because Medicaid is not an entitlement program, individuals are required to demonstrate their eligibility—a process that may be perceived as cumbersome and time consuming, and that may deter some eligible individuals from applying for coverage.

Finally, Medicaid reimbursement rates are lower than physicians receive from most insurance plans. As a result, some physicians refuse to treat Medicaid patients or limit the number they will see, making it difficult for Medicaid recipients in some areas to find a medical home.

SEE ALSO: Age; Disease and Poverty; Disparities, Issues in Cancer; Government; Insurance; Poverty.

BIBLIOGRAPHY. Centers for Medicare and Medicaid Services website, www.cms.hhs.gov (cited December 2006); Centers for Medicare and Medicaid Services, *Medicaid At-a-Glance 2005: A Medicaid Information Source* (Centers for Medicare and Medicaid Services, 2005); G. S. Cooper, et al., "The Utility of Medicare Claims Data for Measuring Cancer Stage," *Medical Care* (v.37/7, 1999); Jonathan Engel, *Poor People's Medicine: Medicaid and American Charity Care Since 1965* (Duke University Press, 2006); E. D. Hoffman, et al., "Overview of the Medicare and Medicaid Programs," *Health Care Financing Review Statistical Supplement* (v.1/348, 2000); Andrew J. Rettenmaier and Thomas Robert Saving, *Medicare Reform: Issues and Answers* (University of Chicago Press, 1999).

SARAH BOSLAUGH
WASHINGTON UNIVERSITY SCHOOL OF MEDICINE

MedImmune (United States)

MEDIMMUNE IS AN American pharmaceutical company that commenced life in 1987 and changed to its current name in 1990. The company is based in Maryland and is listed on the NASDAQ. Its most important product is Synagis, which retards infection from respiratory diseases in children and which provides revenue exceeding $1 billion annually. The company has reached approximately 6 percent of total sales in the pharmaceuticals market overall, although it has posted significant losses in recent years. It has been classified, however, as a company with a low proportion of research-and-development expenditure in the context of the industry. Perhaps this low expenditure is explained by the importance of licensing to the company, in which MedImmune pays another company or patent-holder for the right to manufacture and sell products under its own brand name, sharing the profits.

MedImmune has been involved in a complex court case with another biotechnology firm, Genentech, from which it had bought a license. The case involved the ability of a licensee to sue the licensor for the validity of the patent of the licensed product without first breaking the terms of the license. This case has been connected with the need, accepted by the American government, to reexamine the validity of many registered patents. The case is highly technical but important in principle, in that it could lead to future increases in the financial terms of new licensing agreements that would lead to increased prices being passed on to customers.

MedImmune has been involved in developing or producing pharmaceuticals for combating cancer, including Vitaxin, which aims to create nanoparticles that might be used to transfer agents involved in diagnosing cancer. It has also been involved, with Cerus Corp., with an innovative vaccine treatment aimed at treating cancers of the breast, prostrate, and colon.

Perhaps the most important commercial development will be CAIV-T, an anti-influenza vaccine that is currently undergoing clinical trials. MedImmune also produces FluMist, an alternative product that has not been favored by clinicians on account of both efficacy and price but that has been used when alternative flu-shot products have been in short supply. It seems likely that low supplies of flu shots will recur in the future; hence, FluMist represents an important revenue stream for the company.

SEE ALSO: Clinical Trials; Infection (Childhood, Sexually Transmitted Infections, Hepatitis; Pharmaceutical Industry.

BIBLIOGRAPHY. Stephen Manning, "Flu Shot Shortage May Raise Sales of Flu-Fighting Nasal Spray," Salon.com, www.salon.com/tech/2003/12/08/flu_spray/index.html (cited December 2003); Alex K. Pavlou, "Leading Biotechnology Players, 2002–8: Key Products, Indications and Technologies," *Journal of Commercial Biotechnology* (v.10/2, 2003).

JOHN WALSH
SHINAWATRA UNIVERSITY

Medulloblastoma, Childhood

CHILDHOOD MEDULLOBLASTOMA IS a disease in which malignant (cancer) cells form in the tissues of the brain. The disease originates as a tumor in the cerebellum, the lower back region of the brain responsible for movement, balance, and posture. The spinal cord is the usual site for occurrences of metastasis, with cancer cells then spreading from the cord to other sites. Although cancer is rare in children, brain tumors are the most common type of childhood cancer other than leukemia and lymphoma. Medulloblastoma is the most common pediatric malignant brain tumor, composing 10 percent to 20 percent of all pediatric brain tumors. The disease occurs more frequently in boys than in girls, with peak incidence at age 5 years.

Signs include headache, lethargy, uncoordinated movements, nausea and vomiting, changes in behavior, and unexplained weight loss or gain.

The cause of medulloblastoma, along with that of most other childhood brain tumors, is currently unknown. It is believed, however, that medulloblastoma arises from cerebellar stem cells that have been prevented from dividing and differentiating into their normal cell types.

Diagnosis is typically based on a computed tomography (CT) scan, a type of radiographic imaging that can reveal the presence of an abnormal mass within the cerebellum. When a mass has been identified, magnetic resonance imaging (MRI) is usually performed to delineate better the tumor's size, extent, and location. After the tumor has been located and delineated, a neurosurgeon may remove the mass (or as much of it as possible). A pathologist then examines a sample of the excised tissue under a microscope to identify the mass as benign or malignant. Medulloblastoma has certain features that distinguish it from other brain tumors.

When the diagnosis of medulloblastoma is made, the patient may undergo an MRI of the spine to determine whether the cancer has spread. A spinal tap may also be conducted. In this procedure, a sample of the cerebrospinal fluid is obtained for examination under a microscope to determine the presence of tumor cells. It is extremely rare for medulloblastoma to spread beyond the brain and spinal cord.

Radiation therapy or chemotherapy may be used in conjunction with surgery to treat medulloblastoma in children. If the cancer returns, it is usually within the first five years after treatment.

Certain factors—such as the age of the child when the tumor is found, the location of the tumor, the amount of tumor remaining after surgery, and whether the cancer has spread to other parts of the central nervous system—affect the patient's treatment options and prognosis.

SEE ALSO: American Brain Tumor Association; American Cancer Society; American Society of Pediatric Hematology/Oncology; Chemotherapy; Childhood Brain Tumor Foundation; Childhood Cancers; National Childhood Cancer Foundation; Radiation Therapy; Surgery.

BIBLIOGRAPHY. Raymond D. Adams, et al., *Adams and Victor's Principles of Neurology* (McGraw-Hill, 2005); "Medulloblastoma," www.emedicine.com/neuro/topic624.htm (cited October 2005).

NAVID EZRA
DAVID GEFFEN SCHOOL OF MEDICINE AT UCLA

Melanoma, Intraocular (Eye)

WELL KNOWN TO the general public are cutaneous melanomas of the skin that involve malignant transformation of melanocytes—cells within the epidermis responsible for producing pigment. Melanomas can and do arise anywhere melanocytes exist in the body, however, including the eye. In fact, uveal melanoma is the most common primary intraocular malignancy in adults. The incidence of this tumor increases with age, reaching more than 20 million per year by the seventh decade of life. Although some experts have implicated excessive childhood exposure to ultraviolet radiation as a risk factor, this link is not nearly as clear as it is for cutaneous melanoma.

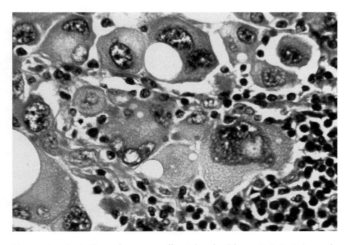

Human metastatic melanoma cells stained with an H & E stain and magnified to 320x.

The uvea includes the iris (the colored part of the eye that alters the amount of light entering the eye), the ciliary body (a muscle that changes the shape of the lens), and the choroid (a layer of tissue that lies next to the retina, which transmits visual information to the brain). Most melanomas of the iris, ciliary body, or choroid are initially completely asymptomatic, although iris melanomas may appear as a dark spot on the iris. As the tumor enlarges, it may cause distortion of the pupil (iris melanoma), blurred vision and glaucoma (ciliary body melanoma), or markedly decreased visual acuity from a secondary retinal detachment (choroidal melanoma). Most melanomas are detected by routine ophthalmic examinations with pupil dilation.

Melanomas situated exclusively in the iris tend to follow a relatively indolent course, whereas melanomas of the ciliary body and choroids are more aggressive. The prognosis of choroidal and ciliary body melanomas is classically related to size, cell type, and proliferative index. By contrast to cutaneous melanomas, large numbers of tumor-infiltrating lymphocytes are associated with an adverse outcome, as are extraocular extension, tumor involvement of the ciliary body, and advanced age of the patient.

When a definite diagnosis of malignant melanoma is made, possible therapies are selected depending on the location and size of the tumor. Small melanomas of the iris or ciliary body sometimes are successfully treated by iridectomy—removal of the part of the iris harboring the tumor. With very large tumors, the only possible option is enucleation, or removal of the eye, followed by placement of an artificial eye in the socket. Plaque therapy is a novel form of radiation therapy effective in treating malignant melanoma of the ciliary body or choroids. The technique involves the localized delivery of radiation to the tumor by a small metallic object containing radioisotopes, sutured to the wall of the eye adjacent to the base of the tumor. In certain situations, laser therapy is used to destroy the tumor with an intensely powerful beam of light. Photocoagulation can also be performed. This procedure uses the laser to destroy the blood vessels that feed the tumor, thus eliminating its nutrient source.

Despite the efficacy of many available therapies in achieving local tumor control, eventual death due to metastases (especially to the liver) may occur in up to 50 percent of patients. Although the 5-year survival rate is approximately 80 percent, the cumulative melanoma mortality rate is 40 percent at 10 years, increasing by 1 percent per year thereafter. Examples of metastases appearing many years after treatment are also well known.

SEE ALSO: Eye Cancer, Retinoblastoma; Radiation Therapy; Surgery.

BIBLIOGRAPHY. R. Folberg, "The Eye," in V. Kumar, et al., eds., *Robbins and Cotran Pathologic Basis of Disease* (Elsevier, Inc., 2005); National Cancer Institute, "Intraocular Melanoma, www.cancer.gov/cancertopics/pdq/treatment/intraocularmelanoma/patient (cited December 2006).

STEPHANIE W. HU
HARVARD MEDICAL SCHOOL

Memorial Sloan-Kettering Cancer Center

THE MEMORIAL SLOAN-KETTERING Cancer Center (MSKCC) is the oldest and largest cancer center in the world. It was founded in 1884 as New York Cancer Hospital.

The MSKCC was originally on the Upper West Side of Manhattan. It moved in 1939 to its present location on York Avenue, where it was built as Memorial Hospital. This site was donated to the hospital in 1936 by John D. Rockefeller.

Construction of a new Memorial Hospital was completed in 1973, and this building is the current location of the MSKCC. Additionally, in 2006 construction of a 23-story research building was completed, and an adjacent 7-story laboratory was begun.

The inclusion of *Sloan-Kettering* in the center's name came about in the 1940s, when Alfred P. Sloan and Charles F. Kettering, both former General Motors Corp. executives, established the Sloan-Kettering Institute (SKI). The SKI was constructed adjacent to Memorial Hospital in 1948, and the two institutions joined in 1980 under the current name.

Several regional outpatient clinics have been constructed since 1980 to expand the reaches of the cancer care offered at MSKCC. Clinics are spread as far as Long Island, New Jersey, and Westchester County.

In 2004 Pediatric Day Hospital was opened for childhood oncology patients.

The MSKCC Breast Examination Center of Harlem has been providing free breast and cervical-cancer screens to female residents of Harlem since 1979. In 2003 the center, via the Ralph Lauren Center for Cancer Care and Prevention, began collaboration with North General Hospital in Harlem. This collaboration brings optimal cancer care and screening to the underserved residents of Harlem.

RESEARCH FACILITIES

In July 2006 the first class of the MSKCC graduate program in cancer biology entered the new Louis V. Gerstner, Jr., Graduate School of Biomedical Sciences at MSKCC. The idea behind this school was that such a program would bring basic science and translational research closer to the clinic.

Research carried out at the MSKCC involves cancer biology and genetics, cell biology, computational biology, developmental biology, immunology, molecular biology, molecular pharmacology and chemistry, and structural biology.

At Memorial Hospital, researchers participate in the Human Oncology and Pathogenesis program as well as clinical research. Research fields are organized by disease and treatment modality, such as infectious diseases, integrative medicine, cancers of the central nervous system, and transplantations.

Education is offered at the MSKCC at several levels. Medical and postdoctoral fellows, as well as medical and graduate students, are trained at the center. Physicians and nurses are encouraged to participate in Continuing Medical or Nursing Education (CME or CNE, respectively), whereby they can stay updated on recent advances in the fields of cancer research and care.

At the MSKCC, care is offered for numerous cancers. Special services are offered to pediatric and international cancer patients. The National Cancer Institute has designed MSKCC a Comprehensive Care Center.

Patients at the center are cared for by a team of specialists. The composition of the team is tailored to the individual patient's needs. Team members may be medical oncologists, pathologists, radiation oncologists, radiologists, and surgeons. Pathologists examine tumor samples to diagnose the tumor and its extent; the radiologists use imaging technology to discern the tumor size and location.

Counseling support groups are available to patients and their caregivers. Specific counseling is targeted to newly diagnosed patients to help them cope with the impact of cancer. Family members and caregivers are also counseled at MSKCC to help them deal with the stresses and concerns of having a loved one with cancer.

CANCER SURVIVORSHIP PROGRAMS

The center also offers resources on cancer survivorship because the journey of cancer treatment continues through the survival process. Support is given in all aspects of a patient's life via counseling for financial, physical, emotional, and other concerns. Special clinics for survivors of adult-onset and childhood cancers offer support, follow-up care, and advice.

The clinics for survivors of adult-onset cancers are disease specific. Each patient has an appointment with a nurse practitioner who performs a physical exam, monitors any long-term needs, recommends further screening and lifestyle habits, and shares this information with the patient's primary-care physician.

The clinic for survivors of childhood cancers is a long-term follow-up program to monitor the health of these patients. A team of physicians (including a cardiologist, neuropsychologist, primary medical oncologist, and radiation oncologist) collaborates to develop a health management plan for each individual. When a patient reaches about 25 years of age, he or she is transitioned to the adult survivor program.

The MSKCC website offers resources for cancer patients and their caregivers. For patients considering coming to the MSKCC, the website offers tips for choosing a doctor, hospital, and cancer-care specialist.

The website also provides information for first-time visitors, such as what to expect at a cancer-care visit. Visitors from out of town can access information about accommodations in Manhattan, as well as travel to and within the city.

Tips are given to patients and their caregivers for optimal communication with the cancer-care team. Sections of the website are targeted to childhood and teenage patients. The teen site includes advice from other teenage cancer patients.

Lately@MSKCC is a monthly e-mail newsletter to which anyone can subscribe to receive information about the center.

Members of the MSKCC give Cancer*Smart* community lectures to educate the public about cancer. These lectures have been recorded and are available on the website.

SEE ALSO: National Cancer Institute; Survivors of Cancer; Women's Cancers.

BIBLIOGRAPHY. James S. Gordon and Sharon Curtin, *Comprehensive Cancer Care: Integrating Alternative, Complementary, and Conventional Therapies* (HarperCollins Publishers, 2001).

CLAUDIA WINOGRAD
UNIVERSITY OF ILLINOIS AT URBANA-CHAMPAIGN

Menarche

MENARCHE IS DEFINED as the first menstrual period or the onset of menstruation. Both socially and medically, menarche is considered to be the pinnacle of female puberty, as it marks the beginning of a woman's reproductive life.

There is a direct association between age at menarche and the risk of various types of cancer, including breast, endometrium, and ovary. Age at menarche, because it marks the onset of estrogen production, is often used in conjunction with many other reproductive and hormone-related factors to determine a woman's lifetime exposure to estrogen. A woman's lifetime exposure to estrogen is a critical risk factor for breast and endometrial cancer, and possibly for other cancers, such as ovarian cancer. Thus, understanding the determinants and variation in age at menarche will help us better understand potential disease risk.

Menarche is an important marker of the start of estrogen production by the ovaries; however, menarche does not mark the initiation of regular ovulation, which can happen up to a few years after menarche. Although regular ovulation does not begin at menarche, age at menarche is a predictor of ovulatory frequency during adolescence such that girls with an earlier menarche regulate their ovulatory cycles more quickly than girls with a later onset. As a result, hormone levels in young adults are correlated with age at menarche, in that earlier onset of menstruation is related to higher levels of various sex hormones throughout adolescence. This effect persists into adulthood; women with an earlier menarche continue to demonstrate higher levels of sex hormones.

Menarche is determined by many factors, including genetics, nutrition, physical activity, and environmental factors. Various physiologic changes prepare the body for the onset of menstruation. One important requirement for menarche to occur is the body's achievement of sufficient body-fat percentage (generally, greater than 17 percent).

MENARCHE AND CANCER RISK

Early age at menarche and other hormonally linked risk factors—such as late age at menopause, exogenous hormone use, decreased parity, and late age at first live birth—contribute to the lifetime estrogen exposure in women. Consequently, these factors have been consistently associated with an increased risk of breast and endometrial cancer in many observational studies. Factors associated with lifetime exposure to estrogen, including menarche, have also been associated, albeit not as consistently, with risk of ovarian cancer.

It is believed that geographic variations in age at menarche and other hormonally related factors help explain differences in rates of breast and endometrial cancer. There exists substantial international variation in the incidence of these hormonally related cancers (such as breast, endometrial, and ovarian cancer), which correlates with many of these nongenetic hormonal factors, such as age at menarche. Because menarche is determined in part by various environmental factors, age at menarche has been shown to vary by geographic location and race and/or ethnicity. In the United States, for example, the average age at menarche is 12.5 years. The average age at menarche is lower not only in the United States, but also in other developed countries compared with developing countries such as India, Bangladesh, and China. Differences in nutrition, physical activity levels, social factors, and genetics help explain these geographic differences.

Rates of hormonally related cancers are highest among white women in Western populations, where there are also a younger age at menarche, more frequent exogenous-hormone use, later age at first live birth, and decreased parity.

Lifestyle interventions that potentially influence the onset of menarche may be beneficial in reducing risk of hormone-related cancers such as those in the breast, endometrium, and ovaries. This is a point worthy of considerable attention in today's society, because not only have Western countries like the United States historically had a lower age at menarche compared with developing countries, but also, the average age at menarche continues to decrease over time. These subtle changes in age at menarche and other hormone-related risk factors may more greatly affect cancer incidence rates in the future. Because age at menarche is related to hormone levels in young adults, an earlier onset of menstruation will increase the lifetime exposure to estrogens, which may lead to an increased risk of breast, endometrial, and ovarian cancer.

EFFECT OF CHILDHOOD OBESITY

The decline in age at menarche in many developed countries is due to changes in various lifestyle factors. As rates of childhood overweight and obesity increase, young girls achieve sufficient body-fat percentage at a younger age and are subsequently physiologically prepared for the onset of menses at a younger age.

The adverse impact of earlier age at menarche in such populations could be influenced through various nutritional and other lifestyle interventions. As previously stated, menarche can occur only after the body has gained a sufficient body-fat percentage. Thus, reducing the rates of childhood overweight or obesity, through nutritional or physical-activity interventions, can favorably affect the onset of menses.

Various studies have shown that high levels of moderate and vigorous physical activity affect markers of ovarian hormone exposure, resulting in delayed menarche, increased likelihood of secondary amenorrhea, and irregular or anovulatory menstrual cycles. These events would result in a reduction of lifetime ovulatory cycles and lower cumulative estrogen exposure, thus potentially lowering the risk of breast, endometrial, and ovarian cancer risk.

The long-term impact of earlier age at menarche will continue to be an area of interest in relation to risk of breast, endometrial, and ovarian cancer. More important, the message of early prevention of breast, endometrial, and other hormone-related cancers through nutrition and physical-activity intervention is critical. By taking measures to improve nutrition and energy expenditure, we can reduce the burden of childhood obesity and subsequently affect disease risk.

SEE ALSO: Estrogens, Steroidal; Obesity; Women's Cancers.

BIBLIOGRAPHY. D. Apter, et al., "Some Endocrine Characteristics of Early Menarche, a Risk Factor for Breast Cancer, Are Preserved into Adulthood," *Journal of Steroid Biochemistry* (v.44, 1989); L. Bernstein, et al., "Ethnicity-Related Variation in Breast Cancer Risk Factors," *Cancer* (v.97, 2003); C. T. Brekelmans, "Risk Factors and Risk Reduction of Breast and Ovarian Cancers," *Current Opinion in Obstetrics & Gynecology* (v.15, 2003); F. De Waard and J. H. Thijssen, "Hormonal Aspects in the Causation of Human Breast Cancer: Epidemiologic Hypotheses Reviewed, with Special Reference to Nutritional Status and First Pregnancy," *The Journal of Steroid Biochemistry and Molecular Biology* (v.97, 2005); "Menarche," www.wikipedia.org (cited October 2006); D. M. Purdie and A. C. Green, "Epidemiology of Endometrial Cancer," *Best Practice & Research. Clinical Obstetrics & Gynaecology* (v.15, 2001); R. Vihko and D. J. Apter, "Endocrine Characteristics of Adolescent Menstrual Cycles: Impact of Early Menarche," *Journal of Steroid Biochemistry* (v.20, 1984).

ALPA V. PATEL, PH.D.
AMERICAN CANCER SOCIETY

Merck & Co. (United States)

MERCK & CO. (Merck) was established in 1891 by George Merck; the company was later run by his son George Merck, Jr. Merck is a leading global researcher and producer of pharmaceuticals in the fields of medicine and vaccine. Merck produces medications that help relieve side effects of cancer treatment, such as osteoporosis, migraines, and nausea.

One drug, EMEND, is used by patients undergoing chemotherapy. This drug is taken before the chemotherapy session to prevent nausea and emesis afterward.

The company's mission is "to provide society with superior products and services by developing innovations and solutions that improve the quality of life and satisfy customer needs, and to provide employees with meaningful work and advancement opportunities, and investors with a superior rate of return." In keeping with this mission, Merck strives to maintain the highest standards of research and work ethics. To this end, employees follow a Code of Conduct, most recently updated in November 2005.

Scientific research is carried out in Merck Research Laboratories (MRL). These labs are across the globe in several countries, including the United States, Canada, France, Italy, Japan, Spain, and the United Kingdom. At MRLs, research is conducted in the fields of Applied Computer Science and Math, Biological Sciences, Biostatistics, Chemical Engineering, Chemistry, Epidemiology, Medicine, Molecular Profiling, Pharmaceutical Science, Pharmacology, and Veterinary Medicine.

Merck invests a large amount of time and money into the development of new drugs. In fact, the company spends approximately $800 million over ten years in the process of bringing one drug from basic laboratory research to patient use. According to the company, for every 10,000 drugs screened, five might be approved for clinical trials; usually only one of those five will be deemed beneficial to a patient.

Merck participates in global initiatives to donate medications, as well as deliver these medications to the people who need them. It also produces vaccines and publishes informational literature on diseases. In addition, the company provides philanthropy via monetary donations to programs and funds. The company provides an online healthcare manual for patients and caregivers: the *Merck Manual of Medical Information Home Edition*. This manual is also available on the company's website. The company also publishes the *Merck Index*, a comprehensive volume outlining information for substances such as biologic agents and other chemicals or drugs. Other Merck manuals cover diagnosis and therapy, health and aging, geriatrics, and veterinary care.

SEE ALSO: Clinical Trials; Education, Cancer; Experimental Cancer Drugs; Vaccines.

BIBLIOGRAPHY. Ahmed F. Abdel-Magid and Stephane Caron, *Fundamentals of Early Clinical Drug Development: From Synthesis Design to Formulation* (Wiley-Interscience, 2006); Anne Clayton, *Insight into a Career in Pharmaceutical Sales* (Pharmaceuticalsales.Com Inc., 2005); Adriana Petryna, Andrew Lakoff, and Arthur Kleinman, *Global Pharmaceuticals: Ethics, Markets, Practices* (Duke University Press, 2006).

CLAUDIA WINOGRAD
UNIVERSITY OF ILLINOIS AT URBANA-CHAMPAIGN

Mesothelioma, Adult Malignant

ADULT MALIGNANT MESOTHELIOMA is a rare form of cancer that attacks the pleural membrane around the lungs. Unlike other lung cancer, mesothelioma develops in the lining that envelops the lungs, not inside the lungs themselves. This disease is caused by the inhalation of asbestos fibers. There is a latency period of 20 to 40 years or more between exposure and symptom manifestation. In the United States, 2,000 to 3,000 people are diagnosed with this disease each year. Ubiquitous and negligent use of asbestos in past decades predicts a rise in mesothelioma cases in the future.

Individuals who develop mesothelioma have usually held jobs in which they came into contact with materials containing asbestos. This group includes employees in virtually all the building trades and many manufacturing industries. Shipyard and powerhouse workers, insulation and linoleum installers, and steamfitters have traditionally been among the highest-exposed employee groups. Secondary exposure to asbestos can also be the cause of mesothelioma. A spouse who washes asbestos-contaminated work clothes, for example, can inhale sufficient asbestos to initiate this cancer. Mesothelioma has also been linked to the use by homeowners of asbestos-containing home-improvement products.

The symptoms of mesothelioma include chronic cough, shortness of breath (dyspnea), painful breathing, fatigue, persistent pain in the chest or upper back, weight loss, and coughing up blood (hemoptysis). Unfortunately, by the time these symptoms appear, the disease has usually progressed to an advanced stage. As a tumor develops on the pleural membrane, the membrane thickens and becomes less flexible. Continued tumor growth makes breathing progressively more difficult. The tumor can invade the chest wall and spread to other parts of the body through the circulatory system.

Mesothelioma does not usually register on a normal X-ray; therefore, this disease can go unnoticed during a routine physical examination. Persons with a history of exposure to asbestos should be evaluated with more advanced imaging techniques, such as computed axial tomography (CAT scan), magnetic resonance imaging (MRI scan), or positron emission tomography (PET scan).

If mesothelioma is suspected as a result of these scans, a biopsy will be preformed by inserting a fine

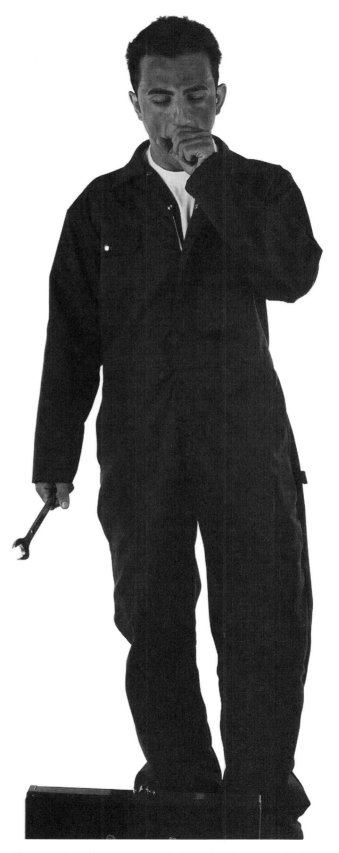

The symptoms of mesothelioma include chronic cough, shortness of breath (dyspnea), painful breathing, and fatigue.

needle through the chest wall to obtain a small sample of tissue. A positive diagnosis of mesothelioma requires the microscopic examination of this tissue sample.

Research efforts are under way to perfect an early-detection tool for mesothelioma. This approach uses the identification of a substance that is present at a higher concentration in mesothelioma patients than in people without this disease. Detection of such a marker in a blood sample, for example, would indicate the presence of mesothelioma.

Malignant mesothelioma may be treated by surgical intervention, radiation therapy, and chemotherapy. Only cases that are determined to be early-stage mesothelioma, in which the tumor is still localized in the pleural membrane, are candidates for surgery. Using a multimodal treatment plan, surgery is often followed by radiation therapy and/or chemotherapy. In the majority of cases, however, mesothelioma has progressed to an advanced stage before it is detected. Therefore, treatment is generally palliative and focuses on pain management, symptom control, and quality-of-life issues. Mesothelioma is often accompanied by an accumulation of fluid or pleural effusion around the lungs. The drainage of this fluid through a tube inserted into the chest can help ease breathing difficulties. This procedure is called thoracentesis. Most victims of mesothelioma survive fewer than 18 months after the disease is diagnosed.

SEE ALSO: Asbestos; Chemotherapy; Pain and Pain Management; Radiation Therapy; Surgery.

BIBLIOGRAPHY. Massachusetts General Hospital Cancer Center, "Learn About Mesothelioma," www.massgeneral.org/cancer/crr/types/thoracic/mesothelioma.asp (cited October 2006); Paul Calabresi and Philip S. Schein, *Medical Oncology* (McGraw-Hill, Inc., 1993).

PAUL J. CLERKIN
SACRAMENTO CITY COLLEGE

Mesothelioma, Childhood

CHILDHOOD MESOTHELIOMA IS a rare cancer that targets the membrane surrounding the lungs. It is an aggressive cancer with a grave prognosis. Although mesothelioma in adults shows a virtually exclusive causal relationship with exposure to asbestos and is characterized by a latency period of 20 to 40 years, the available data for childhood mesothelioma does not appear to support a similar relationship or accommodate such a prolonged timeline.

Childhood mesothelioma is an incompletely understood disease. Current evidence suggests a relationship between this cancer and radiation. A higher-than-normal incidence of childhood mesothelioma has occurred in children following treatment for Wilms's tumor. Wilms's tumor, also known as nephroblastoma, is a cancerous tumor of the kidney. Wilms's tumor occurs most often in children between the ages of 2 and 5 years. A small percentage of children who have received pulmonary radiation for metastasized Wilms's tumor later developed mesothelioma. Although available data do not support a relationship between childhood mesothelioma and exposure to asbestos, the known association between asbestos and adult mesothelioma, along with the ubiquitous nature of asbestos and the possibility of undocumented exposure, suggest that asbestos should not be automatically eliminated as a possible cause of childhood mesothelioma.

Genetic predisposition to cancer, previous cancer diagnosis and/or radiation therapy, exposure to asbestos, and possibly prenatal and postnatal medications might play roles in the occurrence of childhood mesothelioma.

The symptoms of mesothelioma include shortness of breath, chronic cough, and painful breathing. Like adult mesothelioma, childhood mesothelioma should be evaluated with advanced imaging techniques. If these imaging techniques give reason to suspect mesothelioma, a tissue sample is obtained via a needle biopsy. In this procedure, a needle is inserted through the chest wall, and a small sample of tissue is removed. The sample is examined under a microscope to determine whether mesothelioma is an accurate diagnosis. Without documented history of exposure to asbestos, most often present in cases of adult mesothelioma, there may be little reason to suspect the presence of this cancer. In individuals too young to satisfy the latency requirements of adult mesothelioma, history of a previous thoracic cancer successfully treated, in part, with radiation might be an important indicator in the diagnosis of childhood mesothelioma. By the time symptoms become notable and a diagnosis is made, childhood mesothelioma has often progressed to an advanced stage.

There is no cure for mesothelioma, and treatment is palliative in nature. Most victims survive less than a year after this disease is diagnosed. With the development of mesothelioma, there is a thickening of the membrane around the lungs, which renders the membrane less flexible and breathing more difficult. In most cases of mesothelioma, it is common for fluid to accumulate around the lungs. This fluid can be drained by the insertion of a tube through the chest wall. This procedure, called thoracentesis, can make breathing less difficult.

Wilms's tumor, however, has been addressed successfully with a multimodal treatment plan combining the surgical removal of the tumor followed by chemotherapy and radiation treatments. Often, Wilms's tumor is diagnosed and treated before the cancer has spread or metastasized to other parts of the body. When this cancer has metastasized, the lungs are the most common place to which it spreads. In this case, radiation therapy is directed at the lungs.

SEE ALSO: Asbestos; Childhood Cancers; Kidney Cancer, Childhood; Mesothelioma, Adult Malignant; Radiation.

BIBLIOGRAPHY. Joseph Aisner, et al., *Comprehensive Textbook of Thoracic Oncology* (Williams and Wilkins, 1996).

PAUL J. CLERKIN
SACRAMENTO CITY COLLEGE

Mexico

THE SPANISH ARRIVED in Mexico in 1519 and ruled it until independence was declared in 1810 and recognized in 1821, after which Mexico was involved in a series of wars with the United States, losing much territory.

In 1864 Emperor Maximilian was placed on the newly created Mexican throne by European powers, but this empire lasted only until 1867, when it was destroyed in battle and Maximilian was executed. Since then it has been ruled by presidents who have had varying degrees of support from the population,

the Mexican Revolution of 1910 being particularly traumatic. The Republic of Mexico has a population of 107,784,000 (2006), with 186 doctors and 87 nurses per 100,000 people. An example of cancer incidence rates in Mexico includes 144.5 cases of cancer in males per 100,000, according to the International Agency for Research on Cancer.

There are some references in Aztec records that circumcision was used to help prevent penile cancer. This practice was banned by the Spanish, however. During the Spanish period, medical services in Mexico were limited to Europeans and a few wealthy indigenous people. This situation remained much the same after independence until after the Mexican Revolution of the early 20th century, when there was a concerted attempt to improve hospitals and health services.

Hospital de Oncología in Mexico City, established in the 1940s, has been the major clinical cancer-treatment center in the country, with the capacity to treat patients with surgery, radiotherapy, or chemotherapy.

The types of cancer common in Mexico are skin cancer and lung cancer for men, and breast cancer and cervical cancer for women. There is also stomach cancer, possibly from heavy consumption of chili. There is a small prevalence of human T-cell leukemia–lymphoma virus in some black former slave communities and among their descendants in Mexico.

Guillermo Montano from the Hospital General, Unidad de Oncologia, Mexico City, worked on the results of the modifications of hormonal medium associated with radiation in the treatment of advanced cervical cancer. Juan Lopez Cueto, et al., of the same hospital studied radical neck dissection in the treatment of the malignant tumors of oral cavity. Luis Benitez-Bribiesca, et al., from the Departmento de Investigacion Cientifica, Instituto Mexicano del Seguro Social in Mexico City, worked on alkaline phosphatase and regan isozyme in cervical cancer.

Famous Mexicans who died from cancer include Jaime Torres Bodet, poet and novelist, who committed suicide after being diagnosed with cancer; actor Ramón Valdes, who died from lung cancer; and singer Raúl Vale, who died from cancer in Texas.

SEE ALSO: Breast Cancer; Cervical Cancer; Chemotherapy; Gastric (Stomach) Cancer; Lung Cancer, Non-Small Cell; Lung Cancer, Small Cell; Radiation Therapy; Skin Cancer (Melanoma).

BIBLIOGRAPHY. T. Aldrich, et al., "Cervical Cancer and the HPV Link: Identifying Areas for Education in Mexico City's Public Hospitals," *Salud Pública de México* (v.48/3, 2006); C. A. Arce-Salinas, et al., "Classical Fever of Unknown Origin (FUO): Current Causes in Mexico," *Revista de Investigación Clínica; Organo del Hospital de Enfermedades de la Nutrición* (v.57/6, 2005); Limon Noriega, "La Evolución de la Concología en los Tres Últimos Decenios," *Gaceta Médica de Mexico* (v.113, 1977); L. M. Reynales-Shigematsu, et al., "Costs of Medical Care Attributable to Tobacco Consumption at the Mexican Institute of Social Security (IMSS), Morelos [in Spanish]," *Salud Pública de México* (v.47/6, 2005); J. L. Rocha Ramirez, et al., "Hereditary Mixed Polyposis Syndrome. First Report in Mexico [in Spanish]," *Revista de Gastroenterología de México* (v.70/4, 2005); A. V. Schally and D. Gonzalez Barcena, "History of Clinical Studies on Hypothalamic Hormone Analogs in Mexico [in Spanish]," *Gaceta Médica de México* (v.142/4, 2006); Gordon Schendel, *Medicine in Mexico: From Aztec Herbs to Betatrons* (University of Texas Press, 1968); Germán Somolinos D'Ardois, *Historia y Medicina: Figures y Hechos de la Historiografía Médica Mexicana* (Imprenta Universitaria, 1957); "The Cancer Congress of Guadalajara (Mexico)," *Cancer Research* (v.4, 1944); "Bienvenido a la Asociación Mexicana de Lucha Contra el Cáncer," www.amlcc.org (cited November 2006).

JUSTIN CORFIELD
GEELONG GRAMMAR SCHOOL, AUSTRALIA

Migration and Immigration

STUDIES OF THE changes in cancer rates and patterns when groups of people undergo major geographic relocations have been a key element in establishing the dominant role of environmental, rather than genetic, risk factors in the causation (etiology) of cancer. In addition, these studies confirmed observations that environmental exposures influencing the risk of cancer in particular organs of the body may differ and that the period of life when the onset of these exposures occurs can determine their effects on cancer development.

Migration—the movement and resettlement of individuals from one location to another—occurs for economic, political, and social reasons. Migration often occurs between places that differ substantially in their physical and cultural environments. This change can in turn affect the risk of diseases, such as cancer. The migration of large numbers of individuals has provided researchers an unplanned opportunity (a so-called natural experiment) to study the effects of the dramatically changed environment on cancer risks. Most migrations—and consequently, most of the available data on migrants and cancer—relate to movement to more-developed countries from less-developed countries. In particular, the large migrations of people during the 20th century to the United States and Australia, generally for economic opportunities, as well as to Israel, for cultural, political, and economic reasons, have been extensively studied.

Migrant studies of cancer require that cancer incidence rates, which are a measure of cancer risk, be available from the home country, the host (new) country, and for the migrant population residing in the host country. Cancer rates are computed separately by cancer site, such as breast and lung, and by sex, and they are age adjusted to allow comparison between populations with differing age structures. The site-specific cancer incidence rates among the migrant population in the host country are compared with rates for the country of origin, and differences are generally attributed to environmental exposures, as the genetic makeup of these populations is presumably similar (discussed further later in this article). The migrant rates can also be contrasted with the rates of other residents in the host country; here, differences may be attributed to either genetic or environmental (usually, lifestyle related) factors. When appropriate data can be obtained, further comparisons can be made between migrants and their descendants in the host country. Because the offspring of migrants (i.e., second-generation migrants) are likely to have adopted more of the culture of the host country, such comparisons can elucidate the effect of acculturation on cancer risk. Furthermore, within a migrant population, incidence can be compared between immigrants arriving in the country of destination early or late in life, and between immigrants who have lived in the host country for a short or long period. These comparisons can be used to identify the periods of life when exposures have their greatest effect on cancer risk.

The contribution of migrant studies to the understanding of cancer etiology has been substantial. More than any others, studies of migrants established the dominant role of the external environment, including lifestyle factors, in determining cancer risk. The nearly invariable observation is that the cancer rates among migrants can change dramatically after migration and always in the direction of the prevailing rates in the country of destination. Therefore, the cancer risk in first-generation migrants is, as a rule, intermediate between the risks for the home and host populations. Cancer rates among the descendents of migrants have generally moved farther toward the host-country rates, and convergence (equality) of the rates is often observed within a few generations. The number of generations that it takes to reach convergence provides clues to important risk factors, to the timing of relevant exposures, and to the identification of groups that may be more susceptible genetically to the exposures for that cancer. Another important and consistent finding from migrant studies is that the direction and magnitude of the change in risk vary by cancer site for each migrant group, underscoring the specificity of risk factors for cancers of different organs. Several of the points discussed above are illustrated by the findings from migrant studies of particular cancers.

BREAST CANCER

Most studies of breast and prostate cancers have entailed movement from low-risk to high-risk countries. For both sites, the risk among migrants increased progressively through the generations, suggesting an effect of greater acculturation and, thus, higher levels of exposure to the causal factors in the host country. As an example, Japanese female migrants to Hawaii in the early decades of the 20th century experienced a doubling in risk for breast cancer compared with the very low incidence rates in Japan at the time. These first-generation-migrant rates were about 55 percent lower than the rates among whites in Hawaii, and although rates among second-generation Japanese rose further, they remained about 30 percent lower than among whites. These observations suggest that although breast-cancer risk is modifiable, important exposures to risk factors probably occur early in life, possibly related to age at menarche and other reproductive factors.

COLORECTAL CANCER

A striking exception to this observation is the experience with colorectal cancer, in which the rates in first-

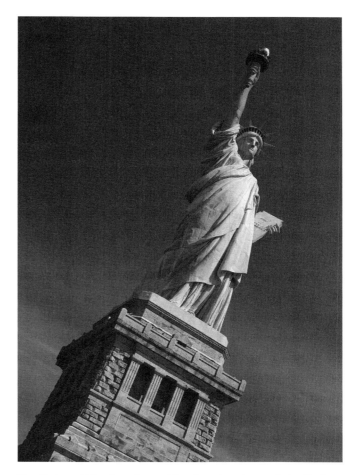

The Statue of Liberty welcomed immigrants, who carried with them their hopes and dreams, but also caused migration of diseases.

generation migrants increased to a level very close to the rates of the host country. This cancer has been studied most fully among Japanese who migrated to Hawaii in the early decades of the 20th century. Their rates of cancer increased threefold to fourfold over the prevailing rates in Japan and, remarkably, reached the same level as that of the host country within a single generation. As most migration occurs among young adults, this immediate full transition to the host country prevailing rates implies that (1) colorectal cancer risk is modifiable, but in this instance, exposure later in life is most critical; and (2) Japanese may have a particular susceptibility to this exposure. Intake of meat is higher among Japanese in the United States compared with Japanese in Japan, and meat has been identified as a risk factor for colorectal cancer. Well-done meat in particular contains potentially carcinogenic heterocyclic aromatic amines, and Japanese may be more susceptible to the effects of these carcinogens than whites because of a higher prevalence of the high-risk alleles of two polymorphic metabolizing genes, *NAT2* and *CYP1A2*. Underscoring the important relationship between the cancer rates among migrants and the general risk of cancer in the host country, it is noteworthy that the colorectal cancer rates among Japanese migrants to Brazil—a lower-risk country for this cancer—remain low.

SKIN CANCER

Another cancer that has been studied mostly in migrants from lower-risk to higher-risk areas is malignant melanoma of the skin. Most studies have been conducted in the high-risk countries of Australia and Israel, where solar exposure is common. Although the changes in risk followed the usual pattern of a gradual increase in the host country, the effect of migration on the risk of melanoma depended on the skin color of the migrants, in that those with darker skin always retained a lower risk than those with lighter skin. Furthermore, individuals migrating early in life (before age 10) had a higher risk of melanoma than did those relocating later in life—another example of the enduring effect of an exposure in childhood (presumably, sun exposure) on risk later in life.

STOMACH CANCER

Stomach cancer represents a site where migrations were generally from high-risk to low-risk countries. Adhering to the general rule that risks move toward those in the host country, rates of stomach cancer (unlike those of breast, prostate, and colorectal cancer) decreased progressively on migration, suggesting an effect of greater acculturation—and, thus, lower levels of exposure to the causal factors—in the host country. To illustrate, the rates among early Japanese migrants to Hawaii decreased approximately 40 percent in the first generation compared with the rates prevailing in Japan. Though the risk declined further in second-generation Japanese, it remained twice as high as the rates in Hawaiian whites. The lack of convergence in risk to that of the host country suggests that an exposure early in life has a lasting influence on the risk of this cancer in adulthood. Infection with *H. pylori* bacteria is a likely possibility, as infection is generally acquired in childhood, and this agent has been identified as a major causal factor for stomach cancer.

NASOPHARYNGEAL CANCER

Another cancer site that has been studied mostly in migrants to a lower-risk setting is nasopharyngeal cancer (NPC), a disease most common in Chinese and some related groups, such as the Inuits of Alaska, the Canadian Arctic, and Greenland. Although the rates of NPC for these ethnic groups are lower in the countries of destination, the rates have remained relatively high. This observation suggests (as was noted for colorectal cancer among Japanese) that these groups may have a greater genetic susceptibility to one or more risk factors for this cancer, such as salted-fish intake, cigarette smoking, and infection with the Epstein-Barr virus.

LUNG CANCER

A final example of what has been learned from site-specific migrant studies pertains to lung cancer. In most populations of the world, the risk of this cancer is determined primarily by the use of tobacco. Thus, tobacco exposure, rather than the prevailing rates in the host country, is the major predictor of lung-cancer risk among migrants. Because cigarette smoking was especially common in some migrant groups (perhaps related to the stresses of migration), the rates of lung cancer in these groups actually exceeded those of either the country of origin or the country of destination. When female migrants from China to other countries were observed to have surprisingly high rates of lung cancer despite low use of tobacco products, further studies led to the identification of cooking fumes from open stoves as an important risk factor for lung cancer in this population.

INTERPRETATION OF FINDINGS

A few caveats are in order with regard to interpreting the findings of migrant cancer studies.

First, caution should be exercised in comparing disease rates among migrants with those of residents of the country of origin. Although it is generally assumed that migrants are representative of the population of the country of origin, they may represent a select group of individuals who differ from the majority of the home population in many respects, including social and cultural behaviors, ethnicity, religion, socioeconomic status, and even certain genetic factors. Thus, at least a portion of the difference in cancer rates observed between a group of migrants and those of the country of origin may reflect such selection bias.

Second, countries differ in the completeness of case ascertainment, diagnostic rules, and screening practices, all of which affect cancer incidence rates and could falsely imply a difference among populations that actually have similar risks. Comparisons of populations within the host country are not subject to this type of bias.

SEE ALSO: Breast Cancer; Colon Cancer; Gastric (Stomach) Cancer; Genetics; Lung Cancer, Non-Small Cell; Lung Cancer, Small Cell; Menarche; Nasopharyngeal Cancer; Prostate Cancer; Rectal Cancer; Skin Cancer (Melanoma); Tobacco Smoking.

BIBLIOGRAPHY. L. N. Kolonel and L. R. Wilkens, "Migrants Studies," in D. Schottenfeld and J. F. Fraumeni, eds., *Cancer Epidemiology and Prevention* (Oxford University Press, 2006).

Lynne R. Wilkens, Ph.D.
Laurence N. Kolonel, Ph.D.
Cancer Research Center of Hawaii,
University of Hawaii

MIT Center for Cancer Research

THE MASSACHUSETTS INSTITUTE of Technology (MIT) has been a leader in science and research since its first class entered in 1865. The purpose of this new school was to foster an independent education to serve an industrializing nation. In 1974 MIT founded the MIT Center for Cancer Research (CCR). The CCR is located on the MIT campus in Cambridge, just outside Boston. It is a Basic Research Center, as designated by the National Cancer Institute. Researchers at the CCR include Nobel laureates, members of the National Academy of Sciences, and Howard Hughes Medical Institute investigators.

Three research programs encompass the investigations at the CCR: Molecular Genetics and Immunology, Genetics and Model Systems, and Cell Biology. The Molecular Genetics and Immunology program looks at how gene regulation and DNA alterations affect cancer. Principal themes of research include signaling

pathways in autoimmunity and cancer, roles of RNA, and effects of DNA modifications such as methylation. The Genetics and Model Systems program researches the genetic aspects of cancer, using the classical model organisms yeast, nematode, fruit fly, zebrafish, mouse, and cell lines. Studies focus on mechanisms of cell death and on parallels and relations between normal-cell and tumor-cell development. Researchers in this program recognize the need to understand normal cell processes to comprehend how these processes are altered in cancer. Finally, the Cell Biology program focuses on cell functions and how they are affected in cancer. Specific areas of focus are cell adhesion, motility, and migration, and how these functions are related to invasion and tumor metastasis; stem-cell biology; and signal transduction and how particular signaling networks are related to mitogenesis (the induction of cell division via mitosis).

CCR scientists collaborate with other researchers in Boston via the MIT-Harvard NanoMedical Consortium in an effort to develop nanotechnology for cancer research and care. Participants in the consortium are based at MIT, Harvard University and Harvard Medical School, Massachusetts General Hospital, and Brigham and Women's Hospital. Along with the applications of nanotechnology in general oncology, the consortium addresses cancers of the brain, colon, lungs, ovaries, and prostate.

Education and training are offered to students in undergraduate and graduate schools, as well as to postdoctoral fellows. Graduate students enter the Center via the Department of Biology. Undergraduates may participate in the MIT Undergraduate Research Opportunity Program, which was established in 1969. Students can receive academic credit or pay for their research, or they may volunteer.

In 1998 and 2001 CCR research culminated in two of the first U.S. Food and Drug Administration-approved anticancer drugs produced via molecular biology: Herceptin and Gleevec. Herceptin was approved in 1998 as part of a multidrug treatment for node-positive breast tumors with cells overexpressing the product of the HER2 gene. Gleevec was approved in 2001 to target chronic myeloid leukemia (CML) and in 2002 for gastrointestinal stromal tumors (GIST). CML patients must be newly diagnosed and must express Philadelphia chromosome-positive CML in the chronic phase.

CCR laboratories are housed in several buildings. The main building is called E17. Additional labs are in the Department of Biology in the Whitehead Institute and Koch Biology Building, the Broad Institute, the Division of Biological Engineering, the Division of Chemical Engineering, and the Department of Chemistry. Researchers benefit from sharing core facilities in bioinformatics and computing, biopolymers, flow cytometry, glassware preparation, histology, media preparation, microarray technologies, microscopy and imaging, shared research resources, transgenic animals, and virus production.

To keep investigators informed of recent advances and achievements of the center, the CCR publishes a quarterly newsletter. Topics include new researchers, awards won by CCR members, novel technologies, and recent publications by investigators at the center.

The CCR has outlined several future directions for research, including the development of novel animal models of cancer and tumorigenesis. Researchers will also use the technology of RNA-interference to determine functions of genes related to cancer. Another research direction will examine the relationship between stem cells and caner. Because stem cells can divide continuously, recent theories suggest that tumors are the products of stem cells that have lost self-regulatory control. Other researchers will focus on the process of metastasis (the invasion of healthy tissue by a malignant tumor).

LUDWIG CANCER CENTER

In 2006 the Ludwig Institute sponsored the foundation of Ludwig Cancer Centers at MIT, Johns Hopkins University, Stanford University, Memorial Sloan-Kettering Cancer Center, Dana-Farber Cancer Institute, Harvard Medical School, and the University of Chicago. At MIT, the center will be called the Ludwig Center for Molecular Oncology at MIT. This new center will study the mechanisms underlying tumor metastasis. It will be housed in a new facility on the MIT campus that will house the CCR as well.

SEE ALSO: Experimental Cancer Drugs; Future of Cancer; Genetics.

BIBLIOGRAPHY. Michael Kahn and Stella Pelengaris, *The Molecular Biology of Cancer* (Blackwell Publishing Professional, 2006); Razelle Kurzrock and Moshe Talpaz, *Molecular Biology in Cancer Medicine*, 2d ed. (Taylor and Francis, 1999); Lauren Pecorino, *Molecular Biology of Cancer: Mechanisms, Targets, and Therapeutics* (Oxford University Press, 2005); D. Rusciano, et al., *Cancer Metastasis: Experimental Approaches (Laboratory Techniques in Biochemistry and Molecular Biology)* (Elsevier Science, 2000).

CLAUDIA WINOGRAD
UNIVERSITY OF ILLINOIS AT URBANA-CHAMPAIGN

Moldova

THIS EASTERN EUROPEAN country was the Principality of Moldavia until it was annexed by the Russian Empire in 1812. In 1918 it became part of Romania, but in 1945 it was annexed by the Soviet Union as the Moldavian Soviet Socialist Republic. On August 27, 1991, it gained its independence as the Republic of Moldova. It has a population of 3,395,600 (2006), with 350 doctors and 874 nurses per 100,000 people—one of the highest ratios in the world. An example of cancer incidence rates in Moldova includes 218.7 cases of cancer in males per 100,000, according to the International Agency for Research on Cancer.

Although some surgical procedures for treating tumors were followed from the late medieval period, much of the knowledge about cancer treatment came from German doctors and others trained in Germany or Russia during the 19th century. Medical services remained extremely limited until after World War II. In 1950 there were only 95 beds for cancer patients in Moldavia, rising to 270 in 1960, remaining the same in the following year.

This number increased heavily in the late 1960s with a major improvement in healthcare throughout the Soviet Union. Since independence, cancer rates in Moldova have continued to rise, as much through people living longer as from vastly improved diagnosis.

It has also come from a rise in lung cancer rates, a problem exacerbated by a massive increase in smoking after B.A.T. and the German manufacturer Reemtsma pushed for the deregulation of the production and sale of cigarettes in the country.

Even though smoking rates were lower in Moldova than in much of the rest of the former Soviet Union,

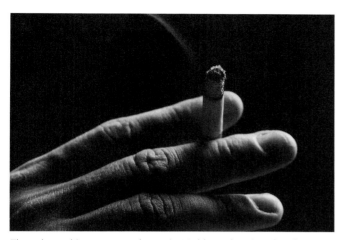

Though smoking rates are lower in Moldova than in other former Soviet Union countries, male lung cancer rates remain high..

male lung cancer deaths was well above the average for the European Union. A recent study concentrated on environmental tobacco smoke.

The Moldovan Academy of Sciences in Kishinev coordinates medical research in the country. Other research on cancer is conducted at the Kishinev States Medical Institute and Moldovan State University.

SEE ALSO: Lung Cancer, Non-Small Cell; Lung Cancer, Small Cell; Russia; Tobacco Smoking.

BIBLIOGRAPHY. O. I. Chernitsa, et al., "S Allele of L-MYC Oncogene Is Associated with Metastatic Lung Cancer in Patients from Moldova," *European Journal of Cancer* (v.34/11, 1998); Anna B. Gilmore, et al., "Pushing up Smoking Incidence: Plans for a Privatized Tobacco Industry in Moldova," *Lancet* (v.365, 2005); L. Negru, "Professorul Iuliu Moldovan Creatorul Primului Instit Oncologic in Romania," *Viata Medicina* (v.30, 1982); I. D. Sorochin, "Razvitie Onkologichcheskof Pomoshchi Naseleniiu Moldavskof SSR za Gody Sovetskoi Vlasti," *Voprosy Onkologii* (v.18, 1972); I. Stepanov, et al., "Analysis of Tobacco-Specific Nitrosamines in Moldovan Cigarette Tobacco," *Journal of Agricultural and Food Chemistry* (v.50, 2002); I. Stepanov, et al., "Uptake of the Tobacco-Specific Lung Carcinogen 4-(methylnitrosamino)-1-(3-pyridyl)-1-butanone by Moldovan Children," *Cancer Epidemiology, Biomarkers & Prevention* (v.15/1, 2006).

JUSTIN CORFIELD
GEELONG GRAMMAR SCHOOL, AUSTRALIA

Morocco

THIS NORTHERN AFRICAN kingdom was ruled by the Moors in medieval times, with the Portuguese capturing and holding some port cities along the coast during the 15th century. These cities were later placed under Spanish rule (when the kingdoms of Spain and Portugal briefly had the same ruler), and by the 1900s the Spanish and French occupied different parts of Morocco. Spain held the northeastern part around Tetuan, the Spanish Sahara, the cities of Ceuta and Melilla (which are still part of Spain), and Ifni. France occupied the remainder of the country except for Tangier, which was an international city.

In 1956 the kingdom of Morocco gained its independence, taking over Ifni in 1969 and the Spanish Sahara when the Spanish left during the 1970s. Morocco has a population of 33,241,000 (2005), with 46 doctors and 105 nurses per 100,000 people. An example of cancer incidence rates in Morocco includes 95.7 cases of cancer in males per 100,000, according to the International Agency for Research on Cancer.

During medieval times, Arab surgeons used the works of Avicenna to treat patients with tumors. With the arrival of the colonial powers, the healthcare system and especially the hospitals became transformed to treat Europeans and wealthy locals, especially Jews and members of the local elite.

Surgical procedures were used extensively for cancer patients. There was also a claim that tocopherols from the alimentary virgin argan oil extracted from an argan tree in Morocco could help prevent prostate cancer, and a recent study has suggested that the oil may have cancer-prevention properties.

After independence, there was a massive increase in money spent on healthcare, with hospitals throughout the country being built or considerably enlarged. With the rise in life expectancy and, hence, more people suffering from cancer, cancer research in the country gained greater urgency.

Recent Moroccans who have suffered from cancer included Said Belqola, an international football referee who died after a long battle with cancer; Laarbi Batma, the leader of the Nass El Ghiwane folk-music group, who died from lung cancer; and Ahmed Yacoubi, an artist and friend of the writer Paul Bowles, who also died from lung cancer. El Haj T'hami el Mezouari el Glaoui, who was better known by his title "Lord of the Atlas," died from stomach cancer. Venezuelan-American immunologist Baruj Benacerraf, the son of Sephardic Jews from Morocco, was involved in cancer research and won the 1980 Nobel Prize in Physiology or Medicine.

SEE ALSO: Breast Cancer; France; Portugal; Prostate Cancer; Spain.

BIBLIOGRAPHY. A. Ainahi, et al., "Study of the RET Gene and His Implication in Thyroid Cancer: Morocco Case Family," *Indian Journal of Cancer* (v.43/3, 2006); A. Drissi, et al., "Tocopherols and Saponins Derived from Argania Spinosa Exert an Antiproliferative Effect on Human Prostate Cancer," *Cancer Investigation* (v.24/6, 2006); R. Duprez, et al., "Molecular Epidemiology of the HHV-8 K1 Gene from Moroccan Patients with Kaposi's Sarcoma," *Virology* (v.353/1, 2006).

JUSTIN CORFIELD
GEELONG GRAMMAR SCHOOL, AUSTRALIA

Mozambique

THIS SOUTHEAST AFRICAN country was a Portuguese possession from about 1500. It was ruled under a variety of jurisdictions until the 20th century, when the whole area became the Portuguese colony of Mocambique. It gained its independence June 25, 1975. Mozambique has a population of 19,792,000 (2005), with 0.76 doctors per 100,000 people and one hospital bed per 1.133 people.

An example of cancer incidence rates in Mozabique includes 140 cases of cancer in males per 100,000, according to the International Agency for Research on Cancer. The main forms of cancer in Mozambique are liver cancer and skin cancer in men, and breast cancer and cervical cancer in women.

During the Portuguese period, healthcare in Mozambique was poor outside the capital, Lourenco Marques (now Maputo). In a 1944 study E.L. Kennaway showed that people working in mines in South Africa who originally came from Portuguese East Africa (as Mozambique was then known) had a rate of liver cancer six times higher than those from other parts of South Africa.

Another study of cancer showed some human T-cell leukemia–lymphoma virus cases in Mozambique.

It is believed that some Mozambique slaves may have suffered from this virus, which was contracted by Portuguese traders in East Africa; the traders took it with them to other parts of the world. After independence, owing to the civil war from 1976 to 1994, health services in the capital and other main cities and towns improved, but there was little or no access to cancer treatment in the countryside.

After the war ended, rates of cervical cancer increased, possibly from higher levels of reporting, and from June 2002 to April 2003 all women with suspected cervical cancer were asked to participate in studies on the distribution of human papillomavirus (HPV) types in cervical cancer. These studies showed that a vaccine targeting HPV-16 and HPV-18 would substantially reduce the rates of cervical cancer in Mozambique.

The Instituto Nacional de Saude (Mozambique Public Health Institute) in Maputo is the official research center. Some research also takes place at the Faculty of Medicine at Universidade Eduardo Mondlane (Eduardo Mondlane University).

SEE ALSO: Breast Cancer; Cervical Cancer; Liver Cancer, Adult (Primary); Portugal; Skin Cancer (Melanoma); Skin Cancer (Non-Melanoma); Vaccines.

BIBLIOGRAPHY. Julie L. Cliff, *Health in Mozambique: A Select Bibliography 1950–1980* (Mozambique Angola and Guinea Information Centre, 1980); Ezekiel Kalipeni and Philip Thiuri, *Issues and Perspectives on Health Care in Contemporary Sub-Saharan Africa* (Edwin Mellen Press, 1997).

JUSTIN CORFIELD
GEELONG GRAMMAR SCHOOL, AUSTRALIA

Multiple Endocrine Neoplasia Syndrome, Childhood

MULTIPLE ENDOCRINE NEOPLASIA (MEN) is made of three genetically distinct groups, each involving adenomatous hyperplasia and malignant tumors within several types of endocrine glands. MENs are inherited autosomal dominant traits, especially from abnormal genetic expression. Specific symptoms and signs can develop at any age. With proper management and surgical removal of the tumors, MEN can be well treated.

SYNDROMES

MEN syndromes are as follows:

Parathyroid adenomas—MEN I, more than 90 percent; MEN IIA, 24 percent; MEN IIB, rare

Pancreatic islet-cell tumors—MEN I, 30 to 75 percent

Pituitary adenomas—MEN I, 50 to 65 percent

Medullary carcinoma of the thyroid—MEN 2A, more than 90 percent; MEN 2B, more than 90 percent

Pheochromocytomas—MEN 2A, 50 percent; MEN 2B, 60 percent

Mucosalneuromas—MEN 2B, 100 percent

Marfanoid habitus—MEN 2B, 100 percent

MEN 1: PARATHYROID ADENOMAS

This disorder (MEN 1) is seen with hyperplasia or adenomas of the pancreatic islets, the auterior pituitary (which secretes prolactin), and the parathyroids. In patients with hyperparathyroidism, the prevalence approaches 100 percent at 50 years but occurs only rarely in children under 18 years of age. In childhood, hyperparathyroidism usually manifests itself by 10 years of age, usually due to a single adenoma.

Symptoms of hyperparathyroidism include muscular weakness, anorexia, nausea, vomiting, constipation, polydipsia, polyuria, loss of weight, and fever. Common are renal calculi, which can produce renal colic and hematuria.

Bone changes can occur, causing back pain, disturbances of gait, fractures, and tumors. Although parathyroid crisis can occur, this is a serum calcium level greater than 5 mg/dL, which can lead to renal failure, stupor, and coma.

In infants, failure to thrive, poor feeding, and hypotonia are very common. After surgical removal of the ademona, pronosis is good.

Primary hypersecretion of pituitary hormone by a suspected adenoma is rare in childhood. Most common secreting pituitary tumors are corticotrophin, prolactin, and growth hormone.

With any pituitary tumors there are various hormonal deficiencies, mainly due to compression of the pituitary tissue. Primary treatment for pituitary tumors is surgical resection; radiation therapy may be more useful in large or recurrent tumors.

MEN 1: PANCREATIC ISLET-CELL TUMORS

Pancreatic islet-cell tumors are the second-most-common MEN I, being found in as many as 75 percent to 80 percent of affected patients over their lifetime. Half the islet-cell tumors are gastrinomas; the rest are B-cell tumors.

Approximately half the patients with MEN I die from a MEN I-related condition, most often from peptic ulcers or other mass effects of a malignant islet-cell tumor. Although insulinomas are frequently multiple, treatment with a partial pancreatectomy may be required.

MEN 2

MEN 2 encompasses three types: MEN 2A, MEN 2B, and familial medullary carcinoma of the thyroid. Each of these types shows a C-cell hyperplasia, which progresses to a multicentric medullary carcinoma of the thyroid. Also, inpatients who develop MEN 2A or 2B generally develop pheochromocytomas (approximately 5 percent of patients).

The C-cells' function is to secrete calcitonin, which causes a lowering of blood calcium. It is believed that C-cells undergo progressive changes, starting with a simple hyperplasia and leading to a full malignancy.

Medullary carcinoma of the thyroid spreads to regional lymph nodes and may metastasize to liver, lung, and/or bone. Death is usually due to distant metastases. Treatment is a total thyroidectomy with a bilateral neck dissection.

Pheochromocytomas are rare but usually develop within the fifth and sixth decades of life, and can be bilateral.

Any child at risk for MEN 2 who develops the symptoms of pheochromocytoma—such as headache, irritability, or hypertension—should have a full examination. Adrenalectomy should precede a thyroidectomy in patients with both pheochromocytoma and medullary thyroid cancer marfanoid habitus and mucosal neuromas, which are part of the MEN 2B subtype. Marfanoid habitus patients have tall stature without the ectopic lenses and aortic abnormalities generally seen in Marfan syndrome. Mucosal neuromas are generally seen in the oral cavity; these lesions are frequently present in the first decade of life.

SEE ALSO: Pancreatic Cancer, Childhood; Pancreatic Cancer, Islet Cell; Thyroid Cancer, Childhood.

BIBLIOGRAPHY. Fima Lifshitz, editor. *Pediatric Endocrinology (Clinical Pediatrics Series), Vol. 9.* (Informa Healthcare, 2003). Dahia P. L. M. and C. Eng editors. *Genetic Disorders of Endocrine Neoplasia, Vol. 28.* (Karger, S. Inc., 2001).

RICHARD E. WILLS
INDEPENDENT SCHOLAR

Myanmar

THIS SOUTHEAST ASIAN country, formerly known as Burma, was an independent kingdom until it was captured by the British. In 1923 Burma was made part of British India, an unpopular move that was reversed in 1937. On January 4, 1948, Burma became independent, and in 1989 the government changed the country's name to Myanmar and the capital's name from Rangoon to Yangon. Myanmar has a population of 50,519,000 (as of 2005), with 30 doctors and 26 nurses per 100,000 people.

During the British period, colonial medical services were largely used by the expatriate European population and the wealthier Indians and Burmese, with most treatment involving surgery. A parallel system using traditional doctors operated in the countryside. Oncologists in Myanmar traditionally trained in the United Kingdom; later, many gained experience in hospitals in India and Thailand. Since independence, medical services have been increased but still remain poor compared with Myanmar's neighbors.

Most male cancer patients in Myanmar suffer from lung cancer and cancer of the larynx, which largely come from smoking or chewing tobacco and from chewing betel nuts, respectively. Both of these diseases affect men from the countryside more than men from the cities. Among women, 16 percent of cancer patients have breast cancer; just under 16 percent have cervical cancer; and 15 percent have lung cancer. Treatment in Myanmar often involves a combination of radiotherapy, chemotherapy, or hormonal therapy, as well as surgery.

The best-known cancer specialist in Myanmar is U Soe Aung, who has written extensively on a variety of medical problems, mainly connected with cancer. Another prominent oncologist, U Myo Tint, was head of the radiotherapy department at Yangon General Hospital.

The most famous political figure since independence to have succumbed to cancer was U Thant, secretary-general of the United Nations from 1961 to 1971, who died from lung cancer in New York. Michael Aris, the husband of Burmese democracy activist Aung San Suu Kyi and a lecturer in Asian history at Oxford University, died of prostate cancer in Britain while his wife was under house arrest in Yangon.

The Central Research Organization in Myanmar coordinates medical research. There are institutes of medicine at the University of Yangon, located in both Yangon and Mandalay.

SEE ALSO: Breast Cancer; Cervical Cancer; India; Laryngeal Cancer; Lung Cancer, Non-Small Cell; Lung Cancer, Small Cell; Thailand; Tobacco Smoking; United Kingdom.

BIBLIOGRAPHY. K. Maung Maung, "Cancer Survivor Tells Tale of Inspiration," *The Myanmar Times* (May 23–29, 2005); Khin Hninn Phyu, "Early Diagnosis, Proper Care Essential for Cure of Cancer," *The Myanmar Times* (May 23–29, 2005); Khin Thet Htar and Mya Tu, *Who's Who in Health and Medicine in Myanmar* (Myanmar Ministry of Health, 2003).

JUSTIN CORFIELD
GEELONG GRAMMAR SCHOOL, AUSTRALIA

Mycosis Fungoides

MYCOSIS FUNGOIDES (MF) is a tumor characterized by patches and plaques on the skin where there is accumulation of cancerous T lymphocytes. MF is a form of cutaneous T-cell lymphoma (CTCL), itself a form of non-Hodgkin's lymphoma that affects the cells of the lymphatic system—the lymphocytes.

There are two main types of lymphocytes: the B cells (B lymphocytes) and T cells (T lymphocytes). B cells help protect the body against bacteria and viruses through production of antibodies. T cells are categorized into T helper cells (CD4+), which help protect the body against viruses, fungi, and bacteria, and cytotoxic cells (CD8+), which digest infected cells or kill them via the production of cytokines.

CTCL represents a spectrum of diseases with a malignancy of the CD4+ cells. MF is the most common type (44 percent) of CTCL. Sezary syndrome is a variant of MF, occurring in about 5 percent of all cases of MF.

MF is described as an enigmatic tumor with an undefined etiology. The risk of MF is increased in men. It is also more common in people of African/Caribbean origin. The disease is more prevalent in middle-aged people, with an average age of onset of 55 years. Occupational exposures have also been implicated in the risk of developing MF. Reports suggest that those working in the glass-forming, ceramics, and pottery industries carry the highest risk.

Early presentation of the disease includes dry patches with a limited distribution mimicking other diseases, such as eczema or psoriasis. Patches may thicken to form cutaneous plaques, which are distributed predominantly in the axillae, breasts, hips, buttocks, and lower half of the body. The plaques may progress to ulcerating tumors over the course of time if left untreated. Itching is the main symptom for many patients. Occasionally, the condition erythroderma presents, where the skin becomes red throughout the body. If this condition is present in the scalp, it may be accompanied by alopecia (loss of hair).

The clinical and histological diagnosis of MF is problematic until the disease is in its advanced stages. As the evolution of MF is slow, it is often a few years before it manifests in the advanced stages. Blood tests and a skin biopsy are often required to confirm the diagnosis.

TREATMENT AND PROGNOSIS

Treatment for the skin includes alleviating symptoms through the use of suitable moisturizers, steroid creams, or ointments to relieve the itching that may occur. If the symptoms are not controlled, other treatments may be considered, such as PUVA, a combination treatment involving administration of psoralen tablets or photo-chemotherapy followed by exposure of the skin to long-wave ultraviolet light. Topical nitrogen mustard (mechlorethamine) and total skin electron-beam therapy are also used as primary therapies, and are associated with long-term disease-free survival in patients presenting with early stages of the disease. Radiotherapy may be used for patients presenting with large, thickened patches concentrated in one area of the body.

The prognosis depends on the extent of skin involvement, metastasis to extracutaneous sites, and the presence of abnormal cells in blood vessels. Survival for patients with disease limited to the skin is generally over 10 years. Those with metastases to extracutaneous disease, however, may have a survival rate of less than one year.

SEE ALSO: Lymphoma, Hodgkin's, Adult; Lymphoma, Non-Hodgkin's, Adult; Sezary Syndrome.

BIBLIOGRAPHY. S. J. Whittaker, et al., "Guidelines for the Management of Primary Cutaneous T-Cell Lymphomas," *British Journal of Dermatology* (v.149, 2003).

FARHANA AKTER
KINGS COLLEGE, LONDON

Myelodysplastic/ Myeloproliferative Diseases

MYELODYSPLASTIC/MYELOPROLIFERATIVE DISEASES (MMD) involve functional abnormalities in the blood and bone marrow. These diseases share characteristics of both myelodysplastic syndromes (MDS) and myeloproliferative disorders (MPD), and result in an overproduction of white blood cells. MMD may progress to acute leukemia.

In myelodysplastic syndromes, the stem cells produced in the bone marrow do not effectively develop into red blood cells, white blood cells, or platelets. Instead, many of the immature cells that are produced are malformed and defective, and often die in the bone marrow or shortly after entering the bloodstream. Blood-count levels are low, which reflects the shortage of cell types. MDS is considered to be a form of cancer, as it is a clonal disease, meaning that a large number of identical abnormal cells is being produced from a single abnormal cell.

In myeloproliferative disorders, there is an overproduction of one or more cell types, which increases the total number of blood cells. Myeloproliferative disorder is accepted as a form of cancer because of the uncontrolled proliferation of cells. There are three main types of MMD: chronic myelomonocytic leukemia (CMML), juvenile myelomonocytic leukemia (JMML), and atypical chronic myelogenous leukemia (ACML).

If the symptoms of an MMD do not match the three main types, it is considered to be myelodysplastic/myeloproliferative disease, unclassifiable (MMD-U). Chronic Myelomonocytic Leukemia (CMML) is a disease in which too many stem cells are directed to become one of two types of white blood cells called myelocytes and monocytes. Some of the cells remain immature white blood cells (blasts); these cells are unable to perform the functions of mature white blood cells. With overproduction of the white blood cells, the red blood cells and platelets are outnumbered, and physical symptoms such as infection, anemia, and easy bleeding may develop.

Juvenile Myelomonocytic Leukemia (JMML) is a rare type of CMML that occurs most often in children under the age of 2. Males and those with type 1 neurofibramotosis have an increased risk of developing this disease. Atypical Chronic Myelogenous Leukemia (ACML) is a disease that occurs when the bone marrow produces too many immature white blood cells in the form of granulocytes. The blasts leave little room for development of red blood cells and platelets in the bone marrow. The cells in ACML appear similar to those in CML, although they possess a chromosomal difference. Symptoms include tiredness, weakness, and easy bruising/bleeding. Like CMML, JMML, and ACML, MMD-U involves cell overproduction. In MMD-U, however, the bone marrow may overproduce red blood cells, white blood cells, or platelets as opposed to primarily white blood cells. The symptoms are similar to those of the other three types of MMD. MMD-U is considered to be very rare.

SEE ALSO: Childhood Cancers; Myelodysplastic Syndromes; Myeloproliferative Disorders, Chronic.

BIBLIOGRAPHY. Nancy Lee Harris, et al., "World Health Organization Classification of Neoplastic Diseases of the Hematopoietic and Lymphoid Tissues: Report of the Clinical Advisory Committee Meeting—Airlie House, Virginia, November 1997," *Journal of Clinical Oncology* (v.17, 1999).

SHAWNA NOVAK
INDEPENDENT SCHOLAR

Myelodysplastic Syndromes

THE MYELODYSPLASTIC SYNDROMES (MDS; previously known as preleukemia) are a heterogeneous group of diseases of the bone marrow, causing failure of production of normal cells. They are uncommon diseases, the treatment of which is often difficult.

MDS was classified into a distinct disease group in 1976. Although these syndromes are not classically defined as malignant, most authorities regard them as behaving in a similar fashion, often progressing to overt leukemia.

MDS results from mutations in the genes of the stem cells, resulting in an abnormal clone that proliferates and replaces the normal cells. This may lead to anemia (due to failure of red cell line), leukopenia (suppression of white cells), or thrombocytopenia (decrease in platelets).

MDS is a rare disease, yet due to increasing awareness and improvements in diagnosis, the incidence appears to be increasing. According to a 2005 survey by the Leukemia and Lymphoma Society (*Facts, 2005–2006*), there were 11,960 total cases in 2005.

MDS is a disease of adults, typically those over 60 years age. However, younger patients, including children, may develop the disease.

MDS may be primary (without any known cause) or secondary. Secondary MDS is often seen in younger patients, maybe due to previous cancer chemotherapy, viral infections, or exposure to toxic chemicals such as benzene. It is postulated that these agents induce mutations in the cells, which suppress healthy cells and promote the growth of abnormal cells.

Two systems are used in the classification of MDS: the French, American, and British (FAB) system, and the World Health Organization system. The categories often overlap as the disease progresses, with increasing marrow arrest and transformation into acute or chronic leukemia.

SYMPTOMS AND DIAGNOSIS

Blood cell counts are usually depressed, with anemia being the most common symptom. Other common symptoms are fatigue, malaise, abnormal bleeding, and recurrent infections.

Occasionally, patients are asymptomatic and are diagnosed by tests. A biopsy of the bone marrow is required for the diagnosis. The marrow shows excess

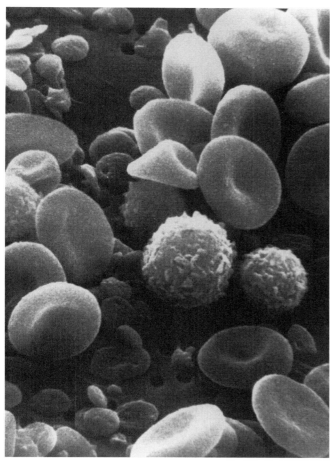

A scanning electron microscope image of normally circulating human blood.

azacidine and decitabine topetecan, immunotherapy, and stem-cell transplantation have been tried with some success. Treatment with growth factors such as erythropoetin may help in increasing cell counts transiently. Supportive therapy with blood transfusions and treatment of infections is often required.

In view of lack of clear-cut guidelines and often-poor response, treatment should be individualized. Conservative therapy should be considered for patients who are older and those with low disease burden; aggressive chemotherapy and stem-cell transplantation should be used in selected patients who are younger, with high disease burden and cytogenetic abnormalities. There are several ongoing trials, the results of which may improve the treatment options available to patients. For more information, search www.ClinicalTrials.gov, keyword myelodysplasia.

SEE ALSO: Antibiotics; Chemotherapy; Clinical Trials; Infection (Childhood, Sexually Transmitted Infections, Hepatitis).

BIBLIOGRAPHY. Mark Heaney and David Golde, "Myelodysplasia," *New England Journal of Medicine* (v.340, 1999).

PRIYA RADHAKRISHNAN
CATHOLIC HEALTHCARE WEST

abnormal cells, often resembling leukemia. The distinction is made based on the number of abnormal cells in the marrow.

Marrow cells are also examined for abnormal chromosomes and mutations. Common abnormalities involve chromosomes 5, 7, and 8. It is postulated that the mutation causes dysregulation of cell development and an increase in cell death of normal elements (apoptosis). The abnormalities combined with clinical evidence of depressed counts lead to the diagnosis of MDS.

It is important, however, to exclude other causes, such as deficiency of vitamin B12 and folate; infection with human immunodeficiency virus (HIV); or exposure to antibiotics or other chemicals, which may lead to abnormalities in bone-marrow cells.

Treatment of MDS with drugs used to treat acute leukemias has been disappointing. Traditional drugs used in the treatment of cancer, newer drugs such as

Myeloma, Multiple

MULTIPLE MYELOMA IS a disorder in which malignant plasma cells accumulate in the bone marrow and produce an immunoglobulin—the M protein—that is usually monoclonal IgG or IgA. It accounts for approximately 10 percent of hematologic malignancies, and more than 15,000 new patients are diagnosed with multiple myeloma in the United States annually.

Multiple myeloma evolves from a premalignant condition clinically known as monoclonal gammopathy of undetermined significance (MGUS). MGUS is the most frequent clonal plasma-cell disorder in the general population, and it transforms into multiple myeloma in 25 percent to 30 percent of patients.

Smoldering myeloma is a loose term for disorders halfway along the spectrum between MGUS and multiple myeloma. The precise mechanisms by which

MGUS transforms into multiple myeloma are unclear. Secondary genetic abnormalities and changes in the bone-marrow microenvironment—such as angiogenesis, suppression of cell-mediated immunity, and alterations in cytokines—are believed to play a role.

In multiple myeloma, a small number of long-lived plasma cells in the bone marrow produce most of the IgG and IgA in the serum. It has been hypothesized that these cells gain immortality because their chromosomes contain many numerical and structural abnormalities that evade apoptosis.

Interleukin-6 is essential for the survival and growth of these immortal myeloma cells. Interleukin-6 also activates osteoclasts in the vicinity of myeloma cells. The activated osteoclasts cause bone resorption, which ultimately leads to osteolytic lesions and bone pain.

The clinical presentation of multiple myeloma is usually that of indolent or localized disease. The median age at diagnosis of multiple myeloma is 68 years, and the most common presenting symptoms are fatigue and bone pain. Clinical findings include osteolytic lesions, anemia, renal insufficiency, and recurrent infections. These clinical findings have a strong diagnostic value if accompanied by more than 10 percent atypical plasma cells in the bone marrow and either a monoclonal immunoglobulin in the serum or light chains in the urine. Light chains appear in the serum only if the patient has severe renal disease. Bone lesions, hypercalcemia, and anemia correlate directly with the presence of the total mass of myeloma mass and have prognostic value.

Common complications of overt multiple myeloma include recurrent bacterial infections, anemia, osteolytic lesions, and renal insufficiency. All these complications—especially infection and renal insufficiency—are major causes of death.

Treatment for myeloma has changed drastically in the past decade and now includes state-of-the-art supportive treatment and infusional chemotherapy courses. Melphalan, cyclophosphamide, and glucocorticoids are the most effective drugs against multiple myeloma. Treatment with high doses of melphalan can induce complete remission, but it sometimes causes irreversible myelosuppression and is limited to patients who no longer respond to the initial low-dose therapy of melphalan plus prednisolone. Transplantation of autologous hematopoietic stem cells accelerates the restoration of hematopoiesis after the

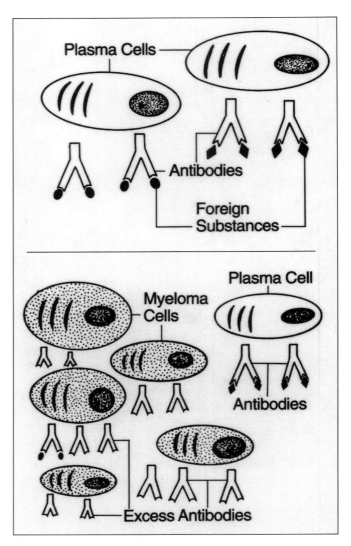

Top: plasma cells producing antibodies. Bottom: too many plasma (myeloma) cells producing antibodies that the body does not need.

addition of melphalan and allows for combination of intensive chemotherapy and total body irradiation or for the use of recurrent high doses of melphalan. Newer studies are exploring the role of interleukin-2, interleukin-4, interferon gamma, and tretinion in the treatment of multiple myeloma. Although median survival is 3 years, some myeloma patients can live longer than 10 years.

SEE ALSO: Chemotherapy; Clinical Trials; Drugs; Genetics; Radiation Therapy.

BIBLIOGRAPHY. M. Boccadoro, "Diagnosis, Prognosis, and Standard Treatment of Multiple Myeloma," *Hematology/*

Oncology Clinics of North America (v.11, 1997); J. Kaufman, "Multiple Myeloma: The Role of Transplant and Novel Treatment Strategies," *Seminars in Oncology* (v.31, 2004).

NAKUL GUPTA
ROSS UNIVERSITY SCHOOL OF MEDICINE

Myeloproliferative Disorders, Chronic

CHRONIC MYELOPROLIFERATIVE DISORDERS (CMD) are an uncommon heterogeneous group of diseases arising in the bone marrow and resulting in the proliferation of malignant haematopoietic cells.

Six disorders are classified as CMD: CML (chronic myelogenous leukemia), PV (polycythemia vera), CIM (chronic idiopathic myelofibrosis), ET (essential thrombocythemia), CNL (chronic neutrophilic leukemia), and CEL (chronic eosinophilic leukemia). Chronic Myelogenous Leukemia (CML) is a type of neoplasm of the blood and bone marrow resulting in abnormal numbers of leukocytes, particularly the neutrophils. The incidence of CML is approximately 1 per 100,000 population per year. CML is associated with a characteristic chromosomal translocation defined by the Philadelphia chromosome.

This is where an exchange of material between breakpoint cluster region q11 on chromosome 22 fuses with the Abelson region q34 on chromosome 9 [t(9;22)(q34;q11.2)]. The BCR-ABL transcript is rendered continuously active and increases cell division, resulting in an increased number of leukocytes. The BCR/ABL molecule has ABL tyrosine kinase activity; thus, selective inhibition of ABL tyrosine kinase activity using the drug imatinib mesylate is possible. The use of imatinib mesylate may be associated with cardiotoxicity, however. If CML is left untreated, the disease may progress to acute-stage leukemia.

Polycythemia Vera (PV) is characterized by increased levels of erythrocytes. The incidence of PV is 0.02 to 2.8 per 100,000 per year. The causes of the increased levels of erythrocytes include a proliferated abnormality of the bone marrow, kidney tumors, excessive increase in erythropoietin level (hormone produced by the kidney), and fluid loss (such as from burns). The excess levels of erythrocytes expose pa-tients to increased risk for thrombo-hemorrhagic complications. Patients may be treated with phlebotomy to achieve hematocrit less than 45 percent in conjunction with a platelet-lowering agent such as anagrelide or hydroxyurea. Low-dose aspirin helps prevent arterial thrombotic complications associated with PV in remission after phlebotomy.

Chronic Idiopathic Myelofibrosis (CIM) has an incidence rate of 0.4 to 0.9 per 100,000 per year. It is characterized by fibrosis development in the bone marrow due to ET or PV. The scarring of the bone marrow hinders production of erythrocytes. To compensate, the liver and spleen begin to produce blood cells, resulting in hepatosplenomegaly.

Essential Thrombocythemia (ET) occurs due to an overproduction of megakaryocytes, leading to an increased number of platelets in the blood. It has an incidence of 0.1 to 1.5 per 100,000 per year. The pathophysiology is undetermined; however, it is known that a mutation of valine to phenylalanine substitution at amino acid position 617 (V617F) within the Janus kinase 2 (*JAK2*) gene of the intracellular tyrosine kinases is associated with essential thrombocytosis. This mutation may also occur in PV. Thrombotic and hemorrhagic events are particularly common in ET. Other risks of the disease include development into leukemia or myelofibrosis.

Chronic Neutrophilic Leukemia (CNL), a rare disorder of undefined etiology, is characterized by a sustained increase in neutrophils. There is a clear absence of the Philadelphia chromosome (Ph1) and BCR-ABL fusion gene. Patients may eventually develop acute-stage leukemia, with a risk of death from progressive neutrophilic leukocytosis or blastic transformation. Chronic Eosinophilic Leukemia (CEL) is a rare disorder characterized by a clonal proliferation of eosinophilic precursors in the bone marrow and blood.

SEE ALSO: Leukemia, Chronic Myelogenous; Myelodysplastic/Myeloproliferative Diseases.

BIBLIOGRAPHY. Jan Jacques Michiels, "Clinical, Pathological and Molecular Features of the Chronic Myeloproliferative Disorders," *Hematology* (v.10/1, 2001).

FARHANA AKTER
KINGS COLLEGE, LONDON

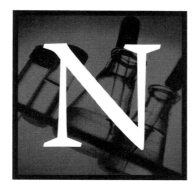

Nasal Cavity and Paranasal Sinus Cancer

CANCERS OF THE nasal cavity and paranasal sinus are rare neoplasms with an incidence of fewer than 1 per 100,000 persons per year. They occur more frequently in places such as Japan and South Africa, although the reasons for this are unclear. The age of onset for the diseases is usually in the fifth decade of life. There are four paranasal sinuses: the maxillary sinuses, located in the upper part of the mandible (jawbone); the frontal sinuses, above the nose; the ethmoid sinuses, behind the upper nose; and the sphenoid sinuses, behind the ethmoid sinuses in the center of the skull. The function of the nasal cavity includes filtering and humidifying the air breathed in. The sinuses are said to give resonance to the voice, contribute to immune defense, and increase mucosal surface area via their ciliated epithelial cells.

The cancers usually begin in the cells that line the oropharynx, with subsequent progression to the different types of cells lining the nasal cavity and paranasal sinuses. Squamous cell carcinoma (arising from squamous epithelial cells) and adenocarcinomas (arising from glandular cells called adenomatous cells) are very common. Other malignancies that can arise include malignant lymphoma, sarcoma, malignant melanoma, esthesioneuroblastoma, and midline granuloma. Among paranasal sinuses, the maxillary sinus is the most affected, followed

by the ethmoid sinuses. Occupational exposures such as wood dust; leather in shoe factories; and chemical agents such as mustard gas, isopropylic alcohol, chromates, nickel compounds, and formaldehyde are thought to increase this risk of acquiring these malignancies. Modern industries often use these agents in a safe manner, however; thus, these risks have decreased over the years. Smoking tobacco and infection are also thought to increase risk.

Symptoms of these diseases include persistent nasal congestion and blockage, which may occur if the neoplasm has become large enough to block the sinuses. The patient may also present with sinusitis (inflammation of the sinuses), epistaxis (acute hemorrhage from the nostrils), trismus (sustained spasm of neck and jaw muscles), proptosis (forward displacement of the eyes), and cranial nerve deficits. Diagnosis is usually made via endoscopic or fiberoptic examination of the entire nasal cavity to rule out benign disease, such as nasal polyposis. Various imaging tests are used to verify the presence or absence of air in the sinuses. Chest X-rays, computerized tomography (CT) scans, and magnetic resonance imaging (MRI) scans help determine metastasis of tumors. A biopsy is indicated when a mass is found; this aids in determining the stage of cancer.

TREATMENT AND PROGNOSIS

Treatment of the cancers depends on the type and locations of tumors. Neoplasms of the nasal cavity are

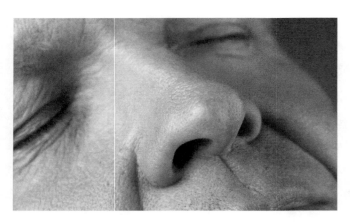

Symptoms of nasal sinus cancer include congestion and blockage, which may occur if the neoplasm has become large enough.

generally treated with surgery and radiation therapy. Maxillary-sinus neoplasms are treated with surgical excision to remove the tumor, as well as radiation therapy. Ethmoid-sinus neoplasms may be treated surgically with rhinotomy (a surgical procedure to drain accumulated pus from the nose), and neoplasms in the sphenoid sinuses are treated with radiation therapy, possibly in combination with chemotherapy.

The prognosis for patients with nasal-cavity cancer is generally poor. The five-year survival rate is approximately 40 percent. The prognosis is worse in patients who have tumors that have metastasized, particularly to the frontal and sphenoid sinuses.

SEE ALSO: Chemotherapy; Head and Neck Cancer; Japan; Radiation Therapy; South Africa; Surgery.

BIBLIOGRAPHY. P.J. Donald, et al., "Cancer of the Nasal Vestibule, Nasal Cavity and Paranasal Sinuses," *B-ENT* (s1, 2005).

FARHANA AKTER
KINGS COLLEGE, LONDON

Nasopharyngeal Cancer

NASOPHARYNGEAL CANCER IS a rare tumor in the nasopharynx of the upper respiratory tract. The nasopharynx is an airspace within the skull that lies behind the nose and above the soft palate. Nasopharyn-

geal cancer has an incidence rate of 1 in 100,000 people per year. It is endemic in southern China, where the incidence is 30 to 50 in 100,000 each year and where it is the third-most-common form of cancer among men. There are three types of nasopharyngeal cancers: keratinizing squamous cell carcinoma, nonkeratinizing carcinoma, and undifferentiated carcinoma.

Studies have reported that the risk of the cancer is increased in individuals who consume preserved salted fish, which contains high levels of carcinogenic N-nitroso compounds. These compounds are the N-nitrosamines and their precursors N-dimethylnitrosamine (NDMA), N-diethylnitrosamine (NDEA), N-nitrosopyrrolidine (NPYR), and N-nitrosopiperidine (NPIP). Cytochrome P450 2E1, an enzyme that subsequently activates the nitrosamines metabolically, forms reactive intermediates capable of damaging DNA, leading to the development of the cancer. The Epstein-Barr virus is also implicated in development of the disease in association with genetic aberrations such as inactivation of the tumor-suppressor genes p16/Ink4, p19/ARF, RASSF1, and Blu. Smoking tobacco and diet also factor as risks for the disease. The virus generally leads to the development of infectious mononucleosis (also known as glandular fever). The pathogenesis of nasopharyngeal tumors may have other genetic origins. The malignancy has been associated with polymorphisms of human leukocyte antigen, which is essential in the immune response to viruses.

Symptoms and signs of the tumor include cervical lymphadenopathy (enlarged lymph nodes), deafness, tinnitus (ringing in the ears), trismus (sustained spasm of neck and jaw muscles), and otitis media (inflammation and infection of the middle ear). Larger tumors may produce nasal obstruction or bleeding.

The disease may be diagnosed via a biopsy. Tumors are characterized histopathologically by an abundant infiltration of lymphocytes, particularly CD4+ T cells. Imaging techniques such as computerized tomography (CT), magnetic resonance imaging (MRI), and positron emission tomography (PET) scans are also employed to diagnose the disease.

Nasopharyngeal cancer is often categorized in stages to determine the most appropriate treatment. If a patient is diagnosed with stage 0/carcinoma in situ, it is suggestive of early-stage cancer, in which the cancer cells are benign and are confined to the lining of the nasopharynx. If the cancer has begun to grow (without metastases), it is classified as stage 1. Stage 2 involves the cancer spreading from nasopharynx to oropharynx and to lymph nodes on one side of the neck (stage 3). If it has spread to both sides of the neck and nearby bones and sinuses, it indicates progression to stage 4. If the cancer is significantly advanced, it may grow into the skull, cranial nerves, eye, or lower part of the throat, and even to the bones, lungs, or brain.

TREATMENT AND PROGNOSIS

Treatment of early-stage cancer is usually radiation therapy. Systemic chemotherapy is often used for high-risk patients, particularly if the tumor has spread to the lymph nodes or other parts of the body. Adjuvant interferon (IFN)-beta therapy is also used to treat this neoplasm.

The prognosis is good, with a long-term survival rate of 50 percent to 80 percent if the cancer is in its early stages and is promptly treated with radiation therapy.

SEE ALSO: Chemotherapy; China; Genetics; Infection (Childhood, Sexually Transmitted Infections, Hepatitis, Etc.); Nasal Cavity and Paranasal Sinus Cancer; Radiation Therapy.

BIBLIOGRAPHY. W. I. Wei and J. S. Sham, "Nasopharyngeal Carcinoma," *Lancet* (v.365/9476, 2005).

FARHANA AKTER
KINGS COLLEGE, LONDON

Nasopharyngeal Cancer, Childhood

NASOPHARYNGEAL CARCINOMA (NPC) is a rare tumor arising from the epithelium that lines the nosopharynx, first described this disease in 1921. Nasopharygeal carcinoma makes up roughly 1 percent to 5 percent of all childhood cancers and less than 30 percent of those cancers specifically affecting the nasopharyx. Males are twice as likely to acquire the disease than females and the most common age group being affected are adolescents. In the United States the incidence is 1 in 100,000 children.

However the incidence varies depending on geographical location and has been noted to be more prevalent among children of Southeast Asian and Northern African descent. Ebstein Barr Virus has been detected in epithelial cells from NPC and is thought to play a role in cell transformation, as well as ethnic background, and environmental carcinogens. Three histological subtypes of NPC have been recognized. Type 1: squamaous cell carcinoma, typically found in the adult population; Type 2: non-keratinizing carcinoma; and Type 3: Undifferentiated carcinoma.

The majority of childhood cases of NPC are Type 3. NPC usually originates in the lateral wall of the nasopharynx, however it may extend laterally or posteriorly to skull base, palate, nasal cavity, or oropharynx. The typical metastatic spread of NPC is to the cervical lymph nodes locally.

Distant metastases may spread to bone, lung, mediastinum, and rarely liver. The most common presenting symptom is cervical lymphadenopathy. Symptoms such as trismus, pain, nasal regurgitation, hearing loss, ottis media, and cranial nerve palsies are also common. Larger tumors may present with nasal obstruction and bleeding.

DIAGNOSIS

Diagnosis is usually made with cervical lymph node biopsy. However further testing such as blood work, nasopharyngoscopy, CT scan, chest x-ray, bone scintigraphy, and EBV viral capsid antigen testing are necessary to determine the extent and severity of the disease. The tumor, node, metastasis (TNM) classification of the American Joint Committee on Cancer is used to determine the tumor staging. The anatomical location and later presentation of NPC makes it less amenable to curative surgical control.

The role of surgery usually lies in obtaining cervical lymph node biopsies. Factors associated with poor prognosis in children include skull base involvement, extent of primary tumor, and cranial nerve involvement. Radiation therapy has been the mainstay of treatment for smaller tumors and less advanced disease, with chemotherapy being reserved for advanced cases.

However, recent studies using concurrent cisplatin, 5-fluorouracil, and radiotherapy have been shown to improve survival. Recent studies have also shown that induction chemotherapy followed by radiation therapy improves local control and progression-free survival rates over radiotherapy alone. St. Jude Children's

Research Hospital reported a 5-year survival rate of 69 percent with the use of chemoradiation therapy.

SEE ALSO: Chemotherapy; China; Genetics; Infection (Childhood, Sexually Transmitted Infections, Hepatitis, Etc.); Nasal Cavity and Paranasal Sinus Cancer; Radiation Therapy.

BIBLIOGRAPHY. C. Rodriguez-Galind, M. Wofford, R.P. Castleberry, G.P. Swanson, et al., "Preradiation Chemotherapy with Methotrexate, Cisplatin, 5-Fluorouracil, and Leucovorin for Pediatric Nasopharyngeal Carcinoma," *Cancer* (2005; 103:850–857); M. Serin, et. al., "Nasopharyngeal Carcinoma in Childhood and Adolescence," *Medical Pediatric Oncology* (1998 Dec; 31(6): 498-505).

FERNANDO A. HERRERA, JR., M.D.
UNIVERSITY OF CALIFORNIA, SAN DIEGO

National Alliance of Breast Cancer Organizations

IN 1986 THE National Alliance of Breast Cancer Organizations (NABCO) was founded as a not-for-profit group to provide information and education to breast-cancer patients, professionals in healthcare, and the public via the media. Although based in New York City, the alliance of over 370 organizations aimed to help cancer patients throughout the United States.

It provided all services free of charge, including resources and referrals. NABCO also campaigned for the legislative rights of cancer patients and survivors. The group worked for 18 years, publishing *NABCO News* quarterly along with information sheets and an annual Breast Cancer Resource List, before shutting down June 30, 1994.

To keep its *NABCO Resource Guide* available, the group recruited the help of 12 organizations, among them the National Coalition for Cancer Survivorship. Thus, information is still provided in three main domains: breast-cancer facts, including general information and risk factors; mammography information and other prevention education; and steps to take after a diagnosis. Another resource provided by NABCO is a list of phone numbers of support groups in every state.

In 1995 the NABCO website was launched as an effort to communicate more effectively with a national audience. Still active, it provides links to information including stages of breast cancer, current research, prevention measures, and living with breast cancer.

NABCO can still receive donations of funds for research and care. In 2000 the alliance partnered with an online donation program to make it easier for people to donate. A related organization is the Sears WNBA Breast Health Awareness Program, whereby the teams of the Women's National Basketball Association reach out to their communities to promote breast-cancer awareness.

SEE ALSO: Breast Cancer; Breast Cancer and Pregnancy; Breast Cancer, Male; Women's Cancers.

BIBLIOGRAPHY. Yashar Hirshaut and Peter Pressman, *Breast Cancer: The Complete Guide* 3rd ed. (Bantam, 2000); Joy B. Kinnon and Zandra Hughes, "Beating Breast Cancer," *Ebony* (October 2002); Elaine Magee, *Tell Me What to Eat to Help Prevent Breast Cancer: Nutrition You Can Live With* (Career Press, 2000); H.W. Lawson, et al., "Implementing Recommendations for the Early Detection of Breast and Cervical Cancer among Low-Income Women," *Morbidity & Mortality Weekly Report. Recommendations & Reports* (v.49/RR-2, 2000); R.M. Henson, et al., "The National Breast and Cervical Cancer Early Detection Program: A Comprehensive Public Health Response to Two Major Health Issues for Women," *Journal of Public Health Management & Practice* (v.2/2, 1996).

CLAUDIA WINOGRAD
UNIVERSITY OF ILLINOIS AT URBANA-CHAMPAIGN

National Breast and Cervical Cancer Early Detection Program

THE NATIONAL BREAST and Cervical Cancer Early Detection Program (NBCCEDP) is a nationwide comprehensive screening program established in response to the Breast and Cervical Cancer Mortality Prevention Act of 1990 (Public Law 101-354, enacted August 10, 1990 [42 U.S.C. 300k through 300n-5]). The NBCCEDP is administered by the Centers for Disease Control and Prevention's (CDC's) Division of Cancer Prevention and Control and is designed to increase awareness, availability, and use of screening tests for breast and cervical cancers among women, particularly low-income, uninsured, and medically underserved women.

As of December 2005, the NBCCEDP had provided over 6.5 million screening tests to over 2.7 million women and diagnosed 26,907 breast cancers, 57,147 cases of mild to severe precancerous cervical lesions, and 1,725 invasive cancers. To date, this program remains the first and only national cancer-screening program in the United States.

The NBCCEDP is implemented primarily through cooperative agreements with state and territorial health departments and with American Indian/Alaska Native tribes or tribal organizations (grantees). Since the program was established in 1991, the CDC has expanded it from 8 state programs initially to all 50 states, the District of Columbia, 13 American Indian/Alaska Native tribes or tribal organizations, and 4 U.S. territories.

At least 60 percent of funds awarded to grantees must be spent on direct patient services, including screening and diagnostic services, as well as essential support services such as case management.

Screening tests include clinical breast examinations and mammograms for the early detection of breast cancer, as well as pelvic examinations and Papanicolau (Pap) tests for the detection of cervical-cancer precursors or of invasive cervical cancer at its earliest stage.

Grantees use the remaining 40 percent of funds to support program management, public and provider education, quality assurance, and surveillance and evaluation activities.

Although Public Law 101-354 does not allow for the reimbursement of treatment services, programs have always been required to find resources to treat breast and cervical cancers detected through the program. To assist programs, Congress subsequently passed the Breast and Cervical Cancer Prevention and Treatment Act of 2000, which allows states the option to provide reimbursement for treatment through Medicaid for women who are screened and diagnosed through the NBCCEDP and found to need treatment for breast or cervical cancer, including precancerous conditions. The Treatment Act was amended in 2001 to include tribal grantees.

SEE ALSO: Breast Cancer; Cervical Cancer; Screening (Cervical and Breast and Colon Cancers); Screening, Access to; Women's Cancers.

BIBLIOGRAPHY. A.B. Ryerson, et al., *The NBCCEDP 1991-2002 National Report* (Centers for Disease Control and Prevention, 2005); H.W. Lawson, et al., "Implementing Recommendations for the Early Detection of Breast and Cervical Cancer among Low-Income Women," *Morbidity & Mortality Weekly Report. Recommendations & Reports* (v.49/RR-2, 2000); R.M. Henson, et al., "The National Breast and Cervical Cancer Early Detection Program: A Comprehensive Public Health Response to Two Major Health Issues for Women," *Journal of Public Health Management & Practice* (v.2/2, 1996).

LISA MARIANI
CENTERS FOR DISEASE CONTROL AND PREVENTION

National Cancer Institute

THE NATIONAL CANCER Institute (NCI) coordinates research on cancer prevention, detection, diagnosis, treatment, rehabilitation, and control in the United States. The NCI is a component of the National Institutes of Health (NIH), one of eight agencies that are part of the Public Health Service within the U.S. Department of Health and Human Services.

The NCI was established as an independent research institute by the National Cancer Institute Act of 1937; its scope and responsibilities were broadened in 1971 with the passage of the National Cancer Act.

In fiscal 2005, the NCI budget was $4.8 billion, the bulk of which was used to fund research activities at the NCI and to award grants and contracts to universities, medical schools, NCI Cancer Centers, research laboratories, and private firms in the United States and around the world. The NCI is located in Bethesda, Maryland, near Washington, D.C.

The NCI coordinates the National Cancer Program, the primary responsibilities of which include the conduct and support of research, training, and information dissemination.

Specific NCI activities include support and coordination of research projects in the United States and abroad; conduct of research in its own laboratories and clinics; support of education and training in fundamental sciences and clinical disciplines related to cancer; support of research projects in cancer control; support of a national network of Cancer Centers;

collaboration with other national and foreign organizations and institutions engaged in cancer research and training; coordination of cancer research by industrial concerns; collection and dissemination of information about cancer; and awarding of construction grants for laboratories, clinics, and related facilities for cancer research. The NCI provides research funding in nearly every state and over 20 foreign countries.

The divisions of the NCI are the Division of Cancer Biology, the Division of Cancer Control and Population Sciences, the Division of Cancer Prevention, the Division of Cancer Treatment and Diagnosis, the Division of Extramural Activities, and the Division of Cancer Epidemiology and Genetics. Its centers are the Center for Cancer Research; the Office of Centers, Training and Resources; the Center for Strategic Science and Technology Initiatives; the Center for Bioinformatics; and the Center to Reduce Cancer Health Disparities.

TRAINING AND CAREER DEVELOPMENT

The NCI supports five extramural and six intramural training programs in basic, clinical, and population sciences. Between 1999 and 2004, the number of persons supported by NCI intramural and extramural programs grew by nearly 26 percent, and the dollar amount awarded more than doubled, from $136.3 million in fiscal 1999 to $281.7 million in fiscal 2004. Detailed information about funding and training opportunities is available from the NCI website.

The Cancer Centers program provides Cancer Center Support Grants (CCSG, also known as P30 grants) to support cancer research programs in 61 institutions (in 2006) in the United States. These programs are located in major academic and research institutions that have broad-based, coordinated, interdisciplinary cancer research programs dedicated to reducing the incidence, morbidity, and mortality of cancer.

Institutions must apply for the program and are subjected to a competitive peer-review process that evaluates the scientific merit of applications. A center that is awarded a CCSG may use it to fund scientific infrastructure and research resources, including scientific leadership, administration, and research technology. Every institution receiving a CCSG is considered to be an NCI Cancer Center, but there are two levels of designation: Comprehensive Cancer Centers and Cancer Centers. Comprehensive Cancer Centers must

integrate research activities across laboratory, clinical, and population-based research. Cancer Centers have scientific agendas that focus on only one or two of these research areas. Most recipients of CCSGs also provide clinical cancer care and services, and many also engage in ancillary activities such as outreach, education, and information dissemination. A list of Cancer Centers is available from the NCI website.

The NCI conducts over 150 cancer clinical trials annually at the NIH Clinical Center in Bethesda. Many more clinical trials are organized and conducted through the NCI's Clinical Trials Cooperative Group Program, which was established in 1955. The purpose of this program is to develop and conduct large-scale clinical trials in multi-institutional settings.

In 2006 over 1,700 individuals and organizations—including community physicians; researchers; and Cancer Centers in the United States, Canada, and Europe—were involved in the program, which enrolls over 22,000 new patients in clinical trials annually.

Information about clinical trials is available from the NCI website.

RESOURCES AND PUBLICATIONS

The NCI website provides basic information for the general public and health professionals about various aspects of cancer, including types of cancer, testing, prevention, treatment options, and clinical trials. A searchable drug dictionary includes basic information about drugs used in cancer treatment, as well as links to active and closed clinical trials using each drug. The NCI also provides information through a toll-free hotline, email, and the LiveHelp online assistance service.

The NCI produces many publications to educate the public about cancer. Information about these publications—which include fact sheets, brochures, and posters—is available through the NCI Publications Catalog on the NCI website.

The *NCI Cancer Bulletin* provides information about NCI programs and initiatives, and other information relevant to cancer research; it may be downloaded from the NCI website.

Many publications are available in multiple languages. Most NCI publications are in the public domain and may be reproduced without permission.

SEE ALSO: Clinical Trials; Disparities, Issues in Cancer; Government.

BIBLIOGRAPHY. National Cancer Institute website, www. cancer.gov (cited December 2006).

Sarah Boslaugh
Washington University School of Medicine

National Cancer Policy Board

FROM 1997 TO 2005 the National Cancer Policy Board functioned within the Institute of Medicine (IOM) of the National Academies and the National Research Council (NRC). The NRC's chairman appointed board members, and each member served a three-year term. The members numbered 20 individuals from outside the federal government, who served to advise the United States in its fight against cancer. These members represented healthcare researchers, providers, and consumers in a variety of fields.

Experts in the field of cancer were consulted to establish goals for raising cancer awareness and promoting prevention, treatment, and research. Additionally, the board had unrestricted funding grants from the National Cancer Institute (NCI) and the Centers for Disease Control and Prevention (CDC).

The board met quarterly to discuss recent advances, gaps in knowledge, and concerns of the public and private sector, and to issue reports and recommendations. It had the license to conduct workshops for more education and research.

NATIONAL CANCER POLICY FORUM

On May 1, 2005, the board was succeeded by the National Cancer Policy Forum, wherein representatives from the government, pharmaceutical industry, academia, and other sectors meet privately for discussion. The forum currently advises the National Academies on initiatives to prevent, treat, and cure cancer.

The forum allows sponsors to participate in discussions. These sponsors include the NCI, the CDC, the U.S. Food and Drug Administration, and other government institutions, along with nongovernment organizations such as UnitedHealth Group. The forum is also licensed to hold symposia and workshops.

Reports on decisions and recommendations made by the forum go to the president of the IOM. The IOM was established in 1970 as part of the National Academy of Sciences. It functions outside the government to maintain an objective approach to research.

Both the IOM and the National Cancer Policy Forum are based in Washington, D.C.

SEE ALSO: Government; National Cancer Institute.

BIBLIOGRAPHY. Karen Adams, Janet M. Corrigan, and Institute of Medicine, *Priority Areas for National Action: Transforming Health Care Quality* (National Academies Press, 2003); American Institute for Cancer Research, *Stopping Cancer Before It Starts: The American Institute for Cancer Research's Program for Cancer Prevention* (Golden Guides from St. Martin's Press, 2000); M. G. Myriam Hunink, et al., *Decision Making in Health and Medicine: Integrating Evidence and Values* (Cambridge University Press, 2001).

Claudia Winograd
Washington University School of Medicine

National Cancer Registrars Association (NCRA)

A CANCER REGISTRAR is a professional working in a cancer registry or a Certified Tumor Registrar (CTR). The National Cancer Registrars Association (NCRA) is a not-for-profit organization that represents these professionals. The NCRA was established as the National Tumor Registrars Association in 1983. This name changed to the current form in 1993. In 2002 the association bylaws were edited to add a Council on Certification to oversee the certification of tumor registrars.

The NCRA's mission is to "serve as the premier education, credentialing and advocacy resource for cancer data professionals." A primary goal of the association is to educate and certify all registrars to ensure that all cancer registries are properly organized and maintained.

The NCRA offers an exam-preparation workshop for members studying for the CTR certification exam. Another service is a constant effort to optimize registrars' work environments. Employment satisfaction is a key concern of the association.

MEETINGS AND RESOURCES

Members attend an annual conference, which keeps them updated on the most recent advances in research and education in the field of cancer registries. On the NCRA website, vendors can advertise their products, and registries can advertise job openings.

SEE ALSO: American Cancer Society; International Association of Cancer Registries; North American Association of Central Cancer Registries.

BIBLIOGRAPHY. Laura Mari Beskow, *Research Recruitment through Cancer Registries: Stakeholder Perspectives* (ProQuest, 2006); Herman R. Menck, *Cancer Registry Management Principles and Practice* (Kendall/Hunt Publishing Co., 2004); R. Sankila, et al., *Evaluation of Clinical Care by Cancer Registries (IARC Technical Publication)* (International Agency for Research on Cancer, 2002).

CLAUDIA WINOGRAD
UNIVERSITY OF ILLINOIS AT URBANA-CHAMPAIGN

National Childhood Cancer Foundation

THE NATIONAL CHILDHOOD Cancer Foundation and the Children's Oncology Group form CureSearch, an organization with the mission to cure childhood cancer. CureSearch's slogan is "Collaboration, Compassion, Research ... Life."

RESEARCH

CureSearch recognizes that research is pivotal to its mission; thus, it maintains a large number of committees dedicated to research in many cancer fields, including cancers that are common in pediatric cancer patients, such as retinoblastoma and acute lymphoblastic leukemia. Other cancers researched by CureSearch are tumors of the bones, central nervous system, and kidneys, as well as Hodgkin's disease, myeloid diseases, neuroblastoma, non-Hodgkin's lymphoma, rhabdomyosarcoma/soft-tissue cancer, and rare tumors. Another focus of research is aspects of childhood cancer rather than specific diseases, such as epidemiology, stem-cell transplantation, nursing, developmental therapeutics, and adolescents and young adults.

Through CureSearch, patients and families can gather information on all stages of the cancer battle. There are resources for patients who are newly diagnosed, undergoing treatment, finishing treatment, or surviving post-treatment. Resources are tailored to cancer types and age groups. Information for newly diagnosed patients includes descriptions and definitions of cancer types, as well as tests, treatments, and therapies. Information is specially written for each audience: parents/family members or patients.

Additional resources are provided for members of communities of children with cancer, including teachers. Pediatric cancer patients and their siblings may require special attention at school; their teachers can gain insight and share experiences via the CureSearch website. Patients and family members can join discussion groups to share their experiences. The website also outlines ways for individuals or companies to donate, whether directly with funds or through stock or vehicle donations.

Clinical trials are important methods to learn about the safety and efficacy of cancer treatments. CureSearch offers counseling and advice regarding clinical trials, as well as information on trial availability and patient eligibility.

SEE ALSO: Childhood Cancers; Clinical Trials; Leukemia, Acute Lymphoblastic, Childhood; Rhabdomyosarcoma, Childhood.

BIBLIOGRAPHY. Gregory H. Reaman and Arnold J. Altman, *Supportive Care of Children with Cancer: Current Therapy and Guidelines from the Children's Oncology Group* (The Johns Hopkins University Press, 2004); Grant Steen and Joseph Mirro, eds., *Childhood Cancer: A Handbook from St. Jude Children's Research Hospital* (HarperCollins Publishers, 2000).

CLAUDIA WINOGRAD
UNIVERSITY OF ILLINOIS AT URBANA-CHAMPAIGN

National Kidney Cancer Association

THE NATIONAL KIDNEY Cancer Association (KCA) was founded in 1990 to ally patients and their families, physicians, health professionals, and researchers. The association collaborates with the National Cancer Institute, the American Society for Clinical Oncology, the

American Urologic Association, and others to promote research and education in the field of kidney cancer.

Founded in Chicago, Illinois, by kidney-cancer patients and their physicians, the KCA has grown as a volunteer organization. It is part of the National Health Council and is currently expanding into the global forum. The association is led by a panel of directors who are members of academia, the pharmaceutical industry, hospitals, and the community. In addition, a team of medical advisers counsels the KCA on strategies for research funding.

To support its international initiatives, the KCA also has offices in Canada and the United Kingdom. Hotline phone numbers are available in many more countries, including Denmark, Estonia, Finland, Germany, Japan, Poland, Brazil, and Sweden.

The KCA funds both private and public research. A major prize provided by the KCA is the Eugene P. Schonfeld Medical Research Award, a two-year award for basic or translational research conducted by young researchers.

EDUCATION AND RESOURCES

The association encourages physicians and clinicians to participate in Continuing Medical Education, whereby licensed professionals remain abreast of new knowledge in their fields. To promote education, the KCA is implementing an "Ask the Experts" podcast in which questions submitted online by anyone involved with kidney cancer are answered. The association's website provides information on current research and clinical trials, treatment options, and patient stories. Patients can register in the association and gain access to private sites such as a patient meeting calendar. The KCA is developing websites in several other languages, including Chinese, French, German, Italian, Japanese, and Spanish. Also planned are patient support groups in Asia, Australia, and the European Union.

SEE ALSO: Kidney (Renal Cell) Cancer; Kidney Cancer, Childhood; Renal Pelvis and Ureter, Transitional Cell Cancer.

BIBLIOGRAPHY. Eric P. Cohen, *Cancer and the Kidney* (Oxford University Press, 2005); Robert A. Figlin, *Kidney Cancer (Cancer Treatment and Research)* (Springer, 2003).

CLAUDIA WINOGRAD
UNIVERSITY OF ILLINOIS AT URBANA-CHAMPAIGN

National Marrow Donor Program (NMDP)

IN THE 1950s it was shown that bone-marrow transplants could be used to treat patients with leukemia and other blood cancers. Because it is difficult to find a suitable donor for a particular patient, Congress established what would become the National Marrow Donor Program (NMDP) to create an international registry of marrow donors. Today, the NMDP maintains the largest directory of donors and units of umbilical-cord blood in the world. The NMDP works to connect patients, physicians, donors, and researchers to resources for marrow donation and transplantation. Umbilical-cord blood is also used to treat patients with leukemia and other blood cancers.

FIRST TRANSPLANTS

The first indications that bone-marrow transplants could help restore defective marrow to health came from experiments performed on mice. These mice with unhealthy marrow received marrow from other mice and were cured.

In the late 1950s in France, a radiation accident caused several people's marrow to become defective. Bone-marrow transplants were attempted on these patients.

In 1958 a French investigator discovered a critical factor in the success of tissue transplants: The human leukocyte antigens (HLA) had to match between donors and recipients.

In the United States, the first successful marrow donation between siblings who were not identical twins took place in 1968 at the University of Minnesota. Five years later, physicians at Memorial Sloan-Kettering Cancer Center performed the first unrelated bone-marrow transplant. The donor was from Denmark.

ESTABLISHMENT OF DONOR DATABASES

People quickly realized that an international database of marrow donors could accelerate the process of matching a donor to a recipient in need. In the early years of this idea, several communities had data on potential donors; most data came from community-wide searches for a specific HLA type.

Tireless work by supporters of a national donor registry came to fruition in July 1986, when Congress charged the U.S. Navy with the task of establishing a national registry of bone-marrow donors. In June 1988 this registry became the National Marrow Donor Program.

The NMDP manages an Office of Patient Advocacy, which educates and counsels patients in need of a transplant. Critical help is provided in the form of financial counseling, as the cost of a bone-marrow transplant is high.

SEE ALSO: Bone Marrow Transplants; Memorial Sloan-Kettering Cancer Center; University of Minnesota Cancer Center.

BIBLIOGRAPHY. Brian J. Bolwell, *Current Controversies in Bone Marrow Transplantation* (Humana Press, 2000).

CLAUDIA WINOGRAD
UNIVERSITY OF ILLINOIS AT URBANA-CHAMPAIGN

National Program of Cancer Registries (NPCR)

IN 1992, THROUGH recognition of a need for more complete local, state, regional, and national cancer incidence data, Congress established the National Program of Cancer Registries (NPCR) at the Centers for Disease Control and Prevention (CDC) by enacting the Cancer Registries Amendment Act (Public Law 102-515).

The NPCR registries are managed by state health departments or other entities designated by the state and cover 96 percent of the U.S. population.

The NPCR has the capacity to monitor the cancer burden in states and nationally; to identify cancer incidence variations by site, race, Hispanic origin, sex, histology, stage of disease, and other patient and tumor characteristics; to describe cancer trends, patterns, and variations for use in cancer-control planning and intervention; to provide data for research; to provide guidance for health-resource allocation; to respond to public concerns and inquiries; to improve planning for future healthcare needs; and to evaluate cancer prevention and control activities.

This program complements the Surveillance, Epidemiology, and End Results (SEER) registries of the National Cancer Institute. The two federal programs together cover 100 percent of the U.S. population.

SERVICES
Before 1992, 10 states had no statewide cancer registry, and others lacked adequate resources and state legislation to collect needed data. Since 1998 CDC has funded 45 states, the District of Columbia, and three U.S. territorial health departments (or other designated entities) at a ratio of $3:$1 to match state support.

The CDC provides technical assistance on registry operations (including guidance for adapting to the electronic medical record) and achieving program standards. The CDC supports patterns of care and linkage studies in selected states. Linkages with the National Death Index, Medicare, Census, and the Indian Health Service patient database enhance the quality and utility of cancer registry data.

INCIDENCE DATA AND RESOURCES
NPCR registries have reported incidence data to CDC since 2001. The first diagnosis year for cancer cases in NPCR is the first year that the registry collected data with the assistance of NPCR funds; 1995 is the earliest diagnosis year in NPCR.

About 1.2 to 1.4 million new invasive cancer cases are added each year. In 2007 CDC anticipated receiving data for more than 13.6 million invasive cancer cases diagnosed from 1995 to 2004.

NPCR and SEER data are combined to provide cancer statistics for the nation in United States Cancer Statistics. Precalculated cancer incidence rates are available for further analysis in two additional formats: a public-use data set in CDC WONDER under Cancer Incidence, and a county-level file that includes selected cancer sites and states.

SEE ALSO: North American Association of Central Cancer Registries; Statistics; Surveillance, Epidemiology, End Results.

BIBLIOGRAPHY. Centers for Disease Control and Prevention website, www.cdc.gov (cited September 2006).

PHYLLIS A. WINGO, PH.D.
CENTERS FOR DISEASE CONTROL
AND PREVENTION

Natural Causes of Cancer

THE CELL IS the fundamental unit of life. It is the smallest structure of the body capable of performing all of the processes that define life. A cancer cell is a cell that has lost the ability to recognize certain signaling pathways and no longer responds properly. Growing in an uncontrollable manner and unable to recognize its own natural boundary, the cancer cells may spread to areas of the body where they do not belong. Research shows that certain risk factors increase the likelihood that a person will develop cancer during their lifetime. In this article we focus on the Natural causes of cancer. These include increased age, diet, obesity, stress, genetic make-up, environmental exposure, and viruses.

INCREASED AGE

Age is a primary risk factor for cancer. According to the American Cancer Society (ACS) 77 percent of all cancers are diagnosed in people age 55 and older. As we age our cells continue to divide and collect genetic errors over time.

DIET AND OBESITY

People who have a poor diet, do not have enough physical activity, or are overweight may be at increased risk of several types of cancer. For example, studies suggest that people whose diet is high in fat have an increased risk of Colon, Uterus, and Prostate cancers. An increased incidence of stomach cancer is seen in certain regions of Japan where a high intake of salty smoked fish is seen. Increased risk for esophageal cancer has been linked to alcohol, tobacco, pickled fermented vegetables, and vitamin A supplements. Liver cancer in China, Africa, Japan, and the U.S. has been correlated with dietary intake of aflatoxin. Lack of physical activity and being overweight are risk factors for Breast, Colon, Esophagus, Kidney, and Uterus cancers. Recent studies indicate that obesity and being overweight may increase the risk of death from many cancers, accounting for up to 14 percent of cancer deaths in men and 20 percent of cancer deaths in women.

PSYCHOLOGICAL STRESS

Although studies have shown that stress factors alter the way the immune system functions, no scientific evidence has proven this to be the case. Some studies have indicated an increased incidence of early death, including death from cancer, among people who have experienced the recent loss of a loved one. A particular area of interest that is currently being studied is the effect of stress on women with a known diagnosis of breast cancer. These studies are looking at whether stress reduction can improve the immune response and possibly slow progression of disease.

GENETIC MAKE-UP

Genetics plays a role in the development of some but not all cancers. Some families have concentrated clusters where several people have cancer, or one individual has multiple cancers. In hereditary cancers, several members of an extended family are affected with the same or related types of cancer. This could be due to an inherited mutation on a particular gene, such as BRCA 1 seen with breast cancer. Genetic counseling is recommended for high-risk families considering genetic testing. Counseling includes a review of the risks, benefits, and limitations of genetic testing.

ENVIRONMENT

Most researchers would agree that roughly 80 percent to 90 percent of cancers are the result of environmental exposure. This is a broad term and includes such exposure as sunlight, smoking, air pollution, ionizing radiation, and other occupational exposures. Substantial increases in cancer risk have been shown in settings where individuals have been exposed to high levels of ionizing radiation, chemicals, metals, and other substances. (i.e. asbestos and mesothelioma)

Strict regulatory control and attention to safe occupational practices, drug testing, and consumer product safety play an important role in reducing risk of cancer from environmental exposures. The U.S. Food and Drug Administration, the Environmental Protection Agency, and the Occupational Safety and Health Administration have developed safety standards and are responsible for enforcing laws aimed at decreasing health risks for the general public.

VIRUSES AND BACTERIA

Being infected with certain viruses can increase the risk or directly lead to development of certain cancers. For instance Human papillomavirus (HPV) is the leading cause of cervical cancer in women,

Hepatitis B and C increase the risk of hepatocellular carcinoma, Ebstein-Barr virus has been linked to nasopharyngeal carcinoma, human immunodeficiency virus (HIV) suppresses the immune system and increases the risk of developing cancers, such as lymphoma and a rare cancer called Kaposi's sarcoma. The bacterium *Helibacter pylori* responsible for stomach ulcers are also capable of causing lymphoma of the small bowel.

The causes of cancer are multifactorial and range from simple diet and lack of physical activity to environmental exposure from secondhand smoke. While we cannot predict with certainty which individuals will develop cancer within their lifetimes, we can assume that the more risk factors present, the higher the chance that cancer will occur.

SEE ALSO: Age; Diet and Nutrition; Genetics; Latitute.

BIBLIOGRAPHY Eugenia E. Calle, Carmen Rodriguez, and Michael J. Thun, "Overweight, Obesity, and Mortality from Cancer in a Prospectively Studied Cohort of U.S. Adults," *The New England Journal of Medicine* (v.348/17, April 2003). Brenda K. Edwards and Holly L. Howe, "Annual Report to the Nation on the Status of Cancer, 1973-1999, Featuring the Implications of Age and Aging on U.S. Cancer Burden," *Cancer* (v. 94/10, May 2002). "What are the Risk Factors for Cancer?" *American Cancer Society*, http://www.cancer.org/docroot/CRI/content.

FERNANDO A. HERRERA, JR., M.D.
UNIVERSITY OF CALIFORNIA, SAN DIEGO

Nepal

THIS LANDLOCKED COUNTRY in southern Asia, located in the Himalaya mountain range, has borders with China to the north and India to the south. It was unified in 1768 and was under British "guidance" until 1955, when it was admitted to the United Nations as an independent country. Nepal has a population of 27,133,000 (2005), with 4 doctors and 5 nurses per 100,000 people. An example of cancer incidence rates in Nepal includes 105.3 cases of cancer in males per 100,000, according to the International Agency for Research on Cancer.

Traditionally, in a country that is extremely poor and has low levels of medical care, many people do not live long enough to suffer from cancer. With increasing life-expectancy rates in the 20th century, however, the number of cancer cases rose. The government is keen to make more people aware of cancer and the benefits of early diagnosis.

The National Council for Science and Technology in Kathmandu, the capital of Nepal, is the official medical research center for the country. Other important work is carried out at the Institute of Medicine at Tribhu-

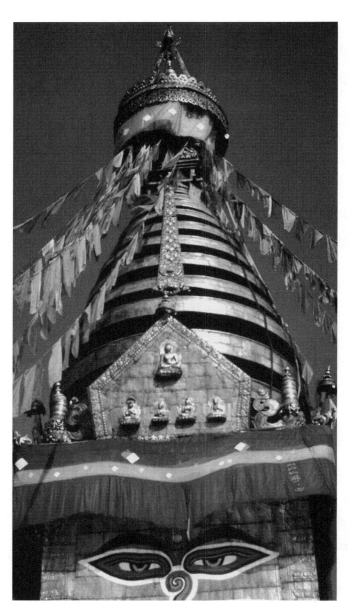

A Buddhist temple in Nepal, where spiritual concerns merge with educating people who are unaware of modern treatment methods.

van University, Kathmandu; at Tribhuvan University Teaching Hospital, Kathmandu; TU Teaching Hospital, Maharajgunj; and the Hospice Nepal, Lalitput.

Recent research has focused not just on different types of cancer, but also on how to alert people who are unaware of modern treatment methods about the success rates from recent medical developments.

SEE ALSO: Poverty; Screening, Access to.

BIBLIOGRAPHY. D.K. Baskota, et al., "Distribution of Malignancies in Head and Neck Regions And Their Management," *Journal of the Nepal Medical Association* (v.44/159, 2005); R. Gongal, et al., "Informing Patients about Cancer in Nepal: What Do People Prefer?," *Palliative Medicine* (v.20/4, 2006); "Screening the Only Option to Prevent Cervical Cancer," *Journal of the Nepal Medical Association* (v.44/159, 2005).

JUSTIN CORFIELD
GEELONG GRAMMAR SCHOOL, AUSTRALIA

Netherlands

THIS EUROPEAN COUNTRY was occupied by the Hapsburg rulers of Austria until 1579, when some of the provinces broke away. Spain finally recognized the Netherlands' independence in 1648. The Netherlands has a population of 16,336,000 (2006), with 251 doctors and 902 nurses per 100,000 people. An example of cancer incidence rates in the Netherlands includes 314.6 cases of cancer in males per 100,000, according to the International Agency for Research on Cancer.

In the 17th century many advances in cancer surgery and treatment were developed in the Netherlands. Much of this research started to contradict the Greco-Roman theories of Galen, arguing along the lines of the iatromechanical school that all physical and chemical processes in the human body are brought about by the motion of atomic particles. One of the leading proponents of this theory was Friedrich Hoffman, a professor of medicine in Halle.

The theory gained support from Francois de le Boe Sylvius, a professor in Leyden, who felt that a change in the nature of lymphatic fluid created a greater acid base, which caused cancer through a system known as acrimony. Claude Deshais Gendron, however, believed that the only cure for cancer was surgery. Nicholas Tulp of Amsterdam recorded a carcinoma of the esophagus in the 17th century. Surgeon Laurence Heisterl performed a mastectomy in 1720.

In the 19th century there were further developments in the Dutch treatment of cancer, many undertaken by Johannes Korteweg at Leyden University. Herman Luhrman, a physician in Leyden, wrote a histological description of a breast carcinoma, and Johanne Schrant described microscopic cancer tissues.

During the 1850s Ludovicus van der Kolk wrote about the discovery of clinically occult cancer cells in healthy tissue some way from a primary breast cancer. In 1880 Richard Volkman suggested that surgery for breast cancer should remove not only the diseased breast, but also palpable nodes nearby.

In 1903 radiotherapy of breast cancer started in the Netherlands, pioneered by D. H. van der Groot, and the Netherlands Cancer Institute was established in Amsterdam in 1913.

Marie Curie visited the Netherlands in 1932, raising the profile of cancer research.

RECENT RESEARCH

Among recent research projects, L. A. Schellekens, et al., of the departments of gynecology and pathology at de Wever Hospital in Heerlen studied the necessity of cervical conization as a diagnostic procedure in patients suspected of cervical cancer.

L. den Engelse of the Chemical Carginogenesis Unit at the Netherlands Cancer Institute researched the metabolism of the carcinogen dimenthylnitrosamine in the rodent and human lung. E. Scherer and P. Emmelot of the same unit performed a related study on the induction of preneoplastic lesions in rat livers by the carcinogen dimenthylnitrosamine.

D. J. Th. Wegener, et al., of St. Radboud Hospital, University of Nijmegen, studied the influence of splenectomy on the in-vitro lymphocyte response to phythohaemagglutnin and pokeweed mitogen in Hodgkin's disease.

One of the most famous Dutch women who suffered from breast cancer was Hendrickje Stoffels, mistress of Rembrandt and the model for his painting *Bathsheba at Her Toilet* (1654). In the painting,

Stoffels is clearly depicted as suffering from breast cancer, to which she succumbed in 1663.

SEE ALSO: Breast Cancer; Cervical Cancer; Esophageal Cancer; Radiation Therapy; Surgery.

BIBLIOGRAPHY. "The Netherlands Cancer Institute," *Cancer Bulletin* (v.11, 1959); Peter Allen Braithwaite and Dace Shugg, "Rembrandt's Bathsheba: The Dark Shadow of the Left Breast," *Annals of the Royal College of Surgeons of England* (v.65, 1983); A. E. de Jong and H. F. Vasen, "The Frequency of a Positive Family History for Colorectal Cancer: A Population-Based Study in the Netherlands," *Netherlands Journal of Medicine* (v.64/10, 2006); Daniel de Moulin, "Historical Notes on Breast Cancer: Emphasis on the Netherlands," *The Netherlands Journal of Surgery* (v.32–34, 1980–1982); C. J. M. Lips, et al., "Central Registration of Multiple Endocrine Neoplasia Type 2 Families in The Netherlands," *Henry Ford Hospital Medical Journal* (v.32, 1984); Kenneth Meyer and William C. Beck, "Mastectomy Performed by Laurence Heister in the Eighteenth Century," *Surgery, Gynecology & Obstetrics* (v.159, 1984); D. M. Parkin, et al., eds., *Cancer Incidence in Five Continents*, vol. VII (International Agency for Research on Cancer and International Association of Cancer Registries, 1997).

JUSTIN CORFIELD
GEELONG GRAMMAR SCHOOL, AUSTRALIA

Neuroblastoma

NEUROBLASTOMA IS A tumor that affects the part of the nervous system that operates without conscious thought (involuntarily), referred to as the autonomic system. Specifically, within the autonomic system the tumor affects the sympathetic nervous system—a system that is ordinarily known to be responsible for the flight-and-fight response, such as increases in blood pressure and heart rate.

The sympathetic system's nerves, located throughout the entire body, are the result of the proliferation and differentiation of neuroblasts (embryonic cells that become nerves during development of the embryo). Unfortunately, it is for this reason that the neuroblastomas may occur in various regions of the body, such as the abdomen, mostly affecting the adrenal glands (40

percent), and the sympathetic nerve clusters next to the spine, known as paraspinal ganglia (25 percent). Additionally, the tumor commonly presents in the thorax (15 percent), pelvis (5 percent), or cervix (3 percent).

Neuroblastoma affects mostly infants and represents 7.8 percent of childhood cancers. In the United States, approximately 650 new cases are diagnosed each year. The disease is virtually nonexistent in patients older than 10 years of age and is increasingly rare after the age of 5.

The specific cause of neuroblastomas is unknown. Scientific literature suggests that neuroblastoma is likely due to some influence during pregnancy. Limited or inconsistent evidence exists on the relationship between neuroblastoma and exposures of, or to, medicines, hormones, previous spontaneous abortion, alcohol, tobacco, and the father's occupational environment.

A recent study suggested that there may be a relationship between the Canadian program of cereal fortification with grain and a decrease in neuroblastoma. However, better studies are needed to confirm this finding.

One-fifth of tumors are diagnosed either before the infant is born or within three months after birth. Prenatal ultrasound has allowed for increased diagnosis of fetal neuroblastoma. In any case, almost all tumors are detected clinically before 5 years of age.

TREATMENT AND PROGNOSIS
Care of children with cancer is usually provided by large multidisciplinary teams. Members of the team

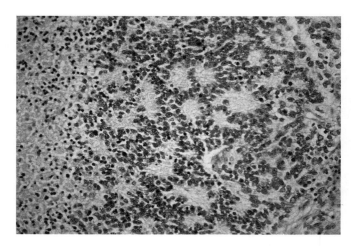

Magnification on a cellular level of Neuroblastoma cells in cell tissue. Magnification is 500X.

include cancer specialists (oncologists), radiation oncologists, surgeons, pharmacists, psychologists, occupational therapists, rehabilitation specialists, and various other providers to address the needs of the patient and their families. Depending on the stage of the tumor, treatment options are diverse, ranging from radiation and chemotherapy to surgery.

The overall five-year survival rate for children with neuroblastoma has improved from 24 percent between 1960 and 1963 to 55 percent between 1985 and 1994. Increased survival rates are attributed in part to earlier detection due to increased technology and awareness, as well as to medical and surgical advances.

The differences in prognosis for patients are quite profound, however, and depend on several factors. Specifically, age, stage, and genetic defects in the tumor cells are three major considerations that determine the prognosis of neuroblastomas.

Generally, patients older than 1 year of age with spreading tumors do not have very good outcomes, whereas patients younger than 1 year of age with spreading tumors and patients with nonspreading tumors of any age are likely to have excellent outcomes. The cancer may spread to various regions, including liver, bone marrow, bone, and lymph nodes. Unfortunately, neuroblastoma spreads very quickly. Thus, children who are diagnosed with neuroblastoma after the age of 1 have a 70 percent to 80 percent likelihood that it has already spread.

The overall five-year survival rate since time of diagnosis is approximately 83 percent for infants, 55 percent for children age 1 to 5, and 40 percent for children older than 5 years.

SEE ALSO: Childhood Cancers; Genetics.

BIBLIOGRAPHY. M. C. Henry, et al., "Neuroblastoma Update," *Current Opinion in Oncology* (v.17/1, 2005).

NAVNEET SINGH
UNIVERSITY OF TORONTO

Neurofibromatosis

NEUROFIBROMATOSIS IS A genetic disease that affects the nervous system by interfering with the development and growth of neural- (nerve-) cell tissues. These disorders cause tumors to grow on the nerves, along with abnormalities of the skin and bones.

Although neurofibromatosis is a genetic disorder, 30 percent to 50 percent of all new cases occur spontaneously as a new gene mutation in individuals with no family history of the disease. When the gene mutation has occurred, however, it will be passed on to the descendents of that individual.

There are two types of neurofibromatosis: neurofibromatosis 1 (NF1) and neurofibromatosis 2 (NF2).

In cases where there is a family history of neurofibromatosis, most families are affected by either NF1 or NF2 and not a combination of both types, because NF1 and NF2 are caused by anomalies on different chromosomes. The effects of both NF1 and NF2 can range from absent to mild symptoms to severe disability and life-threatening complications. Neurofibromatosis increases a child's risk of developing certain types of cancers and requires frequent medical assessment and intervention.

NF1, which occurs when the gene is identified on chromosome 17, is the most commonly occurring type. It is estimated that 1/4,000th of the world population is affected by NF1. This form is typically marked by skin changes, the presence of tumors, and bone abnormalities. Although neurofibromatosis is not in itself cancerous, in 5 percent of affected individuals, cancerous growths occur within the tumors themselves. Many affected individuals have a first-degree relative who is also affected by the disease. Children with NF1 are also at risk to develop juvenile myelomonocytic leukemia (JMML). Although JMML accounts for only 1 percent of all childhood leukemias, 14 percent of the children affected also have NF1.

Many individuals with NF1 symptoms have skin changes evident at birth or pigmentation changes that occur during the first few months of life. Although many individuals are born with or develop benign café-au-lait spots, a skin assessment should be performed.

Most individuals who have NF1 have more than six spots than are at least 5 mm in diameter. In adolescence, the spots must be larger than 15 mm in diameter. The number of spots present does not correlate to the severity of the symptoms.

Symptoms develop at different stages and ages, and not all symptoms may be present during the initial evaluation. Most features occur by adolescence, although many children are diagnosed at an earlier age.

NF1 is always diagnosed by the age of 10. In 25 percent of children, learning disabilities are diagnosed.

Criteria for diagnosis include two or more neurofibromas or one plexiform neurofibroma, freckles under the arm or in the groin area, lisch nodules on the iris of the eye, optic glioma, or characteristic skeletal abnormality. A first-degree relative who suffers from the disease is another criterion used in diagnosis. Although NF1 can become severely painful and debilitating, depending on the extensiveness of the tumors, some children are diagnosed by brown spots on the skin that previously were labeled birthmarks. Children with multiple café-au-lait spots should be reassessed annually to assess for other diagnostic symptoms of the disease.

If there is a family history, genetic screening can be performed; however, individuals with NF1 as a result of a cell mutation cannot be tested through chromosomal studies. Some medical providers may perform a biopsy or X-ray to aid in diagnosis.

NF2, which is the result of an abnormality on chromosome 22, results in the production of a tumor-suppressor protein. NF2 is a rarer form than NF1, affecting 1/40,000th of the world population. Although NF2 is more common in adults, childhood cases are often overlooked or misdiagnosed. The range of ages at diagnosis is 11 to 30 years.

The most common symptoms of NF2 that occur include optical problems, skin changes, and neurological changes. Commonly, symptoms worsen with age; then a correct diagnosis is made.

This type typically presents with bilateral tumors on the eighth cranial nerve, which is responsible for hearing. It is common for the nerve to produce pressure on other nerves and cause additional damage.

Approximately 50 percent of NF2 patients have intracranial meningiomas, which are often difficult to treat, and 40 percent of affected individuals have visual problems.

NF2 diagnosis is based on the presence of symptoms such as hearing loss, tinnitus, visual problems, and poor balance. Headaches, facial pain, and facial numbness can also occur as a result of pressure created by the tumor. An in-depth family history often identifies first-degree relatives who have the disease. Neurofibromatosis can be diagnosed prenatally with amniocentesis or chorionic villus sampling techniques when there is a positive family history. Early testing can also be used when other first-degree relatives are affected. When the disease occurs in an individual without a family history and as a result of a new gene mutation, genetic testing cannot be performed.

Treatment for neurofibromatosis focuses on controlling symptoms.

NF1 treatment frequently focuses on removing bone malformations and painful tumors. Although the tumors may return and worsen, they are generally noncancerous. The incidence of cancerous tumors is 3 percent to 5 percent. If malignancy does occur, treatment consists of surgery, radiation, and chemotherapy.

NF2 tumors can be completely surgically excised, although there is a risk of hearing loss. Partial removal of tumors or radiation can also be used. For slow-growing tumors, some physicians may choose a careful monitoring course with expectant management as needed. NF2 warrants careful monitoring, because tumors that invade other cranial nerves or the brain stem can become life threatening.

SEE ALSO: Childhood Cancers; Genetics.

BIBLIOGRAPHY. Rubenstein, Allan E. and Bruce R. Korf. *Neurofibromatosis.* Thieme Medical Publishers, Incorporated 2005. Riccardi, Vincent M. and June E. Eichner. *Neurofibromatosis: Phenotype, Natural History, and Pathogenesis* (Johns Hopkins University Press, 1986).

MICHELE R. DAVIDSON, PH.D.
INDEPENDENT SCHOLAR

Neutrons

KNOWN TO MAN only within the past 100 years, neutrons have been used in both negative and positive ways that have significantly affected human health.

Soon after their discovery, neutrons became closely linked with cancer. The National Institute of Environmental Health Sciences lists neutrons as known human carcinogens, stating that they could cause cancers due to genetic damage. The institute notes, however, that neutron radiation is not used as much as other forms of radiation and that for the general population, exposure to these particles is mainly from cosmic sources.

The existence of neutrons was proposed in 1920 by Ernest Rutherford. The search for these particles, however, was deterred by their lack of electrical charge. In 1932 the presence of neutrons was finally confirmed by James Chadwick, a physicist at Cambridge University, who gave the particles their name. He was awarded the Nobel Prize in 1935.

Next came the invention of Cyclotron Research. Around the same time in the search for neutrons, Ernest Orlando Lawrence, a physicist at the University of California, Berkeley, invented a device to aid in the study of subatomic particles. This device, called the cyclotron, was patented in 1934, earning its inventor a Nobel Prize in 1939; in addition, his laboratory was renamed the Lawrence Berkeley National Laboratory.

The cyclotron was designed to accelerate atomic particles that were then directed toward a target. The acceleration process energized the particles so tremendously that when they came into contact with a target, the target disintegrated. Thus, the device was designed to reduce other atoms to their subatomic components for research purposes.

Because cyclotrons could be used to disintegrate their targets, scientists considered that this could be a way to destroy malignant cancer cells. It was proposed that via a cyclotron, beams of high-energy neutrons could be directed at tumor cells to disintegrate them, thus curing the cancer patient. This method, termed fast neutron radiotherapy, was put into clinical trial

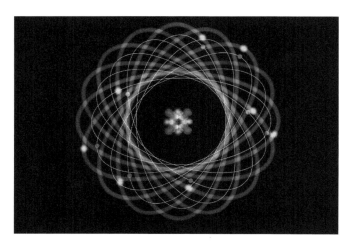

Within the core of an atom, the neutral charged neutrons are held with the positive charged protons. Outer electrons are negative.

in 1938 under the direction of Robert Stone, also from the University of Berkeley, California. Unfortunately, Stone's study resulted in toxic conditions for the patients and did not help cure the cancers. Further research of this method was necessary.

Boron Neutron Capture Therapy (BNCT), initially described in 1936 by Gordon L. Locher, uses boron to capture the neutrons that are being delivered to the targeted cancer cells. Because the boron atoms are attached to molecules that are selectively taken up by the malignant tumor cells, it was proposed that the neutrons would destroy only those cells.

BNCT was studied in the 1950s in clinical trials at Brookhaven National Laboratory and at the Massachusetts Institute of Technology for the treatment of brain tumors—particularly glioblastoma multiforme, a highly malignant tumor. Researchers found, however, that BNCT also damaged normal cells and did not provide a positive therapeutic effect on patients.

Fast Neutron Therapy, on the other hand, has become a significant modality of treatment for certain cancers. In 1965 Mary Catterall conducted clinical trials at Hammersmith Hospital in London, England. In a few years, it was determined that this therapy was beneficial for local control of tumors. Patients began to be treated in the early 1970s at M. D. Anderson Hospital and Tumor Institute in Houston, Texas; the Naval Research Laboratory in Washington, D.C.; and the University of Washington in Seattle.

In the mid-1970s, the Neutron Therapy Facility at Fermi National Accelerator Laboratory (Fermilab), later renamed NIU Institute for Neutron Therapy, was instituted in Illinois. Cancer patients began receiving treatments September 7, 1976. Since then, over 3,100 patients have been treated.

Fast neutron therapy has been more effective at terminating tumors than other methods of conventional radiation therapy. Currently, fast neutron therapy is most beneficial in treating localized salivary-gland tumors, locally advanced prostate cancers, locally advanced head and neck tumors, adenoidcystic carcinomas, and inoperable sarcomas. This therapy may also be appropriate for other localized malignant tumors anywhere in the body that are inoperable or resistant to conventional radiation.

Neutron therapy generally requires shorter treatment periods—only 12 treatments in 4 weeks rather than 30 to 40 treatments in 8 weeks, as in conventional radiation therapy. Due to the complex technology, devices, and operating staff required, however, this therapy has been limited to a small number of facilities and is not available on a widespread basis.

Research is under way on a hybrid form of treatment, in which Boron neutron capture therapy is used to enhance fast neutron therapy.

SEE ALSO: Head and Neck Cancer; Prostate Cancer; Radiation; Radiation Therapy; Salivary Gland Cancer.

BIBLIOGRAPHY. Robert Stone, "Neutron Therapy and Specific Ionization," *American Journal of Roentgenology* (v.59, 1940); National Institutes of Standards and Technology, "World War II," www.100.nist.gov (cited February 2007); National Toxicology Program, "Report on Carcinogens," www.ntp.nieh.nih.gov (cited January 2007); "Neutron Therapy Facility," www.bd.fnal.gov (cited February 2007); Northern Illinois University, "NIU Launches Institute for Neutron Therapy Facility," www.niu.edu (cited January 2007).

SUSANNA N. CHEN
WESTERN UNIVERSITY OF HEALTH SCIENCES

New Zealand

THIS PACIFIC COUNTRY was made a British colony in 1840 and became self-governing in 1907. It was established as an independent country by the Statute of Westminster of 1931, adopted by Parliament in 1947. New Zealand has a population of 4,148,000 (2006), with 218 doctors and 771 nurses per 100,000 people. An example of cancer incidence rates in New Zealand includes 363.1 cases of cancer in males per 100,000, according to the International Agency for Research on Cancer.

With a high life-expectancy rate in New Zealand, there has long been a problem with cancer. In 1867 New Zealand required the registration of all orthodox medical practitioners, which stopped people from offering unorthodox treatments. Since the 1980s the methods of surgical and oncological treatment of colon and rectal cancer have changed dramatically, with the rate of resecting of primary tumors from 1997 to 2003 being 95 percent. A study by J. Borrie, R.J. Rose, G.F.S. Spears, and G.A. Holmes showed that male lung

cancer increased steadily between 1961 and 1971. It is particularly prevalent among Maoris and people of Maori descent. A rising problem in New Zealand is skin cancer, with an increasing number of people suffering from melanomas. Many of those melanomas come from sunburn. Concern about the ozone hole is another factor.

CANCER SOCIETY OF NEW ZEALAND

In 1929 the New Zealand branch of the British Empire Cancer Campaign was formed in New Zealand; in 1963 it was renamed the Cancer Society of New Zealand. The society started clinics around the country, giving advice to people about cancer prevention and early treatment. It also set up research laboratories that used radium treatment and raised funds for hospitals to buy radiotherapy equipment. The national office is in Wellington, with six regional divisions covering different parts of the country.

Many prominent New Zealanders have died from cancer, including artists Henrietta Angus, Catherine Bower, and William Brassington; politicians William Appleton, Frederick Widdowson Doidge, John McKenzie, John Grace, Henry Fish, and Thomas Philip Shand; Michael Joseph Savage, who was prime minister from 1935 to 1940; newspaper proprietor John Balance; aviator Keith Logan Caldwell; journalist

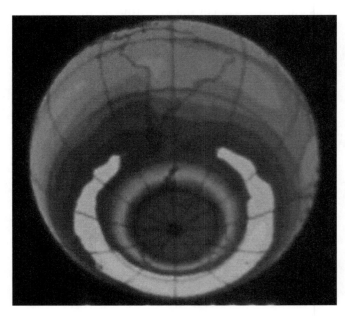

A rising problem of skin cancer in New Zealand may be related to the growing ozone hole over the South Pole (shown in 1990).

Elizabeth Dyson; military pilot and aviation promoter Frederick Patrick Ladd; boxer Edward Morgan; publisher David Blackwood Paul; and novelist Gloria Jasmine Rawlinson.

SEE ALSO: Colon Cancer; Lung Cancer, Non-Small Cell; Lung Cancer, Small Cell; Radiation Therapy; Rectal Cancer; Skin Cancer (Melanoma).

BIBLIOGRAPHY. David Cole, "Doctrinal Deviance in New Zealand Medical Practice: Some Historical Comments," *New Zealand Medical Journal* (v.98, 1985); H. Curry, G. Horne, P. Devane and H. Tobin, "Osteosarcoma in New Zealand: An Outcome Study Comparing Survival Rates between 1981–1987 and 1994–1999," *New Zealand Medical Journal* (v.119/1242, 2006); R. Dunbar, et al., "Melanoma Control: Few Answers, Many Questions," *New Zealand Medical Journal* (v.119/1242, 2006); J. Keating, et al., "Multidisciplinary Treatment of Colorectal Cancer in New Zealand: Survival Rates from 1997–2002," *New Zealand Medical Journal* (v.119/1242, 2006).

JUSTIN CORFIELD
GEELONG GRAMMAR SCHOOL, AUSTRALIA

Nicaragua

THIS CENTRAL AMERICAN republic was part of Spanish America until it gained its independence in 1821 and became part of the United Provinces of Central America. Nicaragua became an independent republic in its own right in 1838. It took over the Mosquito Coast in 1860 and has had no territorial changes since then. The Republic of Nicaragua has a population of 5,488,000 (2005), with 46 doctors and 92 nurses per 100,000 people. An example of cancer incidence rates in Nicaragua includes 140.7 cases of cancer in males per 100,000, according to the International Agency for Research on Cancer. The healthcare system in Nicaragua remained relatively poor until the 1990s.

During the early 20th century the hospitals in Managua and other major cities provided medical services largely for the local elite. Most poor people were unable to pay for the medicines and treatments provided.

With the overthrow of Anastasio Somoza in 1979, the new Sandinista government promised to improve healthcare in the country. This happened in Managua, but a bitter civil war from 1979 to 1990 left much of the infrastructure of rural Nicaragua in ruins.

After the elections of 1990 there was a concerted effort to rebuild medical care in the countryside and improve health education, including cancer awareness. The sheer cost of a dedicated cancer center in Nicaragua meant that the initial plans drawn up by the government were to adapt an existing hospital to allow for the treatment of cervical-cancer patients, rather than building a cancer hospital in Managua.

Nicaragua has one of the highest rates of cervical cancer in the world, approaching 40 percent of all female cancer cases and largely affecting women in their reproductive years. Much of this incidence was because of the lack of screening for many women. In 2003 the Ministry of Health, the Central American Institute of Health, and the Maria Luisa Ortiz Clinic combined their resources to begin a program of cancer education in rural areas. The result was earlier diagnosis and, hence, a better chance of successful treatment.

The other form of cancer that is prevalent in Nicaragua is human papillomavirus (HPV), which has affected many women. The human T-cell leukemia–lymphoma virus has been found in some black former slave communities along the Caribbean coast.

SEE ALSO: Cervical Cancer; Infection (Childhood, Sexually Transmitted Infections, Hepatitis, Etc.); Screening (Cervical and Breast and Colon Cancers); Poverty; Screening, Access to.

BIBLIOGRAPHY. Richard Garfield and Glen Williams, *Health Care in Nicaragua: Primary Care under Changing Regimes* (Oxford University Press, 1992); P. Hindryckx, et al., "Prevalence of High Risk Human Papillomavirus Types among Nicaraguan Women with Histological Proved Pre-Neoplastic and Neoplastic Lesions of the Cervix," *Sexually Transmitted Infections* (v.82/4, 2006); S. L. Howe, et al., "Cervical Cancer Prevention in Remote Rural Nicaragua: A Program Evaluation," *Gynecologic Oncology* (v.99/3, 2005).

JUSTIN CORFIELD
GEELONG GRAMMAR SCHOOL, AUSTRALIA

Nickel Compounds

NICKEL (ATOMIC SYMBOL Ni, atomic number 28) is a hard, ductile transition metal. It makes up only a small percentage of the Earth's crust but is one of the most abundant elements in the Earth's core. Most natural nickel is found in sulfate or oxide form.

Accumulated epidemiologic evidence that stretches back to the 1930s has shown a direct relationship between exposure to high levels of certain nickel compounds and cancers of the nasal sinuses and lungs. This evidence is important to today's society because of the widespread use of nickel. Unfortunately, the mechanisms underlying nickel-induced carcinogenesis are still unclear, and the hazards of working with nickel are still being studied.

The historical use of nickel can be traced back thousands of years. In ancient Syria, it was used to make bronze. In China, it was known as white copper.

Modern understanding of the metal began in 1751, when Baron Axel Fredrik Cronstedt attempted to extract copper from kupfernickel (which means "copper of the Devil" or "false copper"), a compound used to stain glass green. Instead of obtaining copper from this mineral, now called niccolite, he found a white metal that he named nickel.

Today, nickel is ubiquitous. Because of its inertness in air to oxidation and its ferromagnetic properties, nickel is often used in alloys, coins, batteries, ceramics, electroplating, dental fillings and orthodontic appliances, and magnets. The majority of nickel is used to make stainless steel. Nickel cannot be avoided, because it is used in everything from jewelry and buildings to transportation vehicles and electronics.

Nickel is even an essential metal for many plants and microbes because it functions in several enzymes, such as urease, superoxide dismutase, and hydrogenases. A similar function in humans has not yet been noted, but based on studies of microbe and plant enzymes, the World Health Organization has categorized nickel as a "probably essential" metal in humans. Even if humans do not have nickel-containing enzymes, they are exposed to nickel from the plants and microbes they come into contact with.

Exposure to nickel is quite varied. Because nickel is a natural compound in the Earth's crust, it is present in small amounts in water, soil, and air. Nickel compounds can be ingested, come into contact with the skin or mucus membranes, or be inhaled. There are many dietary sources of nickel, including various grains, beans, and legumes, as well as vitamin supplements, chocolate, tea, tuna, shellfish, red wine, and all canned foods and drinks. Food is the most common source of nickel exposure; adults can ingest up to 300 micrograms of nickel per day.

About 10 percent to 15 percent of the population is sensitive to nickel. Ingestion of foods that contain nickel or contact with nickel-containing materials such as jewelry or coins can cause severe allergic reactions in sensitive people, usually in the form of contact dermatitis. Ingestion of high amounts of nickel sulfate or nickel chloride (from contaminated water, for example) can also cause acute gastrointestinal distress and neurological effects.

Acute inhalation of nickel compounds can cause severe lung and kidney damage. Inhalation of a large amount of nickel carbonyl, for example, causes pulmonary fibrosis and renal edema. Chronic inhalation can lead to nickel-induced asthma, bronchitis, and decreased lung function. Generally, the more-soluble nickel compounds (such as nickel acetate) have a greater effect on the lungs. Ingestion of or skin contact with nickel does not increase the risk of cancer. Instead, inhalation seems to be the predominant form of exposure that is associated with cancer.

Airborne Compounds of complex nickel oxides, nickel sulfate, and metallic nickel are present in ambient air at low levels because they are emitted from oil and coal combustion, cigarette smoke, smelting, nickel-metal refining, sewage-sludge incineration, and manufacturing facilities. Nickel is emitted into the air by anthropogenic sources, mostly from burning of residual and fuel oil, followed by nickel refineries, municipal incineration, steel and alloy production, and coal combustion. This is five times the amount that is released from natural sources, such as volcanoes.

In a 1996 air-quality study, the U.S. Environmental Protection Agency (EPA) reported that the average ambient-nickel level in the United States is around 2.2 ng/m3. The United States has no nickel refineries, but the ambient level is higher in urban areas and point sources of emission, such as in Sudbury, Ontario, Canada, where the average intake of nickel is 15 μg per day from air and 140 μg per day from water.

The nickel compounds associated with incinerators, combustion, smelting, and refining are generally nickel sulfate, nickel oxides, and metallic nickel. In more specialized industries, nickel silicate, nickel subsulfide, and nickel chloride are generally emitted.

Water-soluble nickel compounds—such as nickel chloride, nickel sulfate, and nickel nitrate—tend to be more toxic than the less-soluble nickel subsulfide and nickel oxide except in the case of carcinogenesis, in which the nonsoluble compounds are more problematic than soluble compounds at the site of deposition in the body. A 2002 study in Norway, however, showed that water-soluble compounds are associated with a higher risk of lung cancer than previously thought. Nickel carbonyl is also highly toxic but not stable in air, so exposure is generally very limited.

In 1990 the International Committee on Nickel Carcinogenesis in Man compiled data from 10 studies on the effects on workers exposed to high amounts of nickel in industries such as stainless-steel production, nickel mining and smelting, battery production, and nickel-alloy production. A statistically significant increased risk for nasal and lung cancers was found for nickel-refinery workers due to exposure to sulfidic and oxidic nickels.

The only refinery facility that did not show an increase in cancer risk was the one that did not produce high levels of sulfidic and oxidic nickel compounds.

The EPA has estimated that if an individual continuously breathed air containing nickel-refinery dust at an average of 0.004 µg/m3 over his lifetime, he would have a 1 in 1 million increased chance of developing cancer due to the nickel. Continuously breathing air at 0.04 µg/m3 would increase risk by only 1 in 10,000. The risk is even lower when breathing only nickel subsulfide. Nickel-refinery workers tend to breathe in more than these amounts, however, so they are at increased risk for cancer.

The EPA has classified nickel-refinery dust and nickel subsulfide as class A carcinogens, which means that they are known human carcinogens. Nickel carbonyl has been classified as group B2, which means that it is a probable human carcinogen. Metallic nickel has not yet been evaluated by the EPA but is anticipated to be a carcinogen by other groups.

Exposure to cigarette smoke (which contains nickel tetracarbonyl) in addition to refinery dust increases the risk of cancer.

Within the body nickel is usually emitted in particulate form or adsorbs to particles. Inhaled nickel particles deposit in the upper and lower respiratory tracts in a manner dependent on particle size. Larger particles deposit in the nasal sinuses; smaller particles (less than 5 microns in diameter) can travel down to the trachea and bronchi.

About 20 percent to 35 percent of inhaled nickel is retained in the lungs. The more-soluble compounds tend to be absorbed into the blood; less-soluble compounds are removed in phagocytosis by macrophages. Therefore, the less-soluble compounds tend to be retained in the nasal mucosa and lungs longer than the soluble compounds, which may be a factor in the carcinogenic potential of these compounds.

The molecular basis of nickel carcinogenesis is unclear, but many studies have shown various possibilities. It is likely that nickel actually leads to cancer via a combination of many pathways, and new mechanisms are being discovered constantly. Nickel is known, for example, to induce cell proliferation, which would encourage mutated cells to divide and become cancer.

Although nickel has low affinity for DNA, it has high affinity for DNA-associated proteins like histones. Complexing of nickel ions with these proteins can lead to condensation of heterochromatin, DNA hypermethylation, gene silencing, and inhibition of histone acetylation.

Although nickel causes such chromatin damage in vitro, it actually has low mutagenic potential in vivo despite the high carcinogenic activity. Therefore, it is possible that epigenetic effects are important in carcinogenesis.

DNA methylation and inhibition of histone acetylation caused by nickel compounds inactivate gene expression. These patterns can be inherited by daughter cells, leading to cancer.

Reactive oxygen species (ROS) are also very important in cancer development because they lead to cell damage and mutagenesis. Multiple studies have shown that nickel ions lead to an increase in ROS. These ions may specifically oxidatively damage DNA that is genetically inactive.

Nickel may also induce signaling pathways in cells by activating transcription factors that modulate gene expression. Nickel can mimic hypoxic stress in cells, for example, activating expression of hypoxia-inducible factor-1 (HIF-1). This induces formation of proteins that lead to cell proliferation, migration, and invasion, as well as angiogenesis, all of which are hallmarks of cancer. It is possible that one of these cellular targets that lead to cancer will lead to drugs that prevent nickel carcinogenesis in the future.

Perhaps the most famous nickel-refinery town in the world is Port Colborne in Ontario, Canada. This refinery, which stopped producing electrolytic nickel in 1984, was run by International Nickel Company of Canada (Inco, Ltd.). Emissions contaminated soil and air with various metals, including high amounts of nickel. Soil tests by the Ontario Ministry of Environment showed that levels of nickel oxide were 4,000 to 17,000 parts per million (ppm), greatly exceeding the 310-ppm health guideline. Despite the fact that two studies in the late 1990s determined that there were no adverse health effects from the contamination, the Community Based Risk Assessment process was initiated in 2000 by Inco, the city of Port Colborne, the Ontario Ministry of Environment, and the Regional Niagara Public Health Department. The goal was to undertake a risk assessment by determining whether the metal content of the environment was higher than a set level. If so, the area would need to be decontaminated. This process is still going on but is near completion. A class-action lawsuit was filed by residents of Port Colborne in 2001, stating damages to health, property value, and quality of life. The suit failed to be certified, but another suit based on loss of property value was certified in 2005 and will go to trial soon.

SEE ALSO: Genetics; Industry; Lung Cancer, Non-Small Cell; Lung Cancer, Small Cell; Nasal Cavity and Paranasal Sinus Cancer; Tobacco Related Exposures.

BIBLIOGRAPHY. Centers for Disease Control and Prevention, "Toxicological Profile for Nickel," www.atsdr.cdc.gov (cited February 2007); Environmental Protection Agency, "Nickel Compounds," www.epa.gov (cited February 2007); Tom K. Grimsrud, et al., "Exposure to Different Forms of Nickel and Risk of Lung Cancer," *American Journal of Epidemiology* (v.156/12, 2002); Inco, "History of the Port Colborne Refinery," www.inco.com (cited February 2007); Haitian Lu, et al., "Carcinogenic Effects of Nickel Compounds," Molecular and Cellular Biochemistry (v.279, 2005); Stephanie A. Navarro Silvera and Thomas E. Rohan, "Trace Elements and Cancer Risk: A Review of the Epidemiological Evidence," Cancer Causes and Control (v.18/1, 2007).

PREETI A. SUKERKAR
NORTHWESTERN UNIVERSITY

Niger

THIS WEST AFRICAN country was part of the Tuareg kingdom of Takedda and was a French colony from 1899 until it gained its independence August 3, 1960, as the Republic of Niger. It has a population of 13,957,000 (2005), with 3.5 doctors and 23 nurses per 100,000 people. An example of cancer incidence rates in Niger includes 78.3 cases of cancer in males per 100,000, according to the International Agency for Research on Cancer.

During the period of French colonial rule, formal healthcare and hospitals were limited to Niamey, the administrative capital, and major settlements. Medical care was largely available only to the European population and the local elite. There have been significant levels of liver cancer, prostate cancer, and skin cancer among men in Niger, with breast cancer and cervical cancer being the two most prevalent forms affecting women. The Faculty of Health Sciences at the Université de Niamey coordinates much of the medical research in Niger.

SEE ALSO: Breast Cancer; Cervical Cancer; Liver Cancer, Adult (Primary); Prostate Cancer; Skin Cancer (Melanoma); Skin Cancer (Non-Melanoma).

BIBLIOGRAPHY. A. Soyannwo and S.D. Amanor-Boadu, "Management of Cancer Pain—A Survey of Current Practice in West Africa," *The Nigerian Postgraduate Medical Journal* (v.8/4, 2001).

JUSTIN CORFIELD
GEELONG GRAMMAR SCHOOL, AUSTRALIA

Nigeria

THIS WEST AFRICAN country became a British protectorate in 1901. It gained its independence October 1, 1960, and was proclaimed a republic three years later. It has a population of 131,530,000 (2005), with 19 doctors and 66 nurses per 100,000 people.

An example of cancer incidence rates in Nigeria includes 90.7 cases of cancer in males per 100,000, according to the International Agency for Research on Cancer.

Traditional medical treatment in Nigeria involved herbal remedies and pastes, some of which remain quite effective, although they did not solve the problem of dealing with cancerous tumors.

The arrival of European slave traders massively disrupted local societies, with tens of thousands of slaves taken to the Americas. Foreign doctors arrived in the country, the most famous of whom was Mungo Park, who set the scene for British missionaries working in west Africa. By this time, with life-expectancy rates having declined massively, and with malaria and yellow fever devastating the Europeans, there was little concern about cancer.

Before the 20th century, the most prevalent forms of cancer among men were prostate cancer and liver cancer. For women, breast cancer and cervical cancer were the most prevalent. These cancers affected few people because of low life expectancy, however.

A recent study showed that breast cancer is the most common form of cancer in Nigeria (15.9 percent of all deaths from cancer), followed by cervical cancer (15.1 percent), prostate cancer (9.6 percent), liver cancer (8.8 percent), non-Hodgkin's lymphoma (6.6 percent), cancer of the colon and rectum (6.2 percent), Kaposi's sarcoma (4.6 percent), ovarian cancer (2.5 percent), and stomach cancer (2.3 percent).

The recent increase in Kaposi's sarcoma is largely because of a significant rise in human immunodeficiency virus (HIV) infections. Human T-cell leukemia–lymphoma virus is also prevalent in Nigeria.

The main cause of death from breast cancer is late diagnosis, as in many other developing countries. To attempt early mass screening, some regional projects have been launched, including a particularly successful one at Ladoke Akintola University Teaching Hospital in Osogbo.

Some research on cancer takes place at Bloom Cancer Care and Support Centre, Roc Aumadu Bello University Teaching Hospital, and University Hospital.

SEE ALSO: Breast Cancer; Cervical Cancer; Colon Cancer; Gastric (Stomach) Cancer; Infection (Childhood, Sexually Transmitted Infections, Hepatitis); Women's Cancers.

BIBLIOGRAPHY. A.O. Aderounmu, et al., "Knowledge, Attitudes and Practices of the Educated and Non-Educated Women to Cancer of the Breast in Semi-Urban and Rural Areas of SouthWest Nigeria," *Nigerian Postgraduate Medical Journal* (v.13/3, 2006); E.P. Gharoro, et al., "Carcinoma of the Cervix: Aspects of Clinical Presentation and Management in Benin City," *International Journal of Gynecology & Obstetrics* (v.67/1, 1999; Alan S. Rabson, et al. "Morphologic, Cytogenetic and Virologic Studies in Vitro of a Malignant Lymphoma from an African Child," *International Journal of Cancer* (v.1, 1966); Ralph Scram, *A History of Nigerian Health Services* (Ibadan University Press, 1971); T. F. Solanke, et al., Cancer in Nigeria— he Proceedings of the NCS Conference Held in December 1979 (Nigerian Cancer Society, 1982); A. Soyannwo and S.D. Amanor-Boadu, "Management of Cancer Pain—A Survey of Current Practice in West Africa," *The Nigerian Postgraduate Medical Journal* (v.8/4, 2001).

JUSTIN CORFIELD
GEELONG GRAMMAR SCHOOL, AUSTRALIA

Nixon, Richard (War on Cancer)

RICHARD MILHOUS NIXON was born January 9, 1913, in Yorba Linda, California, the son of Francis A. Nixon and Hannah (Milhous) Nixon. Two of his brothers died young from tuberculosis.

Nixon graduated from Duke University School of Law and then returned to California, where he practiced. During that time, he met and married Thelma (Pat), a high-school teacher.

After serving in the U.S. Navy during World War II, he was elected to the House of Representatives in 1946 and to the U.S. Senate in 1950. He was vice president from 1952 to 1960. After losing the 1960 presidential election to John F. Kennedy, Nixon was elected president in 1968. He served as president from 1969 until his resignation in 1974.

As president, Nixon was keen on using the resources of the United States to find a cure for cancer. In his State of the Union speech in January 1971, he made a special request that an additional $100 million be added to the National Cancer Institute budget for cancer research. This request led to the War on Cancer, although Nixon made very little mention of it in his memoirs, referring only to "improving health care."

His commitment was large, however. In October 1971 he converted the U.S. Army's Fort Detrick, Maryland, from a biological warfare facility to the

Frederick Cancer Research and Development Center, which eventually became an internationally recognized laboratory for research on cancer and acquired immunodeficiency syndrome (AIDS).

He signing the National Cancer Act into law December 23, 1971, declaring, "I hope in the years ahead we will look back on this action today as the most significant action taken during my administration."

The money that the Nixon administration spent on cancer treatment allowed scientists to develop massive research projects. A large number of new techniques were tried, and existing procedures were improved. Substantial numbers of the cancer specialists who initially received research grants from the War on Cancer program later were involved in many breakthroughs in treatment, although a single cure eluded them.

Nixon resigned as president and left office August 9, 1974. The funding for cancer research continued, however. His wife, Pat, a longtime heavy smoker, was diagnosed with lung cancer in December 1992. She died six months later. Nixon died April 22, 1994, after a stroke.

SEE ALSO: Government; National Cancer Institute; Tobacco Smoking.

BIBLIOGRAPHY. Richard Nixon, *The Memoirs* (Sidgwick & Jackson, 1978); Richard A. Rettig, *Cancer Crusade: The Story of the National Cancer Act of 1971* (iUniverse, Inc., 2005).

JUSTIN CORFIELD
GEELONG GRAMMAR SCHOOL, AUSTRALIA

Norris Cotton Cancer Center

THE NORRIS COTTON Cancer Center (NCCC) at Dartmouth Medical School in Lebanon, New Hampshire, is affiliated with Dartmouth Medical School, Dartmouth-Hitchcock Medical Center, and the National Cancer Institute (NCI).

Norris Cotton was a U.S. senator from New Hampshire from 1947 to 1974. In 1970 he secured federal funding to build the first regional cancer center in rural New England. The original center opened in 1972 as an underground, two-story building for radiation therapy and related laboratories. In 1973 Cotton obtained more federal support, this time for cancer research at Dartmouth Medical School.

In 1977, two more stories were added to the center, funded by the trustees of Mary Hitchcock Memorial Hospital. The NCI designated the center a Clinical Cancer Center in 1978 and a Comprehensive Cancer Care Center in 1990. The main campus is located in Lebanon. Additional facilities are located in Nashua and Manchester, New Hampshire; and in St. Johnsbury, Vermont. Several hospitals in New Hampshire and Vermont are also affiliated with the NCCC.

The NCCC offers care for breast, brain, colorectal, endocrinal (and thyroidal), esophageal, gynecological, head and neck, lung and chest, oral, pancreatic, pediatric, prostate, stomach, and urologic cancers, as well as for leukemia, lymphoma, melanoma, and sarcoma.

At the NCCC, a clinical oncology team of specialists works with each patient on an individual basis, along with his or her family and primary physician. A team is made up of oncologists, physicians, radiologists, surgeons, specialty nurses, and other professionals.

RESEARCH AND EDUCATION

Some of the research conducted at the center aims to identify factors in a patient's nutrition, environment, or lifestyle that may cause cancer; therefore, an important part of the NCCC practice is to educate members of the community about their risks and how to avoid risk factors. Research is also conducted to develop screening methods which can recognize the first stages of cancer. Another focus of research is to bring improved quality of life to cancer patients.

Several research programs are available at the NCCC: Cancer Control, Cancer Epidemiology and Chemoprevention, Cancer Mechanisms, Molecular Therapeutics, Immunology and Cancer Immunotherapy, and Radiobiology and Bioengineering.

Researchers at the NCCC are privy to shared resources that support their work. These resources include facilities and resources for behavioral science, bioinformatics, biostatistics, clinical and molecular pharmacology, flow cytometry and fluorescence imaging, glassware washing, hybridoma library/monoclonal antibody production, immune monitoring laboratory, irradiation, microarray, molecular biology and proteomics, research pathology, and transgenic mice, as well as a clinical research office.

Graduate students and postdoctoral fellows at Dartmouth University can receive education in cancer biology from clinicians at the NCCC. They can join research labs in basic, clinical, and prevention research. Programs include Autoimmunity/Connective Tissue Biology, Biochemistry and Molecular Biology of Protein Complexes, Cancer Biology and Carcinogenesis, and Immunobiology of Myeloid and Lymphoid Cells. There is a separate postdoctoral training program. Also, graduate and postdoctoral training is offered in cancer biology, supported by a training grant. The Hematology/Oncology Fellowship Program is a three-year program offered to medical fellows, whereby they gain certification in both fields.

Many clinical trials are under way at the NCCC at any time. Patients are extensively screened for eligibility to participate in the trials; furthermore, they receive counseling to prepare them to make the decision to participate.

In an effort to make cancer treatment as comfortable as possible for patients, the NCCC works with local physicians and specialists. An additional patient service is the Familial Cancer Program for members of families with a high history of cancer. Family-history analysis, risk assessment, genetic testing, and genetic counseling are provided, along with advice on cancer-prevention actions patients.

The NCCC has a Haelan Program for Supportive Services. In Old Gaelic, haelan means "to make whole or wholeness." Support is provided for patients and their family members as they deal with their cancer experiences. Core services are stress-reduction classes; seminars; massage; and Reiki, a therapy developed in Japan whereby energy is said to be channeled through the palms of the therapist into the patient. Haelan services are provided at little or no cost.

SEE ALSO: Alternative Therapy: Diet and Nutrition; Alternative Therapy: Alternative Therapy: Manual Healing and Physical Touch; Clinical Trials; National Cancer Institute.

BIBLIOGRAPHY. David Bognar and Walter Cronkite, *Cancer: Increasing Your Odds for Survival — A Resource Guide for Integrating Mainstream, Alternative, and Complementary Therapies* (Hunter House Publishers, 1998); James S. Gordon and Sharon Curtin, *Comprehensive Cancer Care: Integrating Alternative, Complementary, and Conventional Therapies* (HarperCollins Publishers, 2001); Patrick Quil-

lin, *Beating Cancer with Nutrition* (Nutrition Times Press, 2005); Natalie Davis Spingarn, An example of cancer incidence rates in Benin includes 89 cases of cancer in males per 100,000, according to the International Agency for Research on Cancer. (The Johns Hopkins University Press, 1999).

CLAUDIA WINOGRAD
UNIVERSITY OF ILLINOIS AT URBANA-CHAMPAIGN

North American Association of Central Cancer Registries

A NECESSITY FOR examining patient cancer histories to find trends and relevant associations is adequate registering of the data. A standardized method of recording allows clinicians and physicians to scan for relevant data from other institutions. The North American Association of Central Cancer Registries (NAACCR) establishes and enforces uniform protocols for registration of cancer data.

Organized in 1987, the NAACCR is an umbrella organization for U.S. cancer registries, government agencies, private groups, and professional associations. Members of the NAACCR are the central cancer registries of the United States and Canada.

The mission of the association is to "develop and promote uniform data standards for cancer registration; provide education and training; certify population-based registries; aggregate and publish data from central cancer registries; and promote the use of cancer surveillance data and systems for cancer control and epidemiologic research, public health programs, and patient care to reduce the burden of cancer in North America."

The NAACCR is a member of the International Association of Cancer Registries and is sponsored by several institutions, including the American Cancer Society and the National Cancer Registrars Association.

MEETINGS AND PROJECTS

The association holds an annual conference where member registries share strategies and information, and evaluate their compliance with the goals of the NAACCR. These goals are to provide standards for registration, to aid institutions in adopting these standards, to educate institutions in proper data recording and data management, to foster communication among member institutions, to monitor the registrations and give advice for improvement, to establish a set of criteria for registries to earn NAACCR accreditation, and to maintain the organization via establishing a functional infrastructure and financial security.

A major project of the NAACCR is to evaluate the safety and feasibility of maintaining online registries accessible by all members. This project, the NAACCR Call for Data, uses a secure portion of the Association's website. In 1997 the association established a Data Evaluation and Certification Committee, which reviews member registries annually. This review ensures each member's effective adherence to the registration standards established by the NAACCR.

Through its website, the NAACCR provides information to its members regarding proper data collection and recording. The site also provides information on practices to maintain strict patient confidentiality—an important duty of a cancer registry.

SEE ALSO: American Cancer Society; International Association of Cancer Registries; National Cancer Registrars Association (NCRA).

BIBLIOGRAPHY. Herman R. Menck, *Cancer Registry Management Principles and Practice* (Kendall/Hunt Publishing Co., 2004); R. Sankila, et al., *Evaluation of Clinical Care by Cancer Registries (IARC Technical Publication)* (International Agency for Research on Cancer, 2002).

CLAUDIA WINOGRAD
UNIVERSITY OF ILLINOIS AT URBANA-CHAMPAIGN

North Korea

THIS COUNTRY, OFFICIALLY known as the Democratic People's Republic of Korea, is located in northeast Asia. In 1910 the whole Korean peninsula was annexed by Japan, which occupied it until 1945. Following Japan's defeat in World War II, the Soviet Union took control of the northern part of the peninsula, and Kim Il Sung became head of state. In 1950 the Korean War broke out, and although an armistice was agreed on in 1953, no peace treaty has ever been signed.

Healthcare was minimal in Korea before 1945 except for the Korean elite, who were treated in Japanese-run hospitals. Many people relied on herbal cures, and some had access to spa baths and hot springs. There were some improvements from 1945 until 1950, but during the Korean War all cities in North Korea were destroyed by U.S. aerial bombing.

After January 1953, when healthcare was declared to be free to all, efforts were made to rebuild medical services. By the 1970s health services in North Korea were fairly good and were extolled heavily in government publications.

An example of cancer incidence rates in North Korea includes 285.7 cases of cancer in males per 100,000, according to the International Agency for Research on Cancer. Cigarette smoking is very common among men in North Korea. During the Japanese occupation of Korea, the manufacturing of cigarettes was a government monopoly, and this has continued under the North Korean government. With the massive increases in life expectancy during the 1970s and 1980s, it seems likely that the rate of lung cancer has become significant.

Little is known for certain about cancer care in North Korea, although it is known that selenium is used to treat some varieties. Kimchi, the traditional Korean dish made from cabbage and chili, is also believed to reduce the risk of contracting gastric cancer (as does red ginseng), but heavy consumption of it massively increases the risk of stomach cancer.

As in many countries, the healthcare system is considerably better in the nation's capital, Pyongyang, and in some other cities than in most of the countryside. The main hospital in Pyongyang is Red Cross General Hospital of Korea, and throughout the countryside are resorts located around hot springs that have provided health cures over several centuries. The main training hospital is attached to Pyongyang University of Medicine. Doctors at the Academy of Medical Science have been working on a cure for hepatic cancer.

Most of the information about the country that is available outside North Korea centers on the life of Kim Il Sung, the leader of the country from 1948 to his death in 1994. His third wife, Kim Jong-chul, died of breast cancer. He was succeeded in 1994 by Kim Jong Il, whose wife, Ko Yong-hi, also died of breast cancer.

SEE ALSO: Alternative Therapy; Asian Diet; Gastric (Stomach) Cancer; Liver Cancer, Adult (Primary); Lung Cancer,

Non-Small Cell; Lung Cancer, Small Cell; South Korea; Tobacco Smoking.

BIBLIOGRAPHY. "North Korean Leader Marries His Secretary," *The Age* (July 24, 2006); H.R. Shin, et al., "The Cancer-Preventive Potential of Panax Ginseng: A Review of Human and Experimental Evidence," *Cancer Causes Control* (v.11/6, 2000).

JUSTIN CORFIELD
GEELONG GRAMMAR SCHOOL, AUSTRALIA

Norway

THIS SCANDINAVIAN COUNTRY gained its independence from a union with Sweden in 1814 and became the kingdom of Norway. It was invaded by the Germans in 1940 and controlled by the pro-German government of Vidkum Quisling until 1945. It has a population of 4,667,000 (2006), with 413 doctors and 1,840 nurses per 100,000 people. An example of cancer incidence rates in Norway includes 311.5 cases of cancer in males per 100,000, according to the International Agency for Research on Cancer.

Cancer research and treatment in Norway are extensive, with Norwegians enjoying some of the best healthcare in the world. The collection of detailed information on all Norwegian cancer deaths since 1953 has allowed extensive treatment to be carried out for many people.

For men, lung and bronchial cancers are the most common form of cancer, accounting for 34.3 percent of all cases (1988–92 figures), although incidence fell dramatically, to 10 percent, for 30- to 54-year-olds from 1997 to 2001. This drop was attributed largely to a massive fall in the number of people smoking and early treatment. Melanoma of the skin accounts for 11 percent of cases.

For females, melanoma of the skin accounts for 23 percent of cases in 15- to 29-year-olds but for only 8 percent in those over 30, with breast cancer accounting for 37 percent of female cancer cases in that age group. Cervical cancer accounted for 8 percent of cancers among women.

The Norwegian Cancer Society was established in 1948 and has been heavily involved in raising money for cancer research. In 1951 it initiated the Cancer Registry of Norway, along with the Ministry of Health and Social Affairs, Norwegian Radium Hospital, and the Central Bureau of Statistics. The data collected are matched with other information to provide a detailed statistical breakdown of incidence of cancer in the country. The registry has been administered and funded by the Ministry of Health and Social Affairs since 1979. Cancer has claimed numerous famous people in Norway, including Princess Märtha of Sweden, crown princess of Norway; soccer player Roger Albertsen; and Johan Nygaardsvold, prime minister of Norway from 1935 to 1945. King Harald V sought hospital treatment in 2003 and 2004 for urinary cancer.

SEE ALSO: Breast Cancer; Cervical Cancer; Lung Cancer, Non-Small Cell; Lung Cancer, Small Cell; Skin Cancer (Melanoma); Smoking and Society.

BIBLIOGRAPHY. S. K. Helland, et al., "Carcinoid Tumours in the Gastrointestinal Tract—A Population-Based Study from Western Norway," *Scandinavian Journal of Surgery* (v.95/3, 2006); Sören Bloch Laache, *Norsk Medicin i Hundrede Aar* (Syeenske Bogtrykkeri, 1911); T.I. Nilsen, et al., "Recreational Physical Activity and Risk of Prostate Cancer: A Prospective Population-Based Study in Norway (The HUNT Study)," *International Journal of Cancer* (v.119/12, 2006); Cancer in Norway 2002, Cancer in Norway 2003, and Cancer in Norway 2004, www.kreftregisteret.no (cited November 2006).

JUSTIN CORFIELD
GEELONG GRAMMAR SCHOOL, AUSTRALIA

Novartis Group (Switzerland)

NOVARTIS GROUP (SWITZERLAND) is involved in research, development, manufacturing, and marketing of original and generic healthcare products.

Several antineoplastic agents are among Novartis' top-selling pharmaceuticals, including Gleevec/Glivec (imatinib mesylate), used in chronic myelogenous leukemia (CML) and gastrointestinal stromal tumors, with possible application in other types of cancer; Zometa (zoledronic acid), used in hypercalcemia of

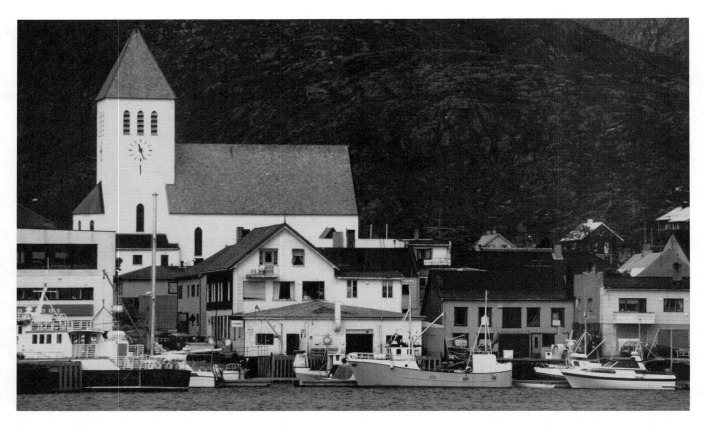

The tranquil life in a Norwegian harbor: Cancer research and treatment in Norway are extensive, with Norwegians enjoying some of the best healthcare in the world. For men, lung and bronchial cancers are the most common form of cancer cases.

malignancy, multiple myeloma, and bone metastases; Sandostatin/Sandostatin LAR (octreotide acetate), used in acromegaly and gastroenteropancreatic neuroendocrine tumors; and Femara (letrozole), used in estrogen-receptor-positive breast cancer.

Novartis' oncology-related portfolio accounts for 25 percent of all pharmaceutical sales. In addition to its cancer products, Novartis' best-known pharmaceuticals are used for organ transplantation; epilepsy; inflammatory bowel syndrome; and vascular, infectious, and neurodegenerative diseases.

Novartis Group was created in 1996 through the largest corporate merger in history, between Ciba-Geigy (Switzerland) and Sandoz (Switzerland), companies with history dating back to the 1800s. Novartis Group employs over 90,000 people and has research, development, and production sites in the European Union, Japan, and the United States, with additional production sites in Brazil and Turkey.

The first Sandoz-Ciba-Geigy group, Basler IG, was established in 1918 but disbanded in 1950. Basler's no-

table inventions included the insecticide dichloro-diphenyl-tricholorethane (DDT) and the psychotropic lysergic acid diethylamide (LSD). Novartis has four divisions: Pharmaceuticals, which develops prescription medications; Vaccines and Chiron Diagnostics, which develop vaccines and blood-testing equipment; Sandoz, which manufactures generic prescription medications; and Consumer Health, which develops nonprescription pharmaceuticals, nutraceuticals, Gerber baby products, and animal products.

Within the pharmaceutical division is an oncology and hematology department with centers in the European Union, Japan, and the United States. Most oncology projects focus on solid-tumor kinase inhibitors. Kinase inhibitors slow the growth of cells, especially rapidly dividing cells, by blocking enzymes crucial to cell functioning.

Gleevec, approved in 2001, is Novartis' second-best-selling pharmaceutical and was the fastest-approved cancer drug in U.S. history. Glivec is the international version. It was the first specific tyrosine kinase inhibitor, targeting an enzyme characteristic of CML rather than inhibiting all cells that divide rapidly. Zometa, approved in 2001 and Novartis' third-best-selling pharmaceutical, is a bisphophonate that slows the abnormal growth or destruction of bone. Other Novartis oncology products include the bisphosphonate Aredia (pamidronate disodium); Desferal (deferioxamine mesylate), and Exjade (deferasirox), used to reduce iron overload due to blood transfusions; Navoban (tropisetron), which prevents chemotherapy-induced nausea and vomiting; Cibacalcin (synthetic human calcitonin), used in Paget's disease of bone; and Lentaron (formestane) and Orimeten (aminglutethimide), used in breast and prostate cancers.

By 2010 Novartis plans to offer several antineoplastics, including PTK787 (vatalanib) for colorectal cancer; AMN107 (nilotinib) for imatinib-resistant CML; and EPO906 (patupilone), RAD001 (everolimus), and LBQ707 (gimatecan) for solid tumors, such as lung, breast, colorectal, and prostate cancers.

SEE ALSO: Breast Cancer; Chemotherapy; Chiron (United States); Colon Cancer; Leukemia, Chronic Myelogenous; Lung Cancer, Non-Small Cell; Lung Cancer, Small Cell; Myeloma, Multiple; Pharmaceutical Industry; Prostate Cancer; Rectal Cancer.

BIBLIOGRAPHY. "Novartis," www.novartis.com (cited 2007).

RISHI RATTAN
COLLEGE OF MEDICINE
UNIVERSITY OF ILLINOIS, CHICAGO

Novo Nordisk (Denmark)

NOVO NORDISK (DENMARK), based in Bagsværd, Denmark, produces pharmaceuticals for diabetes care and also works with cancer pharmaceuticals. Novo Nordisk (NN) provides products for insulin delivery, growth-hormone therapy, hormone-replacement therapy, and homeostasis management. As of 2007 the company had facilities in 79 nations and provided products to nearly 200 countries. Pharmaceutical production is carried out in six countries; the U.S. operations take place in Princeton, New Jersey.

The company stresses decency and ethics in all its activities, and aims to lead pharmaceutical companies in socially responsible behaviors. This aim is reflected in the company charter, which outlines the values that all employees are expected to hold.

In its Research and Development division, NN focuses on cancer and immunobiology. Scientists at NN are experts in both fields, as well as molecular and cellular biology. Close collaborations with other divisions and scientists enable the company to make rapid progress from a molecular or cellular discovery to drug development. An important avenue of research on the safety and efficacy of drugs for cancer therapy is the clinical trial. NN maintains two public registries of its clinical-trial work; one registry discloses all clinical trials under way, and the second provides the results of those trials to the public.

NN operates the Hemophilia Foundation, established in 2005, to address the global need for improved hemophilia care. The foundation is based in Zurich, Switzerland.

SEE ALSO: Clinical Trials; Denmark; Experimental Cancer Drugs.

BIBLIOGRAPHY. Ahmed F. Abdel-Magid and Stephane Caron, *Fundamentals of Early Clinical Drug Development: From Synthesis Design to Formulation* (Wiley-Interscience, 2006); Anne Clayton, *Insight into a Career in Pharmaceutical Sales* (Pharmaceuticalsales.com, Inc., 2005); Rick Ng, *Drugs—From Discovery to Approval* (Wiley-Liss, 2004); Adriana Petryna, et al., *Global Pharmaceuticals: Ethics, Markets, Practices* (Duke University Press, 2006).

CLAUDIA WINOGRAD
UNIVERSITY OF ILLINOIS AT URBANA-CHAMPAIGN

Nuclear Industry

FISSION OCCURS WHEN a neutron hits a large atomic nucleus such as uranium-235 or plutonium-239. The nucleus splits into at least two smaller nuclei, releasing energy as well as additional neutrons that go on to hit other nuclei.

Fusion takes place when small nuclei such as the hydrogen isotopes deuterium and tritium combine under high temperature and pressure to form heavier nuclei, also releasing energy. The nuclear industry employs nuclear fission and fusion in two major areas: weapons and power generation.

Radioactivity is measured in becquerels (Bq), which denote nuclear decays per second. An absorbed radiation dose is measured in grays (Gy); a gray is equal to 1 joule of energy absorbed by 1 Kg of tissue (1 Gy = 100 rad). The biological impact depends on the type of radiation, the location of the absorption, and the duration of the exposure. The equivalent dose is measured in sieverts (Sv), with the same units as the gray (related by a dimensionless radiation-weighting factor). A large dose of radiation within a brief time can cause acute radiation syndrome, which is also known as radiation poisoning or radiation sickness. Light radiation poisoning (about 2 Sv) causes death within 30 days for 10 percent of victims, a lifetime risk of solid cancer of about 20 percent (roughly half of which will be terminal), and a lifetime risk of death from leukemia of 1 percent.

Childhood exposure may double these risks; in particular, children under 5 years old are more than five times more likely than adults to get thyroid cancer. Acute radiation poisoning (over 6 Sv) results in death after 14 days for close to 100 percent of victims. The thyroid gland takes up much of the iodine ingested or inhaled by the body; radioactive iodine, which is a common product of fission, can cause hypothyroidism and thyroid cancer.

Nuclear weapons are explosives that generate their destructive power from uncontrolled nuclear fission or fusion, enabling weapons far more powerful than those made of conventional explosives. Nuclear weapons based on fission are known as A-bombs or atomic bombs; those based on fusion are known as H-bombs, hydrogen bombs, or thermonuclear bombs. When a nuclear weapon explodes, about 50 percent of the total energy is released in the blast. Thermal radiation due to infrared heat radiation accounts for about 40 percent, and ionizing and residual radiation each account for about 5 percent. The primary blast and thermal radiation effects are similar to the mechanisms of conventional explosives but are far more intense; they account for most of the casualties.

The greatest hazard of exposure to ionizing radiation from a large nuclear detonation is caused by fallout: airborne radioactive dust particles 10 nm to 20 μm in diameter. The volume of fallout is proportional to the proximity of the detonation to the ground surface. The dust is carried worldwide by atmospheric winds and may take weeks to years to settle to the ground. Fallout can cause immediate external radiation exposure as well as long-term cumulative internal exposure through contaminated food and water. Atmospheric nuclear tests at the Nevada Test Site have resulted in per-capita thyroid doses across the continental United States ranging from 1 mGy to 100 mGy, depending on location, with a median of 30 mGy. Worldwide atmospheric nuclear testing has resulted in a 5 μSv annual average equivalent dose.

The countries known to have nuclear capability are France, India, North Korea, Pakistan, the People's Republic of China, the Russian Federation (formerly the Soviet Union), the United Kingdom, and the United States. Israel is believed to have nuclear weapons, and South Africa developed nuclear capability but gave it up in the 1990s.

The only hostile uses of nuclear weapons to date were the bombings of Hiroshima and Nagasaki, Japan, by the United States during World War II. In the immediate aftermath 100,000 to 200,000 people died from physical injuries and radiation poisoning. By 1990 hundreds of survivors were known to have died from cancer attributable to radiation exposure.

Dirty bombs, or radiological dispersal devices, are weapons that combine radioactive material with conventional explosives to spread the radioactive material over a wide area. In most cases, however, these devices would be unlikely to cause serious illness or death; consequently, they are considered to be primarily terror weapons.

In 1995 Chechnyan rebels planted a dirty bomb in Moscow, using Caesium-137 from equipment used for treating cancer. They alerted the media without exploding the bomb. In 1998 the Chechen Security Service found and defused a dirty bomb concealed near a railway line in a suburban area 16 km east of the capital.

In 2003 British intelligence determined from evidence found in Afghanistan that Al-Qaeda had constructed a small dirty bomb, but it has not been found. This finding was confirmed by captured Al-Qaeda member Abu Zubaydah.

In 2004 Al-Qaeda member Dhiren Barot was arrested in the United Kingdom and pleaded guilty to plotting to attack the New York Stock Exchange, the International Monetary Fund headquarters, and the World Bank with dirty bombs.

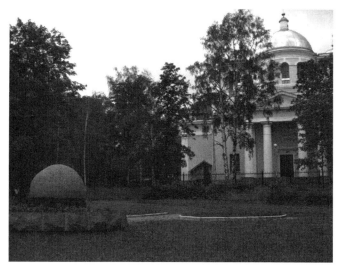

The Cathedral of Alexander Nevsky, with a monument to victims of Chernobyl, in Petrozavodsk, Russia.

POWER GENERATION

Nuclear power generation is the use of a nuclear reactor to release energy in the form of heat from a controlled fission chain reaction using fuel such as uranium-235. This reaction is consequently converted to propulsion by boiling water in a steam turbine. The propulsion may be used directly or to generate electricity. In a uranium reactor, neutrons released through fission travel too fast to sustain the reaction by reliably initiating fission when they hit other uranium-235 nuclei. Consequently, the fission reaction is controlled by slowing these neutrons with moderating materials such as water and graphite control rods. If the temperature of a water moderator rises, its density decreases, reducing the slowing of the neutrons and stabilizing the reaction. Highly enriched uranium or plutonium can be used in fast neutron reactors, which raise the likelihood of fission from fast neutrons by using fuel with a high density of fissile material; the reactions are also controlled by slowing the neutrons with control rods. Nuclear fission was first performed experimentally in Berlin in 1938. The first self-sustaining chain reaction took place in Chicago in 1942. The first reactors were built to create plutonium for weapons like the bomb detonated over Nagasaki.

A nuclear reactor was first used for electricity generation in Idaho in 1951, producing about 100 kW. A 5 MW nuclear power plant in Obninsk in the Soviet Union was the first to provide electricity to a power grid. The first commercial nuclear power generation began in a 50 MW power station in Sellafield, England, in 1956. The first commercial nuclear power plant in the United States opened in Shippingport, Pennsylvania, in 1958. With an installed capacity of 356 GW in 2004, nuclear power today provides 16 percent of the world's domestic electricity production. Thirty countries operate over 400 nuclear reactors. The United States uses most nuclear power, generating 20 percent of its electricity in 104 nuclear power stations for a total of 97.4 GW. The country with the highest proportion is France, which generates 80 percent of its electricity through nuclear power. Over 200 large military submarines and ships such as aircraft carriers and icebreakers use nuclear power plants for propulsion. The use of nuclear power eliminates the need to refuel. Submarines also gain the key advantage of not having to surface regularly to recharge batteries. Rather than employ a reactor, some inaccessible systems such as satellites, space probes, and remote facilities such as unmanned lighthouses use a radioactive power source (typically, plutonium oxide) that gives off heat as it decays naturally. Then the heat is converted to electricity via thermocouples. These power sources can last for decades: Voyager 1, which was launched in 1977 and is now farther from the Sun than any other known solar-system object, was still operating in 2006.

REACTOR ACCIDENTS

Commercial-grade nuclear fuel is insufficiently enriched to cause a nuclear explosion, although if control systems fail catastrophically, a nuclear meltdown may release radioactive products of fission into the environment if the melted, overheated fuel escapes the containment building.

The world's first serious nuclear-reactor accident occurred in Windscale (now also known as Sellafield) in the United Kingdom when the graphite core of a plutonium production reactor caught fire during a maintenance procedure, releasing an estimated 750 TBq of radioactive contamination into the area. There were no immediate casualties. Milk from the surrounding 500 km2 of countryside was destroyed for the following month to prevent the ingestion of radioactive iodine.

The worst nuclear-power accident in the United States occurred in 1979 after a pressurized water reactor at the Three Mile Island Nuclear Generating Station in Pennsylvania experienced a failure of its secondary cooling system pumps. Subsequent operator error led to a loss of coolant and meltdown of about half the core. About 480 PBq of radioactive gas was released into the atmosphere but virtually no radioactive iodine. The largest dose received by any individual was estimated to be 1 mSv. There were no immediate casualties. The projected number of long-term fatalities due to cancer caused by the accident was roughly one.

The worst nuclear-power accident in history happened in 1986 at the Chernobyl Nuclear Power Plant in Ukraine, when operator error during a safety system test led to a steam explosion. The explosion destroyed the top of the reactor and blew off the roof, leading to a graphite fire and the subsequent meltdown of the core. Roughly 10 EBq of radioactive material was released. Fallout spread across the western Soviet Union and Europe, reaching eastern North America. Roughly 60 percent fell in Belarus, with much of Ukraine and Russia also badly contaminated. Subsequently, 336,000 people were evacuated from the region; they had received on average a dose of 33 mSv over the six months following the accident, and some residents received several hundred mSv. A total of 237 people were hospitalized with acute radiation poisoning, of whom 28 died. Three others died of other causes. Nearly 5,000 cases of childhood thyroid cancer have subsequently been reported in Belarus and Ukraine; at least 15 were fatal. Most of these cases are attributable to the accident; however, no other attributable cases of radiation-induced disease are known. The increase in cancer mortality for the 600,000 most highly exposed people is expected to be less than 4 percent; for the next 5 million. it is expected to be less than 1 percent. The increase in total lifetime cancer rates for the wider European population is expected to be 0.01 percent.

SEE ALSO: Electrical Industry; Neutrons; Radiation; Radiation, Gamma; Radiation, Ionizing; Radiation Therapy; Thyroid Cancer; Thyroid Cancer, Childhood.

BIBLIOGRAPHY. United Nations Scientific Committee, "Report of the United Nations Scientific Committee on the Effects of Atomic Radiation to the General Assembly," *Sources and Effects of Ionizing Radiation, vol. II* (United Nations, 2000); International Atomic Energy Agency, "Revisiting Chernobyl: 20 Years Later", www.iaea.org/NewsCenter/Focus/Chernobyl (cited February 2006); International Atomic Energy Agency, "IAEA Publications on Accident Response," www-pub.iaea.org/MTCD/publications/accres.asp (cited February 2006).

MICHAEL R. BAX
STANFORD UNIVERSITY

NYU Cancer Institute

THE NEW YORK University (NYU) Cancer Institute is part of the NYU Medical Center, an academic medical center in the borough of Manhattan in New York City consisting of the NYU School of Medicine and the NYU Hospitals Center. NYU is one of the largest private universities in the United States, with six major centers in New York City, including a main campus in Manhattan.

Outpatient cancer care is provided primarily at the NYU Clinical Cancer Center, which offers cancer-prevention, screening, diagnostic, treatment, and support services, as well as genetic counseling. Treatment provided onsite includes radiation treatment and infusion, injection, and transfusion services. The Center for Women's Cancers at the Clinical Cancer Center includes a dedicated imaging center for radiological procedures, facilities for fine-needle biopsies, a breast-cancer center, a gynecological cancer-care center, and a boutique offering goods and services for women who are undergoing chemotherapy or have had breast surgery. Psychological support services are available, including relaxation workshops; support groups; a creative-arts studio; a drop-in nutrition workshop; smoking-cessation programs; and Look Good . . . Feel Better, a program of the American Cancer Society that helps women maintain their appearance and self-image during chemotherapy and radiation treatments. Support groups are also available for caregivers of cancer patients.

The Lynn Cohen Cancer Screening and Prevention Project for High Risk Women identifies women who have increased risk of women's cancers and offers them early-detection and prevention services. Initial program services are available at no cost. The Cancer Awareness Network for Immigrant Minority Populations, offered in conjunction with the Center for Immigrant Health at NYU, focuses on improving cancer control and outreach activities for members of immigrant groups in the metropolitan area, including immigrants from Korea, China, the Caribbean, and Latin America (primarily Mexico, Guatemala, Ecuador, and Peru). The program focuses on lung cancer, prostate cancer, breast cancer, and cervical cancer.

Research at the NYU Cancer Institute is organized into six scientific research programs: Stem Cell Biology, Cancer Epidemiology and Prevention, Cancer Immunology, Cancer Neurobiology, Environmental and Molecular Carcinogenesis, and Growth Control. In addition, 11 shared core facilities support multiple research programs.

The Stem Cell Biology program is located in the Helen and Martin Kimmel Center for Stem Cell Biology, established in January 2005. The center's mission is to establish a multidisciplinary research center on the basic biology of stem cells in animal models, with the ultimate goal of translating those findings to human embryonic stem-cell research and ultimately creating advanced therapies for human disease.

The Cancer Epidemiology and Prevention program focuses on population research, with the mission of identifying cancer risk factors and developing strategies to reduce their impact and complications. Major research projects include the NYU Women's Health Study, a cohort of 14,000 women followed for 17 years, with particular emphasis on studying breast cancer; and the National Ovarian Cancer Early Detection Program, one of the largest and most comprehensive ovarian-cancer early-detection programs in the world. Program members also conduct research studies on topics such as oral cancer among south Indians who use smokeless tobacco and the usefulness of pregnancy hormonal profiles in assessing breast-cancer risk.

The Cancer Immunology program focuses on understanding immune responses to tumors, and on how those responses may be generated and augmented to be used to inhibit tumor growth. Vaccines currently being evaluated through the program include a dendritic cell vaccine to prevent the recur- rence of melanoma and a vaccine for follicular lymphoma in first remission.

The Cancer Neurobiology program studies brain tumors, including the genetic changes and signal transduction pathways that are responsible for their progression. Areas of focus include the molecular events involved in brain-tumor generation, invasion, and angiogenesis, with the long-term goal of facilitating translational research.

The Environmental and Molecular Carcinogenesis program studies the influence of environmental exposure to carcinogens on the development or inhibition of cancer and methods of preventing exposures that are risk factors for cancer. Program research is conducted in three categories: carcinogenesis and chemoprevention; DNA damage, repair, and mutagenesis; and gene regulation and signal transduction.

The Growth Control program studies intracellular signaling molecules, which regulate cell proliferation, and how perturbations in those processes contribute to cellular transformation. This knowledge is necessary for understanding how a normal cell is transformed into a malignant cell, which facilitates translational research and the development of new cancer therapies.

SEE ALSO: Breast Cancer; Breast Cancer and Pregnancy; Disparities, Issues in Cancer; Education, Cancer; Smokeless Tobacco; Vaccines; Women's Cancers.

BIBLIOGRAPHY. The National Ovarian Cancer Early Detection Program website, www.med.nyu.edu/nocedp (cited December 2006); NYU Cancer Institute website, www.med.nyu.edu/nyuci (cited December 2006); NYU School of Medicine Center for Immigrant Health website, www.med.nyu.edu/cih (cited December 2006); NYU Women's Health Study website, www.med.nyu.edu/womensheathstudy (cited December 2006).

SARAH BOSLAUGH
WASHINGTON UNIVERSITY SCHOOL OF MEDICINE

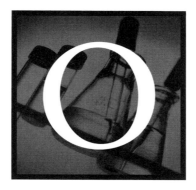

Obesity

THE RISING WEIGHT of the world's population has represented improved health for many centuries. It remained so throughout most of the 20th century until excess body weight started to signify a threat to population health. Steady rises in average body size and obesity rates became a widespread phenomenon in both developed and less-developed regions. At the forefront of this "epidemic" is the United States, where 23.9 percent of adults were obese in 2005—an increase of about 50 percent from the 1995 level (15.6 percent). High prevalence and/or increasing incidence of obesity have also occurred in Eastern Europe, Central and South America (e.g., Argentina, Chile, and Mexico), parts of Western Europe (e.g., the United Kingdom, Germany, Spain, and Finland), the Caribbean, and Southeast Asia.

Fundamentally, excess weight gain occurs when calories consumed exceed calories expended. The various social, economic, and technological characteristics of today's way of living cultivate an environment that encourages such net surplus of energy. Less activity (e.g., sedentary work and transportation, television viewing) and more intake (e.g., large portion sizes, consumption of snacks, consumption of sugar-sweetened beverages) explain the parallel movement of industrialization and obesity.

Health systems around the world are gradually comprehending the sizable burden attributable to obesity, predominantly from diabetes and cardiovascular diseases. Nonetheless, a growing body of evidence since the 1970s establishes a direct association between obesity and cancer. After smoking and alcohol use, overweight/obesity constitutes the third-most-important cause of cancer death—about 2 percent of the 139,000 cancer deaths worldwide. In the United States excess weight was responsible for about 41,000 new cancer cases in 2002—14 percent of all cancer deaths among men and 20 percent of all cancer deaths among women.

The most widely used indicator of adiposity is body mass index (BMI), defined as body weight in kilograms divided by the square of height in meters (kg/m²). The World Health Organization defines normal weight as a BMI between 18.5 and 25, underweight as a BMI below 18.5, overweight as a BMI between 25 and 30, and obese as a BMI above 30. Therefore, a 6-foot-tall individual would be classified as overweight at 184 pounds and as obese at 221 pounds. BMI is widely adopted because it expresses weight adjusted for height, is easy to measure, and is highly correlated with adiposity and disease risks. Nevertheless, BMI is an indirect measure of adiposity because a single BMI value can reflect various degrees of fat versus lean mass—a ratio that varies largely by race, sex, and age. Hence, waist circumference, waist-to-hip ratio (WHR), and the ratio of subscapular to triceps skinfold thickness (S/T ratio) are important in assessing central (visceral) adiposity in addition to overall body size. Accurate but costly measures such as duel-energy X-ray absorptiometry, computed tomography (CT) scans, and magnetic resonance imaging (MRI) are sometimes used in larger-scale studies.

Although randomized trials may provide the best data, studying the link between weight and cancer requires long follow-up and large sample size. Hence, observational studies constitute the core knowledge base on such an association. Several methodological considerations are related to the design and interpretation of these studies. Many factors that are associated with weight are themselves linked to cancer. Failure or incomplete control of these factors confounds the true obesity–cancer relation. Smoking, diet, and physical activity are great examples.

A related issue, often referred to as reverse causation, arises when the direction of causality is unclear. Preclinical cancer may cause weight loss and reduce physical activity rather than the converse, for example, though these mechanisms may be indistinguishable from the data. Further, most studies quantify the difference in cancer risk between obese and nonobese individuals. A conclusion that weight loss can lead to risk reduction should be drawn cautiously. Finally, generalizing study results to a different population can be problematic—not particularly due to genetics but to the strong interaction between body weight and lifestyle factors such as diet and socioeconomic status.

CANCER RISK

Despite methodological challenges, a sufficiently large number of studies consistently shows an association between excess adiposity and cancers of the colon, breast (in postmenopausal women), esophagus, endometrium, and kidney (renal cell). Some evidence also suggests that cancers of the liver, gallbladder, and pancreas; some cancers of blood cells; and aggressive prostate cancer may be related to obesity. On the other hand, obesity is occasionally found to be protective. Before menopause, heavier women appear to experience modest protection from breast cancer compared with leaner women. Lung cancer is also less prevalent among obese individuals, though some investigators speculate that this finding is biased by smoking-related metabolic changes or weight loss due to undetected diseases.

The mechanisms by which obesity induces or promotes carcinogenesis vary by cancer site. The most frequently postulated mechanisms are insulin resistance and altered levels of circulating estrogens.

Adipose tissue regulates the release of free fatty acids and other peptides to modulate energy balance and lipid metabolism. Insulin resistance develops as a metabolic adaptation to free fatty acids, especially from intra-abdominal fat. To compensate, the pancreas increases insulin secretion, resulting in hyperinsulinemia—elevated blood insulin level. Mounting evidence suggests that chronic hyperinsulinemia promotes cancers of the colon and endometrium, and probably other tumors. Adipose tissues and insulin also regulate sex hormones. Excess adiposity, especially in the form of abdominal fat, increases the level of estrogens with insufficient counterbalance from progesterone, which likely leads to the increased risks of cancers of the breast (in postmenopausal women), endometrium, and probably colon.

Following is a brief summary of what is currently known about the association between adiposity and selected cancers.

High BMI increases the incidence of breast cancer among postmenopausal women, whereas heavier premenopausal women have a lower risk (relative risk about 0.7). This relationship remains even after adjusting for known confounders such as physical activity and parity. Poorer detection of small tumors in breasts of leaner women offers only partial, rather than sufficient, explanation for the protective effect in heavier premenopausal women.

The heaviest quarter of postmenopausal women experience a 40 percent greater risk for breast cancer. Substantial weight gain throughout adulthood is also found to increase postmenopausal breast cancer, particularly among those who never used hormone replacement therapy (HRT). Specifically, elevated risk for breast cancer among heavier women is found only for tumors with positive estrogen (ER) and progesterone (PgR) receptors. These findings support the hypothesis that the effect of adiposity on breast cancer is largely driven by endogenous estrogen production.

BMI also affects breast-cancer prognosis, though the effect is generally limited to the early stages (stage I and II) and greatly depends on ER- and PgR-positive status. The risk of recurrence and the risk of dying from breast cancer, on the other hand, are consistently higher among obese women regardless of menopausal status.

Almost all colorectal cancers arise from the precancerous lesions of the colonic epithelium called adenomas; the process takes 10 to 15 years. It is believed that body fatness influences multiple stages of the cancer-forming process, including formation, promotion, and progression. Obesity is associated by a similar magnitude with higher incidence of both colorectal cancer and adenomas. However, the association is stronger for larger adenomas than for smaller adenomas, suggesting that the effect related to adiposity acts predominantly on adenoma growth and promotion to cancer. Further, the association between obesity and colorectal neoplasm is consistently stronger in men (relative risk about 1.5 to 2.0) than in women (relative risk about 1.2 to 1.5), which suggests a likely role of estrogens. The link between adiposity and cancer is more consistent across studies for distal colon than for proximal colon; rectal cancer, however, has shown little evidence of an association with BMI.

Studies conducted in different countries found higher incidence and mortality from renal-cell carcinoma among heavier men and women. Heaviest individuals are found to face risks 1.6 to 2.6 times higher than those of normal weight. A meta-analysis that included 11 studies estimated that for each unit of increase in BMI, the risk of renal-cell cancer increases by 6 percent to 7 percent.

The carcinogenetic effect of BMI is partially mediated through hypertension and diabetes, which are well-established risk factors for renal-cell cancer and closely linked with obesity. However, obesity remains a risk factor independent of blood pressure, indicating that excess adiposity might act on the carcinogenesis pathway through multiple mechanisms. The risk for cancer of the renal pelvis, however, is not affected by body size.

The positive association between BMI and esophageal cancer is limited to adenocarcinoma of the distal esophagus or gastric cardia—the area surrounding the junction of the esophagus and the stomach. Other forms of cancer, such as squamous cell carcinoma, represent biologically different malignancies, and to date no association with obesity has been reported.

In the largest cohort study, conducted in Sweden, the heaviest 20 percent of all subjects experienced a 60 percent to 140 percent higher incidence of cancer. A

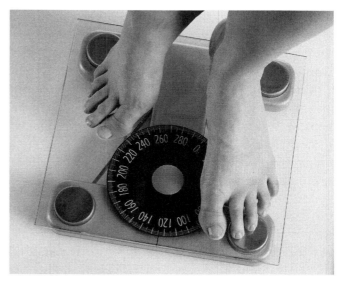

Cancers of the liver, gallbladder, and pancreas; some cancers of the blood cells; and aggressive prostate cancer may be related to obesity.

frequently proposed mechanism is the higher prevalence of gastroesophageal reflux among obese individuals.

Adult overweight/obesity is associated with a twofold to threefold higher risk of endometrial cancer. Studies conducted in North America, Europe, and Asia consistently found a linear increase in endometrial-cancer risk in the presence of significant adult weight gain, irrespective of other risk factors, such as age, HRT use, parity, and cigarette smoking. The increase in risk is stronger among older women and likely additive to the effect of HRT.

Whether central obesity independently raises endometrial-cancer risk beyond BMI is still inconclusive. The lack of definite evidence linking waist circumference or WHR to cancer incidence after controlling for BMI suggests that any added adiposity during adulthood plays a more crucial role than abdominal fat alone.

PREVENTIVE CARE AND WEIGHT MANAGEMENT

As obesity gradually becomes a social phenomenon, often intertwined with other health behaviors, the impact of body size on health may go beyond biology. Weight status increasingly appears in the disparity literature as a possible determinant of access to, and use of, preventive services. Despite their higher risk, obese women in the United States are less likely to undergo screening for breast, colorectal, and cervical cancer, even after adjusting for other known barriers such as income and insurance. This screening disparity is often found in white and sometimes Hispanic women but not in black women or men.

Various explanations have been postulated, such as competing medical priorities, patient reluctance, general health consciousness, and technical difficulties. This area awaits further research to shed light on approaches for improving the delivery of cancer-prevention services.

Although most Americans are aware of the better-known health risks associated with weight gain, weight management receives little attention as a cancer-control strategy. In fact, a recent survey showed that only about 25 percent of individuals know that obesity is also a cancer risk. The International Agency for Research on Cancer and many cancer societies recommend avoiding excess weight gain by establishing habits of healthy eating and performing physical activity for its multiple health benefits, including decreasing the risk of cancer.

SEE ALSO: Diet and Nutrition; Exercise (Lack of); Sedentary Occupations; Western Diet.

BIBLIOGRAPHY. International Agency for Research on Cancer, *IARC Handbook of Cancer Prevention Vol. 6, Weight Control and Physical Activity* (IARC Press, 2002); G. Bray and C. Bouchard, eds., *Handbook of Obesity: Etiology and Pathophysiology* (Marcel Dekker, 2004). T. Byers, et al., "American Cancer Society Guidelines on Nutrition and Physical Activity for Cancer Prevention: Reducing the Risk of Cancer with Healthy Food Choices and Physical Activity," *CA: A Cancer Journal for Clinicians* (v.52, 2002).

Y. Claire Wang
Harvard School of Public Health

Ohio State University Comprehensive Cancer Center

THE OHIO STATE University Comprehensive Cancer Center (OSUCCC) is located in Columbus and affiliated with Ohio State University (OSU). It is a network of 7 interdisciplinary programs, including more than 240 members drawn from 14 colleges at OSU as well as affiliated institutions, including Columbus Children's Hospital and Cincinnati Children's Hospital Medical Center. The OSUCCC has been a National Cancer Institute–designated Comprehensive Cancer Center since 1976; this designation was renewed most recently in 2004.

The mission of the OSUCCC is to reduce cancer morbidity and mortality through conducting basic and clinical research; translate research results to patient care; provide detection, treatment, and rehabilitation services; increase public awareness about cancer; advance the education of healthcare professionals; and promote public-policy changes to improve cancer prevention, detection, and treatment.

The OSUCCC received almost $70 million in research funding in 2003 and 2004. Research OSUCCC is organized into six programs: Cancer Control, Experimental Therapeutics, Immunology, Molecular Biology and Cancer Genetics, Molecular Carcinogenesis and Chemoprevention, and Viral Oncogenesis.

The Cancer Control program conducts research aimed at reducing cancer incidence, morbidity, and mortality. Research concentrates on underserved and minority populations, communication studies, and behavioral-change strategies. The Center for Population Health and Disparities program, part of the Cancer Control program, focuses on health disparities in the Appalachian area of Ohio.

The Experimental Therapeutics program focuses on three areas of research: the mechanisms by which epigenetic alterations contribute to the genesis and chemoresistance of cancer, and the exploitation of such alterations clinically; the use of monoclonal antibody therapy to enhance cell susceptibility to cancer chemotherapy; and the use of novel chemotherapeutic combinations to target survival and chemotherapy resistance pathways in cancer cells.

The Immunology program also focuses on three areas of research: T-cell recognition and cancer therapy, antibody-based cancer therapy, and natural killer cell biology.

The Molecular Biology and Cancer Genetics program focuses on the association between genes and cancer and the exploitation of this association to reduce cancer mortality. Specific aims are to identify genes that predispose individuals to cancer, either through mutations or epigenetic mechanisms; to determine the molecular mechanisms underlying the expression and functions of genes contributing to normal and cancer development; and to promote clinical applications of gene identification for cancer diagnosis, prognosis, surveillance, prevention, and treatment.

The Molecular Carcinogenesis and Chemoprevention program focus on four primary areas: characterization of molecular and cellular changes that contribute to neoplastic transformation and carcinogenesis; development and characterization of novel agents for cancer chemoprevention, and study of their safety, efficacy, and mechanisms of effect; identification of dietary and nutritional components that enhance or inhibit carcinogenesis; and implementation of cancer-prevention studies in humans, emphasizing those at greatest risk due to genetic predisposition, presence of premalignant lesions, or exposure to carcinogens.

The Pediatric Oncology program focuses on children with cancer and blood diseases. The program studies pediatric leukemia/lymphoma gene/cellular therapies, pediatric sarcoma cell signaling, and cancer biology and the microenvironment.

The Viral Oncogenesis program engages in collaborative research to discover mechanisms of virus-related neoplastic disease, identify potential therapeutic agents, and develop novel therapies. The program has three focus areas: discerning molecular and cellular mechanisms associated with HLTV-1 (human lymphotropic virus type I), developing therapeutic virus vectors, and studying lymphoma associated with the Epstein-Barr virus.

The C. James Cancer Hospital and Solove Research Institute, the only freestanding cancer hospital in the Midwest, is the primary location for patient care delivery. Outpatient care is provided at several other locations in the Columbus area, and James Hospital collaborates with other institutions in Ohio, including the Genesis Cancer Unit in Zanesville and the Holzer Center for Cancer Care in Gallipolis.

The hospital provides support groups, services, and classes for cancer patients and their families. Support groups are available for patients with brain tumors, head and neck cancer, leukemia and lymphoma, sarcomas, prostate cancer, and gynecological cancers; there are also groups for families of individuals who are in cancer treatment or have completed treatment. Other services include massage therapy and music therapy. Specialized programs are available for children with cancer or who have family members with

cancer. Classes offered include the Look Good…Feel Better program, which helps women manage their appearance during cancer treatment; the Prepared Family Caregiver program for individuals who will be providing home care for members of their families; and smoking-cessation classes.

SEE ALSO: Cervical Cancer; Disparities, Issues in Cancer; Education, Cancer; Screening (Cervical and Breast and Colon Cancers); Screening, Access to; Smoking and Society; Tobacco Smoking.

BIBLIOGRAPHY. The Ohio State University Comprehensive Cancer Center website, www.osuccc.osu.edu (cited December 2006).

SARAH BOSLAUGH
WASHINGTON UNIVERSITY SCHOOL OF MEDICINE

OHSU Cancer Institute

THE OREGON HEALTH and Science University (OHSU) Cancer Institute is part of Oregon Health and Science University in Portland, the only health-sciences academic center in Oregon. It was designated a Clinical Cancer Center by the National Cancer Institute in 1997. Although the institute is located in the largest metropolitan area in Oregon, outreach to people living in rural areas, including the development of cancer education and control programs, is a priority because half the population of Oregon and southwestern Washington is rural. The institute collaborates with OHSU Hospital, the OHSU outpatient clinics, and the Portland Veterans Administration Medical Center.

The OHSU Cancer Institute has four primary research programs, each of which interfaces with clinical care: Cancer Biology, Hematological Malignancies, Solid Tumors, and Cancer Prevention and Control. Research is supported by 11 shared resources: biostatistics, cell culture media, clinical research management, flow cytometry, gene microarrays, informatics, molecular biology, pathology, pharmacokinetics, proteomics, and transgenics.

The Cancer Biology program has two focus groups. The signal transduction group investigates signal transduction mechanisms relevant to the regulation of normal- and cancer-cell growth, the function of growth factors and their receptions, kinase-mediated signaling phenomena, and the regulation of transcription. The Carcinogenesis/Genetic Instability Focus group studies cell cycle control, regulation of apoptosis, and the relationship of both to genetic instability and cancer. The Hematological Malignances program has three primary areas of interest: hematopoiesis, molecular leukemogenesis/lymphomagenesis, and human immunodeficiency virus/acquired immunodeficiency syndrome (HIV/AIDS).

The Solid Tumors program focuses on gastrointestinal malignancies, prostate cancer, and other solid tumors (in particular, skin malignancies, breast cancer, gynecologic malignancies, and bone and soft-tissue sarcomas).

The Cancer Prevention and Control program has three focus areas: survivorship and symptom management; surveillance, epidemiology, and prevention; and clinical breast-examination training. The program's Underserved Populations group focuses on cancer control in Native American populations, stem-cell matching in patients from underrepresented populations, and tobacco control.

The institute offers cancer care using a multidisciplinary team approach. In addition, four OHSU Cancer Multidisciplinary Centers integrate cancer care and research on several common types of cancer.

The Breast Health Education program was developed in 1999 to improve the quality of clinical breast exams for women in Oregon to increase early detection of breast cancer. The program also teaches women, particularly those in high-risk and underserved communities, how to perform breast self-exams and educates the public about the need for proper breast exams.

Many support services are available for patients and their families. Cancer social workers help patients and their families cope with treatment and assists with the coordination of community and financial resources. Cancer counselors provide patient and family counseling, and run cancer support groups. Pediatric cancer social workers and counselors provide similar services to children with cancer and their families. Counseling concerning end-of-life care is also available through the institute.

SEE ALSO: Breast Cancer; Disparities, Issues in Cancer; Screening (Cervical and Breast and Colon Cancers).

BIBLIOGRAPHY. The Oregon Health Sciences University Cancer Institute website, www.ohsucancer.com (cited December 2006).

SARAH BOSLAUGH
WASHINGTON UNIVERSITY SCHOOL OF MEDICINE

Oncology Nursing Society

THE ONCOLOGY NURSING Society (ONS) is a professional organization open to registered nurses and interested professionals in the areas of nursing research, education, patient care, and administration.

In 1973 the American Nurses Association and the American Cancer Society cosponsored the first National Cancer Nursing Research Conference. Following this meeting, a group of nurses discussed the need for a professional organization specific to their occupation. The ONS was formed two years later. The mission of the society is to "promote excellence in oncology nursing and quality cancer care." The ONS is based in Pittsburgh, Pennsylvania, and has international efforts for education and dissemination of information. Members advocate at all levels, from local to international.

The ONS has many chapters and special-interest groups (SIGs). Members of chapters can communicate with one another as well as with the ONS via the virtual communities accessible from the ONS website. SIGs publish newsletters and maintain websites.

PUBLICATIONS, AND MEETING AND EVENTS

As a membership benefit, society nurses receive subscriptions to three journals: *Clinical Journal of Oncology Nursing, Oncology Nursing Forum,* and *ONS News.*

National conferences recognize fields within oncology nursing, such as nursing research and advanced-practice nursing. Also, the ONS has declared May to be Oncology Nursing Month and an opportunity to educate the public about oncology nursing.

SEE ALSO: American Cancer Society; European Oncology Nursing Society.

BIBLIOGRAPHY. Jessica Corner and Christopher Bailey, *Cancer Nursing* (Blackwell Publishers, 2001); Connie Henke Yarbro, et al., *Cancer Nursing: Principles and Practice (Jones and Bartlett Series in Oncology)* (Jones and Bartlett Publishers, 2005).

CLAUDIA WINOGRAD
UNIVERSITY OF ILLINOIS AT URBANA-CHAMPAIGN

Ono Pharmaceutical (Japan)

ONO PHARMACEUTICAL, INC., is an international pharmaceutical company specializing in "ethical drugs" at the forefront of international medical standards. It has a research-and-development (R&D) focus on drugs that treat painful diseases, including those that are side effects of cancer treatments. Other R&D initiatives are cellular signaling, enzyme inhibitors, neuroscience, and prostaglandins. Ono pharmaceuticals are distributed to nearly 40 countries.

The company was started in 1717 by Ichibei Fushimiya, an apothecary who opened a shop in Osaka. In 1934 the company Ono Ichibei Shoten was established; it became Ono Pharmaceutical in 1947.

The head office of Ono is located in Osaka. Branches, sales offices, research institutes, manufacturing plants, and distribution facilities are located throughout Japan. The overseas branch is in Seoul, South Korea; overseas subsidiaries are in the United Kingdom and the United States.

In 1968 a laboratory at Ono was the first in the world to synthesize a prostaglandin. Prostaglandins are lipid derivatives of fatty acids that have many roles in the body, including cell-growth control and regulation of inflammatory reactions.

SEE ALSO: Experimental Cancer Drugs; Japan.

BIBLIOGRAPHY. Ahmed F. Abdel-Magid and Stephane Caron, *Fundamentals of Early Clinical Drug Development: From Synthesis Design to Formulation* (Wiley-Interscience, 2006); Rick Ng, *Drugs—From Discovery to Approval* (Wiley-Liss, 2004); Adriana Petryna, et al., *Global Pharmaceuticals: Ethics, Markets, Practices* (Duke University Press, 2006).

CLAUDIA WINOGRAD
UNIVERSITY OF ILLINOIS AT URBANA-CHAMPAIGN

Oral Cancer, Childhood

ORAL CANCER IS any abnormal growth and spread of cells in the mouth cavity, including the lips, the insides of the lips and cheeks, the tongue, the gums, and the floor of the mouth, and the roof of the mouth. Oral cancer generally refers to squamous cell carcinoma—cancer of the thin, flat cells lining the mouth, tongue, and lips. Rarer types include oral malignant melanoma, mucoepidermoid carcinoma, and adenoid cystic carcinoma. Although oral cancer is the most common type of a group of cancers referred to as head and neck cancer, it is extremely rare in children.

Adults over the age of 40, especially longtime users of tobacco or alcohol, are typically those at risk for oral cancer. Oral cancer is extremely rare in children, with the great majority of tumors in the oral cavity found to be benign (not cancerous). In childhood, oral cancers often reflect congenital disease or a malignancy of developing tissues, such as rhabdomyosarcoma, a rare cancer arising from skeletal muscle tissue. Adolescents with oral squamous cell carcinoma should be screened for Fanconi's anemia, an inherited disorder affecting primarily the bone marrow.

Symptoms of oral cancer include a mouth sore that lasts longer than two weeks, swelling or growth of lumps anywhere in the mouth or neck, red or white patches in the mouth or on the lips, repeated bleeding from the mouth, difficulty swallowing, loose teeth, an earache, and persistent hoarseness. Often, these same symptoms indicate an infection or another problem but should be checked by a doctor or dentist to allow for early diagnosis and treatment.

If the doctor or dentist suspects oral cancer, he or she may remove a small sample of tissue to determine whether the tissue is in fact cancerous—a procedure referred to as a biopsy. If the biopsy indicates cancer, the doctor needs to determine the stage of the cancer to decide the best possible treatment. The size of the tumor and its spread indicate the stage of the cancer.

While treatment of benign oral tumors is surgical, treatment of malignant tumors in children may include surgery, chemotherapy, and radiation therapy. Surgical treatment can be debilitating, depending on the size of the tumor, with removal of significant amounts of tissue, including tissue of the tongue, palate, and cheek. In these cases, reconstructive surgery may be desirable.

It is particularly important to maintain oral health during treatment for childhood cancer to prevent tooth decay and infection. Children with very low blood counts should use toothbrushes with very soft bristles and should take care not to cut the gums with dental floss. Older children should use a fluoride mouth rinse to prevent the severe tooth decay that can result from reduced saliva flow because of radiation to the head and neck. Though necessary dental work may have to be delayed during cancer treatment, it should not be neglected.

Often, oral cancer is not detected early enough, which leads to a high fatality rate. If it is detected early, it is highly curable, with an 80 percent survival rate.

SEE ALSO: Childhood Cancers; Head and Neck Cancer; Oral Cavity Cancer, Lip and; Oropharyngeal Cancer; Rhabdomyosarcoma, Childhood.

BIBLIOGRAPY. C. D. Llewellyn, et al., "Risk Factors for Squamous Cell Carcinoma of the Oral Cavity in Young People—A Comprehensive Literature Review," *Oral Oncology* (v.37, 2001).

HARLEEN KHANIJOUN
UNIVERSITY OF ALABAMA

Oral Cavity Cancer, Lip and

ORAL-CAVITY CANCERS ARE diseases in which oral-cavity cells grow and replicate uncontrollably. They account for 30 percent of head and neck cancers in the United States. The American Cancer Society estimated approximately 5,000 deaths and 22,000 new diagnoses in 2006 (not including pharyngeal cancers). The incidence of female cases has increased significantly in recent decades. Oral-cavity cancers are the most prevalent cancers in Southeast Asian countries where chewing tobacco and betel nuts is a widespread habit.

The oral cavity includes the lips, the gums, the front two-thirds of the tongue, the roof and floor of the mouth, the inside lining of the lips and cheeks, and the area behind the wisdom teeth. Benign or malignant tumors can develop in any of these locations, and both types require treatment.

Oral-cavity cancers have a variety of signs, symptoms, and behaviors. In the United States, cancers of the lip, tongue, and floor of the mouth have the highest incidences. They can present as ulcers, cauliflowerlike growths, or flat red or white patches. Wounds that do not seem to heal or that bleed easily should be examined immediately. Tumors such as tongue cancers tend to cause pain; others, such as cancers of the floor of the mouth, do not. Other signs and symptoms include numbness in the oral cavity; loosening teeth; dentures that no longer fit; and difficulties in speech, chewing, and swallowing. Many cancers can spread to the neck lymph nodes, significantly decreasing survival rates.

The connections between oral-cavity cancers and the use of tobacco and alcohol are firmly established; 90% of patients use some form of tobacco, and many drink alcohol as well. Tobacco and alcohol are synergistic, meaning that the combination is more deleterious than the individual effects added together. Chronic irritants such as poor oral hygiene, ill-fitting dentures, and certain viral infections are also risk factors. Risk of oral-cavity cancer increases with age, which is a concerning implication for our aging society.

Treatment options include surgery, radiation therapy, and chemotherapy. Surgical resection of cancerous tissues and a ring of surrounding normal tissues is the treatment of choice for early-stage cancers. Surgery is often followed by radiation therapy for advanced malignancies. Because large resections may compromise the physical and functional integrity of the oral cavity, facial reconstruction and speech and swallowing rehabilitation are integral aspects of the treatment process. Advanced, inoperable tumors are managed by chemotherapy and irradiation. Survival rates are clearly superior in cancers detected at earlier stages, making early diagnosis essential. Quality of life has become an important focus in treatment of oral-cavity cancer. Recent advances in oral-cavity reconstructive surgery have allowed better functional and aesthetic outcomes after large surgeries. Ongoing research in oral-cavity-cancer biology and clinical trials will provide further insights into optimal treatment and management of the cancer.

SEE ALSO: Alcohol; Head and Neck Cancer; Oral Cancer, Childhood; Oropharyngeal Cancer; Tobacco Smoking.

BIBLIOGRAPHY. National Institutes of Health, *What You Need to Know about Oral Cancers* (NIH Publication No. 03-1574, 2003).

YOSHIHIRO YONEKAWA
WEILL MEDICAL COLLEGE OF CORNELL UNIVERSITY

Organization of European Cancer Institutes

THE 50 UNITED States each face unique challenges with regard to cancer care, just as each European country does. In Europe, another challenge is present: a language barrier. Thus, many cancer institutes in Europe joined together in the Organization of European Cancer Institutes (OECI)–European Economic Interest Group to share information and foster international collaboration. Membership is composed of universities and institutes. The OECI is based in Brussels, Belgium.

Pierre Denoix, director of the International Union Against Cancer (UICC), called a meeting of institute directors October 26, 1977, at the Emperor's Castle in Vienna, Austria. Sixty representatives of European and other international cancer institutes attended this gathering, where the OECI was established. The first general-assembly meeting was held in Rodos, Greece, May 18–20, 1980.

The mission of the OECI is to improve cooperation and collaboration among the various cancer institutes across Europe. From the start, the organization has worked closely with the UICC Cancer and its Committee on International Collaborative Activities.

A major project of the OECI is Transfog (Translational and Functional Onco-Genomics), which seeks to identify and characterize the genes involved in breast, colon, and lung cancers for purposes of diagnosis and therapy. The project also aims to establish a standard procedure for evaluation of potential genes for cancer therapy. A subsection of the OECI is the Pathobiology Working Group (PWG), which establishes standards of procedure in pathology in the participating institutes. One initiative of the PWG is TuBaFrost, a European tumor-tissue bank. Any participating cancer center can deposit frozen tissue specimens. The ultimate goal is to establish a tissue collection large enough to supply multicenter translational research.

SEE ALSO: European Association for Cancer Research; European Cancer Prevention Organization; National Cancer Institute.

BIBLIOGRAPHY. A. J. M. Vermorken, et al., *Towards Coordination of Cancer Research in Europe* (Ios Pr. Inc., 1994).

CLAUDIA WINOGRAD
UNIVERSITY OF ILLINOIS AT URBANA-CHAMPAIGN

Oropharyngeal Cancer

OROPHARYNGEAL CANCER IS a tumor found in the oropharynx of the upper respiratory tract. The oropharynx abuts structures in the oral cavity such as the soft palate, the tonsils, and the posterior pharyngeal wall located in the back wall of the throat.

Oropharyngeal cancer arises in the oropharyngeal epithelium—in particular, the squamous cell epithelium. Tumors that arise in the posterior wall of the oropharynx are often associated with metastases to the retropharyngeal lymph nodes, which may provide patients a worse prognosis. The etiology of the cancer is unknown; however; there are many predisposing factors for developing oropharyngeal cancer. The greatest risk factor is high exposure to tobacco smoke from cigarettes and cigars or passive smoking. Smokers are six times more likely than nonsmokers to develop this form of cancer. As more men are current smokers than women, oropharyngeal cancer is more common among men.

Alcohol consumption similarly increases the risk of developing this cancer; drinkers have six times the risk of nondrinkers. Alcohol may also cause damage of DNA, initiating the growth of tumor cells, which if left untreated may metastasize to other organs.

Cigarettes and alcohol contain nitrosamines and other chemicals that damage the oropharyngeal epithelium lining.

The human papillomavirus type-16 infection may contribute to the development of oral-cavity and oropharyngeal cancers in around 20 percent of people.

People taking immunosuppressive drugs to treat certain immune-system diseases or to prevent rejection of transplanted organs may be also at increased risk for cancers of the oropharynx.

The diagnosis of oropharyngeal cancer is made through recognition of symptoms such as difficulty in swallowing, numbness of the tongue, and aberrations in voice production. These symptoms are common to many other diseases; hence, other diagnostic methods are employed, such as panendoscopy, in which fiber-optic endoscopes are used to examine the oropharynx. Diagnosis is also made through microscopic examination of cells using exfoliative cytology.

Imaging studies also have an important role in defining the extent of oropharyngeal tumors. Chest X-rays, computed tomography (CT) scans, and magnetic resonance imaging (MRI) are used to detect metastases. If the cancer has metastasized to the lymph nodes, positron emission tomography (PET) may be used. Barium swallows are also employed to detect any aberrations in swallowing.

Treatments for oropharyngeal cancers include surgery, chemoradiation, and neck dissection for tumors that have metastasized to retropharyngeal lymph nodes. Any difficulties in swallowing and chewing can be treated with a gastrostomy tube to help feeding. Complications of surgical treatment include wound infection, which may result in functional morbidity and prolonged hospitalization.

The prognosis for a benign oropharyngeal cancer is poor. Less than 60 percent of patients are likely to survive after five years. Metastatic disease has a worse prognosis, with only 30 percent of patients surviving following treatment. Reducing exposure to risk factors, however, can prevent the cancer in approximately two-thirds of all cases. Reduction or elimination of tobacco and alcohol is essential, although the latter may be difficult, as patients often present with chronic alcoholism.

SEE ALSO: Alcohol; Head and Neck Cancer; Infection (Childhood, Sexually Transmitted Infections, Hepatitis); Oral Cavity Cancer, Lip and; Tobacco Smoking.

BIBLIOGRAPHY. V. Strnad, "Treatment of Oral Cavity and Oropharyngeal Cancer. Indications, Technical Aspects, and Results of Interstitial Brachytherapy," *Strahlentherapie und Onkologie* (v.180/11, 2004).

FARHANA AKTER
KINGS COLLEGE, LONDON

Ovarian Cancer, Childhood

TUMORS OF THE ovary are uncommon in children, with an incidence of about 2.6 per 100,000 annually. Approximately one-third of pediatric ovarian neoplasms are malignant, representing about 1 percent of all childhood malignancies. The incidence increases in children at the age of 8 or 9 and peaks at age 19.

In contrast to ovarian cancer in adults, in which tumors of epithelial origin predominate, germ-cell tumors represent about two-thirds of ovarian cancer in children. In order of decreasing frequency, the categories of malignant germ-cell tumors in children are dysgerminoma, endodermal sinus tumor (yolk-sac carcinoma), immature teratoma, mixed germ-cell tumor, and embryonal carcinoma. The level of malignancy is determined by the morphological stage of differentiation. Sex-cord stromal tumors include thecoma-fibroma, Sertoli-Leydig cell tumors, and granulose cell tumors. Malignant epithelial tumors, including cystadenomas, are common in adult women but rare in children. Small-cell carcinoma of the ovary is extremely rare in children but has been reported.

Although the exact etiology of ovarian cancer in children is unknown, evidence indicates that hormonal factors play an important role in ovarian germ-cell tumorogenesis. The most common symptom of ovarian cancer in children is acute or chronic abdominal pain, present in up to 80 percent of cases. The pain often mimics acute appendicitis. A palpable abdominal mass is present in about half of children with ovarian cancer. Nonspecific gastrointestinal symptoms are frequently reported, including constipation, nausea, and vomiting, as well as urinary symptoms.

About 10 percent of patients demonstrate isosexual precocious puberty, in which girls begin to develop sexual characteristics before the age of 8-1/2 years. Isosexual precocity is especially prevalent in children with granulosa-theca tumors. Symptoms related to childhood ovarian cancer often warrant the initial use of ultrasonography, which can differentiate cystic masses from solid masses. Computed tomography (CT) imaging of the abdomen and pelvis is essential in determining the size of the tumor and the presence of calcifications or fat, and to identify whether metastases are present.

Levels of specific proteins produced by tumors, including alpha-fetoprotein (AFP) and beta-human chorionic gonadotropin (β-HCG), are elevated in children with ovarian germ-cell cancer and therefore are an essential aid in diagnosis. Tumor staging for ovarian cancer, as defined by the International Federation of Gynecology and Obstetrics, is dependent on clinical, surgical, and pathologic findings.

TREATMENT AND PROGNOSIS

Treatment of childhood ovarian cancer—which includes complete tumor resection, chemotherapy, and occasionally radiotherapy—has yielded excellent long-term results. Following complete resection of the affected ovary and associated uterine tube (salpingo-oophorectomy), patients with rapidly decreasing levels of serum tumor markers and no detectable metastases often do well without the need for additional therapy. Metastatic disease to any site, however, requires further intensive chemotherapy.

Because radiotherapy therapy in childhood ovarian cancer carries a high risk of late sequelae, including potential infertility, use of radiotherapy is restricted to tumors that have relapsed despite second-line surgery and chemotherapy.

With the use of platinum-based regimens, including PEB (cisplatin, etoposide, and bleomycin) and JEB (carboplatin, etoposide, and bleomycin), most patients experience a complete cure and maintain fertility. Five-year survival rates as high as 97 percent have been reported, even in patients with advanced disease. Long-term survival and rates of recurrence of childhood ovarian cancer need to be evaluated further, however.

SEE ALSO: Childhood Cancers; Germ Cell Tumor, Extracranial, Childhood; Ovarian Epithelial Cancer; Ovarian Germ Cell Tumor; Ovarian Low Malignant Potential Tumor.

BIBLIOGRAPHY. Antoine De Backer, et al., "Ovarian Germ Cell Tumors in Children: A Clinical Study of 66 Patients," *Pediatric Blood Cancer* (v.46, 2006); C. Ross Pinkerton, "Malignant Germ Cell Tumours in Childhood," *European Journal of Cancer* (v.33, 1997); Philip A. Pizzo and David G. Poplack, *Principles and Practice of Pediatric Oncology: Ovarian Tumors* [electronic resource] (Lippincott Williams & Wilkins, 2002); Kris Ann Shultz, et al., "Pediatric Ovarian Tumors: A Review of 67 Cases," *Pediatric Blood Cancer* (v.44, 2005).

Shaun E. Gruenbaum
Ben-Gurion University of the Negev and
Columbia University Medical Center
Benjamin F. Gruenbaum
University of Connecticut

Ovarian Epithelial Cancer

OVARIAN EPITHELIAL CANCER is a neoplasm of the ovaries. It is one of the most common gynecological malignancies and is associated with considerable morbidity and a high mortality rate in women. Ovarian cancer is the fifth-leading cause of cancer death in women. Reproductive factors are the dominant markers of risk—the longer a woman ovulates, and the more ovulatory cycles she has, the greater her risk of ovarian cancer. The molecular pathology of ovarian carcinomas is heterogeneous and involves a high number of prognostic markers and multiple pathways of development.

TYPES OF OVARIAN CANCER

Ovarian cancers are named after the tissue from which they develop. There are three types of ovarian cancers: germ-cell tumors, stromal tumors, and epithelial tumors.

Epithelial tumors are characterized by several histological features, including the serous, mucinous, endometrioid, and clear-cell types. Serous carcinoma, which is associated with a high risk of mortality, may arise due to germ-line mutations in the BRCA1 (breast cancer 1, early onset) and BRCA2 (breast cancer 2, early onset) genes. BRCA1 and BRCA2 are tumor-suppressor genes located on chromosome 17q21 and 13q12, respectively.

When mutated, they are associated with some instances of inherited ovarian and breast cancer. The mutation of the p53 tumor suppressor gene may also lead to the development of a high-grade serous carcinoma. By contrast, low-grade (minimally invasive) serous carcinomas may be due to somatic mutations in BRAF (v-raf murine sarcoma viral oncogene homolog B1) genes or aberrations in the KRAS (K-ras signaling pathway), such as a single amino-acid substitution that may develop via an adenoma–borderline–carcinoma (benign disease progressing to a tumor) sequence.

Mucinous carcinoma also arises due to KRAS mutations developing via an adenoma–borderline–carcinoma sequence. Endometrioid carcinoma, associated with a high risk of mortality, has similar changes to high-grade serous carcinomas. Low-grade endometrioid carcinomas, which generally have a good prognosis, are characterized by alterations in the CTNNB1 (beta-catenin) pathway. CTNNB1 is an adherens junction protein; adherens junctions are vital for the maintenance of epithelial layers. PTEN (phosphatase and tensin homolog) mutations and microsatellite instability may also play a role in a development of low-grade endometrioid tumors.

Clear-cell carcinomas are characterized by mutations of TGFbetaR2 (transforming growth factor beta receptor II), which is a modulator of cellular proliferation and extracellular matrix deposition. The overexpression of HNF-1 beta (hepatocyte nuclear factor -1 beta) is a good molecular marker for ovarian clear-cell tumors.

The risk factors for developing ovarian cancer include higher education, family history of ovarian cancer, BRCA-1 and BRCA-2 genes, and talc exposure. Factors that prevent ovarian cancer include oral contraceptives, multiple pregnancies, prolonged lactation, hysterectomy, and a diet high in vegetables and fruits. Symptoms of the disease are nonspecific and include vaginal bleeding, pelvic pain, and abdominal distension. Advanced disease may present with a pelvic/abdominal mass.

Ovarian epithelial cancer is treated surgically, followed by standard postoperative chemotherapy with the agents cisplatin, carboplatin, and paclitaxel.

The disease is associated with recurrences in most patients, and the overall prognosis for the disease is poor, with a five-year survival rate of 50 percent.

SEE ALSO: Breast Cancer; Genetics; Ovarian Cancer, Childhood; Ovarian Germ Cell Tumor; Women's Cancers.

BIBLIOGRAPHY. M. Christies and M. K. Oehler, "Molecular Pathology of Epithelial Ovarian Cancer," *Journal of British Menopause Society* (v.12/2, 2006).

Farhana Akter
Kings College, London

Ovarian Germ Cell Tumor

OVARIAN GERM-CELL TUMOR is a rare form of ovarian cancer. The tumors arise from the germ (egg) cells of the ovary that become cancerous and often occur in teenage girls or young women, usually affecting just one ovary. The majority of ovarian germ-cell tumors are benign (usually, dermoid cysts), and the malignant form can be derived from dermoid cysts or primitive malignant germ-cell tumors. About 50 percent to 75 percent of the malignant tumors are detected in an early stage.

There are several types of malignant ovarian germ-cell tumors: dysgerminoma, endodermal sinus tumor, embryonal carcinoma, choriocarcinoma, and immature teratomas. Dysgerminoma is the most frequent malignant germ-cell tumor; it occurs primarily in women younger than 35, but a small percentage of these tumors occurs in prepubertal girls. Approximately 15 percent of the dysgerminoma affects both ovaries. Endodermal sinus tumors or yolk-sac tumors are the second-most-common germ-cell tumors; most are malignant, often occurring as part of mixed germ-cell tumors along with dysgerminoma, immature teratoma, or choriocarcinoma. Endodermal sinus tumors are usually present in children and women younger than 20.

Embryonal carcinomas and choriocarcinomas are both rare and usually diagnosed in patients younger

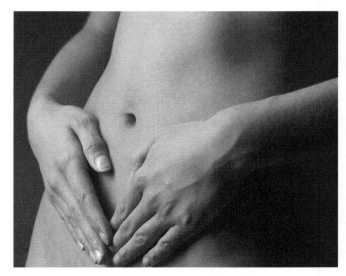

Education on ovarian cancer and self examination may be helpful, however gynecological examinations are a necessity.

than 20. Immature teratomas contain cancer cells that look like those from a developing baby and can be either pure or mixed. Because there are often no symptoms early in the disease progression, ovarian germ-cell tumors can be difficult to diagnose. Nevertheless, tumors can be found during regular gynecological checkups. Additional tests, such as ultrasound or computed tomography (CT) scans, might be used for diagnosis.

Blood tests are used to measure the levels of alpha-fetoprotein (AFP) and human chorionic gonadotropin (HCG) in the blood; when elevated, these levels may indicate the presence of ovarian germ-cell tumors. Most patients with ovarian germ-cell tumors can be treated with combination chemotherapy, but the prognosis and treatment for individual patients depend on the type, size, and stage of cancer. Patients receiving combination chemotherapy after initial surgery often have an improved prognosis.

SEE ALSO: Germ Cell Tumor, Extracranial, Childhood; Germ Cell Tumor, Extragonadal; Ovarian Cancer, Childhood; Women's Cancers.

BIBLIOGRAPHY. Raymond E. Lenhard, Jr., et al., eds., *Clinical Oncology*, 1st ed. (American Cancer Society, 2001); Mark H. Beers, et al., eds., *The Merck Manual of Diagnosis and Therapy*, 18th ed. (Merck Research Laboratories, 2006).

STEPHEN CHEN
UNIVERSITY OF TORONTO

Ovarian Low Malignant Potential Tumor

OVARIAN CANCER IS one of the most common gynecological cancers. It begins as a malignant tumor or as an abnormal growth of cells surrounding normal cells. The tumor may originate in one or both ovaries and eventually moves to other parts of the body. In the United States ovarian cancer is the second-most-common gynecological cancer (affecting about 1 in 70 women) and is the deadliest; 1 percent of all women die of it. Ovarian cancer is the fifth-leading cause of cancer overall and is responsible for more deaths than any other reproductive-organ cancer. Ovarian cancer most commonly occurs in women in their 50s. Over half of all ovarian cancers are found in women over the age of 65.

TYPES OF CANCER

Ovarian tumors are identified by where the cells are found within the ovarian tissue. There are three specific classifications: epithelia (surface of ovary), germ cell (middle of ovary), and stromal cell (sex-cord-stromal-inner). Eighty percent of ovarian tumors originate within the epithelium; the remaining 20 percent are germ and stromal cells.

The causes of ovarian cancer are still being looked at, but there are factors that can affect its development, including menstrual history, age, fertility or birth-control drugs, family history, diet, breast cancer, hysterectomy, and pregnancy. Nulliparity (no childbirth); delay in childbirth; delay in menopause; and/or a family history of endometrial, colon, or breast cancer can also increase the risk. Major symptoms are abdominal swelling (gas, bloating, indigestion, or long-term stomach pain), bleeding between periods or just after menopause; pelvic pain, with a general feeling of pressure within the pelvis; and deep leg pain. Only 25 percent of all ovarian cancers are detected in the early stages. The best prevention is early detection, with yearly pelvic examinations starting at age 18.

SEE ALSO: Breast Cancer; Colon Cancer; Endometrial Cancer; Women's Cancers.

BIBLIOGRAPHY. Philip M. Parker, *The Official Patient's Sourcebook on Ovarian Low Malignant Potential Tumors: A Revised and Updated Directory for the Internet Age* (Icon Health Publications, 2002).

RICHARD E. WILLS
INDEPENDENT SCHOLAR

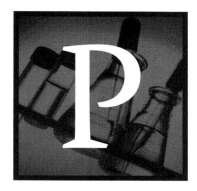

Pain, Cancer, and Management of

IT IS ESTIMATED that more than 9 million people in the world experience pain as a result of cancer. Pain, both caused by cancer itself and occurring as a consequence of cancer diagnosis and treatment, is a burden for patients and represents a major obstacle for healthcare providers. Although the vast majority of cancer pain is treatable using analgesic therapy, surgery, radiation, and other adjuvant therapies, various educational and socioeconomic barriers separate cancer patients from effective assessment and treatment for their pain. Current legislative, scientific, and social efforts may be effective in reducing these barriers and facilitating more effective treatment for cancer pain.

THE PROBLEM OF CANCER PAIN

Pain is one of the most common reasons patients seek the care of a physician. One-third of cancer patients have pain at the time of diagnoses, and approximately three-quarters have pain during the advanced stages of their disease. Cancer patients have been shown to experience moderate to severe cancer pain more often than not as their disease progresses. Often, cancer pain is so severe as to limit functional ability, and the vast majority of both pediatric and adult cancer pa-

tients die from cancer without ever having achieved adequate pain relief.

The most common cause of cancer pain is direct tumor involvement, comprising two-thirds of cases of pain from metastatic cancer and occurring in the vast majority of patients on inpatient pain services and over one-half of patients seen in outpatient pain clinics. Pain also develops secondary to diagnostic therapies and occurs in more than 20 percent of patients who undergo surgery, radiation therapy, or chemotherapy. Pain can also be a result of poor blood circulation, blockage of an organ or vessel, infection, inflammation, psychological distress, or inactivity because of disease. In children with cancer, pain is commonly associated with procedures and is reported to occur in up to 50 percent of children who receive active therapy.

Cancer patients may also experience a qualitative variety of pain including somatic, visceral, and neuropathic pain. More than three-quarters of patients report two or more distinct complaints, and more than one-third report three types of pain, the most common combination being that of somatic and neuropathic pains. Somatic pain is most often a result of bone pain resulting from metastases, and it is usually described by patients as dull, sharp, aching, or throbbing. It is well-localized and often constant. Visceral pain is vaguer and more poorly defined than somatic pain. It is often a result of abnormal stretching of internal organs or irritation of the serous membranes that line the viscera. Visceral pain is commonly described as dull, aching, or a sensation of increased pressure. Neuropathic pain has several subtypes and can be caused by cancer invasion of the nervous system or by injury from cancer therapy. It is described as burning, shock-like, or shooting and may be sporadic or constant. Neuropathic pain may include allodynia, which is pain from a nonpainful stimulus, or hyperalgesia, which is increased pain from a painful stimulus. Somatic and visceral pains generally respond to analgesic therapy. Neuropathic pain is more challenging to treat but has been responsive to treatment with tricyclic antidepressants, certain anticonvulsants, and more invasive procedural and surgical interventions.

Effective pain management begins with accurate diagnosis. An initial assessment for pain levels in a patient should involve a detailed history, physical examination, and psychological assessment. Assessments should be performed at regular intervals, as well as at the time of any medication change or report of new pain. Various methods for diagnosing pain exist, many of which employ standardized methods and tools including pain scales. One-dimensional pain scales ask patients to rate pain intensity on a numerical rating or visual analog scale between no pain and the worst pain imaginable. Pain intensity is sometimes assessed in children or people with cognitive impairments using a faces pain scale, which matches increasing pain intensities with facial expressions indicating emotional states. Multidimensional pain scales assess aspects of pain in addition to intensity, such as location, quality, and effect on emotional state. These measures include the McGill Pain Questionnaire (MPQ), the Memorial Pain Assessment Card, and the Brief Pain Inventory (BPI). The Treatment Outcomes of Pain Survey (TOPS) is a pain-enhanced version of the gold standard health-related quality-of-life (HRQoL) instrument known as the Medical Outcomes Study Short Form 36 (MOS SF-36, or SF-36). This instrument incorporates additional dimensions such as functional limitations, life control, and objective work disability.

PHARMACOTHERAPY FOR CANCER PAIN

One of the primary methods for treating cancer pain involves the use of analgesics, or pain-relieving medications. Perhaps the most widely used guideline for pain management is the World Health Organization's (WHO's) analgesic ladder, developed in 1986 to address the inadequacy of cancer pain management. It involves the use of a three-step analgesic ladder that corresponds to three categories of pain. Step 1 is for mild to moderate pain and calls for the use of nonopioid pain medications such as aspirin or other NSAIDS. Most mild to moderate cancer pain can be safely and adequately controlled with nonopioid medications; however, aspirin is of concern in cancer patients because of its tendency to increase bleeding and cause gastrointestinal side effects. If a patient continues to have mild to moderate pain while taking a nonopioid analgesic, the dosage may be increased to the maximum safe dose while adding a step 2 opioid analgesic such as codeine. For patients who are still in pain while taking a step 2 opioid, the dose of the step 2 medication should be increased, or a step 3 opioid such as morphine or fentanyl may be substituted for the step 2 opioid.

Step 3 opioids may be increased until the desired outcome is achieved. All medication changes should adjust for the opioid tolerance level of the patient. The three-step analgesic ladder allows for the use of adjuvant therapies at any of the three steps. In moderate to severe cancer pain, clinicians may elect to begin analgesic therapy at the second step. In addition to the use of the stepwise approach, clinicians are advised to be sure of proper dosing. Oral administration of analgesics is the preferred route, though many drugs may also be given parenterally. Coanalgesic therapy may be considered at any phase of treatment, and the side effects of analgesics should be closely monitored, as they are a common barrier to adequate treatment for pain. Adjuvants may serve to enhance analgesic therapy by one or more of the following: increasing the efficacy of opioids, treating adverse symptoms associated with analgesic therapy or symptoms that exacerbate the cancer-related pain, or producing independent analgesia. Adjuvants include medications such as antidepressants, corticosteroids, and anticonvulsants.

Morphine is the most common opioid used for the treatment of cancer pain. It is widely available, is produced in a variety of formulations, is easily administered, and has a low cost. Patients are commonly assessed for adequate pain control using every-4-hour dosing and then converted to sustained-release morphine, which allows for administration every 12 hours. Rescue doses of immediate-release morphine are prescribed for breakthrough pain and are generally equivalent to the 4-hour dose. Morphine may be administered by sublingual, parenteral, or rectal dose in patients where oral administration is not an option. Oxycodone and hydromorphone are alternatives to morphine with similar efficacy, bioavailability, and side effects. Each is available in normal and modified-release formulations and may also be given orally or parenterally. Fentanyl and methadone are synthetic opioids that have also been shown to be effective in the treatment of cancer pain. Fentanyl is administered continuously via transdermal patch for up to 72 hours, making it particularly useful in patients with stable levels of pain who cannot take oral medications. Methadone may be administered orally, parenterally, or rectally, similar to morphine, but may take longer than morphine to achieve stable blood levels. Methadone is an effective alternative to morphine, with a similar side effect profile and analgesic efficacy. Conversion from morphine to methadone should be initiated with caution, as the toxic effects of methadone may not be apparent for up to 5 days.

Side effects of opioids are common and often must be addressed as a part of a patient's treatment plan. As much as two-thirds of all patients who begin opioid therapy experience nausea during the first week of treatment. This nausea commonly subsides with stabilization of the dose. Other common side effects of opioids include constipation, respiratory sedation, and itching. Side effects of methadone in addition to the spectrum of opioid side effects include excess sweating and flushing. Patients may develop a tolerance to the side effects of an opioid with continued use.

Tolerance, physical dependence, and addiction may occur as a result of opioid usage. Tolerance and physical dependence are both physiological processes, whereas addiction is psychological in nature. Tolerance is the progressive decline of the potency of an opioid with continued use. Tolerance can develop as a normal result of opioid use, and dose escalation is all that is usually required for additional pain control. When a physiologic tolerance to a particular opioid has been developed, the patient may have a cross tolerance to other opioids. Physical dependence is characterized by withdrawal manifestations after an abrupt discontinuation, the administration of an opioid an-

tagonist, or a dose reduction of an opioid in a patient who has been using the drug for an extended period of time. Typical signs of withdrawal include agitation, tachycardia, diaphoresis, and insomnia. Patients who have been using an opioid for an extended period of time often develop physiological dependence. Opioid therapy should be gradually reduced or discontinued, rather than changed abruptly. Addiction is a psychological and behavioral syndrome characterized by drug-seeking behavior. Addiction is rare among patients being treated in palliative care.

Surgery may be an effective form of pain control in patients with advanced metastatic disease. Surgical palliation aims to improve the quality of life of patients and to reduce their adverse symptoms and is indicated when less-invasive means of pain control have failed or when therapeutic interventions are the source of the pain. Surgery has also been shown to be particularly effective at reducing neuropathic pain. Significant cost may be associated with surgery for pain relief, and patients with advanced metastatic disease must weigh the risks of the procedure against the desired benefits.

Complementary therapies including massage therapy, mind–body techniques, music therapy, acupuncture, and dietary supplementation also may have a role in reducing the burden from cancer pain. Patients receiving hypnosis and cognitive behavioral therapy have been shown to experience greater pain relief than controls, as well as less anxiety and distress. Relaxation and imagery training have been found to be effective in reducing pain, as well as analgesic side effects. Alternative treatments such as exercise, electrical nerve stimulation, imaging techniques, and psychotherapy also have been shown to have some benefits in the treatment of neuropathic pain.

ROLE OF PALLIATIVE CARE

WHO regards palliative care as an essential part of cancer treatment and has affirmed its role early in the disease process. Palliative care aims to relieve pain and suffering and to promote an increased quality of life for patients and their families. Although palliative care does not aim to hasten death, it accepts dying as a normal process and serves to help patients and their families cope with illness and through the bereavement process. Palliative care may be initiated at the time of diagnosis, rather than in the late stages of the disease. The palliative care process begins with establishing the goals of the patient, which may be used to established advanced directives regarding the types of care the patient will receive. Palliative care can help to achieve these goals via pain management and symptom control and by providing spiritual, psychosocial, and bereavement support to patients and their families.

BARRIERS TO PAIN MANAGEMENT

Barriers to effective pain management in cancer patients include inadequate assessment, whether from a failure of patients to report their pain or from physician inaccuracy; inadequate treatment; poor access to care; lack of financial resources; and minority bias. Inadequate pain assessment has been stated by health professionals to be the number one potential barrier to optimal pain care. Inaccurate or inadequate assessment may be caused by patient underreporting of pain, which may stem from fear of being labeled as seeking drugs, by cultural stoicism, or by misconceptions about the normalcy of their pain levels. All cancer patients should be screened for the presence of pain using standardized diagnostic techniques at regular intervals. Patients should also be educated on the importance of reporting pain to their providers. Even in the presence of patient reporting of pain and the benefit of standardized assessment tools, physicians have been shown to underassess pain as well as underestimate the level of pain-related interference with activities, including sleep. Language disconcordance and socioeconomic variation also may increase the difficulty of effective patient–physician communication and further exacerbate the problem of accurate pain assessment. Lack of effective translation can impede the informed consent process, cause physicians to adopt a more conservative style of medical management, and lead to poor outcomes for patients who do not speak English as their primary language.

Despite recent innovations in pain control, patients continue to report that one of their greatest fears is unrelieved pain, and up to 70 percent of patients die with unrelieved cancer pain. Even when cancer pain is accurately assessed and an adequate treatment regimen has been established, access to medications and continuing care remains a problem for too many patients. For example, low-income patients who live in rural areas may have difficulty traveling to a pharmacy for their medications. The inability to access a pharmacy may be of particular concern for those cancer patients who are the most ill or who are suffering from severe side effects. Pain control techniques outside of the traditional analgesics, many of which are often only performed in major medical centers, are also unavailable to many patients, including racial and ethnic minorities, low-income groups, patients living in rural areas, and patients without access to transportation.

Healthcare coverage and reimbursement policies create yet another barrier to cancer pain management. In the United States, access to medical services and prescription drugs is based on a person's ability to pay, either through personal resources or through third-party private or government health insurance. Many people have either little or no health insurance, with minorities representing a disproportionate number of the uninsured and underinsured. It is reasonable to assume, then, that their access to healthcare services, including pain management, is impaired. Adequate prescription drug coverage is essential for cancer patients, as drug therapy is the primary method of cancer pain management. This problem is particularly serious for people over the age of 65 years who are on Medicare. Patients are sometimes admitted to an inpatient facility so that their prescription drug costs can be covered. Thus, the lack of prescription drug coverage by Medicare has led to a shift to more expensive and intensive care, including the use of a catheter and long-term intravenous or subcutaneous drug administration via a pump. The Medicare hospice option allows eligible patients to receive care, including outpatient prescription drug coverage, but only from a Medicare-certified hospice.

Low-income patients eligible for Medicaid have access to healthcare services, including prescription drugs. However, coverage and reimbursement restrictions vary by state. In addition, restrictions may discourage appropriate use of medication and encourage more expensive forms of pain management. Private health insurance and health maintenance organizations also vary in their coverage of pain-related services. Patients may be limited by lack of outpatient prescription drug coverage, copayments, deductibles, exclusions, and caps. In addition to individual costs, there are great institutional costs that may pose a barrier to effective cancer pain management. Healthcare institutions may not adopt the guideline-based treatment strategies because they are less cost-efficient than the usual care patients receive. However, using guideline-based strategies to manage cancer pain is much more effective than using the usual care approach and leads to better treatment outcomes.

The Center for Studying Health Systems Change has found that significant gaps in access to care among Latinos, African Americans, and Caucasians have persisted over the past decade, with Latinos and blacks consistently reporting lower levels of access than whites. The same trend holds true for low-income families of all races, who are more likely than any other group to report decreased access to healthcare over time. This disparate pain epidemic has consequences that reach beyond the physical health of patients. Cancer patients in pain have been shown to be less engaged in pleasant activities, have more sleep problems and greater fatigue, need more assistance with physical care, and experience greater hopelessness and more anger. Pain management investigations have found widespread disparities in cancer treatment as a function of patient race or ethnicity. Many studies have reported that ethnic minorities are prescribed lower doses of analgesic than nonminority patients with similar clinical manifestations of pain. This indicates that physician bias may be a factor. Race concordance between the physician and patient, particularly for African Americans, is associated with higher patient satisfaction and greater participatory decision making. This in turn can result in greater compliance and improved health outcomes. African-American patients who have African-American physicians are more likely to report having received counseling about preventive care and cancer screening, which can be vital to effective pain management, as a significant number of patients in the United States have misconceptions about cancer.

In the case of cancer pain, primary prevention is a difficult option to pursue because such a high percentage of cancer patients experience pain and because opioids are not given as prophylaxis. Secondary prevention of cancer pain rests on adequate assessment and efficient management of the pain and associated symptoms. Attempts by public health organizations to institute behavioral health changes at the regional or local level are often implemented via a community, school system, or workplace. Classical models aimed at a community have included mass media–based educational programs, which have been shown to be effective in improving community health related to various conditions, such as cardiovascular disease.

Pain has long been recognized as an important issue in public health. In 1998, the World Health Institute declared pain a world medical emergency. Because a significant percentage of cancer patients experience pain as part of their disease, cancer pain has been a consistent subset of research on pain. Although pain is experienced on an individual basis, its effects affect families, communities, and the nation as a whole. Unrelieved pain has been estimated to cost the United States more than $61 billion annual dollars in lost productivity. Despite advances in the prevention of cancer, numerous studies on the etiology of cancer pain, and recognized guidelines as to proper pain assessment and treatment, cancer pain remains an unsolved public health problem. Various public health organizations exist to increase awareness of cancer pain, encourage further education of physicians and other healthcare providers regarding effective cancer pain management, and further research efforts regarding methods of pain management.

Many of these organizations have released formal guidelines or recommendations as to the management of pain, such as the American Cancer Society, WHO and the American Pain Society. In 2000, The Joint Commission on Accreditation of Healthcare Organizations mandated adoption of policies for pain education, screening, follow-up, and measurement. Thousands of hospitals and outpatient clinics across the United States have implemented these policies, yet numerous studies have demonstrated a continued deficit in pain management practices across the country as well as a lack of standardization in the management of pain by physicians. It has been demonstrated that implementation of protocols standardizing the medical management of pain can lead to decreased levels of pain in patients if properly executed. The question remains as to where the accepted model of pain management falls short within the clinical setting. It has been suggested that the training of physicians and their daily care of patients may hinder their appreciation for the population-based models of public health. Few studies have attempted to answer the question of where the public health and medical models have failed to coincide.

In June 2006, the Susan G. Komen Breast Cancer Foundation, the Lance Armstrong Foundation, and the American Cancer Society announced the joint funding of a nationwide project to evaluate pain management policies in all 50 United States. This study comes almost 5 years after its predecessor, Achieving Balance in State Pain Policy, published in 2003 by the University of Wisconsin Pain and Policy Studies Group (PPSG). The PPSG developed their research program to improve U.S. drug control and professional practice policies regarding pain management and other forms of palliative care. The program contained various items, including national surveys of medical board members, educational workshops for medical board members, evaluation of federal and state policies, guideline development, monitoring adoption of regulatory policy, and policy databases and resources available on the Internet. The initial PPSG research helped the Federation of State Medical Boards in 1998 to develop "Model Guidelines for the Use of Controlled Substances for the Treatment of Pain." One preference of the Federation of State Medical Boards is that adequate pain relief be promoted by medical regulators and practitioners rather than by state legislatures. Since its inception, 22 states have either adopted or adapted the model guidelines. In 2004, a revised edition of the guidelines was adopted, which more clearly addresses the issue of inadequate treatment of pain.

The quality of state policy that governs medical practice directly affects medial decision making and patient care. Policies that encourage pain management can support physicians who use opioids and other pain medications to treat pain. Conversely, policies that are restrictive can influence physicians to not prescribe pain mediations, thus making it hard for patients to receive adequate care. The integration of government regulations with the realities of medical attempts to control pain is an essential step in reducing the disparities in cancer pain management. This issue is of particular importance for racial and ethnic groups who are at increased risk of public scrutiny for drug usage.

SEE ALSO: Alternative Therapy: Mind, Body, and Spirit; Drugs; Hospice.

BIBLIOGRAPHY. C. Quigley, "The Role of Opioids in Cancer Pain," *British Medical Journal* (v.331, 2005); G. W. Hanks, F. de Conno, N. Cherny, et al. "Morphine and Alternative Opioids in Cancer Pain: The EAPC Recommendations," *British Journal of Cancer* (v.84, 2001); J. D. Toombs and L. A. Kral, "Methadone Treatment for Pain States," *American Family Physician* (v.71, 2005); R. S. Morrison, Diane E. Meier, "Palliative Care," *New England Journal of Medicine* (v. 350, 2004); Ian Gilron, C. P. Watson, Catherine M. Cahill, and Dwight E. Moulin, "Neuropathic Pain: A Practical Guide for the Clinician," *Canadian Medical Association Journal* (v.175, 2006); E. Bruera and H. N. Kim, "Cancer Pain," *Journal of the American Medical Association* (v.290, 2003).

LISA MCELROY
MICHIGAN STATE UNIVERSITY

Paint

PAINT HAS BEEN used to protect and adorn surfaces from the time of the cave paintings of the prehistoric humans. The materials used to make paint have, until the advent of modern chemistry, been composed only of natural materials. Modern paints, however, are often combinations of natural and artificial materials. They are usually composed of at least one finely ground pigment and a liquid vehicle or carrier.

Paints are applied to a huge variety of surfaces as a thin veneer. Most paints are applied as a liquid and then allowed to dry as a thin film. Pigments and the vehicle also contribute to the surface bonding that is needed if the paint is to adhere to the surface.

Paint vehicles are made of at least one resin and a solvent. Resins are sticky materials that are produced from a number of sources. Resins used comprise acrylics, alkyds, epoxies, and vinyls. These include natural organic materials and chemicals manufactured by the chemical industry from a number of compounds in a variety of chemical reactions. Resins act as the adhesive that bonds the paint to the surface being painted. The characteristics of the resins used in paint determine its hardness as a paint, its gloss, its drying time, and its adhesive quality.

Solvents make paint liquid. The solvent used depends on the resin used. Water is the most commonly used interior solvent used in household paints. Other paints may be oil based. Other commonly used solvents include mineral spirits, naphtha, and xylene. It is also common to use solvents as paint thinners.

Extenders or inert pigments also may be added to a paint to increase its resistance to wear. Common materials used as inert pigments are mica, clay, powdered marble, and talc. Some paint extenders are used on metal surfaces to protect them from rusting. Read lead and zinc chromate are commonly used rust inhibiters.

The colors in paints come from the pigments used. White paint may use titanium dioxide, whereas lead chromate may be used to get orange or yellow.

Paints are classified by chemists according to the type of "cure" or drying mechanism that is used. Some pains cure through simple evaporation, and other paints require a chemical reaction to cure. This occurs when a catalyst triggers a reaction to bond the resins together.

Many surfaces are prepared for painting with the use of primers, sealers, or undercoats. These are paints that fill in porous surfaces like bare wood. Others create a coat that bonds to the surface that is being painted. Then the overcoats or paint is applied to this surface and, in turn, bonds with the undercoating much better than it could to the raw surface.

Household paints used in household interiors are usually water-based latex paints. The solvent is water, and the resin is a form of latex or rubber. Historically, natural rubber was used, but today polyvinyl acetate or acrylic resins are the resins used in latex paints, making the term *latex* a misnomer. Latex paints are easily applied, have little odor, and are not flammable. In addition, once dried they can be easily cleaned.

Household exterior paints are usually latex based, but some are oil based to gain additional properties that can withstand outdoor weathering. The solvent used in oil-based paints may be a natural oil, such as linseed oil, or an oil derived from the petroleum industry. The most commonly used paint vehicle is linseed oil. It has properties that make the paint more fluid (and therefore easier to apply), transparent, and glossy. It is available in several forms such as cold pressed, alkali, sun bleached or thickened, and polymerized (called *stand oil*).

Oil-based paints cure by means of oxidation. As the solvent evaporates, the paint reacts with oxygen in the air to form a hard oxide on the painted surface.

Industrial paints are used on consumer goods, industrial goods, and in buildings. The paint used on automobiles, refrigerators, washing machines, dryers, and many other household appliances is usually baked on in an oven. The baking produces an extremely hard, finished surface. Commonly, bake-on paints are acrylic resin paints.

Paints used on metal surfaces usually use a metal primer as a rust inhibitor. Metal surface paints are also designed to withstand high temperatures or to withstand exposure to water or other chemicals, as in industrial plants. The aerospace industry and the airline industry use special paints to withstand temperature extremes.

Paints can contain a variety of chemicals that can pose a number of health hazards, from irritants to carcinogens. Lead was used for decades in household paints. However, it was discovered to be toxic to children, who upon being attracted to peeling paint, ate it and got lead poisoning. The use of significant quantities of lead in paint has been outlawed. The solvents used in paints can continue to emit fumes for years as the paint slowly completes its final evaporation. However, more dangerous are the carcinogenic chemicals that can occur in paints.

Many metal surface paints use chromate compounds that contain hexavalent chromium, which is a known carcinogen. For industrial workers, the use of spray painting equipment creates an opportunity for inhaling particles of paint that can lodge in the upper portion of the lungs, exposing the workers to a carcinogen. Because the size of the paint particles is relatively large, the risk is less than it would be if the spayed paint were atomize to much finer particles.

Carcinogenic compounds in paints include pigments in paints that are potentially carcinogenic, such as lead, cadmium, and chromium, and solvent carcinogens include methylene chloride. Studies of workers exposed to these materials have shown an increased risk of pancreatic and liver cancer.

Tests of paints on laboratory animals have produced skin tumors in mice and laboratory rats. Chemicals such as benzoyl peroxide, 7,12-dimethylbenz(a)anthracene, N-methyl-N'-nitro-N-nitrosoguanidine, and 12-O-tetradecanoylphorbol-13-acetate produced skin tumors in mice, indicating that these substances are probably carcinogenic in humans as well. Other probable carcinogens include perchloroethylene and polychlorinated biphenyls.

Some paints, most often water-based paints, also use biocides to prevent fungal growth, and sometimes the biocide used is formaldehyde, which is a potential carcinogen.

SEE ALSO: Chemical Industry; Solvents; Vinyl; Wood Preserver.

BIBLIOGRAPHY. John Brazinski, *Manual on Determination of Volatile Organic Compound (VOC) Content in Paints, Inks and Related Coating Products* (American Society for Testing and Materials, 1993); Vincent M. Coluccio, ed., *Lead-Based Paint Hazards: Assessment and Management* (Van Nostrand Reinhold, 1994); R. Lambourne and T. A. Strivens. *Paint and Surface Coatings: Theory and Practice* (SciTech Publishing, 1999); World Health Organization, ed., *Some Organic Solvents, Resin Monomers and Related Compounds, Pigments and Occupational Exposures in Paint Manufacturing: The Evaluation of Carcinogenic Risks to Humans* (World Health Organization, 1990); Royal Society of Chemistry Staff, *Long Term Neurotoxic Effects of Paint Solvents* (Royal Society of Chemistry, 1990); G. P. A. Turner, *Introduction to Paint Chemistry and Principles of Paint Technology* (Chapman and Hall, 1988).

ANDREW J. WASKEY
DALTON STATE COLLEGE

Pakistan

THIS SOUTH ASIAN country was formed with the partition of India in 1947. Before that, Pakistan made up two parts of British India, West Pakistan being on the western border of India, and East Pakistan, in the east, almost entirely surrounded on land by India. East Pakistan became Bangladesh in 1971. The population of Pakistan was 165,804,000 is 2004, and there are 57 doctors and 34 nurses per 100,000 people. An example of cancer incidence rates in Pakistan includes 130 cases of cancer in males per 100,000, according to the International Agency for Research on Cancer.

During the British colonial period, healthcare in hospitals for the European population and the wealthy elite was good, with surgery available for cancer sufferers. However, the cost of medical care was well beyond the ability to the vast mass of the population, most of whom died young, who therefore had a lower risk of succumbing to cancer.

After independence, there was a major impetus to increase the healthcare available throughout the whole country. Medical care in the main city Karachi, as well as Rawalpindi and the new capital Islamabad, has been relatively good, although it still is extremely problematic in remote parts of the country.

The founder of Pakistan, and its first governor-general, Mohammed Ali Jinnah (1876–1948) succumbed to lung cancer and tuberculosis just over a year after the creation of the country. Jinnah had been a heavy smoker and had actually been diagnosed with cancer several years earlier. However, he managed to keep this diagnosis secret. He became intractable during the negotiations for partition, with some historians suggesting that had his condition been known, Indian politicians might have delayed the whole process to achieve a better bargaining position upon Jinnah's death.

The most common cancers in Pakistan for men are lung cancer and oral cancer. For women, breast cancer and cervical cancer are the most prevalent. As a result, there has been an impetus in recent years to encourage people to seek early diagnosis for problems, and also to get more women screened regularly. This should result in earlier treatment and a greater success rate.

At independence, the largest city in the country was the port of Karachi, and this city was initially Pakistan's capital. As a result, the Karachi Cancer Registry was the first established in the country. On December 3, 1966, the postal authorities in Pakistan issued a postage stamp commemorating the Arab medieval cancer surgeon Avicenna (980–1037). In an important study of cancer in the North-West Frontier Province in 2000–04, A. Zeb, A. Rasool, and S. Nasreen found that reported cancers were more prevalent in men (61 percent) and that the largest occupational group reporting cancers were farmers (43.8 percent), followed by housewives (33.8 percent). Laborers and civil servants had the lowest rates of cancer incidence.

After retiring from cricket, Imran Khan, probably the best known Pakistani cricketer, has devoted much of his time to the Shaukat Khanum Memorial Cancer Hospital and Research Center, which he established in Lahore in memory of his mother, Mrs. Shaukat Khanum, who died from cancer. Funds were first raised in 1989, and the hospital was opened on December 29, 1994. It has since treated many patients.

A number of prominent Pakistanis have suffered from cancer. Altaf Gauhar (1923–2000), a civil servant and later a prominent journalist and author, died from cancer, and Anwar Hussain Khokhar (1920–2002), a member of Pakistan's first test cricket team, died from liver cancer in Lahore.

The Pakistan Council for Science and Technology, Islamabad, advises the Pakistan government on science and technology policy and has worked with the Pakistan National Institute of Health, which also located in Islamabad, in coordinating cancer research in the country. There is also research being undertaken by the Cancer Support Group of the Aga Khan University Hospital and by several other organizations in the country. The Ministry of Health, Pakistan, and the Pakistan Atomic Energy Commission are both members of the International Union against Cancer.

SEE ALSO: Asian Diet; India.

BIBLIOGRAPHY. P. Akhter, K. Rahman, S. D. Orfi, and N. Ahmad, "Radiological Impact of Dietary Intakes of Naturally Occurring Radionuclides on Pakistani Adults," *Food and Chemical Toxicology* (v.45, 2007); T. S. Ali and S. Baig, "Evaluation of a Cancer Awareness Campaign: Experience with a Selected Population in Karachi," *Asian Pacific Journal of Cancer Prevention* (v.7/3, 2006); Y. Bhugari, "Karachi Cancer Registry Data—Implications for the National Cancer Control Program of Pakistan," *Asian Pacific Journal of Cancer Prevention* (v.5/1, 2004); S. Jamal, N. Mamoon, S. Mushtag, and M. Luqman, "Pattern of Childhood Malignancies: Study of 922 Cases at Armed Forces Institute of Pathology (AFIP), Rawalpindi, Pakistan," *Asian Pacific Journal of Cancer Prevention* (v.7/3, 2006); A. Zeb, A. Rasool, and S. Nasreen, "Occupation and Cancer Incidence in District Dir (NWFP), Pakistan, 2000–2004," *Asian Pacific Journal of Cancer Prevention* (v.7/3, 2006).

JUSTIN CORFIELD
GEELONG GRAMMAR SCHOOL, AUSTRALIA

Palestinian Hemophilia Association

THE PALESTINIAN HEMOPHILIA Association (PHA) is a nongovernmental, not-for-profit organization, the purpose of which is to improve the condition of hemophiliacs and persons with other bleeding disorders. The association was created by hemophiliacs, their families, and professionals who are concerned that comprehensive medical and social care is not currently available for hemophiliacs, and it was officially registered as a nongovernmental organization with the Palestinian Interior and Health Ministries in May 2006.

The planned activities of the PHA include organizing the hemophiliac community, advocating for the availability of appropriate treatment for hemophiliac, conducting human rights and public awareness campaigns, working to integrate hemophiliacs within their communities, collecting data about hemophilia and bleeding disorders, and disseminating information to professionals and the general public about hemophilia and how new cases may be prevented or minimized. The temporary national office of the PHA is located in Ramallah, Palestine.

Specific medical goals of the PHA include increasing the availability of clotting factor (blood products that constitute the primary treatment for hemophilia) within Palestine, ensuring proper diagnosis and medical care through medical institutions and mobile clinics, establishing a treatment protocol for hemophilia, and establishing a national database for hemophiliacs and carriers of hemophilia. Educational goals include increasing awareness of hemophilia among medical personnel and the general public, educating family members and the community at large, further integration of hemophiliacs within Palestinian society, advocating for the rights of hemophiliacs to move freely within Palestine to seek medical treatment, and establishing a national office that will offer around-the-clock reference and referral services.

The PHA was established partly in response to the fact that treatment of hemophilia is not a priority within Palestinian governmental or private sectors, with the result that treatment is not regularly available and is not always provided following a standardized protocol. In addition, knowledge and understanding of hemophilia is low among the Palestinian general public. The roots of the PHA date back to 1996, when the first Hemophilia Association was formed in Palestine. This organization conducted an epidemiologic study of hemophilia in Palestine and surveyed the knowledge of hemophilia and the availability of healthcare for the disease. At present, the PHA has records for over 350 hemophiliacs and estimates that there may be over 1,000 hemophiliacs and several thousand hemophilia carriers in Palestine. Other key findings of this survey were that 65 percent of hemophiliacs in Palestine were younger than age 20 years and that a number of families had more than one hemophiliac member, indicating a possible lack of understanding of the genetic cause of hemophilia.

SEE ALSO: Education; Cancer.

BIBLIOGRAPHY. Palestinian Hemophilia Association, www. hemophilia.ps/ (cited November 2006).

SARAH BOSLAUGH
WASHINGTON UNIVERSITY SCHOOL OF MEDICINE

Pancreatic Cancer

PANCREATIC CANCER IS the fourth leading cause of cancer death in the United States and is often a lethal disease because of limited early detection and late clinical presentation. In some cases of familial pancreatic cancer, early detection can improve survival. The majority of pancreatic cancer cases are ductal adenocarcinomas—malignant glandular tissue that is derived from the pancreatic ducts that drain the pancreatic juice into the small intestine. Most patients are in their seventh decade of life when diagnosed and die within 6 months of diagnosis. Risk factors for developing pancreatic cancer include tobacco usage, alcohol usage, pancreatitis (inflammation of the pancreas), recent diagnosis of diabetes mellitus, and previous partial gastrectomy (partial removal of the stomach). Up to 10 percent of all pancreatic cancer may be inherited or related to a cancer syndrome, such as Peutz-Jeghers syndrome, Familial Adenomatous Polyposis, a *BRCA2* germline mutation, cystic fibrosis, ataxia telangiectasia, hereditary pancreatitis (caused by a mutation in the *PRSS1* Gene), or Familial Pancreatic Carcinoma syndrome.

Prevailing evidence indicates that local pancreatic environmental stress caused by items such as alcohol, tobacco, or germline mutation of *PRSS1*, a gene that encodes a protective protein for inflammation, triggers inflammation in the pancreas. The inflammation ulti-

mately causes damage to pancreatic ductal cell DNA, which drives the cell toward a cancer phenotype, and then ultimately to cancer. The genetic damage is thought to occur in a stepwise fashion, first forming precursor histological lesions called pancreatic intraepithelial neoplasia at a microscopic level. These lesions progress to frank cancer through alterations and mutation of the DNA and, in particular, through *K-RAS* (an oncogene found mutated in over 90 percent of pancreatic cancers), *p16* (a cell cycle antagonist found mutated in over 95 percent of pancreatic cancers, *p53* (a tumor suppressor found mutated in 75 percent of cancers), and loss of the tumor suppressor *SMAD4*, a key suppressive intracellular signal transduction molecule.

Patients often will present initially with vague symptoms, such as nonspecific abdominal or back pain, weight loss, and fatigue. Jaundice (yellowing of the skin) can occur in up to 50 percent of patients when the pancreatic cancer obstructs the bile ducts that normally drain bile into the small intestine.

DIAGNOSIS AND TREATMENT

Abdominal computed tomography, often with subsequent endoscopic ultrasound of the pancreas, is generally the main tool used to diagnose pancreatic cancer. Magnetic resonance cholangiopancreatography and endoscopic retrograde cholangiopancreatography, techniques that visualize the pancreatic ducts, may also be used for the diagnosis. In addition, elevated levels of a tumor marker, CA 19-9, may aid in differentiating benign from malignant pancreatic tumors.

The only hope for cure is surgical resection, typically with the Whipple procedure (removing the pancreas and surrounding tissues), but only 15 percent of patients will meet respectability guidelines after the determination of the extent of local invasion and spread of the pancreatic tumor. Chemotherapy is used as an adjunct or for palliation, but it is not curative. Chemotherapy often involves use of the drugs 5-fluorouracil and gemcitabine.

PROGNOSIS AND PREVENTION

Pancreatic cancer carries a poor prognosis. Five-year survival after resection is 25 percent for those who undergo surgery and less than 5 percent for those who cannot undergo surgery.

There is no current strategy for preventing nonfamilial pancreatic cancers, except to not use tobacco.

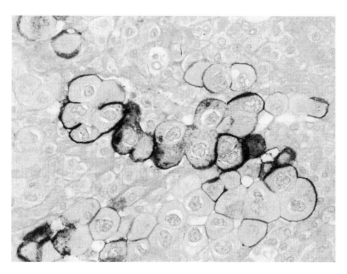

The majority of pancreatic cancer cases are ductal adenocarcinomas—malignant glandular tissue derived from the pancreatic ducts

In patients and family members with familial forms of pancreatic cancer, surveillance with abdominal computed tomography and endoscopic ultrasound should proceed by age 40 years, or younger if there are younger afflicted members in the family. Prevention is focused on surgically removing lesions that are detected at surveillance.

SEE ALSO: Pancreatic Cancer, Childhood.

BIBLIOGRAPHY. A. Jemal, R. Siegel, E. Ward, et al., "Cancer Statistics, 2006," *CA: A Cancer Journal for Clinicians* (v.56, 2006); J. Kleeff, C. Michalski, H. Friess, and M.W. Buchler, "Pancreatic Cancer: From Bench to 5-Year Survival," *Pancreas* (v.33, 2006).

JIMMY Y.C. CHOW, PH.D.
UNIVERSITY OF CALIFORNIA, SAN DIEGO
JOHN M. CARETHERS, M.D.
UNIVERSITY OF CALIFORNIA, SAN DIEGO

Pancreatic Cancer, Childhood

PANCREATIC TUMORS RARELY occur in childhood. Although pancreatic cancer is the fifth leading cancer in adults in the United States, childhood pancreatic cancers represent less than 5 percent of all malignancies in children under age 15 years. Cancers of the pancreas may be classified by pathology as adenocarcinomas, squamous cell carcinomas, acinar cell carcinomas, liposarcomas, lymphomas, papillary-cystic carcinomas, pancreatoblastomas, malignant insulinomas, glucagonomas, and gastrinomas. Malignant tumors often mimic their benign counterpart with similar clinicopathologic features. Mucinous cystadenocarcinomas are solitary, large, unilocular cysts composed of mucin-secreting epithelial cells. However, this type of tumor invades locally in the same way as a ductal adenocarcinoma. There is a strong female predominance, and the prognosis is excellent if resection is complete.

Adenocarcinoma of the pancreas (ductal or acinar) is also a rare neoplasm of the pancreas. Genetic studies indicate an increased incidence of pancreatic adenocarcinoma in patients with hereditary pancreatitis, patients with Peutz-Jeghers polyposis, and patients with celiac disease (although this increased risk is only observed in adult celiac patients). In addition, epidemiology studies have suggested an increased risk in pancreatic adenocarcinomas with higher socioeconomic class, higher consumption of animal fat and protein, wine consumption, and exposure to degreasers. Women who smoke or had oophorectomies (surgical removal of the ovaries) were also found to have an increased risk. Trisomy 21 (Down syndrome) also shows an increase risk for pancreatic tumors as well. Prognosis is poor in these patients, and chemotherapy is provided for palliation.

Ductal adenocarcinomas are usually located in the head of the pancreas and are often positive for carcinoembryonic antigen. Molecular analysis of tissue and pancreatic fluid in these patients have shown loss of chromosome 18q and may either activate oncogenes (*Kras, C-erB12*) or inactivate tumor suppressor genes (*SMAD4, TP53, MTS1*). This cancer requires aggressive surgical management with the Whipple procedure, which removes the pancreas and surrounding structures. The 3-year survival rate is approximately 2 percent, with a mean survival after surgery around 4–6 months. Because delay in prognosis is common in pancreatic tumors in the child, 85 percent of pancreatic adenocarcinomas will have metastasized (spread to other organs) at the time of presentation.

Acinar adenocarcinomas generally present after metastasis has occurred and has been described in children as young as 3 years of age. Some of these patients present with a constellation of findings including polyarthralgia (joint aches), extrapancreatic fat necrosis, and eosinophilia (elevation in the blood of a type of white blood cell). These tumors frequently demonstrate allelic losses on chromosome 11p and alterations in the APC-βcatenin pathway. Treatment is direct excision, and prognosis is more favorable than that for ductal adenocarcinoma.

Pancreatoblastoma is more common in boys than in girls and presents often as an incidental abdominal mass. A number of patients will secrete antidiuretic hormone from their tumors. Serum alpha-feto protein will be elevated and can be useful for following the course of disease. Primary resection is the treatment for this cancer, and prognosis is good in these children. Islet cell carcinomas arise from functional pancreatic lesions and are associated with hypoglycemia, or they can be part of the Zollinger-Ellison syndrome (caused by a tumor that secretes the hormone gastrin). These cancers are usually associated with multiple endocrine neoplasia type I syndrome. There is also an association between von Hippel Lindau (VHL) disease and islet cell carcinoma, caused by a germline mutation of the VHL gene on chromosome 3p25.

A variety of nonepithelial tumors of the pancreas have been described, although they are rarely found in children. Rhabdomyosarcomas and lymphomas and primitive neuroectodermal tumors can sometimes present as primary tumors of the pancreas. Secondary involvement of the pancreas by tumors can result from hematogenous spread in malignant melanoma, renal and lung tumors, and leukemia.

SEE ALSO: Childhood Cancers; Pancreatic Cancer.

BIBLIOGRAPHY. W. Allan Walker, Olivier Goulet, Ronald E. Kleinman, Philip M. Sherman, Barry L. Shneider, and Ian R. Sanderson, *Pediatric Gastrointestinal Disease*, 4th ed. (Decker, 2004); Albert B. Lowenfels, Pascale Maisonneuve, Eugene P. DiMagno, et al., "Hereditary Pancreatitis and the Risk of Pancreatic Cancer," *Journal of the National Cancer Institute* (v.89/6, 2006).

SHERRY C. HUANG, M.D.
UNIVERSITY OF CALIFORNIA, SAN DIEGO
JOHN M. CARETHERS, M.D.
UNIVERSITY OF CALIFORNIA, SAN DIEGO

Pancreatic Cancer, Islet Cell

ISLET CELL CANCER, a rare cancer, is a disease in which cancer (malignant) cells are found in certain tissues of the pancreas. The pancreas is about six inches long and is shaped like a thin pear, wider at one end and narrower at the other. The pancreas lies behind the stomach, inside a loop formed by part of the small intestine. The broader right end of the pancreas is called the head, the middle section is called the body, and the narrow left end is the tail.

The pancreas has two basic jobs in the body. It produces digestive juices that help break down (digest) food, and hormones (such as insulin) that regulate how the body stores and uses food. The area of the pancreas that produces digestive juices is called the exocrine pancreas. About 95 percent of pancreatic cancers begin in the exocrine pancreas. The hormone-producing area of the pancreas has special cells called islet cells and is called the endocrine pancreas. Only about 5 percent of pancreatic cancers start here.

The islet cells in the pancreas make many hormones, including insulin, which help the body store and use sugars. When islet cells in the pancreas become cancerous, they may make too many hormones. Islet cell cancers that make too many hormones are called functioning tumors. Other islet cell cancers may not make extra hormones and are called nonfunctioning tumors. Tumors that do not spread to other parts of the body can also be found in the islet cells. These are called benign tumors and are not cancer. A doctor will need to determine whether the tumor is cancer or a benign tumor.

A doctor should be seen if there is pain in the abdomen, diarrhea, stomach pain, a tired feeling all the time, fainting, or weight gain without eating too much. If there are symptoms, the doctor will order blood and urine tests to see whether the amounts of hormones in the body are normal. Other tests, including x-rays and special scans, may also be done. The chance of recovery (prognosis) depends on the type of islet cell cancer the patient has, how far the cancer has spread, and the patient's overall health.

Once islet cell cancer is found, more tests will be done to find out if cancer cells have spread to other parts of the body. This is called staging. The staging system for islet cell cancer is still being developed. These tumors are most often divided into one of three groups:

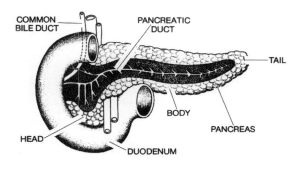

Line drawing showing detail of pancreas. The pancreas lies behind the stomach, inside a loop formed by part of the small intestine.

1) islet cell cancers occurring in one site within the pancreas,

2) islet cell cancers occurring in several sites within the pancreas, or

3) islet cell cancers that have spread to lymph nodes near the pancreas or to distant sites.

A doctor also needs to know the type of islet cell tumor to plan treatment. The following types of islet cell tumors are found:

Gastrinoma. The tumor makes large amounts of a hormone called gastrin, which causes too much acid to be made in the stomach. Ulcers may develop as a result of too much stomach acid.

Insulinoma. The tumor makes too much of the hormone insulin and causes the body to store sugar instead of burning the sugar for energy. This causes too little sugar in the blood, a condition called hypoglycemia.

Glucagonoma. This tumor makes too much of the hormone glucagon and causes too much sugar in the blood, a condition called hyperglycemia.

Miscellaneous. Other types of islet cell cancer can affect the pancreas and/or small intestine. Each type of tumor may affect different hormones in the body and cause different symptoms.

Recurrent. Recurrent disease means that the cancer has come back (recurred) after it has been treated. It may come back in the pancreas or in another part of the body.

SEE ALSO: Pancreatic Cancer; Pancreatic Cancer, Childhood.

BIBLIOGRAPHY. Timothy Canavan and Donna Cohen, "Vulvar Cancer," *Journal of the American Academy of Family Physicians* (v.66/7, October 2002); W. Allan Walker, Olivier Goulet, Ronald E. Kleinman, Philip M. Sherman, Barry L. Shneider, and Ian R.Sanderson, *Pediatric Gastrointestinal Disease* (Decker, 2004); Albert B. Lowenfels, Pascale Maisonneuve, Eugene P. DiMagno, et al., "Hereditary Pancreatitis and the Risk of Pancreatic Cancer," *Journal of the National Cancer Institute* (v.89/6, 2006).

NATIONAL CANCER INSTITUTE
WASHINGTON, D.C.

Paper Industry

THE INVENTION OF paper is considered one of the greatest achievements of mankind. Today, countries that lead in the production and consumption of paper are also the most advanced. The word *paper* is derived from the ancient Egyptian writing material called papyrus, which was formed from beaten strips of papyrus plants. The Egyptians sold papyrus to the ancient Greeks and Romans, but the establishment of the library at Alexandria in Egypt meant greater demand for the product and greater pressure on papyrus manufacturers. Because the plants could not be grown in temperate environments of Europe, an alternative was invented—vellum. Invented by the Greeks, vellum, or parchment, was made of processed sheepskin. At the same time, while the Egyptians and Greeks were using papyrus and vellum, respectively, the Chinese had discovered how to make paper. It is said that the Chinese court official Cai Lun, inspired by wasps and bees, first described the modern method of papermaking from wood pulp in 105 B.C.E. However, recent discoveries indicate that the ancient Chinese military was using paper for communication as early as 8 B.C.E.

It is believed that papermaking was a Chinese discovery, the knowledge of which slowly filtered from China to the Middle East, to southern Europe, to northern Europe, and finally to the rest of the world. However, the production of paper as a writing material exceeded the use of vellum during the 15th century. By the time the Europeans began to colonize other parts of the world, papermaking had become thoroughly integrated into European culture and was carried overseas by the colonists. In the United States, the first paper mill was built in Germantown,

Pennsylvania, in 1690. In short, making paper from plant fibers is a very old art that goes back well over two thousand years.

MODERN METHODS OF PAPERMAKING

Modern methods of making paper using machinery came of age in 1799. Before this date, paper was largely made by hand, with rags as the main source of fiber. With the invention by the turn of the 19th century of machines to make paper, wood became the main source of fiber. The use of cloth in the process has always produced higher-quality paper, and today, a large proportion of cotton and linen fibers in the mix create many excellent papers for special uses from wedding invitation paper to special paper for ink drawings. By the 1850s, the modern paper industry, based on the production of pulp from wood, had reached maturity. Since then, the paper industry has experienced many technological advancements that have resulted in the invention of modern machinery capable of producing continuous sheets of paper at the rate of over 20 miles per hour.

The making of paper is a two-stage process. First, wood must be turned into pulp, which is then used to make paper. Two main processes are used to convert logs to wood pulp. The first is the mechanical process in which logs are tumbled to remove the bark. Once the bark is removed, the logs are sent to grinders, which break the wood down into pulp by pressing it between huge, revolving slabs. The pulp is then filtered to remove foreign objects. The second method is the chemical process. In the chemical process, the harvested logs are cut into small wood chips, which are then poured into huge vats known as digesters, where chemicals are added, and the mixture is cooked at high pressure to release lignin, the natural glue that bonds wood fiber. Sodium hydroxide and sodium sulfide are the preferred chemical solution for this process. The pulp is washed to remove the chemicals and lignin and then bleached to remove the dark color and residual lignin. The end product is whiter, more resistant, and absorbent. The pulp is then dried and shipped to paper mills, where it is used to produce different types of paper.

In making the final product, paper, the pulp is spread onto a moving belt of fine wire mesh, through which water is drained from above and below to produce a smooth sheet of paper. The semidry sheet is then run through heated drying cylinders to evaporate the remaining water. Once dried, the sheet of paper passes between heated rolls to ensure uniform thickness and surface smoothness. The Fourdrinier machine, which was invented in England in 1807, is one type of machine that turns pulp into paper. Finally, the dried paper is wound onto large reels. Each jumbo roll holds over 50 tons of paper that can be cut into smaller rolls, wrapped, and either supplied to customers or converted into office paper, coated paper, tissue, and a myriad of other products. For example, in the modern economy, paper is used for money or banknotes, books, magazines, newspapers, packaging, cleaning, construction, and so on. Paper has become an omnipresent item that modern man would not know what to do without.

The bulk of the fiber used in the papermaking process today comes from wood harvested specifically for that purpose. However, fiber from sawmills wood chips, recycled newspaper, recycled cloth, and vegetable matter are also used. Coniferous trees, such as spruce and fir (also known as "softwoods"), are preferred for papermaking because the cellulose fibers in the pulp of these species are longer, which results in stronger paper. However, because of the great demand for paper products and because of improved pulp-processing technologies, almost any species of tree can now be harvested for paper, including hardwood trees such as poplar and elm. Where trees are scarce, other plants such as bamboo, straw, sugarcane, flax, hemp, and jute have been used to produce paper. Cotton and linen rags—usually cuttings and waste from textile factories—are used in fine-grade papers such as letterhead and resume paper and for bank notes and security certificates.

LOCATION AND GLOBAL GEOGRAPHY OF PAPERMAKING

The locating of pulp mills is constrained by the availability of paper's raw materials—the world's stands of timber. The wood from which pulp is made is usually cut into standard lengths of 6–8 feet, close to the point where the trees are felled. Often the felling of trees occurs close to waterways or seacoasts so the wood can be floated downstream or rafted along the coast to the pulp mill. The pulp mill is often located close to the paper mill and the consuming markets. This means that for the industry to be profitable it

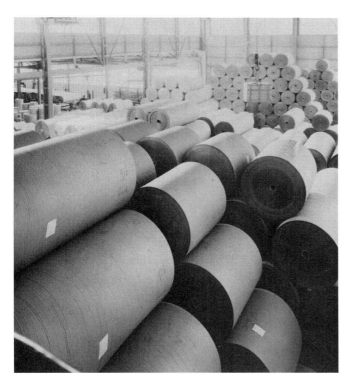

The dried paper is wound onto large reels. Each jumbo roll holds over 50 tons of paper that can be cut into smaller rolls.

and will likely play a significant role in the industry's growth over the next few years. A closer look at the statistics narrows the field to essentially two countries, the United States and Canada. For example, according to PricewaterhouseCoopers's annual Global Forest and Paper Industry Survey, of the top 20 forest and paper products companies in the world, U.S. companies grossed 57 percent of the proceeds from the sale of paper products in 2002. In 2004, the same survey by PricewaterhouseCoopers showed the continued dominance of the United States and Canada.

ENVIRONMENTAL AND HEALTH CONCERNS

The paper industry consumes a huge amount of trees that are cut down for the purpose of making paper. Environmentalists have long argued against the industry as being environmentally destructive in destroying mature and high-value trees that have taken generations to grow. Even if companies planted new trees in place of those they cut down, it is argued, new trees cannot replace the value of older trees. One solution to the destruction of woodlands for the paper industry has been to recycle used paper, and particularly newspapers. Today, recycling is a major industry in the United States that is alleviating the need for wholesale destruction of precious woodlands.

The fact that the paper industry requires huge amounts of water is itself a disadvantage in terms of human health, as the chemical stew that comes from the processing of pulp and paper must be disposed somewhere. Often the effluent is released back into local rivers or lakes. In some circumstances, the chemicals used might seep into ground aquifers that provide drinking water. Given that many chemicals harmful to human and animal life are used, the paper industry has been of great concern among the scientific community. Indeed, such chemicals as dyes, inks, and bleach can be extremely toxic and harmful to the environment when they are released into water supplies and nearby land after use. Aquatic ecosystems and fauna such as fish are often compromised by these chemicals.

Of greater significance is the possible effect of these chemicals on human health. Although scientific studies have not conclusively shown the relationship between chemicals used in the paper industry and cancer, it is a fact that pulp and paper production workers are constantly exposed to a complex mixture

needs to be close to its markets. Countries that rely solely on the exploitation of natural reserves thus operate at a loss, as the sites of tree felling must shift outward and away from markets when the nearby tree stands are depleted. In contrast, countries that maintain a careful program of cut and replenish continue to make paper at ever-increasing profits, as production is done in areas not far from densely settled areas. The most preferred site for the manufacturing of pulp and paper would therefore be one where wood is readily available in addition to markets, labor, inexpensive power, and water. Water is a vital component in the production of both pulp and paper. The paper industry cannot thrive in areas where water freezes or recurrent droughts are common.

The global geography of the paper industry clearly shows the dominance of the technically advanced nations. The global pulp and paper industry is dominated by the United States, Canada, Finland, Sweden, and a few East Asian countries such as Japan and Indonesia. Australasia and Latin America also have significant pulp and paper industries. Russia and China are rapidly catching up to these nations, however, of hazardous substances, including known or suspected carcinogens such as wood dust, various wood extracts and associated bioaerosols, reduced-sulfur compounds, talc, formaldehyde, combustion products, epichlorohydrin, acid mists, auramine and other benzidine-based dyes, and a range of chlorinated organic compounds. The specific chlorinated organic compounds that these workers are exposed to daily include volatile chlorinated hydrocarbons such as trichloroethylene, perchloroethylene, dichloromethane, and trichloromethane and nonvolatile organochlorine compounds such as chlorophenols and their salts (pentachlorophenol), polychlorinated biphenyls, and polychlorinated dibenzodioxins or polychlorinated dibenzofurans. The International Agency for Research on Cancer has classified the volatile organochlorines trichloroethylene and perchloroethylene as being probably carcinogenic to humans, based on sufficient evidence for carcinogenicity in animals.

Other epidemiological studies conducted from the 1980s to the present have indicated increased risks of gastrointestinal cancers, respiratory system cancers, and certain lymphatic and hematopoietic neoplasms in pulp and paper industry workers. Some studies have concentrated on examining the cancer mortality risks of workers in the pulp and paper industry who are exposed to sulfur dioxide and other volatile chemicals. Many of these studies indicate that occupational exposure to sulfur dioxide in the pulp and paper industry may be associated with an increased risk of lung cancer. In short, although there is uncertainty in the scientific community about the exact nature and extent of cancer risks, the slew of chemicals used in this industry is known to be hazardous to human health. When these chemicals are allowed to seep into ground aquifers important for human consumption, then the risks to human health become amplified.

In conclusion, it can be said that the discovery of paper has been an important ingredient for the advancement of society in the developed part of the world. Paper is an important part of daily life, with so many uses that without it, Western society would not have advanced to the level it has. However, the future of the paper industry is currently in question for being environmentally destructive. The paper industry does not only cause the loss of trees but has also raised health concerns for the workers, who are constantly exposed to dangerous, cancer-causing chemicals. Not only that, but when these chemicals find their way into rivers and ground aquifers, they may destroy ecosystems and put people in danger of ingesting carcinogens. With increasing environmental concerns, the industry is investing heavily in programs to clean up environmental pollution. Today, the U.S. government has put in place requirements that demand pollution-free paper production. Unfortunately, the heavy cost of such clean-up efforts is ultimately passed on to the consumer.

SEE ALSO: Chemical Industry; Chlorine; Solvents.

BIBLIOGRAPHY. D. Berryman, F. Houde, C. DeBlois, et al., "Nonylphenolic Compounds in Drinking and Surface Waters Downstream of Treated Textile and Pulp and Paper Effluents: A Survey and Preliminary Assessment of Their Potential Effects on Public Health and Aquatic Life," *Chemosphere* (v.56/3, 2004); Rosanne Ellis, Michael Heuvel, Murray Smith, et al., "Effects of Maternal versus Direct Exposure to Pulp and Paper Mill Effluent on Rainbow Trout Early Life Stages," *Journal of Toxicology and Environmental Health Part A* (v.68/5, 2005); Richard Morgan Highsmith and John Granville Jensen, *Geography of Commodity Production* (Lippincott, 1963); Kjell Toren, Bodil Persson, and Gun Wingren, "Health Effects of Working in Pulp and Paper Mills: Malignant Diseases," *American Journal of Industrial Medicine* (v.29/2, 1996); Kjell Toren, Stig Hagberg, and Hakan Westberg, "Health Effects of Working in Pulp and Paper Mills: Exposure, Obstructive Airways Diseases, Hypersensitivity Reactions, and Cardiovascular Diseases," *American Journal of Industrial Medicine* (v.29/2, 1996); Hilde Langseth and Aage Andersen, "Cancer Incidence among Women in the Norwegian Pulp and Paper Industry," *American Journal of Industrial Medicine* (v.36/1, 1999).

EZEKIEL KALIPENI
UNIVERSITY OF ILLINOIS AT URBANA-CHAMPAIGN

Papua New Guinea

PAPUA NEW GUINEA, a Melanesian country that occupying the eastern half of the island of New Guinea, was occupied by the Germans (New Guinea) and the British (Papua) until World War I. In 1914, an

Australian force captured New Guinea and merged it administratively to form Papua and New Guinea, which was a mandated territory of the League of Nations. In 1975, the territory became an independent country as Papua New Guinea. It had a population of 5,887,000 in 2005 and 7.3 doctors and 67 nurses per 100,000 people. An example of cancer incidence rates in Papua New Guinea includes 148 cases of cancer in males per 100,000, according to the International Agency for Research on Cancer.

Healthcare in Papua New Guinea was underdeveloped until recent years. Indeed, access to much of the country was difficult until the 1970s, and even nowadays some areas remain extremely remote, with the main means of transport to these places being by plane and, more recently, by helicopter or, to some of the offshore islands, by boat. Until recently, hospital care in Port Moresby, the capital, and other towns such as Wau were largely for Australian, American, or European expatriates, with a large focus on tropical diseases rather than cancer.

The cancer registry in Papua New Guinea was established in 1958, with the official title being the Tumour Registry of Papua New Guinea. Much of the early interest in cancer in Papua New Guinea was because many of the people had been isolated in the central highlands and other areas for many centuries, and as a result, their lifestyles and healthcare system operated in total isolation from advances in medical practices elsewhere in the world. Initially, few deaths were reported to the cancer registry, possibly because of misdiagnosis or even nondiagnosis. However very quickly figures started to show levels of oral cancer, skin cancer, liver cancer, and penile cancers, as well as Burkitt's lymphoma, in many parts of the population. With women, breast and cervical cancer were also found. For oral cancer, it was initially assumed to have come from chewing substances other than tobacco, particularly the areca nut with lime. However, some medical researchers have queried this conclusion. Overall cancer rates in Papua New Guinea are below those in nearby places such as Fiji and New Caledonia.

In 1989, an extensive study was conducted into all malignant tumors reported from 1958 until 1988 to try to work out the geographical spread of particular types of cancers. The most dramatic finding was a massive rise in carcinoma of the oral cavity, which is believed to be associated with the increase in the chewing of betel nuts in the highlands. There has also been a 300 percent increase in reported cases of cervical cancer, with a 600 percent increase seen in the highlands. These figures are likely to be caused by nonreporting in the early years of the registry, as well as a change in lifestyles and people living longer and therefore being at greater risk of cancer. The study also showed a decline in stomach cancer and hepatocellular carcinoma, with both Burkitt's lymphoma and non-Hodgkin's lymphoma remaining rare in the highlands; Burkitt's lymphoma tends to occur in people along the coastal regions of the country, which are also the areas with a higher rainfall and a more intense malaria transmission rate. The study also observed a decline in the incidence of squamous carcinoma of skin as better medical techniques were used to deal with tropical ulcers.

The Tumor Registry has shown that there has been a 200 percent rise in breast cancer, with little regional variations across the country. This resulted in several studies on the nature of the symptoms and their treatment, showing that the most likely age for sufferers was in the 45–54-year range, with 83.9 percent of women with breast cancer aged 54 years or less, 55.7 percent being under 45 years old, and 15 percent being under age 35 years. During the 1960s, J. Kariks of the Department of Health worked with V. J. McGovern of the Royal Prince Alfred Hospital in Sydney, Australia, on hepatoma in New Britain. In 1988, a secessionist revolt broke out on the island of Bougainville, largely because of worry about pollution from the Panguna Copper Mine, which many believed may have caused deformities in children and small animals.

Several famous people connected with Papua New Guinea have died from cancer, including Sir Francis Chichester (1901–72), who suffered from lung cancer in 1958–59 but recovered to go around the world on the *Gypsy Moth*.

Papua New Guinea's official research center remains the Institute of Medical Research.

SEE ALSO: Australia; Oral Cavity Cancer, Lip and.

BIBLIOGRAPHY. L. Atkinson, R. Purohit, P. Reay-Young, and G. C. Scott, "Cancer Reporting in Papua New Guinea: 1958–70 and 1971–78," *National Cancer Institute Monograph* (v.62, 1982); Anirudh Halder, Jacob Morewya, and

David A. K. Watters, "Rising Incidence of Breast Cancer in Papua New Guinea," *ANZ Journal of Surgery* (v.71, 2001); B. E. Henderson and G. H. Aiken, "Cancer in Papua New Guinea," *National Cancer Institute Monograph* (v.53, 1979); W. M. Martin, S. K. Sengupta, D. P. Murphy, and D. L. Barua, "The Spectrum of Cancer in Papua New Guinea. An Analysis Based on the Cancer Registry 1979-1988," *Cancer* (v.70/12, 1992).

JUSTIN CORFIELD
GEELONG GRAMMAR SCHOOL, AUSTRALIA

Paraguay

PARAGUAY, A LANDLOCKED South American country, was a Spanish colony until 1811, when it gained its independence as the Republic of Paraguay. From then until the early 20th century, much of the health services in the country remained underdeveloped, with the best medical care available in Asunción, the capital. An example of cancer incidence rates in Paraguay includes 157 cases of cancer in males per 100,000, according to the International Agency for Research on Cancer.

In the late 19th century, a few foreign doctors started to move to Paraguay, and some local doctors were also trained in oncology. Apart from herbal treatments used in the countryside, most of the medical treatment for cancer sufferers and for those with tumors relied on surgery. The low rates of cancer during this period were largely a result of the country's low life expectancy, with the vast majority of the adult male population of the country being killed during the War of the Triple Alliance (1864–70).

Many people in Paraguay consume a drink made out of an infusion of yerba, a local plant that is related to holly. This infusion is brewed into yerba mate, a drink not dissimilar from strong tea, that is said to show some ability to fight cancer. Yerba mate was one of the largest exports from Paraguay until the War of the Triple Alliance, and recent research by scientists at the University of Illinois has shown that yerba is rich in phenolic constituents, which can inhibit the proliferation of oral cancer cells.

However a 1995 study by P. A. Rolon, X. Castellsague, M. Benz, and N. Munoz of the Laboratorio de Anatomia Patolgica y Citologia in Asunción shows that there is some increased risk of esophageal cancer with the use of yerba mate, although the authors show that this is because high mate consumption is often undertaken by people who also smoke tobacco and who are heavy consumers of alcohol. There have also been recent studies of mate consumption at the Oncology Institute of Montevideo, Uruguay, that tend to confirm a link to an increased esophageal cancer risk. Mention should also be made that there has been found to be a noticeable prevalence of human t-cell leukemia–lymphoma virus in some black former slave communities located on the outskirts of Asunción.

In the early 20th century, as life expectancy in Paraguay increased, so did the prevalence of cancer, with the number of cases rising massively from the 1970s on. One of the specialists in Asunción at the time, specializing in thyroid cases, was Dr. Anibal Estigarribia from the Facultad de Ciencias Médicas. Another was Manuel Riveros, who produced a lymphadenography study in cancer for the Maria and Josefa Barbero National Cancer Institute.

The National Cancer Institute is located in Asunción and still coordinates health services for cancer sufferers in the country. It provides a teaching center for medical staff and also is a focus for the Ministry of Public Health and Social Welfare. It also performs work with insurance companies and private charities. In addition, there is a Paraguayan Anti-Cancer League, which raises awareness of cancer in schools and also raises money for cancer research and for treatment of cancer sufferers and their family.

SEE ALSO: Argentina; Brazil; Colombia; Venezuela.

BIBLIOGRAPHY. Alyn Brodsky, *Eliza Lynch & Friend* (Cassell, 1976); P. A. Rolon, X. Castellsague, M. Benz, and N. Munoz, "Hot and Cold Mate Drinking and Esophageal Cancer in Paraguay," *Cancer Epidemiology Biomarkers and Prevention* (v.4/6, 1995); Vikash Sewram, Eduardo de Stafani, Paul Brennan, and Paolo Boffetta, "Maté Consumption and the Risk of Squamous Cell Esophageal Cancer in Uruguay," *Cancer Epidemiology Biomarkers and Prevention* (v.12, 2003).

JUSTIN CORFIELD
GEELONG GRAMMAR SCHOOL, AUSTRALIA

Parathyroid Cancer

PARATHYROID CANCER IS a rare disease in which parathyroid gland cells grow and replicate uncontrollably. The parathyroid glands are four pea-sized glands located at the base of the neck, typically on the back surface of the thyroid gland. They secrete an essential hormone called parathyroid hormone (PTH or parathormone), which controls calcium metabolism.

Parathyroid glands can develop benign or malignant tumors, both of which require treatment. Benign tumors are local growths, not cancers. Conversely, malignant tumors are what we have termed cancers, and they have the potential to invade the surrounding tissues and metastasize to distant sites. Both benign and malignant tumors cause the parathyroid glands to become overactive in a condition called hyperparathyroidism.

Although parathyroid cancer is rare, hyperparathyroidism itself is a common condition that affects one in every 500–1,000 people in the United States. Benign parathyroid tumors cause the majority of hyperparathyroidism cases, whereas cancers account for less than 0.5 percent of the incidences. Overactive parathyroid glands secrete excess PTH in both benign and malignant conditions. PTH signals calcium to be released from the bones, as well as signalling the intestines to absorb more calcium from the diet. Hyperparathyroidism thus results in an abnormal elevation of blood calcium, a condition called hypercalcemia. It is a fatal situation that warrants immediate medical attention, because our body's nerves and muscles are dependent on a narrow range of calcium concentrations.

The symptoms of hyperparathyroidism and hypercalcemia include weakness, fatigue, nausea, constipation, excess urination, thirst, and loss of appetite. Compared to patients with benign hyperparathyroidism, parathyroid cancer patients are also likely to have neck masses, bone diseases, kidney diseases, and extremely high calcium and PTH levels in the blood. The chances of recovery depend on the stage of the cancer, on whether it is operable, on whether calcium concentrations are controllable, and on the patient's general health.

Risk factors for parathyroid cancer are not well established. However, recent studies indicate that an inheritable mutation in the *HRPT2* tumor suppressor gene can play a critical role in parathyroid cancer development. Tumor suppressor genes are DNA sequences that encode proteins that restrain cell proliferation. Cells can grow and divide uncontrollably when mutations disrupt such genes.

The goal of parathyroid cancer treatment is to lower PTH levels to control blood calcium concentrations. Before any curative attempts, hypercalcemia is first controlled by drugs and hydration because, as parathyroid cancer is typically slow growing, hypercalcemia does more harm than the cancer itself.

The definitive treatment for parathyroid cancer is surgery. It involves the careful removal of the cancerous gland in operations called parathyroidectomies. Parts of the thyroid gland, thymus, and other surrounding tissue are often removed as well. If the cancer has metastasized to other organs such as the lymph nodes, lungs, bones, and liver, these tumors are surgically removed in the same manner. Radiation therapy and chemotherapy are still in their investigational stages. They are administered if the cancer is inoperable and if calcium-controlling drugs have failed.

It is important for patients to have regular follow-up appointments with physicians to closely monitor blood calcium and PTH levels to detect any early signs of recurring parathyroid cancer. The standard treatment for recurring parathyroid cancers is repeated surgical resections. About one-third of all patients are cured after the initial treatment; one-third encounter aggressive forms, unfortunately leading to short survival; and one-third experience recurrence of curable, slow-growing tumors.

SEE ALSO: Head and Neck Cancer; Surgery; Thyroid Cancer.

BIBLIOGRAPHY. National Cancer Institute, "Parathyroid Cancer (PDQ®): Treatment," www.cancer.gov (cited December 2006).

YOSHIHIRO YONEKAWA
WEILL MEDICAL COLLEGE OF CORNELL UNIVERSITY

Passive Smoking

PASSIVE SMOKING (ALSO known as secondhand smoking, involuntary smoking, or exposure to environmental tobacco smoke) describes the inhalation of a mixture of sidestream smoke given off by a smolder-ing cigarette and the mainstream smoke exhaled by a smoker. Worldwide, approximately 1.3 billion people currently smoke cigarettes or other products (more than 1 billion men and 250 million women) [Guidon 2003]. Over fifty percent of children in the world are exposed to secondhand smoke in their homes (UCETS and Child Health). In the United States, more than 126 million nonsmokers are exposed to secondhand smoke annually, and of these, almost 22 million are children [Surgeon General 2006].

The extremely high prevalence of passive smoke exposure and the mounting evidence of its harmful, even deadly, health effects demand the attention of policy makers, scientists, industry, and the popula-tion in general. Although passive smoke exposure has decreased in developed countries since the publica-tion of the Surgeon General's Report on *The Health Consequences of Smoking* in 1982 [Surgeon General 1982], many developing countries around the world have reported increases in smoking and passive smoke exposure among both children and adults. As such, exposure to passive smoke remains a global public health hazard.

STUDIES ON PASSIVE SMOKING

Every year, the scientific community understands more about the harmful effects of tobacco on nonsmokers. In the 1972 Surgeon General's report, also titled *The Health Consequences of Smoking*, Dr. Jesse Steinfeld reported that "smoking in enclosed places could lead to high levels of cigarette smoke components in the air." This was the first time public health officials ad-dressed passive smoking in the United States. The first conclusive evidence on the danger of passive smoking, Takeshi Hirayama's study on the increased risk of lung cancer in Japanese women married to smokers, was published in 1981 [Hirayama 1981].

Dozens of studies have since confirmed the link between passive smoking and lung cancer over the past decades. In May 2006, the Surgeon General Dr. Richard Carmona stated that, "the health effects of secondhand smoke exposure are more pervasive than we previously thought. The scientific evidence is now indisputable: secondhand smoke is not a mere an-noyance. It is a serious health hazard that can lead to disease and premature death in children and non-smoking adults." The California Environmental Pro-

tection Agency currently estimates that secondhand smoke exposure causes approximately 3,400 annual lung cancer deaths (in addition to 22,700–69,600 heart disease deaths) among adult nonsmokers in the United States. This conclusion extends to all passive smoke exposure in the home, workplace, or public places such as bars and restaurants.

The threat from passive smoke exposure extends be-yond the lung. The 2004 Surgeon General's Report pro-vided strong evidence of the adverse impact of smok-ing and concluded that smoking harms nearly every organ in the body by causing disease and worsening health. To date, investigators have provided evidence that smoking is associated with acute myeloid leuke-mia, bladder cancer, cervical cancer, esophageal can-cer, gastric cancer, kidney cancer, laryngeal cancer, oral cavity and pharyngeal cancer, and pancreatic cancer in smokers. According to the World Health Organiza-tion, nonsmokers who are exposed to passive smoking are exposed to the same carcinogens as active smok-ers [IARC 2002]. Because of this fact, many investiga-tors have hypothesized that passive smoke exposure is the cause of many cancers in addition to lung cancer. Researchers continue to investigate the role of passive smoke in the development of other cancers, such as nasopharyngeal cancer or cervical cancer.

Passive smoke is currently classified as a group 1 cacinogen, or a carcinogen which has demonstrated *sufficient evidence* of carcinogenicity in humans. Side-stream smoke contains 69 known carcinogens includ-ing formaldehyde, lead, arsenic, benzene, and radioac-tive polonium 210 [IARC 2002]. Several carcinogens have been shown to be present at higher concentra-tions in sidestream smoke than in mainstream smoke, because sidestream smoke is generated at lower tem-peratures and under different combustion conditions than mainstream smoke.

Population-based study of the adverse health ef-fects caused by passive smoke depend on its accu-rate measurement in the environment. There are many issues that complicate the measurement of the dose of passive smoke inhaled; both types of smoke change as they get diluted and distributed in the en-vironment and with time. The direct measurement of passive smoke exposure is subsequently compli-cated as the quantity of secondhand smoke inhaled involuntarily varies and its composition depends on smoking patterns and cigarette type. Furthermore,

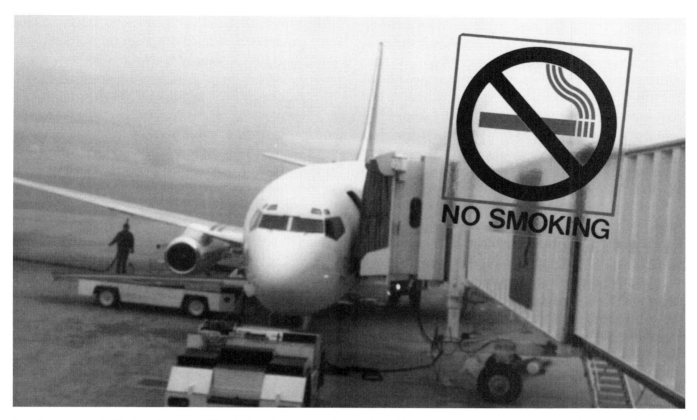

Despite successes in Western Europe and North America, interventions and smoking bans have not received support throughout the rest of the world and most countries have not yet implemented public health measures to control passive smoke exposure.

the individual capacity to detoxify carcinogens after passive smoke is inhaled varies from individual to individual, making the epidemiological study of the health effects of passive smoke exposure difficult. There are biological markers, such as DNA adducts and serum cotinine levels that are currently employed by investigators to objectively detect smoke exposure. However, the presence of measurement error in scientific studies makes it more difficult to detect an effect (such as an increased risk of lung cancer). As limitations in exposure measurement are minimized, future studies will have more power to clearly delineate the health impact of passive smoke exposure on cancer outcomes.

Thanks to the research detailing the harmful impact of passive smoke, the case for smoke-free environments has grown much stronger. Tobacco control efforts have pursued smoking bans in the past decades to decrease nonsmoker exposure to passive smoke. Banning smoking in public and work places protects the health of non-smokers. Workplace

smoking bans have demonstrably reduced exposure to passive smoking. The research in this area has also demonstrated that smokers who are employed in workplaces with smoking bans consume fewer cigarettes per day, consider quitting, and quit at a greater rate than smokers employed in workplaces where smoking is not prohibited.

SMOKING LEGISLATION

Workplace bans in bars and restaurants have received a lot of attention in recent years and have been strongly debated. The first general ban on smoking in all establishments serving food and drink, including restaurants, cafés, and nightclubs, was introduced in Norway on June 1, 2004, and in Sweden on June 1, 2005, and now many parts of the United States, including Florida, Delaware, California, Connecticut, Ohio, and New York, have similar legislation in place. The bans have grown in scope as many states in the United States and countries around the world now prohibit smoking in public buildings as well as private businesses.

A study frequently cited in the literature as evidence of the protective impact of smoking ban on the health of a community was published by Sargent et al. in the *British Medical Journal* in 2004 [Sargent 2004]. The study was conducted in Helena, Montana and demonstrated how the introduction of a smoke-free policy positively impacted hospital admissions. More specifically, hospital admissions for acute myocardial infarction (AMI) dropped significantly (by 40 percent) during a 6-month period during which a local ban on workplace and public smoking was enforced. After the ban was suspended, admissions returned to baseline levels. The geographic areas surrounding Helena, which did not institute the 6-month ban, showed no change in admission rates for AMI. The investigators concluded that a smoking ban in workplaces and public places may be associated with an effect on morbidity from heart disease.

Despite the accumulating evidence of a relationship between smoking bans and improved health, lawmakers continue to face strong resistance to implementation of smoke-free legislation. A major concern of those opposed to smoking bans is economic loss in bars and restaurants. Researchers are finding, however, that the economic losses predicted by those opposed to smoking bans have not been observed. In fact, recent evidence suggests that business has improved in states with smoking bans in bars and restaurants in the years following the implementation of a ban.

A study of the impact of the smoking ban in restaurants in California provided evidence of the favorable trend. Specifically, first quarter sales in 1996 in the State of California were $2.0 billion in 1996 and 1997 (the 2 years before ban), $2.1 billion in 1998 (year smoking banned), and continued to increase to $2.3 billion in 1998, to $2.6 billion in 2000, and $2.7 billion in 2001. Similar effects have been observed in New York City.

Despite successes in Western Europe and North America, interventions and smoking bans have not received support throughout the rest of the world and most countries have not yet implemented public health measures to control passive smoke exposure. Statistics demonstrate that the overall percentage of smokers has decreased in developed countries, but the prevalence is still increasing in developing countries and among women. In 1995, more smokers lived in low- and middle-income countries (933 million) than in high-income countries (209 million). About 35 percent of men in developed countries smoke, compared with almost 50 percent of men in developing nations and almost two-thirds of Chinese men [Jha, P 2000]. The geography of smoking and subsequent passive smoke exposure continues to shift from the developed to the developing world. It is clear that current tobacco control efforts and the control of passive smoke exposure are insufficient to mitigate the future health burden in the developing world due to tobacco.

As such, there is evidence that passive smoke exposure is hazardous to human health and has been associated with cancer. The mounting evidence has resulted in the grouping of passive smoke as a class I human carcinogen. More research is currently being conducted to further assess the risk of passive smoke exposure on an array of different health outcomes. The ability to point to even more evidence of the adverse consequences of smoke exposure will demand that policy makers around the world address strategies to prevent the harmful exposure currently experienced by nonsmoking adults and children worldwide.

SEE ALSO: Smoking Cessation (Nicotine Replacement Therapy).

BIBLIOGRAPHY. U.S. Department of Health and Human Services, "The Health Consequences of Smoking: Cancer: A Report of the Surgeon General." Public Health Service, Office of Smoking and Health, 1982. DHHS(PHS) 82-50179; U.S. Department of Health and Human Services. "The Health Consequences of Involuntary Exposure to Tobacco Smoke: A Report of the Surgeon General." www.surgeongeneral.gov/library/secondhandsmoke/report (cited September 2006); "International Consultation on Environmental Tobacco Smoke (ETS) and Child Health." W.H.O.; G. E. Guidon, D. Boisclair (cited November 2006). "Past, Current And Future Trends In Tobacco Use." Vol 2003: The World Bank. www1.worldbank.org/tobacco/publications.asp (cited 2003); P. Jha, F. Chaloupka (cited January 2007), R. P. Sargent, R. M. Shepard, S. A. Glantz, eds., "Reduced Incidence of Admissions for Myocardial Infarction Associated With Public Smoking Ban: Before and After Study," BMJ 2004 (v. 328).

BRISEIS KILFOY
YALE UNIVERSITY

Penile Cancer

THERE ARE MANY different forms of penile cancer, with the severity depending on the extent to which the cancer has spread. Early detection offers many advantages, and there are many treatment options, including surgery, radiation therapy, biological therapy, and laser therapy.

Penile cancer usually begins as a small lesion on the penis and tends to spread very slowly. Malignancies are usually found in the head of the penis (the glans), with the foreskin (or prepuce) the next most common site. Tumors in the shaft of the penis are uncommon.

Penile cancer usually involves squamous cell carcinomas (cancer not involving melanomas). One common type of penile cancer is epidermoid carcinoma (where the cancer develops in the skin of the penis). Another is verrucous carcinoma (a low-grade malignancy that may spread into surrounding tissue). Approximately 5 percent of penile cancers are caused by melanomas from pigment-producing skin cells, basal cell penile cancer (i.e., cancer not caused by melanomas), and sarcomas (cancers of the connective or supportive tissue such as muscles and blood vessels). HPV (human papillomavirus) was classified as a cause of penile cancer by the International Agency for Research on Cancer in 1995. Another rare form of cancer, which develops in the sweat glands in the skin of the penis, is called adenocarcinoma.

The severity of penile cancer depends on whether the cancer is detected at the earliest stage (known as carcinoma in situ) and whether the carcinoma is localized or has spread to other areas. Early treatment can cure penile cancer. However, penile cancer may be emotionally devastating, embarrassing, and shameful for men, which may lead them to delay seeking treatment. Such delays may exacerbate the problem.

Typically, penile cancer is treated with surgery, such as local resection for superficial carcinomas (partial amputation of the affected part of the penis, possibly treated with a penile reconstruction), in which a small incision is made until the surgeon reaches normal skin tissue. Such surgery usually does not prevent patients from being able to have sexual intercourse. However, in some cases, surgical removal of the penis and perhaps a lymph node may be necessary. In addition to surgery, chemotherapy, radiation therapy, biological therapy, and laser therapy are other possible treatment options.

Penile cancer usually affects older men (those over 60 years of age), although a small proportion of the disease occurs in younger men. Malignancies of the penis are rare among circumcised men, and those circumcised as babies almost never develop penile cancer. The interaction between various viruses and penile cancer is an area still being investigated, particularly the effects of sexually transmitted diseases such as the herpes and human papilloma viruses.

The risk of mortality associated with penile cancer varies greatly according to whether there is carcinoma in situ (the earliest stage of squamous cell cancer) and whether the carcinoma is localized to a specific area. The overall 5-year survival rate from penile cancer is approximately 50 percent. This type of cancer is generally uncommon in Western countries. The American Cancer Society estimates that approximately 260 men died from penile cancer in 2006. However, penile cancer is much more common in less developed countries and accounts for approximately a quarter of all cancers diagnosed in men in Asia and Africa.

SEE ALSO: American Cancer Society; Biologic Therapy; Chemotherapy; Radiation Therapy; Sarcoma, Soft Tissue, Adult; Surgery.

BIBLIOGRAPHY. Bin K. Kroon, Simon Horenblas, and Omgo E. Nieweg, "Contemporary Management of Penile Squamous Cell Carcinoma," *Journal of Surgical Oncology* (v.89/1, 2005).

MARK SHERRY
UNIVERSITY OF TOLEDO

Perfume

PERFUME IS A mixture of aroma compounds, solvents, and fragrant essential oils that are applied to the human body, living spaces, and objects. The use of perfumes, colognes, and products that contain fragrance dates back several centuries and has increased in popularity in recent decades. Although perfume makers and manufacturers strive to make perfumes appealing to customers, there are documented health risks to perfume ranging from dermatitis to carcinogenic ingredients in fragrances. Many perfumes have floral, woody, and fresh scents. Plants have long been used in perfumery because of their essential oils and aroma compounds. Animal and synthetic sources are commonly used as well.

The word perfume comes from the Latin *per fume*, meaning "through smoke." The art of making perfume dates back to ancient Egypt. The art was later refined by the Romans and the Arabs. Islamic cultures in Asia played a pivotal role in modern perfumery before the 14th century. They used steam distillation and other distillation technologies that were later used by the Europeans as early as the 14th century. By the 18th century, aromatic plants were being grown in the Grasse region of France, and France remains the center of European perfume trading and design today.

PERFUME REGULATION

The U.S. federal government has some authority over fragrances, but this power is seldom used. In the United States, fragrances that are considered cosmetics are placed under the authority of the Food and Drug Administration. This responsibility is shared with the Consumer Products Safety Commission, with some input from the Environmental Protection Agency. Cosmetic safety in Canada falls under the jurisdiction of Health Canada. The European Commission supervises fragrances in Europe.

The Cosmetic, Toiletry, and Fragrance Association is the leading U.S. trade association for the personal care products industry, with more than 500 member companies. Founded in 1894, CTFA works to promote fair trading and to protect industry interests. The Research Institute for Fragrance Materials gathers data on the safety of fragrance ingredients, and the International Fragrance Association then reviews this information and formulates guidelines for use. The International Fragrance Association also regulates the toxicity levels of fragrances in perfume.

There are no warning labels on perfumes. The only ingredient that must be listed on the perfume label is "fragrance." This "fragrance" may include over 100 small portions of materials, and the perfume industry is generally very secretive about the ingredients put in their products. Much of the data on perfume safety focuses on skin allergies. The excessive use of perfume is associated with skin aller-

gies, and chemicals such as acetophenone, ethyl acetate, and acetone are found in many perfumes and are known for their effect on those with potential respiratory allergies.

The materials in fragrances quickly get into the air and pose health issues for those with allergies, asthma, chronic lung disease, migraines, and other ailments. Over 70 percent of asthmatics report that their asthma is triggered by fragrances. This sensitivity can affect job performance and can impede daily activities because of the widespread use of perfumes and other scented products.

HEALTH RISKS

Approximately 5.6 million people living in the United States have skin allergies to fragrances, including those found in perfumes. Synthetic musks have a number of effects. They are known to accumulate in breast milk and are able to cross the placenta between mother and baby. These compounds also contaminate waters and can affect environments at even higher levels than pesticides can. Some of these materials also may be carcinogens or cocarcinogens.

FRAGRANCE FOR HEALTH

There is a free program sponsored by the Cosmetic, Toiletry, and Fragrance Association, the American Cancer Society, and the National Cosmetology Association called, "Look Good ... Feel Better." It teaches *cancer* patients how to deal with changes to their appearance as a result of radiation or chemotherapy. At workshops across the United States, women who are undergoing radiation or chemotherapy receive instruction from trained cosmetologists, hairstylists, and other experts.

The program also offers individual teaching and makeup sessions and distributes instructional books and videos for women to learn beautifying techniques on their own. In addition, cosmetics companies give away about $16 million worth of products each year. Serving over 40,000 women, counterparts to this program exist in 10 other countries.

Researchers continue to unlock the mysteries of perfume ingredients as they relate to health hazards. There are a number of journals and organizations committed to educating the public on the benefits and risks of using perfumes. The major organizations associated with perfume have been mentioned, but relevant peer-reviewed academic journals include *Regulatory Toxicology and Pharmacology* and the *Flavour and Fragrance Journal.*

SEE ALSO: Cosmetics; Deodorizers; Detergents.

BIBLIOGRAPHY. Betty Bridges, "Fragrance: Emerging Health and Environmental Concerns," *Flavour and Fragrance Journal* (v.17, 2002); Research Institute for Fragrance Materials, RIFM Database, www.rifm.org (cited January 2007); D. T. Salvito, M. G. H. Vey, and R. J. Senna, "Fragrance Materials and Their Environmental Impact," *Flavour and Fragrance Journal* (v.19, 2004).

VERONICA OUMA, PH.D.
HOFSTRA UNIVERSITY

Peru

PERU, A LATIN American country, was ruled by the Incas until the arrival of the Spanish conquistadors in 1531. The conquistadors established Spanish rule over much of South America, with Peru being the administrative center of their possessions. In the late 1810s, as various parts of Spanish America tried to gain independence, Peru remained loyal to the Spanish crown. The government was attacked by republicans led by José de San Martín, becoming independent on July 28, 1821. Peru had a population of 27,968,000 in 2005, with 93 doctors and 115 nurses per 100,000 people. An example of cancer incidence rates in Peru includes 210 cases of cancer in males per 100,000, according to the International Agency for Research on Cancer.

During the Spanish colonial period, medical services were largely restricted to Europeans and a handful of the local elite. It was not until the late 19th century that health services were considerably enlarged, and many treatments, including for cancer, remained out of the financial reach of most of the Peruvians until the second half of the 20th century.

In 1955, work started at the Laboratory for Cancer Research in Lima; this research became the basis of the study by Pablo Mri-Chavez of the Instituto de Investigaciones de la Altura, Universidad Peruana Cayetano Heredia, Lima, on the observations on the effect of high altitude on neoplastic growth.

The establishment of cancer registries was another important move. The Registro de Cancer de Lima Metropolitana, run by Dr. Eduardo Caceres and Maribel Almonte, and the Registro de Cancer de Base Poplacional de Trujillo, from Trujillo, under the direction of P. F. Albujar, both collect important data.

Other recent studies of cancer in Peru include that by G. F. Gonzales and L. G. Valerio of the Department of Biological and Physiological Sciences, Faculty of Sciences and Philosophy and Instituto de Investigaciones de la Altura, Universidad Peruana Cayetano Heredia, Lima. These researchers worked on the possibility of finding anticancer treatments in natural products. Other projects include one at the Instituto de Medicina Tropical Alexander von Humboldt, and another at the Universidad Peruana Cayetano Heredia, on Kaposi's sarcoma. Another study noticed the prevalence of human t-cell leukemia–lymphoma virus in some black former slave communities in Peru. Ernesto Bustamante, who was born in Lima in 1950, was awarded the Breast Cancer Concept Award by the U.S. Department of Defense on the recommendation of the Medical Research Programs in 2002.

The Instituto de Enfermedades Neoplásicas, Peru; the Liga Peruana de Lucha Contra el Cáncer, Peru; the Oncosalud, Peru; the Sociedad Peruana de Cancerología, Peru; and the Sociedad Peruana de Oncología Médica, Peru, are members of the International Union Against Cancer.

SEE ALSO: Argentina; Brazil; Venezuela.

BIBLIOGRAPHY. D. M. Parkin, S. L. Whelan, J. Ferlay, L. Raymond, and J. Young (eds.), *Cancer Incidence in Five Continents Volume VII* (International Agency for Research on Cancer and International Association of Cancer Registries, 1997); Juan B. Lastres y Quinones, *Historia de la medicina peruana* (Imprenta Santa Maria, 1951); G. F. Gonzales and L. G. Valerio, "Medicinal Plants from Peru: A Review of Plants as Potential Agents Against Cancer," *Anticancer Agents in Medicinal Chemistry* (v.6/5, 2006); S. Mohanna, V. Maco, A. Gown, D. Morales, F. Bravo, and E. Gotuzzo, "Is Classic Kaposi's Sarcoma Endemic in Peru? Report of a Case in an Indigenous Patient," *American Journal of Tropical Medicine and Hygiene* (v.75/2, 2006).

JUSTIN CORFIELD
GEELONG GRAMMAR SCHOOL, AUSTRALIA

Pesticide

THERE IS WIDESPREAD public concern that exposure to pesticides may increase humans' cancer risk. The public health issue is truly global, as 45 percent of the world's working populations (approximately 1.8 billion people) are farmers, and most of these people, as well as many other individuals, are occupationally exposed to pesticides. Indeed, the National Nutrition Examination Survey has shown that residues of pesticides and their metabolites have been found in the blood and urine of most of the general population in the United States, leading some to conclude that nearly everyone on earth has had some exposure to pesticides. At present, the available data are insufficient to estimate the pesticide-related cancer risk for those occupationally exposed or for the general population. However, excesses of certain types of cancer among occupations that use pesticides and in animal studies show significant excesses of cancer resulting from exposure to some pesticides. These observations have led the International Agency for Research on Cancer to conclude that "occupational exposures in spraying and application of non-arsenical insecticides" is classified as a probable human carcinogen.

The U.S. Environmental Protection Agency estimated that more than 5 billion pounds of pesticides were used worldwide in 2001. The general population may be exposed to pesticides through ingestion of residues on treated foods; by skin exposure after applications in home, garden, and public space applications; and by inhalation during the application process. The most important exposure route for those who apply the chemicals is through the skin, particularly through dermal exposure to the hands.

It is postulated that pesticides may operate through either a genetic or an epigenetic mechanism, resulting in cancer. Genotoxic effects causing pathological changes to DNA or RNA have been observed in several biomonitoring studies. Epigenetic mechanisms cause carcinogenic effects by mechanisms other than direct genetic damage; for example, cellular proliferation, peroxisome proliferation, generation of reactive oxygen species, modulation of signal transduction pathways, inhibition of intercellular communication, and hormonal and immune perturbations.

Cancer risk within a population may be quite diverse. Pesticide metabolism studies can help identify individuals within a population that are at a particular risk to cancer. For example, recently, chlorpyrifos (an organophosphate insecticide) was reported to stimulate fivefold a form of the CYP gene found in some, but not all, members of the general population. CYP genes are an important family of enzymes involved in xenobiotic metabolism. This stimulation may explain pesticide–pesticide or pesticide–drug interactions related to cancer development. The importance of these preliminary findings to human carcinogenesis is not yet known.

At present, arsenic and arsenical compounds are the only pesticides classified by the International Agency for Research on Cancer as having sufficient evidence of being carcinogenic to humans, based on a number of positive epidemiological associations with lung and skin cancer. There is some—still inconclusive—evidence that selected organochlorine insecticides, phenoxyacetic acid herbicides, triazine herbicides, and organophosphate insecticides, play an important role in certain human cancers.

Organochlorine compounds are generally insecticides and are the most widely studied compounds in relation to cancer. They have been reported to be associated with non-Hodgkin's lymphoma and cancers of the central nervous system, prostate, pancreas, breast, and liver in occupational populations, but the results have not linked specific pesticides to cancers in a consistent fashion. DDT, one of the most widely used organochlorine chemicals, and its metabolites have been associated with increased risk of breast cancer in some studies, but recent findings, including the largest study published so far, does not support a causal association. The other organochlorines, such as chlordane, lindane, methoxychlor, and toxaphene, have been associated with excess lymphoma or leukemia. Some organochlorine insecticides are still being used in developing countries to control disease vectors, although the use of organochlorine pesticides was prohibited in developed countries because of their environmental persistence, adverse effects on the environment, and concern regarding potential adverse human health effects.

Phenoxyl acid herbicides include 2,4-D, 2,4,5-T, MCPA, and other related compounds that are widely used in agriculture and lawn and garden application. Farmers or manufacturing workers exposed to these chemicals from several countries have been reported to show increased risk of non-Hodgkin's lymphoma,

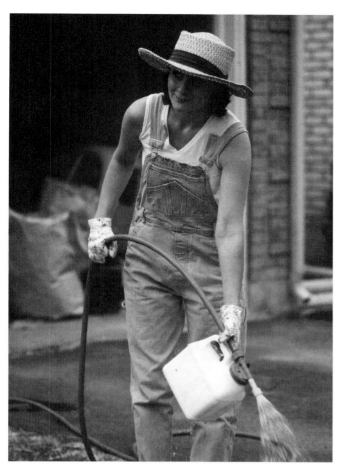

The U.S. Environmental Protection Agency estimated that more than 5 billion pounds of pesticides were used worldwide in 2001.

study in the United States, did not find any significant associations between atrazine use among pesticide applicators and either prostate or ovarian cancer, but the study did suggest a trend for non-Hodgkin's lymphoma, multiple myeloma, and lung and bladder cancer. These analyses highlighted the need for further investigation into the associations. Several animal studies have found that atrazine induced mammary gland adenocarcinomas and increased occurrence of uterine adenocarcinomas.

Some individual organophosphates have shown excess leukemia risks among farmers exposed to crotoxyphos, dichlorvos, and famphur and excess non-Hodgkin's lymphoma risk among those exposed to diazinon, dichlorvos, and Malathion. These associations from case–control studies, however, have not appropriately considered multiple pesticide exposures. Use of chlorpyrifos, one of the most widely applied organophosphate insecticides, showed a significant exposure–response relationship with lung cancer incidence while controlling for the effect of smoking and other pesticide exposures in the cohort of U.S. farmers, although the mechanism of action is not known. A number of organophosphate insecticides were associated with prostate cancer risk among farmers with a family history of prostate cancer in the Agricultural Health Study, including fonofos and phorate.

Carbofuran, a widely used carbamate insecticide, was found to be a risk factor for non-Hodgkin's lymphoma, brain cancer, and lung cancer among farmers, although carbamate insecticides are considered less hazardous than organochlorine and organophosphate pesticides. Alachlor, an acetanilide herbicide categorized as probable human carcinogen by the U.S. Environmental Protection Agency, has been reported as having a possible association with incidence of leukemia among U.S. pesticide applicators.

The major limitation of pesticide studies historically has been inadequate exposure assessment. Multiple pesticide exposures make it difficult to identify any one pesticide causally linked to a specific cancer. Long-term prospective cohort studies such as the Agricultural Health Study are designed to evaluate the relationship between individual pesticide exposures and cancer and other diseases among farmers and their families. This study has assembled detailed information on pesticide use by 57,311 licensed pesticide applicators and 32,347 spouses, for a total of 89,658 individuals before cancer

soft tissue sarcoma, leukemia, and prostate cancer in some, but not all, studies. International differences in study results might depend on the type of phenoxyl acid herbicides used and the levels of dioxin contaminants, mainly 2,3,7,8-TCDD. A number of epidemiologic studies of phenoxyl herbicides and non-Hodgkin's lymphoma have revealed significant exposure–response relationships. In experimental animals, however, phenoxyl acid herbicides do not appear to be genotoxic or carcinogenic.

Triazine herbicides are a group of compounds with a triazine group, and they include atrazine, simazine, propazine, terbutylazine, and cyanzine. Exposure to atrazine has been reported to be associated with ovarian cancer among farmers and with prostate cancer in manufacturing; however, these associations were not consistent in all studies. Recent results from the Agricultural Health Study, a large prospective cohort development, and has been updating the participants' exposure and lifestyle information every 5 years. Long-term prospective studies are costly, but they afford the best opportunity to identify links between a specific pesticide and a specific cancer.

Exposure to pesticides may also be a contributing factor in the pathogenesis of childhood cancer. Parental pesticide use was fairly consistently associated with acute lymphocytic leukemia and central nervous system tumors, and less consistently with Wilms' tumor, Ewing's sarcoma, and soft tissue sarcomas. Children are particularly vulnerable to the effects of pesticides because children may be physiologically more susceptible to the toxic effect of pesticides, have a greater ratio of surface area to body mass, and have greater energy demands compared with adults, which accounts for their greater potential for dermal or respiratory exposure to pesticides.

Most commercial pesticide formulations include carrier substances and other chemicals, usually mentioned as inert ingredients. Career substances, for example, allow the active ingredient to be mixed with water in a suspension or emulsion, so that a more dilute product can be effectively applied to the crop. It has been suspected that inert ingredients may be toxic and may enhance or supplement the toxic effects of the active pesticide ingredient.

Some evidence from animal testing indicates that the commercial formulation of a pesticide may cause a greater biological effect on the animal than does the pure active ingredient. However, the exact composition and nature of a pesticide formulation are generally proprietary and, therefore, are designated as confidential business information. This situation has complicated the evaluation of pesticide carcinogenicity.

Diet is also popularly perceived as an important source of exposure to pesticide in the general population. Although a National Research Council report issued in 1989 on diet and cancer concluded that there is no evidence that pesticides or natural toxicants in food contribute significantly to cancer risk in the United States, another study from the United States, performed in 2000, estimated that exposure to several pesticides including arsenic, chlordane, DDT, dieldrin, and dioxin, in the average diet of adults and children exceeded benchmark concentrations for cancer effects. The cancer risk estimates are based on limited available food consumption data and, therefore, are somewhat inconsistent.

The major studies of pesticide exposure and cancer risk are being conducted in highly developed countries, where population-based cancer registries, health insurance records, and better documentation of pesticide exposure are available. Migrant or seasonal farm workers, who are mostly minorities from low-income families, are generally harder to study epidemiologically.

In less developed countries, several factors contribute to higher exposure experiences, and possibly to greater cancer risks; these include widespread misuse of pesticides, lax regulatory enforcement of pesticide label instructions, lower literacy rates impeding compliancy with label instructions, and a general pressure to grow food. From a public health and ethical perspective, therefore, it is imperative that once specific links are firmly established between specific pesticide exposures and cancer risk in developed countries, these results need to be translated into regulatory action for both developed and developing nations.

Assessing cancer risk associated with pesticides in humans has been a challenging scientific task, both toxicologically and epidemiologically. Pesticides are frequently a complex mixture of compounds, and these mixtures change with time to address the emerging needs of farms and other users. In addition, farmers and other pesticide applicators use a variety of compounds during the course of their work life, making the accurate documentation of exposures problematic in many studies. Nonetheless, considerable progress is being made, particularly in studies where there is attention to accurate exposure assessment and integration of the sciences of toxicology and epidemiology. Until more reliable answers are provided by scientific studies, a precautionary action principal is recommended to control exposure, but effective, scientifically sound regulatory action is needed as soon as the data are available.

SEE ALSO: DDT; Herbicide; Insecticides; International Agency for Research on Cancer.

BIBLIOGRAPHY. Michael Alavanja and Matthew Bonner, "Pesticides and Human Cancers," *Cancer Investigation* (v.23/8, 2005); International Agency for Research on Cancer, *Occupational Exposures in Insecticide Application, and Some Pesticides* (IARC, 1991); Misa Kishi and Joseph Ladou, "International Pesticide Use," *International Journal of Occupational Environmental Health* (v.7/4, 2001).

WON JIN LEE, M.D., M.P.H., PH.D.
KOREA UNIVERSITY
MICHAEL C.R. ALAVANJA, PH.D.
NATIONAL CANCER INSTITUTE

Pfizer (United States)

PFIZER, INC. (PFIZER) is famous for its popular drugs such as Viagra, to treat erectile dysfunction; and Lipitor, for high cholesterol. The pharmaceutical company, based in New York, produces several cancer drugs as well. These include Aromasin and Ellence for breast cancer and Camptosar for colorectal cancer.

Pfizer was founded in 1849 by a pair of cousins. Charles Pfizer and Charles Erhardt opened Charles Pfizer and Company in Brooklyn, New York. The company's first product was an antiparasitic known as Santonin. With the Civil War and its demands for medicinal products, the mid-19th century brought fortune and success to Pfizer. The company produced cream of tartar which served as a diuretic, tartaric acid for its laxative properties, camphor, iodine, morphine, and more.

Pfizer's name is primarily recognized for its contributions to the pharmaceutical industry; however, the company has also made products that branched into other fields. For example, mercurials were also used for photography. Citric acid became a staple for soft drink companies. In fact, the production of citric acid for beverages supported Pfizer well into the twentieth century.

The company's mission is to "become the world's most valued company to patients, customers, colleagues, investors, business partners, and the communities". In achieving this mission, the company has a purpose statement to "dedicate [itself] to humanity's quest for longer, healthier, happier lives through innovation in pharmaceutical, consumer, and animal health products". Additionally, Pfizer has outlined nine values to which each employee ascribes. These values are of community, customer focus, innovation, integrity, leadership, performance, quality, respect for people, and teamwork. To achieve its purpose of improving health of people and their animal companions, the company has a four-part addendum: discovering new medicines, educating consumers, providing highest quality medications, and setting a global standard for corporate responsibility.

Pfizer corporate headquarters are located in New York, New York. Research and development sites are based in the states of California, Connecticut, Massachusetts, Michigan, Missouri, and the nations of Japan and the United Kingdom.

The company slogan is "Working for a healthier world." Over the years, the company has earned numerous accolades that highlight its successes in following the mission statement. For example, in the year 2006, Pfizer received its eighth recognition from *Working Mother Magazine* as one of the 100 Best Companies for Working Mothers. Additionally, in August 2006, Pfizer was named the Top Corporate Giver by the *Chronicle of Philanthropy*. The company has also been recognized for participation in international endeavors to provide better access to healthcare for those people and animals living in impoverished areas.

In order to help the Food and Drug Administration continue monitoring Pfizer drugs after marketing, the company has declared a Post Marketing Commitment (PMC). A PMC is used to survey the use of a particular drug and gather information on its safety and efficacy, at a scale much larger than prior clinical trials. A subset of the PMC studies is focused on pediatric care.

SEE ALSO: Clinical Trials; Experimental Cancer Drugs.

BIBLIOGRAPHY. Ahmed F. Abdel-Magid and Stephane Caron, *Fundamentals of Early Clinical Drug Development: From Synthesis Design to Formulation* (Wiley-Interscience, 2006); Anne Clayton, *Insight into a Career in Pharmaceutical Sales* (Pharmaceuticalsales.Com Inc., 2005); Rick Ng, *Drugs—From Discovery to Approval* (Wiley-Liss, 2004); Adriana Petryna, Andrew Lakoff, and Arthur Kleinman, *Global Pharmaceuticals: Ethics, Markets, Practices* (Duke University Press, 2006).

CLAUDIA WINOGRAD
UNIVERSITY OF ILLINOIS AT URBANA-CHAMPAIGN

Pharmaceutical Industry

THE PHARMACEUTICAL INDUSTRY began to grow on a large scale in the last two decades of the 19th century, when a combination of different industries matured to enable the production and distribution of products to a much greater extent than had been previously possible. This meant that economy of scale started to assume more importance in the competitiveness of companies, and this, of course, encouraged growth and consolidation within the industry. Even when new sectors came into being within the pharmaceutical industry, such as the biotechnology sector in the 1970s and 1980s, the commercial imperative for the industry to become larger has witnessed numerous examples of mergers and acquisitions and joint ventures in terms of research and development and in licensing and patenting of intellectual property.

Before the development of rapid and cheap computational power, most pharmaceutical research was significantly labor intensive, and as many of those involved in research are highly qualified and, hence, command significant salaries, the overall cost of research was also necessarily high. To this factor must be added the length of time necessary to develop concepts and then conduct clinical trials, in laboratory conditions, with laboratory animals and then with human volunteers. These trials are generally required before state-level licensing authorities (such as the U.S. Food and Drug Administration) are prepared to allow pharmaceuticals to be marketed openly. The result is that some products spend decades in preproduction before they can be brought to market and even begin to claw back their development costs; indeed, many products do not make it onto the market at all, as they may be found insufficiently effective, may be superseded by subsequent innovations, or may not be found profitable at the scale at which demand exists. As a consequence, pharmaceutical companies set their products at expensive price points to try to cover the development costs of the products involved, as well as that of the unsuccessful products, and, also, earn what is deemed to be a suitable profit margin, bearing in mind the cost of capital borrowed over the long term and still representing a cost decades later. This means that many products on the market are more expensive than most people can afford, which would

seem to defeat the point of manufacturing them from a commercial point of view. This is where health insurance becomes involved; on a public or privately funded basis, the insurance companies provide funds for drugs for people who need them from contributions of all who are members. Clearly, there are incentives working in different directions in a system such as this. Pharmaceutical companies have little if any incentive to reduce their costs, especially as there are high barriers to entry in the industry; that is, it is difficult for new companies to enter the drugs market and compete with large existing companies without having access to qualified researchers and laboratory equipment and the capital necessary to support these assets until such time as they can become profitable. In contrast, insurance providers wish to minimize the cost of the drugs to them. In such cases, it is usually appropriate for the government to institute a regulatory scheme to supervise the industry. The ability of government to establish such a scheme depends in part to its ability to withstand (willingly or not) the lobbying and fundraising efforts of industry players. This strength is more difficult to achieve in countries such as the United States, in which democratic elections depend on personality and possession of money to a much greater extent than they do on coherent and commonly held ideology.

There has been a great deal of debate, therefore, concerning the extent to which pharmaceutical companies are justified in maintaining the generally very high prices of the products that they bring to market. It has been argued that the costs pharmaceutical companies claim it is necessary for them to bear are in fact subsidized by government, as much research is conducted by or in collaboration with universities, whereas the near-monopoly like conditions that are attached to insurance programs encourage swollen and unjustified costs. Needless to say, pharmaceutical companies resist these charges. Whatever the truth, it is apparent that, especially in recent years, when companies have been able to obtain leverage from new discoveries related to DNA and genetic manipulation, the profitability of the larger companies has become enormous in many cases. A company such as Amgen, for example, which was only created in 1980, achieved a profit of US$12.4 billion in the year 2005 while reinvesting less than 20 percent of that profit in research and development.

The cost of pharmaceutical products is brought into much sharper relief when they are exported to less-developed countries, where people are much less able to afford them and governments have much less capacity and capital to organize an efficient and well-regulated social insurance program. At the same time, people in such countries are likely to have greater need for drugs for diseases that are still endemic, or else infection rates will remain very high (such as for HIV/AIDS) as a result of poor information and preventative regimes. Governments of such states face the dilemma that they cannot organize effective health interventions for their people because the cost of medicines is too high. Because of the issue of patents and intellectual property rights (IPR), it has been deemed illegal for states to license their own firms to reverse engineer the drugs, effectively copying them, and then market this new version of the medicine under a generic brand name. The original inventors of the drugs seek, generally aggressively, to maintain the IPR of their inventions through patenting and international registration of their property. This includes the use of international trade negotiations at the World Trade Organization and the formation and promulgation of the Agreement on Trade-Related Aspects of Intellectual Property Rights (TRIPS). Developing states have observed that recent international forums have seen developed countries seeking to push TRIPS throughout the world (ignoring persistent tariffs in their own markets, particularly in agricultural markets) and seeking to extend protection to forms of property for which patenting is not fair or suitable (e.g., types of fruit or cereal).

Developing country governments face the quandary that they must either let many of their people suffer—and perhaps die—or else permit domestic drug companies to manufacture generic-label, low-cost copies of drugs and be in contravention of international trade norms. Some countries, notably South Africa and India, have tended toward the latter stance and, faced with the potential unraveling of the IPR system, have developed country governments and the drugs companies they support to have permitted special circumstance deals to be licensed.

The pharmaceutical industry is dominated by firms in North America and in Europe, where industrialization occurred the earliest and permitted the growth of such firms at an earlier age. Few companies from coun-

tries that industrialized at a later stage have been able to break into the first rank of such firms. Even so, those firms must constantly invest in innovation and new products to tackle emergent demand and substitute products or methods. The research indicates that attempting to use merger-and-acquisition-style activity as a primary driver of industry growth is, as in the case of other industrial sectors, not a sustainable strategy.

SEE ALSO: Drugs.

BIBLIOGRAPHY. Sandy Campart and Etienne Pfister, "Technology, Cooperation and Stock Market Value: An Event Study of New Partnership Announcements in the Biotechnology and Pharmaceutical Industries," *Economics of Innovation and New Technology* (v.16/1, 2007); Alfred D. Chandler, Jr., *Shaping the Industrial Century: The Remarkable Story of the Evolution of the Modern Chemical and Pharmaceutical Industries* (Harvard University Press, 2005); Oliver Gassmann, Gerrit Reepmeyer, and Maximilian von Zedtwitz, *Leading Pharmaceutical Innovation: Trends and Drivers for Growth in the Pharmaceutical Industry* (Springer, 2004); Merrill Goozner, *The $800 Million Pill: The Truth behind the Cost of New Drugs* (University of California Press, 2005).

JOHN WALSH
SHINAWATRA UNIVERSITY

Phelps, Michael E.

A NEUROSCIENTIST SPECIALIZING in nuclear medicine, Michael E. Phelps was the joint winner, with David E. Kuhl, of the Charles F. Kettering Prize of the General Motors Cancer Foundation in 2001 for "research in the development of positron emission tomography (PET) scanning and the use of this technology to study normal and abnormal cellular function."

Michael Edward Phelps was born on August 24, 1939, in Cleveland, Ohio, and gained his B.S. in chemistry and B.S. in mathematics at Western Washington University in 1965 and his doctorate in chemistry at Washington University in 1970. In 1971, Phelps was appointed assistant professor of radiation science at the School of Medicine at Washington University, later being promoted to associate professor. Phelps was also assistant professor, and later associate professor, in electrical engineering from 1974 until 1975 and associate professor in radiology and biophysics at the Medical School of the University of Pennsylvania from 1975 until 1976. He was concurrently a member of the Computing and Biomathematics Study Section at the National Institute of Health from 1974 until 1978, an adviser to the Laboratory of Cerebral Metabolism beginning in 1977, and cochairman of the instrumentation session for the Society of Nuclear Medicine in 1977. From 1976 until 1992, Phelps was professor of radiology and biophysics at the School of Medicine, University of California, Los Angeles, and beginning in 1980 was the division chief of nuclear medicine and professor of biomathematics, also at the School of Medicine. In 1983, he was appointed Jennifer Jones Simon Professor, and in 1992 he was appointed professor and chairman of the department of molecular and medical pharmacology.

In 1981, Phelps established the use of imaging technologies now known as brain mapping to show how particular parts of the brain are used for images, hearing, thinking, working, and remembering. Phelps's invention, positron emission tomography (PET) massively advanced human knowledge for everybody interested in this field. PET has subsequently been used to study the early stages of Parkinson's and Huntington's diseases as well as epilepsy. It was used in cancer research to study reaction to abnormal cells. With Dr. Simon Cherry and Dr. Arion Chatziioannou, Phelps developed a miniaturized PET scanner, known as microPET, which has been used for imaging mice in biological and pharmaceutical research. With a colleague, Dr. Henry Huang, Phelps also developed a software-based Kinetic Imaging System (KIS), which has been extremely useful in performing tracer- and pharmacokinetics and pharmacodynamics with PET.

Active in many other areas, Phelps, was chairman in 1982, and again in the following year, of the Neurological Section—and then chairman of the Computer Tomography Section—of the World Federation of Nuclear Medicine and Biology; was chairman of the Instrumentation Section of the International Society for Cerebral Blood Flow and Metabolism in 1983; and was on the commission of the Association for Research into Nervous and Mental Disorders in 1983. Beginning in 1981, Phelps was also a principal investigator at the Department of Energy.

Phelps has received numerous honors including the Gold Medal Award from the Society of Nuclear medicine in 1977; the Von Hevesy Prize in 1978 and again in 1982; the Certificate for Excellence from the Society for Cerebral Blood Flow and Metabolism in 1979; the Oldendorf Award from the Society of Computer Tomography and Neurology Imaging and the S. Weir Mitchell Award from the American Academy of Neurologists in 1981; the Paul Aebersold Award in 1983; the Ernest O. Lawrence Presidential Award, the Sarah L. Poiley Award, and the Special Award for Individual Distinction from the American Nuclear Society in 1984; the Rosenthal Award in 1987; the Landauer Award in 1988; the Ted Block Award in 1989; the Robert J. and Claire Pasarow Foundation Award in 1992; and the Distinguished Scientist Award from the Institute of Clinical Positron Emission Tomography in 1995. In 1998, Phelps received the Enrico Fermi Presidential Award, which was given to him by President Clinton. After receiving the Charles F. Kettering Prize in 2001, Phelps was also awarded the Benedict Cassen Memorial Prize from the Society of Nuclear Medicine in 2002, having been the Benedict Cassen Memorial Lecturer in 1983. Phelps has published nearly 700 peer-reviewed scientific articles, books, and chapters in books and has been cited in over 410,000 other publications. He has also been the principle or coprinciple investigator in projects that collectively have received $225 million in grants and has been given $21 million in private donations to support his research. Phelps is chairman of the board of the Norton Simon Foundation, chairman of the board of the Norton Simon Research Foundation, and a member of the board of the Norton Simon Art Foundation, which together hold $2.5 billion in assets.

SEE ALSO: Technology, Imaging

BIBLIOGRAPHY. *American Men and Women of Science* (R.R. Bowker/Gale Group, 1971–2003); *Notable Scientists from 1900 to the Present* (Gale Group, 2001); *Who's Who in America* (Marquis Who's Who, 1984–2004); *Who's Who in Medicine and Healthcare* (Marquis Who's Who, 1997–2000); *Who's Who in the West* (Marquis Who's Who, 2001–2002).

JUSTIN CORFIELD
GEELONG GRAMMAR SCHOOL, AUSTRALIA

Pheochromocytoma

PHEOCHROMOCYTOMAS ARE CATECHOL-AMINE-PRODUCING neuroendocrine tumors arising from chromaffin cells of the adrenal medulla or extraadrenal paraganglia. These rare tumors can have a highly variable clinical presentation but most commonly present with episodes of headaches, sweating, palpitations, and hypertension. These tumors are important because they give rise to surgically correctable forms of hypertension. If the removal of pheochromocytoma is timely, prognosis is excellent. However, prognosis is poor in patients with metastases, which especially occur in patients with large, extraadrenal tumors.

The prevalence of pheochromocytoma is not precisely known, though studies have shown that the prevalence of pheochromocytoma in patients with hypertension is 0.1–0.6 percent. Hereditary pheochromocytomas occur in multiple endocrine neoplasia type 2, von-Hippel Landau syndrome, neurofibromatosis type 1, and the familial paraganglionomas. Sporadic forms of pheochromocytoma are usually diagnosed in individuals aged 40–50 years, whereas hereditary forms are diagnosed earlier, most often before age 40 years.

Clinical presentation of pheochromocytoma can vary greatly, with similar signs and symptoms produced by many other clinical conditions. Most, but not all, the clinical signs and symptoms of pheochromocytoma are a result of the direct actions of secreted catecholamines. The most common set of symptoms comprises attacks of headaches described as intense and global, palpitations, and diaphoresis. Hypertension is often paroxysmal in nature, occurring in some patients on a background of sustained hypertension, although others can have normal blood pressure between paroxysms. Hypertensive episodes can be severe and result in hypertensive emergencies.

Despite improved diagnostic techniques that can bring about an earlier diagnosis of pheochromocytoma, there still usually remains a delay of 3 years between initial symptoms and a final diagnosis. The most obvious reason for this delay is that in daily clinical patient care, the individual symptoms are quite nonspecific—especially headaches, palpitations, and sweating, which are the most frequent symptoms seen. Advances in genetics and recognition of the high prevalence of pheochromocytoma in certain fa-milial syndromes, such as endocrine neoplasia type 2, led to mandatory routine screening in patients with identified mutations.

All patients with suspected pheochromocytoma undergo biochemical testing. Biochemical tests include measurements of urinary and plasma catecholamines, urinary metanephrines (normetanephrine and metanephrine), urinary vanillylmandelic acid (VMA), and plasma-free metanephrines (normetanephrine and metanephrine). Evidence indicates that measurement of metanephrines, either in the urine or plasma, is the most sensitive test for diagnosis. Use of clonidine, an α-adrenergic blocker, to suppress catecholamine release from the sympathoadrenal system provides a dynamic pharmacological test to distinguish increased catecholamine release caused by sympathetic activation from increased release resulting from pheochromocytomas. Failure to suppress plasma normetanephrine is highly indicative of pheochromocytoma.

If a pheochromocytoma is suspected, computed tomography scans of the entire abdomen (including the pelvis), both with and without contrast, are most often used for the initial localization of adrenal or possible extraadrenal abdominal pheochromocytomas. Once a pheochromocytoma is located and localized, laparoscopic removal is the preferred surgical technique. Pretreatment with an α-adrenergic blocker can usually be undertaken on an outpatient basis and is safe in most patients. At present, after adequate medical preparation, operative mortality is less than 1 percent if the procedure is undertaken by an experienced anesthesiologist and a skilful surgeon. The long-term prognosis of patients after resection of a solitary sporadic pheochromocytoma is excellent, although hypertension might persist after surgery in nearly 50 percent of patients.

SEE ALSO: Surgery.

BIBLIOGRAPHY. E. Bravo, "Pheochromocytoma: State-of-the-Art and Future Prospects," *Endocrine Reviews* (v.24, 2003); E.E. Edstrom, "The Management of Benign and Malignant Pheochromocytoma and Abdominal Paraganglioma," *European Journal of Surgical Oncology* (v.29, 2003).

NAKUL GUPTA
ROSS UNIVERSITY SCHOOL OF MEDICINE

Philippines

THE PHILIPPINES COMPRISES 7107 islands off the east coast of southeast Asia and was occupied by the Spanish beginning in 1565. Gradually, the Spaniards expanded their rule over the whole archipelago but lost the Philippines in a war with the United States in 1898. During World War II, the Philippines were occupied by the Japanese. They gained their independence in 1944. The Republic of the Philippines had a population of 85,237,000 in 2005, with 123 doctors and 418 nurses per 100,000 people. An example of cancer incidence rates in Philippines includes 190 cases of cancer in males per 100,000, according to the International Agency for Research on Cancer.

During the Spanish colonial period, hospital services were largely restricted to Europeans and to wealthy Chinese and local elites, with a combination of European and Chinese practices used for treating tumors.

In the 1890s, when the Philippines was trying to achieve independence from the Spanish, the great hero of the nationalist movement was José Rizal (1861–96) who was, by training, a physician. Although he never advocated independence himself, his writings urged a social renewal, and his first novel, written in 1886, was called *Noli me tangere* (*The Social Cancer*), a passionate critique of the evils of Spanish rule in the Philippines, comparing the Spanish to a cancer that was killing the spirit of the nation. During the 1960s, Manuel D. Navarro of the Faculty of Medicine and Surgery at the University of Santo Tomas, Manila, worked on immunologic tests for cancer based on observations by Engel in 1930 on the presence of human chorionic gonadotrophin (HCG) in malignant urine.

A number of prominent Filipinos and people connected with the Philippines have suffered from cancer, including boxer Pedro Adigue (1943–2003); Father Horacio de la Costa (1916–77), the first Filipino Provincial General of the Society of Jesus in the Philippines; actor Nestor de Villa (1928–2004), who died from prostate cancer; and lawyer Marcelo Briones Fernan (1927–99), who was Chief Justice from 1988 to 1991.

On October 5, 1970, the postal authorities in the Philippines issued three postage stamps highlighting the campaign against cancer, with each stamp showing a crab drawn by Alexander Calder superimposed on a map of the Philippines. On April 14, 1980, another

other two stamps were issued to commemorate anti-smoking efforts for World Health Day.

The Institute of Public Health in Manila is the official body in the country for coordinating medical research, with the Philippine Cancer Society being the main anticancer organization. The Philippine Cancer Society was established in 1956, and 11 years later it was certified as a science foundation by the National Science Technology Authority in Manila. It does not receive any government subsidy and is financed entirely by membership dues, donations, and public contributions to annual fund-raising campaigns. It publishes information on cancer in the Philippines. The Philippine Cancer Society is a member of the International Union Against Cancer.

SEE ALSO: International Union Against Cancer.

BIBLIOGRAPHY. José Policarpio Bantug, *A Short History of Medicine in the Philippines During the Spanish Regime 1565–1898* (Colegio Médico-Farmacéutico de Filipinas, 1953); D. M. Parkin, S. L. Whelan, J. Ferlay, L. Raymond, and J. Young (eds.), *Cancer Incidence in Five Continents Vol VII* (International Agency for Research on Cancer and International Association of Cancer Registries, 1997); X. S. Wang, A. V. Laudico, H. Guo, et al., "Filipino Version of the M. D. Anderson Symptom Inventory: Validation and Multisymptom Measurement in Cancer Patients," *Journal of Pain and Symptom Management* (v.31/6, 2006); T. Y. Wu and J. Bancroft, "Filipino American Women's Perceptions and Experiences with Breast Cancer Screening," *Oncology Nursing Forum* (v.33/4, 2006); "The Philippine Cancer Society," philcancer.com (cited November 2006).

JUSTIN CORFIELD
GEELONG GRAMMAR SCHOOL, AUSTRALIA

Photodynamic Therapy

PHOTODYNAMIC THERAPY (PDT) is a special form of phototherapy, a term that includes all treatments that use light to induce reactions in the body that are of benefit to patients.

PDT is a developing technique that can potentially destroy unwanted tissue while sparing normal tissue. First, a drug called a photosensitizer is administered to the patient, usually by injection. The photosensitizer alone is harmless and has no effect on either healthy or abnormal tissue. However, when light (often from a laser) is directed onto tissue containing the drug, the drug becomes activated and the tissue is rapidly destroyed precisely where the light has been directed. Thus, by careful application of the light beam, the technique can be targeted selectively at the abnormal tissue.

Some of the drugs being developed also have the desirable property of building up a concentration in tumors (and certain other kinds of proliferating tissue) relative to the surrounding healthy tissue, which also helps in targeting. There is only one potentially adverse effect of this type of treatment—the use of some drugs can result in skin photosensitivity, which means that patients must stay out of bright light for some time following the administration of the drug.

PDT, using the drug Photofrin, has now been approved as a therapy for a limited number of applications in various parts of the world, and it is now clear that there are some instances in which PDT is at least as good as—and possibly better than—alternative treatments. However, it has to be emphasized that PDT is still largely an experimental therapy and is currently only applicable to a very small range of patients. More research is needed to further develop and assess PDT with different drugs in different clinical situations. Nevertheless, there is growing confidence that PDT will soon become an added weapon in the fight against cancer and other diseases.

MECHANISM OF ACTION

PDT combines the preferential accumulation of the photosensitizer in the target tissue with precise illumination to provide the selectivity of the treatment. The light penetrates the tissue and causes excitation of the photosensitizers.

Activation of the photosensitizers by light is a prerequisite to successful PDT. The transmission of light through tissue is low at 400 nm because of scattering and absorption by natural chromophores. Light penetration increases with increasing wavelength up to 800 nm. A particular wavelength of light is needed for each photosensitizer to maximize both penetration through the tumor and excitation of the photosensitizer.

PDT light delivery systems have improved in the last 20 years. Tuneable dye lasers are frequently used in investigative studies because they allow maximum

flexibility; however, for clinical use they are not ideal because of their size and mobility restraints.

Licensing of specific photosensitizers, using one particular wavelength, has led to the development of small compact lasers, such as diode lasers and light-emitting diode array lasers, which are more convenient to use in clinical situations. However, superficial lesions also can be easily treated with lamps such as the xenon arc lamp. The further development of light applicators compatible with endoscopes and the use of several optical fibers in interstitial therapy of larger tumors has overcome the penetration difficulties encountered in earlier studies.

Photosensitizers have a stable electronic configuration, which is in a singlet state in their lowest or ground-state energy level. Following absorption of a photon of light of a specific wavelength, a molecule is promoted to an excited state, which is also a singlet state and is short lived. The photosensitizer returns to the ground state by emitting a photon (fluorescence) or by internal conversion with energy loss as heat. It is also possible that the molecule may convert to the triplet state via intersystem crossing, which involves a change in the spin of an electron. The triplet state photosensitizer has a lower energy than the singlet state but has a longer lifetime (typically more than 500 ns for photosensitizers), which increases the probability of energy transfer to other molecules.

The tendency of a photosensitizer to reach the triplet state is measured by the triplet state quantum yield, which measures the probability of formation of the triplet state per photon absorbed (depending on the interaction of the singlet species with other substrates producing fluorescent quenching). The triplet state lifetime influences the amount of cytotoxic species produced by collision-induced energy transfer to molecular oxygen and other cellular components. A high intersystem crossing probability will produce an effective population of excited triplet state photosensitizer molecules, the energy of which can then be transferred by the two mechanisms described below. In addition, the photosensitizer is not destroyed but returns to its ground state without chemical alteration and is able to repeat the process of energy transfer to oxygen many times.

There are two mechanisms by which the triplet state photosensitizer can react with biomolecules; these are known as type I and type II reactions. Type I reactions involve electron/hydrogen transfer directly from the photosensitizer, producing ions, or electron/hydrogen abstraction from a substrate molecule to form free radicals. These radicals then react rapidly, usually with oxygen, resulting in the production of highly reactive oxygen species (e.g., the superoxide and the peroxide anions). These radicals then attack cellular targets.

Type II reactions produce the electronically excited and highly reactive state of oxygen known as singlet oxygen. Direct interaction of the excited triplet state photosensitizer with molecular oxygen (which, unusually, has a triplet ground state) results in the photosensitizer returning to its singlet ground state and the formation of singlet oxygen.

In PDT, it is difficult to distinguish between the two reaction mechanisms. There is probably a contribution from both type I and type II processes, indicating that the mechanism of damage is dependent on oxygen tension and photosensitizer concentration.

PDT produces cytotoxic effects through photodamage to subcellular organelles and biomolecules. These sites of photodamage may reflect the localization of the photosensitizer in the cell. A variety of cellular components such as amino acids (particularly cysteine, histidine, tryptophan, tyrosine, and methionine), nucleosides (mainly guanine), and unsaturated lipids can react with singlet oxygen. The diffusion distance of singlet oxygen is relatively short (about 0.1 micron); therefore, the photosensitizer must associate intimately with the substrate for efficient photosensitization to occur. Although the type II process is considered the more relevant reaction mechanism in PDT, cytotoxic species generated by the type I reaction process can also act in a site-specific manner.

Many factors determine the cellular targets of photosensitizers. The incubation parameters and mode of delivery, as well as the chemical nature of the photosensitizer, can all influence subcellular localization, creating a number of potential targets for photodamage. In cell culture studies with porphyrin-based photosensitizers, short incubation times (up to 1 hour) before illumination leads primarily to membrane damage, whereas extended incubation periods followed by light exposure results in damage to cellular organelles and macromolecules.

Hydrophobic (lipophilic) compounds preferentially bind membranes and will target structures such

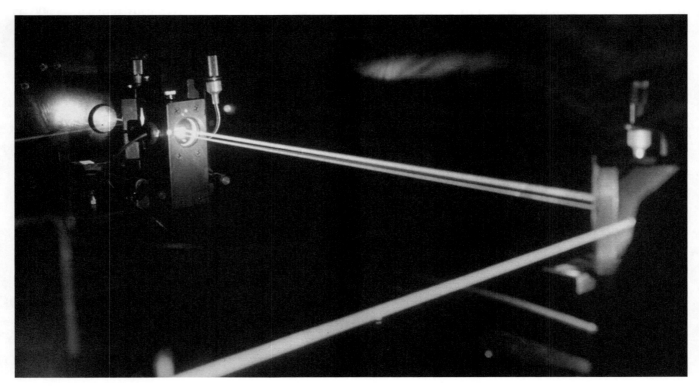

In Photodynamic Therapy (PDT), a light (often from a laser) is directed onto tissue containing a photosensitizer drug. The drug becomes activated and the tissue is rapidly destroyed precisely where the light has been directed.

as the plasma membrane, mitochondria, lysosomes, endoplasmic reticulum, and nucleus. Oxidative degradation of membrane lipids can cause the loss of membrane integrity, resulting in impaired membrane transport mechanisms and increased permeability and rupturing of membranes. Cross-linking of membrane-associated polypeptides may result in the inactivation of enzymes, receptors, and ion channels.

The mitochondrion has been shown to be a critical target in PDT. Lipophilic porphyrins have demonstrated intimate intracellular association with mitochondrial membranes, whereas cationic compounds such as rhodamines and cyanines may accumulate in these organelles because of mitochondrial membrane potential. Much work has focused on photosensitization of mitochondria because these organelles perform vital functions in the cell. ATP is synthesized by oxidative phosphorylation in the mitochondria and is necessary for energy-requiring processes such as replication, protein synthesis, DNA synthesis, and transport. Mitochondrial photosensitization may cause the uncoupling of respiration and phosphorylation, resulting in the impairment of ATP synthesis and subsequent loss of cellular function. At the molecular level, several mitochondrial enzymes and carriers involved in ATP synthesis have displayed sensitivity to mitochondrial photosensitization. Following PDT, the loss of mitochondrial integrity has been observed to occur before the loss of plasma membrane integrity, underlining the importance of the mitochondria as targets for PDT. Mitochondrial damage can also induce nuclear chromatin condensation and has been linked to the induction of apoptosis.

Lysosomal localization has been observed for a number of photosensitizers. Initially, it was thought that cell death was a result of the release of enzymes following lysosomal membrane photodamage; however, cell survival has since been observed following photodamage to 80 percent of cellular lysosomes. Recent studies have demonstrated that photosensitizers are redistributed from the lysosomes to other cellular sites on light exposure.

At the level of the nucleus, PDT has been shown to cause single-/double-stranded breaks and alkali-labile sites in DNA, as well as induction of sister chromatid exchanges and chromosomal aberrations. However, further studies have indicated that nuclear damage or repair is not generally a dominant factor in PDT-mediated cytotoxicity

USES

PDT may be used to treat cancers of the skin (but not melanoma) or cancers that are on, or near, the lining of internal organs, such as cancers of the head and neck area, lining of the mouth, lungs, esophagus, stomach, bladder, and bile ducts.

Doctors are working to identify the types of cancer for which PDT is most effective, and research trials are taking place to look at new photosensitizing agents, new laser and nonlaser light treatments, and ways of reducing the side effects.

In cancers that are treated at an early stage, the aim of treatment may be to try to cure the cancer. The aim of PDT for advanced cancer is usually to reduce symptoms by shrinking the tumor. PDT cannot cure advanced cancer. Photodynamic therapy treatments for some cancers, such as prostate and pancreatic, are still the subjects of research. Some research studies have used PDT to treat conditions that may develop into cancers, including a condition that affects the vulva, known as vulval intraepithelial neoplasia.

PDT can safely be given to patients who have had other cancer treatments such as surgery, radiotherapy, and chemotherapy.

LIMITATIONS

The light needed to activate most photosensitizers cannot pass through more than about one-third of an inch of tissue (1 cm). For this reason, PDT is usually used to treat tumors on or just under the skin or on the lining of internal organs or cavities. PDT is also less effective in treating large tumors because the light cannot pass far into these tumors. PDT is a local treatment and generally cannot be used to treat cancer that has spread (metastasized).

ADVERSE EFFECTS

As with all kinds of treatment, the experience of PDT can vary from person to person. How the treatment is given and the side effects that it may cause vary according to the area of the body affected by the cancer, the type of photosensitizing drug given, the time between giving the drug and applying the light, and the amount of skin sensitivity to light following treatment.

Porfimer sodium makes the skin and eyes sensitive to light for approximately 6 weeks after treatment. Thus, patients are advised to avoid direct sunlight and bright indoor light for at least 6 weeks.

Photosensitizers tend to build up in tumors, and the activating light is focused on the tumor. As a result, damage to healthy tissue is minimal. However, PDT can cause burns, swelling, pain, and scarring in nearby healthy tissue. Other side effects of PDT are related to the area that is treated. They can include coughing, trouble swallowing, stomach pain, painful breathing, and shortness of breath; these side effects are usually temporary.

FUTURE OF PDT

Photodynamic therapy may be used to treat other cancers and diseases in the future. Studies are now in progress to test the use of PDT for several types of cancer and precancerous conditions, including cancers of the skin, cervix, bladder, prostate, bile duct, pancreas, stomach, brain, and head and neck. Newer photosensitizing agents now being studied may have several advantages over the ones now being used. They may be able to treat tumors that are deeper under the skin or in body tissues; they may be more selective for cancer cells, as opposed to normal cells; they may collect in cancer cells more quickly, reducing the time needed between getting the drug and receiving the light therapy; and they may be removed from the body more quickly, reducing the time people need to worry about photosensitivity reactions.

Researchers are also looking at different types of lasers and other light sources. Some newer agents may respond to small doses of radiation as well as to light, which could allow doctors to use smaller amounts of radiation than the doses used in conventional radiation therapy, which could lead to fewer side effects.

Another exciting area of research is in the use of PDT as an adjuvant (addition) to current therapy to make it more effective. One way to do this may be to use PDT intraoperatively (during surgery) to help prevent the recurrence of cancer on large surface areas such as the pleura (lining of the lung) and the peritoneum (lining of the abdomen), which are common sites of spread for some types of cancer.

Eventually, PDT may be used to help treat larger solid tumors as well. A technique known as interstitial therapy involves using imaging tests (such as computed tomography scans) to guide fiberoptics directly into tumors, using needles. This technique may be especially useful in areas that would require extensive surgery. Early results of studies of interstitial therapy in head and neck tumors are promising.

SEE ALSO: Skin Cancer (Non-Melanoma); Technology: New Therapies.

BIBLIOGRAPHY. D. Dolmans, D. Fukumura, and R. K. Jain, "Photodynamic Therapy for Cancer," *Nature Reviews Cancer* (v.3/5, 2003); B. C. Wilson, "Photodynamic Therapy for Cancer: Principles," *Canadian Journal of Gastroenterology* (v.16/6, 2002); M.B. Vrouenraets, G. W. M. Visser, G. B. Snow, G. A. M. S. van Dongen, "Basic Principles, Applications in Oncology and Improved Selectivity of Photodynamic Therapy," *Anticancer Research* (v.23, 2003); T. J. Dougherty, C. J. Gomer, B. W. Henderson, et al., "Photodynamic Therapy," *Journal of the National Cancer Institute* (v.90/12, 1998); Robert Souhami, Ian Tannock, Peter Hohenberger, and Jean-Claude Horiot, *Oxford Textbook of Oncology,* 2nd ed. (Oxford University Press, 2001); Robert L. Souhami and Jeffrey Tobias, *Cancer and Its Management* (4th ed.) (Blackwell Scientific, 2003); Derek Raghavan, Martin L. Brecher, David H. Johnson, Neal J. Meropol, Paul L. Moots, and J. T. Thigpen, *Textbook of Uncommon Cancers* (2nd ed.) (Wiley, 1999); *British National Formulary* (50th ed.) (British Medical Association and Royal Pharmaceutical Society of Great Britain, 2005).

QURATULAIN MASOOD
NATIONAL UNIVERSITY OF SCIENCES AND TECHNOLOGY

Pineoblastoma and Supratentorial Primitive Neuroectodermal, Childhood

PINEOBLASTOMA AND SUPRATENTORIAL primitive neuroectodermal tumors (PNET) are high-grade, relatively undifferentiated tumors arising from the pineal regions and the cerebral hemispheres, respectively. Although they are histologically very similar to medulloblastoma, supratentorial PNETs have markedly different clinical behavior and are generally considered to represent a more aggressive tumor than medulloblastoma, with a frequently massive tumor burden and a higher incidence of disseminated dis-

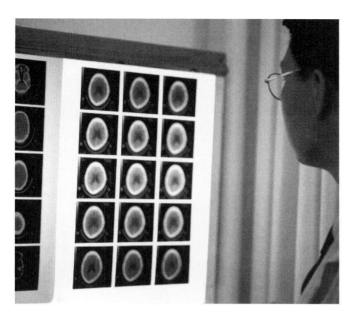

Supratentorial PNETs are generally considered to represent a more aggressive tumor than medulloblastoma,

ease at diagnosis. Supratentorial PNET's account for approximately 2-3 percent of all childhood brain tumors, and pineoblastomas are even more infrequent. The majority of supratentorial PNETs arise from the cerebral hemispheres with the frontal, parietal, and temporal lobes most frequently involved.

SYMPTOMS

The symptoms of childhood supratentorial primitive neuroectodermal tumors and pineoblastoma vary and often depend on the child's age, where the tumor is located, and the size of the tumor. Patients usually present with nonspecific symptoms such as headaches, nausea, vomiting, and seizures. Intracranial or spinal subarachnoid dissemination is estimated to be present in 20–40 percent of patients at the time of diagnosis. The overall five-year survival rate in patients with pineoblastoma and supratentorial PNETs is approximately 18 percent, with younger children having a worse prognosis.

MANAGEMENT

Complete surgical resection is the primary mode of treatment when possible. Postoperative radiation is also favored due to the propensity of these tumors to spread throughout the subarachnoid space. However with very young patients the dose of radiation

should be decreased to avoid long-term neurological complications. Chemotherapy may be warranted if complete resection is not possible, young patient age, and recurrence. Children's Cancer Group are underway, evaluating varying combinations of chemotherapy with and without radiotherapy. The best results, so far, have come from the Children's Hospital of Pennsylvania study, reporting a five-year event-free survival rate of 80 percent.

SEE ALSO: Medulloblastoma, Childhood.

BIBLIOGRAPHY. Victor A. Levin *"Primary CNS Tumors of the Supratentorial Compartment: Cancer in the nervous system* (Oxford: Oxford University Press, *2002);* Peter B. Dirks "Supratentorial primitive neuroectodermal tumors in children," *Journal of Neuro-Oncology* (v. 29, 1996);

FERNANDO A. HERRERA, JR., M.D.
UNIVERSITY OF CALIFORNIA, SAN DIEGO

Pinkel, Donald P.

AN AMERICAN PEDIATRICIAN, Donald P. Pinkel was the winner of the Charles F. Kettering Prize of the General Motors Cancer Foundation in 1986 for "the development of a curative treatment for acute lymphocytic leukemia, the most common cancer in children."

Donald Paul Pinkel was born on September 7, 1926, in Buffalo, New York, the son of Lawrence William Pinkel and Ann (née Richardson). He served with the U.S. Navy in World War II from 1944 to 1945 and gained his B.S. from Canisius College in 1947 and his M.D. from the University of Buffalo in 1951, getting his diplomate from the American Board of Internal Medicine, the American Board of Oncology, National Board of Examiners. Starting at the Children's Hospital, Buffalo, as an intern in 1951, when he left in 1954 he was a resident. After a year in the U.S. Army as a 1st lieutenant, Pinkel then worked as a research fellow at the Children's Hospital Medical Center, Boston, from 1955 until 1956, when he was appointed chief of pediatrics at the Roswell Park Memorial Institute in Buffalo, holding that position until 1961, when he became medical director of St. Jude's Children's Research Hospital, Memphis, remaining there until 1973. He was then chairman in pediatrics at the Medical College of Wisconsin, Milwaukee, from 1974 until 1978, and was also pediatrician-in-chief at the Milwaukee Children's Hospital and associate director of the Wisconsin Clinic Cancer Center, Madison. Moving to California in 1978, Pinkel became chief of pediatrics at the City of Hope Medical Center, Duarte, remaining there until 1982, when he became chairman of pediatrics at Temple University School of Medicine, Philadelphia, from 1982 until 1985.

In 1985, Pinkel moved to Texas and became professor of the Kana Research Center and chairman and director of the pediatric leukemia program at the University of Texas System Cancer Center and the M.D. Anderson Hospital and Tumor Institute of Houston until he retired in 1993 and became professor emeritus at the University of Texas–M.D. Anderson Cancer Center. Pinkel has been clinical professor in pediatrics at the University of South California, Los Angeles, since 2002.

Pinkel has contributed extensively to professional journals, and his major works include *Treatment of Acute Lymphocytic Leukemia* (Leukemia Research Fund, 1973) and, as coeditor with Roberta A. Gottlieb, *Handbook of Pediatric Oncology* (Little, Brown, 1989). He has also written many scholarly papers. Pinkel was on the board of directors of Lee County Cooperative Clinic, Mariana, Arkansas, from 1972 to 1974. In 1972, he was given the Albert Lasker Award for Medical Research from the Lasker Foundation, and 2 years later he was given the Windermere Lectureship by the British Pediatric Association. Pinkel has also received the David Karnofsky Award from the American Society of Clinical Oncology in 1978, the Zimmerman Prize for Cancer Research from the Zimmerman Foundation in 1979, and the Charles F. Kettering Prize in 1986. Two years later, he received the Clinical Research Award from the American Cancer Society, and 4 years later he received the Return of the Child Award from the Leukemia Society of America. He won the Pollin Prize for pediatric research from New York Presbyterian Hospital in 2003. A member of many professional associations, he is a member of the American Pediatrics Society, the American Association for Cancer Research, the Society for Experimental Biology and Medicine, and the American Society of Hematology.

SEE ALSO: American Cancer Society; Leukemia Society of America.

BIBLIOGRAPHY. *American Men and Women of Science* (R.R. Bowker/Gale Group, 1971–2003); *Who's Who in America* (Marquis Who's Who, 1988–2004); *Who's Who in the South and Southwest* (Marquis Who's Who, 2000).

JUSTIN CORFIELD
GEELONG GRAMMAR SCHOOL, AUSTRALIA

Pituitary Tumor

PITUITARY TUMOR IS a tumor of the pituitary gland. It is one of the most common types of brain tumors, found predominantly in young or middle-aged adults. The pituitary gland is located in a depression of the base of the skull called the sella turcica. It lies immediately below the hypothalamus, which regulates its functions. The gland produces hormones responsible for various endocrine functions and is composed of two parts: the anterior (adenohypophysis) and posterior (neurohypophysis) lobes. The anterior lobe produces various hormones, including prolactin, adrenocorticotropic hormone (ACTH), growth hormone (GH), thyroid-stimulating hormone (TSH), leuteinizing hormone (LH), and follicle-stimulating hormone (FSH). The posterior lobe contains neurons that secrete the hormones oxytocin and vasopressin.

The majority of tumors that arise in the pituitary are adenomas. An adenoma is a benign tumor that develops from epithelial tissue. Pituitary adenomas may be classified by their size: microadenomas are tumors less than 10 mm in size that often secrete anterior pituitary hormones; macroadenomas (which are greater than 10 mm in size) do not secret hormones, but they often cause compression of the optic nerves and gradual loss of vision by compressing nearby brain or cranial nerve structures.

Pituitary adenomas are also classified by the hormones they produce. The majority of pituitary tumors produce excess amounts of pituitary hormones. Excess secretion of prolactin (prolactinomas) causes menstrual aberrations in females and impotence in males. Adenomas resulting from abnormal secretion of ACTH result in Cushing's syndrome, which can cause hypercortisolism. GH-producing adenomas cause acromegaly (e.g., enlargement of extremities) in adults and gigantism in children; these adenomas are usually characterized by an increase in the levels of insulin-like growth factor 1 (IGF-1), produced by the liver, found in the blood. TSH adenomas may produce an abnormal metabolism; however, they are extremely rare. LSH/FSH adenomas are also very rare but may cause infertility. Tumors in the posterior lobe of the pituitary are rare, but if they do occur, they usually lead to symptoms of diabetes insipidus, *characterized by an increased thirst.* The etiology of pituitary tumor is undefined. However, the incidence of pituitary tumors may be increased if they are associated with other diseases such as multiple endocrine neoplasia type I (MEN I). MEN I is a familial syndrome that may affect multiple endocrine glands including the pituitary, parathyroid, and pancreas. Although this disease is uncommon, those individuals who inherit the gene for MEN1 have an increased susceptibility to developing pituitary tumor.

Pituitary tumor is often diagnosed using various endocrine function tests such as the urine cortisol test. Imaging tests such as computerized tomography and magnetic resonance imaging, as well as visual field tests used to measure an individual's entire scope of vision, are frequently employed for diagnosis.

The prognosis for pituitary tumor following treatment is favorable. Treatments depend on the type of tumor, symptoms, and metastatic spread. Microadenomas are usually treated with a neurosurgical procedure called transsphenoidal microsurgery. This procedure is also effective in lowering GH levels. Macroadenomas are treated surgically and medically. Medical therapies for prolactin-secreting tumors include dopamine agonists such as cabergoline and bromocriptine, which work by suppressing prolactin production. They are also used alongside somatostatin analogs and GH receptor antagonists to treat GH tumors that have recurred after surgery. Other tumor types are usually treated with surgery followed by medical therapy to alleviate symptoms.

SEE ALSO: Multiple Endocrine Neoplasia Syndrome, Childhood.

BIBLIOGRAPHY. B. W. Scheithauer, T. A. Gaffey, R. V. Lloyd, et al., "Pathobiology of Pituitary Adenomas and Carcinomas," *Neurosurgery* (v. 59/2, 2006).

FARHANA AKTER
KINGS COLLEGE LONDON

Plastics Industry

PLASTICS ARE SYNTHETIC materials that can be designed and shaped to fit a wide range of needs. They are made from hydrocarbons and are malleable enough to form films, fibers, or other objects. The word *plastic* comes from a Greek word *plastikos*, which means something that can be molded. The first plastic-like materials were made in the 1840s from natural materials. Lac, gutta-percha, and cemented asbestos were bonded and molded to make handles, knobs, brush handles, and other objects. Celluloid was the first synthetic plastic. It was made from camphor and pyroxylin (cellulosed nitrate), which is a form of gun cotton. Celluloid was invented by John W. Hyatt and was capable of being molded into many products such as clock cases, combs, and eventually, celluloid film.

In 1884, Hilaire Chardonnet, a French chemist, invented viscose rayon. This invention was followed by the discovery of cellophane in 1908. Around this time, Bakelite was invented by combining carbolic acid and formaldehyde. The resin produced was very difficult to control and produced violent reactions until Leo H. Baekeland developed a method for controlling the reaction. Other chemists then used Bakelite in combination with other materials to produce plastic materials that were excellent for making telephones and pot handles as well as electrical parts. From this time on, the 20th century saw chemists inventing a growing list of plastic materials and making innovative developments in the uses of plastics.

There are now hundreds of plastics and synthetic materials, which have a wide range of properties that can be used by industrial designers to manufacture all kinds of useful objects. Plastics can range from very hard to very soft, and they may be clear or have coloring. Hard plastics may be used to make dinner plates, football helmets, or other parts that resist hard wear. Some common hard plastics are melamines, phenolics, epoxy, and alkyds. In addition, similar to using metal bars to reinforce concrete, fibers or other filler materials can be mixed with a plastic material to give greater strength. Filler materials may be metal powders or strips, glass fibers, wood dust, or other fillers that add strength.

Plastic can also be formed into sheets. The sheets can be made into a kind of plyboard by laminating them together. Laminates are often made from decorative plastics, as each layer can be colored differently to create unusual effects. They can also be bonded to other materials such as paper, wood, or marble to make useful articles.

Plastic fibers can be spun from liquid solutions of plastic materials. Nylon, which is a hard plastic that can be made into solid objects, can be spun through eyelets in a manner similar to that by which a spider spins its silk. The resulting nylon fibers can then be woven into nylon fabrics. Other plastic materials such as acrylic or polyester also can be spun into fibers that can then be spun into yarn and woven into cloth. They can also be blended with natural fibers, such as cotton or wool, to make polyester blends.

Soft plastics are usually made from polyethylenes, silicones, soft vinyls, and urethanes. Everything from children's toys and laundry baskets to washable bowls for dogs has been made from these types of plastics. They can also be formed into spongy materials such as pillow cushions or further softened with the addition of other chemical plasticizers. Resistant plastics succumb less to extremes of heat, cold, or other stresses. The nose cones of rockets, storage containers for chemicals, pipes, event table tops, and kitchen counter tops, laminated from resistant plastics, have been made for modern use. Transparent plastics are made for compounds such as polystyrenes, vinyls, acrylics, and polyethylenes and can be clear or colored. Everything from bottles for medicines, water, food wrapping, cups, and contact lenses are made from these plastics.

Plastics can be classified in a number of ways. Common ways of classifying do so in terms of the basic polymers involved, in terms of the materials' reaction to heat, or in terms of the polymerization method used or by other taxonomic schemes. The classification based on the way in which the plastic material reacts to heat groups the substances into thermoplastic or thermosetting categories. Hundreds of plastics can be made from by adding other chemicals to these basic two types. Thermosetting plastic include alkyd, allylic, epoxy, melamine and urea, phenolic, polyester, silicone, and urethane. These materials often are used to make rugged, weather-resistant hard plastics. Thermoplastic materials include acrylonitrile-butadiene-styrene, acetal, acrylic, nylon, polycarbonate, polyvinyl chloride, tetrafluoroethylene, and cellulose acetates. These materials can be formulated to make tough, lightweight materials that can be used as optical lenses, fabrics, electrical parts, packaging, or heat- and chemical-resistant substances.

The use of plastics to make plates, cups, eating utensils, food containers, and food wraps puts plastics into close contact with humans in a very wide variety of ways. In addition, plastics have found numerous uses in medicine, such as in making containers for medicine. Unbreakable in ordinary use, plastics have also been used to make parts for internal use in the human body. The plastics used to make screws, rivets, plates, suture thread, heart and artery stints, and other parts do not react with the body or with its chemicals to harm it. Artificial limbs and even plastic skins find very effective use in humans.

There have, however, been plastics that have been withdrawn from public use. The softer plastics are the more likely for this possibility is to occur. White school glues have been withdrawn because the polyvinyl acetate used to make them had been contaminated with vinyl acetate, which is a suspected carcinogen.

Although plastic materials per se are probably not carcinogenic, many of the chemicals from which they are made are. In addition, there are claims being made from various sources that microwave heating of plastic contains causes the release of dioxin, which is a known carcinogen.

Scientific investigation of these claims in important not only because they affect human health but also because journalism driven by viewer ratings, combined with incomplete information, creates and has created a large body of urban legend or misinformation about the dangers of plastic products. Of real concern are the issue of traces of a carcinogenic compound remaining in a plastic product that can affect human health and the issue of the migration of chemicals, because they react with other chemicals to become or release carcinogens.

Because of these legitimate, though in many cases unfounded, concerns about a connection between cancer and plastics and about the potential for carcinogens to be released by leaching or migration of chemicals, the plastics industry has had to wage an information campaign to refute claims that various chemicals are carcinogenic when there are, to date, no scientific studies to support such a claim.

The plastics industry must work with an enormous array of chemicals to manufacture the huge variety of plastic material and items that are sold to industry, the military, and the public. Many of these original chemicals such as benzene and vinyl chloride are known carcinogens. Thus, in manufacturing, with these and all other carcinogenic chemicals, great care has to be taken to ensure that there are no fugitive emissions in the workplace. In addition, because the chemical reactions that make the final plastic material may be less than 100 percent complete, there may be traces of vinyl chlorine, for example, in the final product. These traces might mean, for instance, that polyvinyl chloride is fine for sewer pipe but should not be put into use where it will is contact with food or drinking water. However, there is also evidence that disputes the claim that this substance can leach into water or food products.

The gravest danger for carcinogenic exposure to humans is not to the public at large but to workers in the plastics industry. In many cases, however, no threat has been found. For example, in studies that were etiological studies, made over 45 years, of workers using styrene (vinyl benzene), no evidence of carcinogenic activity was found. In addition, numerous studies performed on laboratory animals conducted according to internationally recognized standards have been made that also show no signs of carcinogenicity in animals. In fact, styrene is a naturally occurring chemical in many foods such as fruits, nuts, vegetables, and meats. Its industrial production is devoted to the making of plastic materials.

SEE ALSO: Chemical Industry.

BIBLIOGRAPHY. John A. Brydson, *Plastics Materials* (Elsevier Science and Technology, 1999); Robert A. Charyvat, ed., *Coloring of Plastics, Fundamentals* (Wiley, 2003); Nicholas P. Cheremisinoff, *Hazardous Chemicals in the Polymer Industry* (Marcel Dekker, 1994); Charles A. Harper, *Handbook of Plastic Processes* (Wiley, 2006); Charles A. Harper, *Handbook of Plastic Technologies: The Complete Guide to Properties and Performance* (McGraw-Hill, 2006); Jeffrey L. Meikle, *American Plastic: A Cultural History* (Rutgers University Press, 1995); Richard P. Pohanish, *Handbook of Toxic and Hazardous Chemicals and Carcinogens* (Noyes Publications, 2002); Gerd Potsch and Walther Michaeli, *Injection Molding: An Introduction* (Hanser-Gardner, 1995); Werner Rasshofer, Eckehard Weigand, Kurt C. Frisch, and Daniel Klempner, *Advances in Plastics Recycling: Automotive Polyurethanes* (CRC Press, 2001).

ANDREW J. WASKEY
DALTON STATE COLLEGE

Pleuropulmonary Blastoma

APPROXIMATELY 30 PERCENT of all childhood cancers are characterized by a defect occurring during the embryonic development. One such disease is pleuropulmonary blastoma (PPB), a rare, aggressive, dysontogenetic neoplasm of childhood. It is a disease associated with poor outcome and a high chance of recurrence and metastases, particularly to the central nervous system.

PPB accounts for less than 1 percent of all primary malignant lung tumors in children. It is commonly seen in children between the ages of 3 and 4 years. It may also be seen in adults, but this is extremely rare.

PPB may arise in the pulmonary parenchyma, the mediastinum, and pleura, giving rise to symptoms of respiratory distress, fever, chest pain, cough, recurrent pulmonary infection, anorexia, and malaise. PPB may also present with pneumothorax (collection of air in the space surrounding the lungs). It is also often associated with cystic lung lesions and may metastasize to the brain, bone, lymph nodes, liver, pancreas, kidney, and adrenal glands.

The disease typically presents as a pulmonary or pleural-based tumor with cystic, solid, or combined features. This has led to a classification of PBB into types I, II, or III. Type I is a predominately cystic type, type II is a combination of cystic and solid types, and type III is a predominately solid type. Histological features of the tumor include a neoplastic population of undifferentiated small round cells, larger spindle-shaped cells, and primitive mesenchymal cells. These features are analogous to those of other dysontogenetic tumors, such as Wilms tumor in the kidney, and embryonal rhabdomyosarcoma. These neoplasms have a strong familial association with PPB. Many patients suffering from PPB have close relatives with a history of cancer. The familial association is often referred to as PPB family cancer syndrome, and it arises in approximately 25 percent of children with PPB. There is no known cause for the familial link; however, a thorough family history is usually pursued and all family members examined if possible.

The cause of PPB is not known. Most cases are sporadic. There are cytogenetic reports indicating that PPB is characterized by several chromosomal imbalances, and polysomy of chromosome 8 appears to be related to the development of PPB. This chromosomal aberration is found only in the mesenchymal elements that undergo clonal proliferation; however, it is absent in the epithelial components. Other cytogenic findings include trisomy of chromosome 2 and aberrations on chromosome 11 involving the WT2 (Wilms tumor 2) gene. However, these findings are not all specific to PPB, and strong evidence of gene mutation is still lacking.

Diagnosis of the disease is often delayed, as its occurrence is so rare. There is no cure for the disease; surgical resection is the current mainstay treatment. Radiotherapy and chemotherapy may be employed for PBB types II and III. Chemotherapeutic agents may include vincristine, cyclophosphamide, dactinomycin, and doxorubicin. The prognosis for PPB is poor, particularly for patients with advanced-stage disease and for those with types II and III disease, as these types are often associated with metastases to extrapulmonary sites. Less than 50 percent of patients survive beyond 1–2 years of age. Children with type I PPB have a greater prognosis for survival. Other favorable prognostic factors include a small size of the mass (less than 5 cm) and the complete excision of the tumor during surgical treatment.

SEE ALSO: Childhood Cancers; Wilms tumor.

BIBLIOGRAPHY. Gerald L. Mandell, *Atlas of Infectious Disease: Pleuropulmonary and Bronchial Infections* (Elsevier Health Sciences, 1996); "Pleuropulmonary Blastoma: A Case Report," www.ispub.com (cited September 2006).

FARHANA AKTER
KINGS COLLEGE LONDON

Poland

POLAND IS AN eastern European country that traces its origins back to medieval and early modern times, when it covered vastly more territory than today. In 1740, Poland covered present-day Lithuania, Belarus, and some of the Ukraine, but it was partitioned between Prussia, Russia, and Austria in 1772, 1793, and 1795. Recreated briefly by Napoleon (as the Grand Duchy of Warsaw), it was only reestablished as an independent country after World War I. During World War II, it was occupied by Germany and then,

with different boundaries, reestablished in 1945. It had a population of 38,128,000 in 2005, with 236 doctors and 527 nurses per 100,000 people. An example of cancer incidence rates in Poland includes 301 cases of cancer in males per 100,000, according to the International Agency for Research on Cancer.

There is clear evidence of cancer in medieval Poland. In 1977, an archaeological excavation of an 11th-century burial ground at Czersk, in the north of Poland, the skeleton of a man showed clear signs of malignant bone tumor in the jaw. There is also a reference, by French writer Ambroise Paré, from January 20, 1269, in which Countess Margaret of Cracow was said to have given birth to 36 live infants and also to have had a "mole of the uterus," probably an early description of a hydatidiform mole.

During the 18th and early 19th centuries, there occurred major developments in surgical procedures and medical treatments. A Polish doctor, Samuel Thomas von Soemmering, in 1795, noticed a link between lip carcinomas and people who smoked pipes. Martin Heinrich Rathke (1793–1860) was born in Danzig and was involved in scientists being able to describe congenital tumors that arose from craniopharyngeal ducts between the pharynx and the pituitary. An early Polish doctor involved in oncology was Julius Cohnhem (1839–84), who born in Pomerania, which was at the time occupied by Germany. Cohnhem studied in Kiel, Breslau, and Leipzig. His work showed that malignant tumors could develop from immature embryonic cells left in tissues.

The Polish surgeon Johannes von Mikulicz-Radecki (1850–1905), pioneered some developments in modern surgery, assisting Theodor Billroth at the University of Vienna and then serving as professor of surgery at the University of Cracow from 1882 to 1887, Konigsburg from 1887 to 1890, and Breslau (Wroclaw) from 1890 to 1905. During that time, von Mikulicz-Radecki worked on surgical procedures dealing with cancer of the digestive tract, being the first, in 1885, to suture a perforated gastric ulcer; surgically restore part of the esophagus of a patient in 1886; and cut away a malignant portion of the colon in 1903. Much of this innovative surgery was performed with improved models of the esophagoscope and gastroscope. Indeed, at the same time, Walery Jawoski (1849–1924) worked on cures for gastric disease including cancer, becoming the pioneer for gastroenterology in Poland.

Mention must also be made of Marie Curie (1867–1934), who was born in Warsaw as Marie Sklodowskiej, moving to Paris in 1891, where she met and married Pierre Curie. In Paris, Madame Curie worked on radioactivity and twice won the Nobel Prize—in 1903, jointly with her husband, for physics, and in 1911 for chemistry. Marie Curie was responsible for the establishment in 1932 of the Radium Institute in Warsaw, built with the encouragement of the president Ignacy Moscicki. A Radiation Department was built in the following year. After World War II, the name of this department was changed to the Marie Sklodowskiej-Curie Oncological Institute; it remains the main cancer research and treatment center in the country today.

In 1918, Poland regained its independence, and there followed a vast improvement of the medical services in the country, including for cancer treatment. The Polish Anti-Cancer Society was founded in 1929 and ran until World War II, being an important educational and fund-raising group for 10 years. For some years, the society worked in conjunction with the Committee for Combating Cancer in Poland, which was particularly active between 1931 and 1936.

The 1920s and 1930s were a period when some Polish doctors and medical researchers were involved in following up the research of the Japanese researcher Katsusaburo Yamagiwa in working out the causes of cancer in animals. Stefan Banach (1892–1945), born in Krakow, which was then in the Austro-Hungarian empire, was a prominent mathematician who was involved in the founding of modern functional analysis and who also helped develop the theory of topological vector spaces. During the German occupation of Poland, Banach worked on lice during his studies of infectious diseases; he died from lung cancer just after the end of the war in Europe. Another scientist from this time who was involved in oncology was Ludwika Hirszfelda, who studied tumor serology.

The medical services available in Poland were devastated in World War II but were rebuilt during the late 1940s and 1950s, with much money devoted to cancer research. From 1947 to 1948, the Institute of Oncology, established in Warsaw at the department of pathology, started publishing extensively about cancer in Poland. The Centralne Laboratorium Ochrony Radiologicznej in Warsaw works under the aegis of the Ministry of Energy and Atomic Energy in various fields of radiological protection. There was also a Provincial Oncological Center in Posnan and the ORL Clinic at the Silesian Medical Academy. A Department of Pulmonary Illness operated at the Krakow Special Hospital, which from 1956 until 1977 treated many patients for lung and bronchial carcinomas.

At the oncology department of the faculty of medicine at Akademia Medyczna w Bialymstoku, Professor Andrzej Klepacki was involved in the diagnostic value of the immunochemical method of determination of the mammary carcinoma antigen, the fibrin stabilizing factor activity of skin carcinoma. Bozena Sablinska, Ludwika Tarlowska, and Zofia Drozdzewska also worked at the institute on the results of long-term (10–15 years) observation of 2,800 patients with carcinoma of the cervix who were treated with radiotherapy between 1950 and 1955; Tadeusz Koszarowski, Anna Madejczyk, and Danuta Gajl researched the broader indications for radical mastectomy by preoperative radiotherapy in breast cancer; and J. Buraczewski studied malignant bone tumors arising from bone dysplasias.

Zygmunt Albert, Anna Stelmachowska, and Antonia Harlozinska, from the Department of Experimental Oncology at the Institute of Immunology and Experimental Therapy at the Polish Academy of Sciences in Wroclaw, worked on the autoimmunologic findings in transplantable Crocker sarcoma. Z. Olszewski, of Clinic I of Obstetrics and Gynaecology of Cracow Academy of Medicine, researched the results of hemotherapy and chemotherapy in cases of gynecological cancer that were deemed to be incurable. At Lodz, Boguslaw Krawczyk of the Department of Obstetrics and Gynecology at the M.S.W. Hospital worked on the treatment of early cases of uterine cervix cancer.

Mention must also be made of Albert Bruce Sabin (1906–93), born at Białystok, who moved to the United States, where he became a prominent physician and microbiologist who was best known for his work on the oral polio vaccine. Sabin also conducted some experiments into the treatment of some cancers. In recent years, there has been controversy over claims by Lublin-born biochemist Stanislaw Burzynski (b. 1943) to have used antineoplasms for curing cancer patients.

The most famous cancer researcher of Polish ethnicity remains Philip Strax (1909–99), whose parents came from Poland while it was still a part of the Russian Empire, moving to New York, where Strax was born. Strax was the joint winner, with Sam Shapiro, of the Charles F. Kettering Prize of the General Motors Cancer Foundation in 1988.

A 1977 study of cancer in Poland showed that the rise in lung cancer coincided with a rise in smoking. After the collapse of communism, there was a massive increase in cigarette advertising in Poland, but with greater health awareness, the number of people suffering from lung cancer has started to fall.

The Polskie Towarzystwo Onkologiczne helps with the public education campaign in making people aware of the problem of cancer and supports clinical research and treatment. The Jakuba Potockiego Foundation also provides help. The International Hereditary Cancer Centre and the Polish Oncological Society are both members of the International Union Against Cancer. The Terry Fox Run, which raises money for cancer research, had its first race run in Poland in 2004.

The great hero of the Polish revolution, and the first head of state of Poland from November 1918 until 1922, Józef Piłsudski (1867–1935), died from liver cancer. Other important Poles who died from cancer include Zahava Burack (1932–2001), holocaust survivor and philanthropist; Tad Danielewski (1921–91), film director; Kazimierz Gorski (1921–2006), famous soccer coach; Tadeusz Kutrzeba (1885–1947), general captured during the siege of Warsaw in 1939; F. Romauld Spasowski (1921–95), Polish Ambassador to Washington, D.C., who defected in 1981; and Aleksander Zawadzki (1899–1964), communist head of state from 1952 to 1964.

SEE ALSO: Strax, Philip

BIBLIOGRAPHY. M. Bebenek, "EUROCARE Study Underestimated the Curability of Breast Cancer in Poland," *Annals of Oncology* (v.18, 2007); H. Gadomska, "Ocena cze,estosci wyst e,epowania osteosarcoma na tle innych postaci nowotdworow zosliwych kos'sci, Warsawa 1963–1974," *Nowotwory* (1979); J. Gladykowka-Rzeczyska, "Mandibular Tumor in a Male Skeleton from a Medieval Burial Ground in Czersk," *Folia Morphologica* (v.37, 1978); H. Kolodziejska, "Onkologia polska w XXX-lecie Polskiej Rzeczypospoliteudowej," *Nowotwory* (v.24, 1974); T. Koszarowski, "Rozwoj onkologii w Polsce w latach 1932–1944 i 1948–1973; szkic historyczny z okaji rocznicy 25-lecia Instytutu Onkologii im. Marii Sklodowskiej-Curie w Polskiej Rzecypospolitej Ludowej," *Nowotwory* (v.21, 1973); J. Rutkowski, "Dzieje walki z rakiem na terenie Lodzi," *Archiwum Historii Medycyny* (v.32, 1969); J. Supady. "Udzial lekarzy polskich w krajowych I miedzynarodowych zjazdach onkologicznych w latach 1918–1938," *Nowotwory* (v.29, 1979).

JUSTIN CORFIELD
GEELONG GRAMMAR SCHOOL, AUSTRALIA

Polishes

POLISHES ARE PREPARATIONS used on a variety of surfaces, including leather, wood, and metal, that are applied to produce a glossy finish. Polishes can be found in nature: Apples can be polished by simply rubbing their surface, as the natural wax coating found in their skin will shine after polishing.

Normally, surfaces are polished with a preparation that smoothes and finishes the surface so that it can be shined to a bright finish. Polishing is the action that cleans and then removes all excess polish preparation as the physical action of "shining" creates a smooth shiny surface. The majority of polishes are made of waxes that are mixed into a liquid or salve form. Other polishes are used on metals to remove tarnish. In cases such as that of the apple, a rubbing action produces the shine. In other cases, a chemical reaction causes the shine.

First, the polish is spread over a surface. The solvent in which the wax is mixed then evaporates, leaving only the wax behind. The polish then creates a coating on the surface, which protects it and that, in the case of some polishes, can also be shined. Polishes are used widely on metal, leather, clay, and wood surfaces and on the finger- and toenails of some individuals.

Nail polishes are cosmetics used to lacquer the nails of the hands and feet. This custom of human decoration is at least five thousand years old. In ancient Egypt, henna was used to decorate the hands and feet, and in Egypt and ancient China, the color placed on the nails of the hands was used to identify social rank. The chemicals used in modern nail polishes, however, are similar to those used in paint. Pigments, solvent nitrocellulose, formaldehyde, and other compounds are combined to form the polish. Once painted on the nail, the polish is then left to dry.

Nitrocellulose (cellulose nitrate), a major constituent of nail polish, is popularly known as flash paper or, when used as an explosive, as guncotton. Nitrocellulose is a very flammable compound formed by nitrating cellulose with chemicals such as nitric acid.

The resulting nitrocellulose is then dissolved in a solvent to create a clear polish, to which pigments in all the basic colors of the rainbow can be added. Basic colors can be mixed to form additional colors, or they may be tinted by the addition of white pigment. Tinting creates an even greater range of colors. Shading the basic colors can also be done by adding black. For example, with a little addition of black to the color blue, ever-darker shades of blue can be made. The range of colors available to consumers on the market is very broad.

Although there are nail polishes intended for use by men, women wear nail polishes the most. Traditional nail polish colors are red, pink, and flesh colored, although darker colors have gained some influence in fashion from popular cultures, such as those following a "Goth" culture wearing black or dark red polish.

Formaldehyde, also called methanal, is a carcinogenic agent that found in some fingernail polishes. It is the most basic of the aldehyde compounds and has a chemical formula of H_2CO. First synthesized by the Russian chemist Aleksandr Butlerov in 1859, formaldehyde is made by the incomplete combustion of organic carbon compounds. It occurs naturally in the atmosphere and in some metabolic processes in many organisms.

Formaldehyde is very toxic and is also a known carcinogen. The International Agency for Research on Cancer has classified it as a Group xx carcinogen. The U.S. Environmental Protection Agency has classified it as a probable human carcinogen because existing evidence has been deemed sufficient to conclude that formaldehyde causes nasopharyngeal cancer. To counter the carcinogenic dangers of formaldehyde, many nail polish companies have turned to other compounds that currently are considered to be much safer. Their goal is to eliminate carcinogenic exposure.

Wood polishes are used to create a bright or smooth finish to wood, especially to wooden furniture. An older technique for polishing wood is French Polishing. This does not involve a specific polish compound but polishes successive layers of shellac with a rubber pad to create a high gloss. In the 19th century, when labor was cheap, this polishing technique was often used on mahogany. Since the 1930s, an abrasive buffing of a nitrocellulose lacquer applied to furniture has been used. Wood polishes are most commonly applied to wooden floors and to wooden furniture. The polish may be applied as a spray or as an aerosol. Although floor polishes are among the easiest polishes to use, they so usually contain silicon oils, which can damage furniture lacquers or varnishes.

There are two basic types of liquid wooden polishes in current use. The emulsion polishes are composed of waxes, oils, and organic solvents. Oil wood polishes may be either drying oil polishes or nondrying oil polishes. They achieve their best results if used as a final finish. The nondrying oil polishes may contain paraffin, lemon oil, or mineral oil. With these products, some of the oil polish remains on the furniture and may collect dust. The drying oil wood polishes use linseed oil and walnut oil. These polishes dry by oxidation, which can build up over a long period of time.

Semisolid polishes are commercially called paste waxes. They require considerable labor during application. Some furniture polishes use petroleum distillates, which have been linked to both skin and lung cancer. Those that contain nitrobenzene are extremely toxic and carcinogenic. In addition, some wood polishes use petroleum distillates, which also are associated with cancer. However, to date, mineral spirits have not been linked to mutant cellular changes or to carcinogenic effects.

Nitrobenzene, also called nitrobenzol or oil of mirbane, is an organic compound that smells like almonds and has been in the past used as a mild perfume in soap. It is toxic and has a chemical formula of $C_6H_5NO_2$. It has a number of uses: It is used as a solvent for other chemicals, it is used as a mild oxidizing agent, it is used in the manufacture of other chemicals, it is used in the manufacture of polishes for shoes and wood and for leather dressing, and its primary use is as a wood polish on flooring.

Studies of rats and mice exposed to nitrobenzene have been performed, indicating that it can be absorbed by contact with the skin as well as through inhalation. The exposed rats developed a variety of tumors in many sites including the liver, lungs, breast, and thyroid gland. This result has been used as a basis for a recommendation to classify nitrobenzene as a Group B2 (probable) human carcinogen. To date, no information is available on its carcinogenic toxicity to humans.

Shoe polishes contain also coloring. Black shoe polish contains a dye that reacts with the leather to restore its color. These polishes use a waxy paste or cream to shine or waterproof leather shoes or boots. Tallow and other waxes or greases also have been used to polish footwear for centuries. Modern formulas for shoe polish do not seem to pose a carcinogenic risk.

Burnishing is a polishing technique used to decorate pottery. To burnish a piece of pottery, its surface is polished with a tool that may be made of wood, bone, or some other material. The surface is smoothed while the clay is still in a semidry or leathery "green state." The pottery object is then fired in a kiln. After firing, the pottery's burnished surface will be very shiny. There exist ceramic traditions that use pattern burnishing on either the outside or the inside of pottery to create shiny pattern. Metal polishes use the atomic structure of the surface of the metal to achieve a polished surface. As such, different metals use different compounds. Brass polish and silver polish are formulated to remove oxides and to create a bright surface. A natural acid such as lemon juice can also remove the tarnish. In some metal polishing operations, silicon compounds also are used as the polishes; silicon pads, or even pads with diamond dust in solution, can be used.

Automobile polishes also have been examined, and most have not been found to be associated with carcinogens that are known, nor have they exhibited carcinogenic effects in human or animal studies.

SEE ALSO: Chemical Industry; Paint.

BIBLIOGRAPHY. J. C. S. Brough, *Staining and Polishing: Including Varnishing and Other Methods of Finishing Wood, with Appendix of Recipes* (Read Books, 2006); R. Colin Garner et al, eds., *Human Carcinogen Exposure: Biomonitoring and Risk Assessment* (Oxford University Press, 1999); American Society for Testing Materials, ed., *1999 Annual Book of ASTM Standards: Soaps and other Detergents: Polishes; Leather; Resilient Floor Coverings* (American Society for Testing and Materials, 1999); American Society for Testing Materials, ed., *Soap, Polishes, Leather, Resilient Floor Coverings* (American Society for Testing and Materials, 2005); Icon Group International Staff, *2000 Import and Export Market for Polishes and Creams for Footwear, Furniture and Floors in N. American and Caribbean* (Icon Group International, 2000).

ANDREW J. WASKEY
DALTON STATE COLLEGE

Pollution, Air

AIR SUPPLIES US with *oxygen*, which is essential for our bodies to survive. Humans probably first experienced harm from air pollution when they built fires in poorly ventilated caves. Since these days, as a result of the industrialization of society, the introduction of motorized vehicles, and the explosion of the population, there has been a steady change in the composition of the atmosphere.

Air pollution is a major environmental health problem affecting developing and developed countries alike. The effects of air pollution on health are very complex, as there are many different sources of pollution, and their individual effects vary from one source to another. It is not only the ambient air quality in cities but also the indoor air quality in rural and urban areas that cause concern. Inhaled air pollutants have a serious effect on human health by affecting the lungs and the respiratory system; they are also taken up by the blood and pumped throughout the body. These pollutants are also deposited on soil and plants and in the water, further contributing to human exposure.

OUTDOOR AND INDOOR AIR POLLUTANTS

Air pollution consists of a chemical, physical, or biological agent that modifies the natural characteristics of the atmosphere. The primary air pollutants found in outdoor air of most urban areas are carbon monoxide, nitrogen oxides, sulfur oxides, hydrocarbons, carbon dioxide, chlorofluorocarbons, hazardous air pollutants, lead, ozone, nitrogen oxide, particulate matter, and volatile organic compounds. Among these pollutants, particulate matter, organic matter, or nitrogen dioxide have been discovered to have the strongest links to increased risk factors and the development of cancer.

Particulate matter consists of microscopic particles less than one-seventh the width of a human hair. Because of its small size, some particulate matter can bypass the body's natural defenses and penetrate deep into the lungs. Some of these pollutants can have direct harmful effects, but the main problem comes from other cancer-causing chemicals that are stuck to their surfaces. Among these by-products of combustion and incomplete burning of fuels are dioxins and polycyclic organic matter. Polycyclic organic matter consists of over 100 compounds, including polycyclic aromatic hydrocarbons, polychlorinated biphenyls, and benzo(a)pyrene, which may affect the development of the fetus and increase cancer risks later in life. Volatile organic compounds, such as benzene and 1,3-butadiene, also link with the development or the risk of cancer.

The two most important types of indoor air pollution are environmental tobacco smoke, often called secondhand smoke, and radon gas. Environmental tobacco smoke contains about 4,000 chemicals, including 200 known poisons, such as formaldehyde and carbon monoxide, as well as 43 carcinogens. Environmental tobacco smoke causes an estimated 3,000 lung cancer deaths and 35,000 to 50,000 heart disease deaths in nonsmokers per year. Some people may not be used to thinking about secondhand smoke as air pollution, but in terms of cancer, this smoke has a larger effect than traffic fumes or industrial emissions.

The other indoor air pollution related to cancer is Radon-222, which can decay quickly and give off tiny radioactive particles. When inhaled, these radioactive particles can damage the cells that line the lungs. Long-term exposure to radon can lead to lung cancer. As with air pollution, radon has a tiny effect on cancer risk compared to smoking, but it is the second leading cause of lung cancer in the United States. Scientists estimate that approximately 15,000 to 22,000 lung cancer deaths per year are related to radon.

On the basis of the findings of estimated toxic chemicals in air from local communities gathered by the U.S. Environmental Protection Agency Cumulative Exposure Project, the Environmental Defense Fund reported that more than 220 million Americans breathe air that is 100 times more toxic than the goal set by Congress 10 years ago. Also, the cancer risk from breathing air in certain neighborhoods is more than 1,000 times higher than the established goal.

The exact causes of pollution for each city may be different depending on the region's geographical location, temperature, wind, and weather factors. For example, a temperature inversion can cause the dispersion of pollutants in air, and cities surrounded by mountains also experience trapping of pollution.

SOURCES OF POLLUTANTS

More and more data have accumulated to indicate that long-term exposure to air pollution in some of America's biggest metropolitan areas significantly raises the risk of lung cancer. In addition, epidemio-

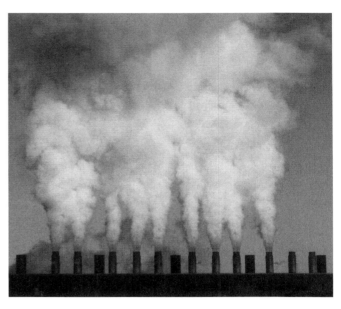

Air pollution consists of a chemical, physical, or biological agent that modifies the natural characteristics of the atmosphere.

logical studies have shown an increased rate of lung cancer when humans are exposed to broader mixtures of air pollutants for a long period of time. In experimental laboratory studies, animals, through inhalation exposure to air pollutants, exhibited respiratory tract tumors, lung tumors, and leukemia.

Researchers from Brigham Young University and New York University reported that the number of lung cancer deaths increased 8 percent for every increase of 10 μg per cubic meter of fine particulate matter, based on a study that involved a population of 500,000 adults. This risk primarily comes from combustion-related soot emitted by cars and trucks, coal-fired power plants, and factories. Of the cancer risk calculated by the Environmental Defense Fund for the United States as a whole, 60 percent is from mobile sources and 26 percent from small business sources, with the remaining 14 percent from identifiable industrial sources.

Nitrogen dioxide, primarily from automobile exhaust, has also been examined for its link to cancer. The National Institute of Cancer indicated that nitrogen dioxide can cause genetic changes, but no evidence has shown that the compound causes cancer. The Department of Health and Human Services, the International Agency for Research on Cancer, and the Environmental Protection Agency have not classified nitrogen oxides for potential carcinogenicity. However, Richters and Kuraitis reported that inhalation of ambient levels of nitrogen dioxide could influence the frequency of blood-borne cancer cell metastasis to the lungs. Nitrogen dioxide also may affect cells of the immune system, which might, in part, account for its contribution to cancer cell metastasis.

The development and progression of cancer is a very complex process. From a mechanism point of view, different air pollutants can act at different sites in the sequence of cancer causation and progression. Certain air pollutants could participate in the process of carcinogenesis, and others in the process of cancer dissemination and metastasis. With respect to carcinogenesis, Richters and Kuraitis proposed that noxious air pollutants could act as initiators or complete carcinogens, cocarcinogens, or promoters leading to the development of cancer.

Despite the well-documented evidence supporting the hypothesis about the link between long-term exposure to air pollution and lung cancer, Katsouyanni and Pershagen have pointed out the problems inherent in adequately assessing the exposure effect. Routinely measured air pollutants do not include, as a rule, established carcinogens, and air pollution measurements usually come from fixed-site monitors, making it difficult to estimate individual exposure, especially long-term.

REGULATION, MONITORING, AND REDUCTION OF AIR POLLUTANTS

The purposes of regular monitoring are to assess air quality and ensure conformity with air-quality standards set by law. These standards exist to protect the public health from known or anticipated adverse effects associated with the presence of specific pollutants in the air. Several common air pollutants are regulated under state and federal Clean Air Acts and are known as criteria air pollutants. Two of the most widespread criteria pollutants are particulate matter and ozone. Other criteria pollutants include nitrogen dioxide, carbon monoxide, lead, sulfur dioxide, sulfates, and hydrogen sulfide. However, carcinogens among air pollutants are not monitored routinely in most places where air pollution monitoring has been established. Among these compounds, benzo(a)pyrene concentrations have been measured sporadically as an index of air carcinogenicity, but there is a lack of data on long

time-trends. Diesel exhaust also has attracted attention, but studies so far have been conducted mostly on persons occupationally exposed.

Air pollution does not discriminate between young and old; it is therefore essential to work from every angle to minimize pollution levels. A number of ways exist for the government, industry, and individuals to reduce the air pollution that contributes to the risk of cancer: first, bringing tobacco products under the regulation of the U.S. Food and Drug Administration through congressional legislation would allow national regulations to dramatically reduce the harm done by secondhand smoke; second, legally mandating controls and regulations limiting automobile tailpipe and industrial smoke-stack emissions that would cover existing and new coal fired plants; third, imposing a carbon tax to promote conservation and the development of alternative, renewable clean energy sources; and the expansion and use of existing mass transit and car pooling and bicycling as people movers, along with the voluntary cessation of discretionary wood-burning activities. All of these actions would reduce the danger of contracting lung cancer and other respiratory related diseases.

SEE ALSO: Pollution, Water.

BIBLIOGRAPHY. J. Lewtas, C. Lewis, R. Zweidinger, R. Stevens, and L. Cupitt, "Sources of Genotoxicity and Cancer Risk in Ambient Air," *Pharmacogenetics* (v.2, 1992); F. Nyberg, P. Gustavsson, Lars Jarup, et al., "Urban Air Pollution and Lung Cancer in Stockholm," *Epidemiology*, (v.11/5, 2000); A. Richters and K. Kuraitis, "Air Pollutants and the Facilitation of Cancer Metastasis." *Environmental Health Perspectives*, (v.52, 1993); The Department of Health and Human Services, "ToxiFact," www.astdr.cdc; A. J. Cohen and A. Pope III, "Lung Cancer and Air Pollution," *Environmental Health Prospect* (v.103, 1995); Environmental Defense Fund, "Most Americans Face Cancer Risk from Toxic Air Pollution," healthandenergy.com; National Institutes of Health, "Radon and Cancer," www.cancer.gov; Environmental Protection Agency, "Polycyclic Organic Matter," www.epa.gov; K. Katsouyanni and G. Pershagen, "Ambient Air Pollution Exposure and Cancer," *Cancer Causes and Control* (v.8, 1997); *U.S.A. Today*, "Study: Air Pollution, Lung Cancer Are Linked," www.usatoday.com (cited March 2002); Campaign for Tobacco-Free Kids, "FDA Regulation of Tobacco Products: Why It's Needed and What It Will Do," www.tobaccofreekids.org/reports.

H. Jeng
Old Dominion University

Pollution, Water

WATER IS SECOND only to air in importance for human life on Earth. Our water is made up of surface water, such as rivers, lakes, and seas, and groundwater. Two primary sources of drinking water are surface water and groundwater. As Takeshi One pointed out, surface waters receive large quantities of wastewater from industrial, agricultural, and domestic sources, including municipal sewage treatment plants. Groundwater also can be contaminated by leakage from underground storage tanks and landfills. Because water is a superb solvent, it serves as a potential medium for human exposure to a large number and variety of carcinogens.

The U.S. Environmental Protection Agency's Toxic Release Inventory for 2001 reported that more than 100,000 metric tons of chemicals are released into surface waters, and 762,000 metric tons of chemicals are emitted into the atmosphere annually by industries in the United States. Large quantities of toxic materials are routinely released, either directly or indirectly, into surface water and groundwater. Of particular concern are the 800 metric tons of chemicals released into surface waters and 60,000 metric tons of chemicals emitted into the atmosphere that are cancer causing (carcinogens). These carcinogens are categorized into two types: persistent compounds and volatile compounds. The persistent compounds include metals such as arsenic and lead and polycyclic aromatic compounds. The volatile compounds are mostly volatile organics.

A large body of research supports a link between water pollution and cancer, but there are also those who disagree—and who have research data to support their position. The predominant view is that there is a definite link between water pollution and cancer, but this link has not been adequately defined or quantified yet. Additional research in this area is required to ascertain the causation of specific cancers from specific pollutant carcinogens, but a correlation has been definitively established.

CARCINOGENIC CONTAMINANTS

The information for quantifying risk between carcinogenic compounds in water and cancer is limited to epidemiologic data, occasionally with support from metabolic or biomarker studies. The reasons for the lack of toxicological evaluation of water contaminants stem from either unavailable and appropriate animal models or the fact that surface water and groundwater are complex mixtures with a chemical composition that varies temporally and from place to place.

Source water contaminants of concern include arsenic, asbestos, radon, agricultural chemicals, and hazardous waste. Arsenic has the strongest evidence for posing substantial cancer risk, particularly for liver, lung, bladder, and kidney cancer. Asbestos is a proven carcinogen, but the risk of causing cancer associated with asbestos in drinking water appears to be unfounded. Radon is also a known carcinogen, but there is little evidence linking consumption of radon-contaminated water to human cancer.

Source waters can easily be contaminated by farm runoff of insecticides, fungicides, rodenticides, herbicides, and fertilizers, all of which contain phosphorous or nitrogen. Some pesticides are proven carcinogens; however, drinking water contamination with pesticides has not been conclusively associated with cancer. The inconclusive findings are controlled by the concentrations of pesticide in water bodies, the amount absorbed from water or other sources, the duration of exposure to the chemical, and the speed that the compound is metabolized and excreted from the body. Some epidemiological studies do suggest that fertilizers, and particularly nitrate fertilizers, may pose a risk. Studies among populations in China that have been exposed to high levels of nitrates in drinking water have correlated nitrate contamination and stomach and liver cancer. Brain cancer, non-Hodgkin's lymphoma, and gastric mucosal changes have also been linked to nitrate exposure.

In addition to runoff, leakage from hazardous waste sites presents another matter of great concern related to the contamination of drinking water from groundwater sources. Contaminated drinking water from hazardous waste sites in 75 towns in northern New Jersey affected the health of people in the communities; however, no link to cancer was determined. Because the development of cancer takes a long period of time, however, the study may not project the risk of affected persons developing cancer later in life. Trichloroethylene, the second most common chemical found at Superfund sites, has been examined for its link to cancer. Epidemiological studies have shown inconsistent or inconclusive findings; however, animal studies have reported increases in lung, liver, kidney, and testicular tumors and lymphoma. The U.S. Environmental Protection Agency is currently reassessing the cancer classification of the compound.

Another source of potential contamination is water treatment. Chlorine has been added to drinking water since the early 1900s in the United States as an essential element to prevent waterborne diseases. However, chlorination does pose a potential carcinogenic risk. When a large concentration of organic matter is present in chlorinated water, by-products such as trihalomethane can form. These by-products have been associated with bladder, colon, and rectum cancer. An important note from a public health perspective is that the amount of disease prevented from chlorinating drinking water vastly outnumbers the correlation found between chlorination by-products and cancer. If the amount of organic matter is controlled in the treatment system, however, chlorinated by-products are as prevalent.

Exposure can also occur via distribution systems. The pipes, joints, and fixtures that make up the water treatment and distribution systems include materials made from iron, copper, lead, plastics, asbestos, and concrete. Trichloroethylene (one of the plastics) has been shown to contribute to leukemia, but direct evidence of a causal relationship is still lacking.

The only conclusive epidemiologic evidence for a certain link between a contaminant and cancer is for arsenic. The rest of the epidemiologic evidence is inconclusive, and further research is necessary to ensure accurate results.

EXPOSURE ROUTES

The primary exposure to water pollution comes from ingestion via drinking water. Volatile organic compounds and radionuclides have the potential to become airborne and get inhaled, and some of the same volatile compounds also have potential for dermal ex-

posure, but the most common exposure route by far is ingestion. Because of this, drinking water quality and adherence to the Safe Drinking Water Act are of utmost concern. Additional legislation dealing with carcinogens in drinking water might be necessary once conclusive epidemiological evidence exists defining correlations between specific carcinogens and the cancers they cause.

REGULATION AND ENVIRONMENTAL POLICY

During the 1970s, a decade that witnessed the birth of the U.S. environmental movement, Congress approved the two main federal laws governing water quality: the Clean Water Act and the Safe Drinking Water Act, signed in 1972 and 1974, respectively. The Clean Water Act set a goal of eliminating all pollution discharges into U.S. water by 1985. The Safe Drinking Water Act allows the federal government to regulate drinking water contaminants suspected of causing chemical poisoning or noncommunicable diseases. The Clean Water Act authorized the Environmental Protection Agency to establish national standards for known or suspected drinking water contaminants. A reauthorization of the Safe Drinking Water Act came about in 1986 and laid out mandatory guidelines for regulating key contaminants. Based on assessing risk of cancer development during a 70-year water consumption period, the agency determined criteria for contaminants in drinking water. The act required the monitoring of unregulated contaminants, established benchmarks for water treatment technologies, strengthened enforcement, and promoted protection of groundwater sources.

The 1990s showed a growing awareness of water pollution and mounting concern about waterborne disease. This concern sparked demands for more effective ways of ensuring drinking water safety. In 1991, the Environmental Protection Agency issued a revised standard for lead in tap water that many critics condemned as inadequate. The litany of historical attention to water pollution and clean water in the United States is impressive—but still inadequate. When compared to other places in the world that are still struggling to prevent waterborne diseases, the United States is definitely much more advanced in the area of water quality. However, that does not diminish the immediate attention needed from responsible officials at every level to prevent carcinogenic contamination of source waters and remove the carcinogens that abound in the existing surface and groundwater supplies of our country.

SEE ALSO: Pollution, Air; Water Treatment; Water, Drinking and Arsenic.

BIBLIOGRAPHY. Robert D. Morris, "Drinking Water and Cancer," *Environmental Health Perspectives* (v.103, 1995); Kenneth P. Cantor, "Drinking Water and Cancer," *Cancer Causes and Control* (v.8, 1997); Takeshi One, Tetsushi Watanabe, and Keiji Wakabayashi, "Mutagens in Surface Waters: A Review," *Mutation Research* (v.567, 2004). www.epa.gov (accessed January 2007); Nancy M. Trautmann and Keith S. Porter, "Pesticides: Health Effects in Drinking Water," pmep.cce.cornell.edu; Environmental Research Foundation, "Rachel's Hazardous Waste New #370," www.ejnet.org.

H. Jeng
Old Dominion University

Portugal

PORTUGAL, LOCATED ON the Iberian Peninsula and neighboring Spain, gained its independence in 1128 with the defeat of the Moors in Lisbon. Since then, Portugal has maintained its independence and has largely remained uninvolved in most recent European wars, although it was invaded by Napoleon during the Napoleonic Wars and was on the Allied side in World War I. Portugal maintained a large colonial empire, of which it divested itself in 1976. It had a population of 10,606,000 in 2006 and has 312 doctors and 379 nurses per 100,000 people. An example of cancer incidence rates in Portugal includes 285 cases of cancer in males per 100,000, according to the International Agency for Research on Cancer.

Portugal has one of the lowest rates of cancer in the world, with the result that many cancer specialists have studied the population. In spite of its large colonial possessions, Portugal was not a wealthy country until its acceptance as a member of the European Economic Community (now the European Union). Portugal had public and private hospitals throughout the country, as well as the *santas ca-sas da misericórdia* (charity hospitals) to help poor people. In Lisbon, the capital, there is a cancer hospital and a cancer research unit. The English prince, Edward (1330–76), known as the "Black Prince" and son of Edward III, fought in Portugal during this period. When he died, it was thought that he had been suffering from fever; it is now believed, however, that the Black Prince had a type of cancer. There is also another early connection between Portugal, England, and the diagnosis of cancer: A prominent surgeon who treated tumors in Elizabethan England was Roderigo Lopez Gallo, who was born in Crato, Portugal, in 1525. He studied at the University of Coimbra and then in Spain before going to England where he, as Dr. Lopez, ran a successful medical practice. In 1594, he was executed for high treason, and the character of Shylock in William Shakespeare's *The Merchant of Venice* is largely based on him, although heavily exaggerated.

Fernando Goncalves Namora (1919–89), the famous Portuguese writer and poet, was also trained at the University of Coimbra. He then established a medical practice in the Beira Baixa region of north-central Portugal, about which he wrote some of his early works of fiction. During the early 1960s, he moved to Lisbon to work at the Lisbon Cancer Institute, resigning in 1965 to take up writing full-time. In 1988, he received the Order of Henry the Navigator, Portugal's highest civilian award.

Professor Iberico Nogueira, also from Coimbra, researched the role of the Centre de Coimbra de l'Instituto Portugues de Oncologia Francisco Gentil in its dealing with gynecologic tumors and collaborated with Dr. D. Freire de Oliveira, who worked on benign and malignant lesions in the uterus.

In recent years, there have been studies performed in Portugal of the role of pesticides in the rise of the prevalence of cancer in the Oporto region, conducted by C. Costa, J. P. Teixeira, S. Silva, J. Roma-Torres, P. Coelho, J. Gaspar, M. Alves, B. Laffon, J. Rueff, and O. Mayan of the National Institute of Health, Center of Environmental and Occupational Health. There has also been another study into gastric cancer by N. Lunet, C. Valbuena, F. Carneiro, C. Lopes, and H. Barros of the Department of Hygiene and Epidemiology at the University of Porto Medical School.

Among the Portuguese citizens who have died from cancer are Vitor Damas (1947–2003), soccer goalkeeper; Antonio Dias Cardoso (1933–2006), Angolan nationalist; and José Maria Pedroto (1928–84), soccer player. Simone de Oliveira (1938–), a singer and actress, has experienced remission from breast cancer after seeking treatment.

The Instituto Português de Oncologia de Francisco Gentil and the Liga Portuguesa Contra o Cancro are members of the International Union Against Cancer. Research into cancer continues to be undertaken at the Faculties of Medicine at the Universidade de Coimbra, Universidade de Lisboa, and Universidade do Porto. The Terry Fox Run, raising money for cancer research, had their first marathon race in Portugal in 1994.

SEE ALSO: International Union Against Cancer

BIBLIOGRAPHY. C. Costa, J. P. Teixeira, S. Silva, et al., "Cytogenetic and Molecular Biomonitoring of a Portuguese Population Exposed to Pesticides," *Mutagenesis* (v.21/5, 2006); N. Lunet, C. Valbuena, F. Carneiro, C. Lopes, and H. Barros, "Antioxidant Vitamins and Risk of Gastric Cancer: A Case-Control Study in Portugal," *Nutrition and Cancer* (v.55/1, 2006); M. do Rosario Giraldes, "Health Projections in Portugal," in *Health Projections in Europe: Methods and Applications* (World Health Organization Regional Office for Europe, 1986); A. D'O. Maximiano, *História da medicina em Portugal* (M. Gomes, 1899).

JUSTIN CORFIELD
GEELONG GRAMMAR SCHOOL, AUSTRALIA

Poverty

IN 1991, THE Director of the National Cancer Institute proclaimed poverty to be a carcinogen (i.e., a cancer-causing agent). Population (epidemiologic) studies have identified associations between being poor, as well as living in a poor neighborhood, and the development of certain cancers.

PLAUSIBLE MECHANISMS

There are plausible reasons why cancer may bear a greater burden (in terms of cancer development or survival) among poorer populations. Individuals growing up in poor households may be less informed than those raised in richer households about behavioral risk factors for specific cancers including poor diets, lack of exercise, and smoking, and thus may be more likely to engage in these behaviors. Such behavioral patterns by levels of income have in fact been observed. For instance, in national surveys in the United States, 36.5 percent and 52.7 percent of men below the federal poverty line were current smokers and engaged in no leisure-time exercise, as compared to 22.6 percent and 44.8 percent of men at more than 200 percent above the poverty line, respectively.

Furthermore, poor individuals are more likely to live in poor neighborhoods, which may be stocked with fewer resources and amenities (e.g., large supermarkets, green spaces) that make it easier for healthy behaviors to be adopted. Poor individuals are less likely to have access to healthcare and cancer screening and to receive the same quality of healthcare and treatment as rich individuals. In addition, poor individuals are more likely to work in occupations that may expose them to potential carcinogens.

RISKS, SCREENING AND TREATMENT

There is some evidence that poorer individuals (versus richer individuals) are more likely to develop and die from certain cancers, including colorectal cancer and lung cancer. In one study, those with incomes less than $10,000 per year were 1.8 times and 1.2 times more likely to die from lung cancer and cancer at other sites combined than those with incomes $10,000 or more per year, respectively, after taking into account one's age and other personal factors including smoking and cholesterol. However, the direction of the association appears to be reversed for breast cancer. This association for breast cancer may in part be a result of poor women being more likely to have more children and to have them at a younger age (both protective factors against breast cancer), as compared to women with higher incomes.

Both women and men at the lower end of the income spectrum are less likely to receive cancer screening, including for colorectal cancer. Low-income women have been found to have lower rates of both Papanicolaou smear screening (for cervical cancer) and mammography screening (for breast cancer) in their respective recommended age groups for screening, as compared to higher-income women. These patterns are partly driven by the fact that poor individuals less likely to have health insurance in countries that lack national health insurance programs, such as the United States. Being uninsured can affect the level of cancer treatment received following diagnosis, as a result of the costs involved. Some evidence indicates that poor individuals are less likely than richer individuals to receive recommended treatments for cancer, including for colorectal cancer and breast cancer.

Between 2 and 5 percent of all cancer deaths in the United States are estimated to be related to occupational exposures. Key forms of occupationally related cancers include lung cancer (e.g., related to arsenic, asbestos, and radon exposures), bladder cancer (e.g., related to benzidine exposure), and mesothelioma (primarily caused by asbestos exposure). Poor individuals are more likely to be working in manual and industrial labor occupations that may expose them to such carcinogens.

NEIGHBORHOOD POVERTY AND CANCER RISKS

There is also growing evidence to support the notion that the lack of resources and amenities in poor neighborhoods may shape risk factors for cancer and contribute to the development of cancer, even after considering one's personal income and education.

For example, using data from national surveys, young and middle-aged adults living in federal poverty areas (based on U.S. Census data on the percentage of families with low income, substandard housing, children in single-headed households, unskilled males in the labor force, and adults with low educational attainment) were twice as likely to die from cancer at all sites combined after accounting for one's demographic and socioeconomic characteristics and behavioral risk factors. In a study of four urban communities in the United States, women in the poorest neighborhoods (based on median household income) were more likely to eat low intakes of vegetables, controlling for one's age, income, and total caloric intake.

Furthermore, screening behaviors may be influenced by living in a poor neighborhood. For instance, in a study of black women, those living in poor neighborhoods had 1.2 times higher odds of not obtaining a Papanicolaou smear within the previous 2 years, controlling for socioeconomic characteristics, smoking, and body mass index. Poverty both at the individual and neighborhood level appears to be an important risk factor for certain cancers. Future studies for the relationship

of poverty with particular cancers will help to better establish these associations. In so doing, healthcare workers and policy makers may more effectively address the health of poor individuals and poor neighborhoods and reduce the overall burden of cancer.

SEE ALSO: Breast Cancer; Cervical Cancer; Colon Cancer; Education, Cancer; Screening (Cervical and Breast and Colon Cancers).

BIBLIOGRAPHY. H. C. Bucher and D. R. Ragland, "Socioeconomic Indicators and Mortality from Coronary Heart Disease and Cancer: A 22-Year Follow-Up of Middle-Aged Men," *American Journal of Public Health* (v.85, 1995); A. V. Diez Roux, F. J. Nieto, L. Caulfield, et al., "Neighbourhood Differences in Diet: The Atherosclerosis Risk in Communities (ARIC) Study," *Journal of Epidemiological Community Health* (v.53, 1999); G. D. Datta, G. A. Colditz, I. Kawachi, et al., "Individual-, Neighborhood-, and State-Level Socioeconomic Predictors of Cervical Carcinoma Screening among US Black Women: A Multilevel Analysis," *Cancer* (v.106, 2006); B. G. Link, M. E. Northridge, J. C. Phelan, and M. L. Ganz, "Social Epidemiology and the Fundamental Cause Concept: On the Structuring of Effective Cancer Screens by Socioeconomic Status and Cancer Prevention," *Milbank Quarterly* (v.76, 2002); N. J. Waitzman and K. R. Smith, "Phantom of the Area: Poverty-Area Residence and Mortality in the United States," *American Journal of Public Health* (v.88, 1998); E. Ward, A. Jemal, V. Cokkinides, et al., "Cancer Disparities by Race/Ethnicity and Socioeconomic Status," *CA Cancer Journal for Clinicians* (v.54, 2004).

DANIEL KIM
HARVARD UNIVERSITY

Prevention, Health, and Exercise

THERE IS A growing body of evidence associating physical activity with a reduced risk of cancer and cancer progression. Current research has looked at the relation of physical activity and cancer prevention by examining the effects of exercise at specific cancer sites. The majority of studies looking at the association between physical activity and prevention of cancer have studied the colorectum, breast, prostate, lung, and ovary. Of these cancers, colorectal, breast, and prostate have the greatest amount of information regarding the effects of physical activity on cancer risk. Fewer studies have been conducted looking at this relationship with other cancer types.

COLORECTAL CANCER

Colorectal cancer is the second most common cancer in both men and women in the United States. This form of cancer affected almost 145,000 men and women and caused 56,000 deaths in 2005. Modifiable risk factors for colorectal cancer include smoking, heavy alcohol use, obesity, physical inactivity, and a diet involving high amounts of red meat and low amounts of fruits and vegetables. It is estimated that approximately 90 percent of all cases and deaths related to colorectal cancer are preventable. However, signs and symptoms associated with the disease are rarely seen, increasing the importance of medical screenings.

The majority of research studies show that physical activity has an inverse correlation with the risk of colorectal cancer in men. Unlike most cancers, high-intensity exercise training shows the most reduction in colorectal cancer risk. High-intensity exercise is defined as greater than 60 percent of a person's maximal oxygen consumption or maximal heart rate. However, women have shown inconsistent results pertaining to the association between physical activity and colorectal cancer. The risk reduction with physical activity normally ranges between 40 and 90 percent. A dose–response has also been shown between increasing levels of physical activity and decreasing incidence of colorectal cancer. Possible mechanisms for the inverse association between physical activity and colorectal cancer include reduced body fat and associated endocrine changes, decreased gut transit time, hyperinsulinemia (higher than normal insulin levels), change in prostaglandin ratio, lowered bile acid secretion, and altered gut flora (microorganisms living in the digestive tract that aid in digestion).

Physical activity has been associated with a decrease in obesity. Obesity, especially visceral (fat around organs) obesity, is associated with increased insulin resistance and lipid levels. Increases in lipids, along with the metabolic effects of insulin, can lead to an increase in intracellular energy substrates and growth factors, which may stimulate cell growth and increase the risk of cancer. A potential mechanism for the physical activity–related reduction in colorectal cancer is the decrease in insulin resistance, plasma insulin levels, lipid levels, and enhanced insulin sensitivity.

Physical activity also decreases gut transit time, the time it takes for substances to pass through the intestinal tract. The rapid transit reduces the contact time of colonic mucosa with carcinogens, like bile acid, giving a possible explanation for the protective effects of physical activity. The increased gut transit time is possible because of increased parasympathetic nervous system innervation and subsequent increased intestinal peristalsis. High levels of prostaglandin E2 (PG E2), a hormone-like substance that is released in response to infection or inflammation, are associated with increased risk of colorectal cancer through increased cell proliferation and decreased colonic motility. Physical activity has been shown to lower PGE2 levels, possibly through an exercise-induced lowering of insulin or insulin-like growth factor 1 (IGF-1).

Both insulin and IGF-1 receptors are located in colorectal tumor tissue, and elevated levels of these molecules have been associated with an increased risk of colorectal cancer. IGFs regulate cell differentiation, proliferation, and apoptosis, and their actions are important in the production of new tumors. The insulin–colon cancer relationship is based on the hypothesis that insulin resistance can induce colorectal cancer through the growth promoting effects of insulin, glucose, and triglycerides on colorectal cancer cells. Physical activity may help decrease the risk of colorectal cancer, in this case by increasing insulin sensitivity and decreasing plasma insulin levels.

Physical activity has been shown to enhance immune function and inflammatory response. Physical activity is thought to increase the number and activity of components of immune function (e.g., natural killer cells, neutrophils, macrophages, and regulating cytokines), thus increasing tumor cytolytic activity (tumor destruction). These increases are important because they enhance immunomodulation, a change in the body's immune system, allowing for the identification and destruction of cancerous cells before they have the chance to proliferate and metastasize. The proposed relationship between immune function and the intensity of physical activity is shown as an inverted J-shaped curve, with the lowest risk among people who engage in regular physical activity.

Physical activity has also been shown to modify prostaglandin metabolism; in particular, strenuous physical

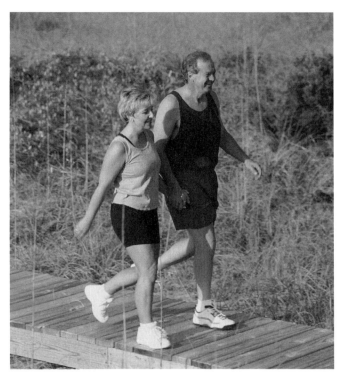

Physical activity is shown to have potential beneficial effects on reducing the risk of most cancer types.

activity increases levels of prostaglandin F2α, a cancer inhibitor, and decreases levels of prostaglandin E2, a known cancer promoter. These effects are particularly important for colorectal cancer, in which prostaglandins play a significant role in colonic cell proliferation.

BREAST CANCER

Breast cancer is the most commonly occurring cancer in women, excluding skin cancer. Breast cancer accounts for approximately one of every three women diagnosed with cancer in the United States. Incidence and death generally increase with age, as 95 percent of new cases, and 97 percent of breast cancer deaths, occur in women over the age of 40 years. Even though breast cancer primarily affects women, this disease also affects men, although males account for less than 1 percent of the total cases. The American Cancer Society lists the following as modifiable risk factors for breast cancer: postmenopausal obesity, use of post-menopausal hormones, alcohol consumption, and physical inactivity.

Physical activity has been shown to have a protective effect on the risk of breast cancer. This risk reduction averages to 30–40 percent for the most physically active women when compared with the least active women. As with most cancers, the exact duration, intensity, and frequency of physical activity needed to elicit a risk reduction or protective effect is not currently known. Most studies show an association of physical activity and decreased risk of breast cancer as the subject reaches moderate-intense levels of exercise. Moderate-intensity physical activity is defined as from 40 to 60 percent of a person's maximal oxygen consumption or maximal heart rate. However, a dose response is shown, with higher risk reductions associated with increasing physical activity intensities. Several potential mechanisms have been suggested to explain the relationship between physical activity and reduced breast cancer. These include decreased endogenous estrogens, decreased insulin and insulin-like growth factors, decreased obesity, increased weight control, alterations in menstrual cycle patterns, delayed age of menarche, and increased natural immune mechanisms.

Physical activity is associated with a decrease in time exposure to endogenous sex hormones. These hormones include estradiol, estrone, testosterone, and androgens. Increased levels of these hormones have been associated with an increased risk of breast cancer. Decreased time exposure to the hormones is accomplished by delaying the age of menarche and reducing the number of ovulatory cycles. Increased physical activity has been associated with decreased serum concentrations of estrone, estradiol, testosterone, and androgens.

Obesity has been linked to an increase in insulin resistance, increased levels of IGF factors, increased number of total life ovulatory cycles, increased levels of estrogens, increased levels of unbound estradiol, increased progesterone levels, and immunosuppression, each of which is a biomarker of increased risk for breast cancer. Obese women are shown to have a 35 percent increase in estrogen concentrations and a 130 percent increase in estradiol concentrations when compared with nonobese women. Further, obese postmenopausal women are at an increased risk of breast cancer when compared with premenopausal women. This increased risk is likely caused by an increased exposure to estrogen produced from increasing adipose or fat tissue, which is associated with aging and a decrease in physical activity. Physical activity lowers concentrations of fat-produced estrogens and may also decrease estrogens by increasing the production of sex hormone binding globulin (SHBG). Because physical activity increases the production of SHBG, it is associated with a decrease in estrogen and androgen bioavailability.

In addition to total obesity, body fat distribution seems to be just as important as the level of obesity. Visceral body fat is shown to be a significant risk factor of breast cancer through its association with increased insulin resistance, increased levels of unbound androgen and estrogen, and decreased levels of SHBG. Natural killer cells play an important role in the immune system by destroying both tumor and virally infected cells. Research has shown that high levels of estrogen decrease natural killer cell activity, a condition commonly seen with breast cancer. Physical activity can be beneficial by lowering levels of estrogen, helping to increase natural killer cell activity and immune function, thus reducing the risk developing breast cancer.

PROSTATE CANCER

Prostate cancer (PrCa) is the most common solid-tumor cancer diagnosed in men, accounting for 30 percent of all male cancer cases, and is the second leading cause of cancer mortality in the United States. Cases of PrCa are most pronounced between the ages of 45 and 74 years. One in 10 men will be diagnosed with PrCa in their lifetime. Further, men who die from PrCa live an average of 9 years fewer than men who do not. The majority of PrCa cases are seen in Western countries, where high caloric intake from an energy-dense diet and a sedentary lifestyle, which often leads to obesity, has been consistently linked as a risk factor for PrCa. Research has shown that physical activity has an inverse association with the risk of PrCa. The exact amount and intensity to cause a decreased risk is currently unknown. However, most studies show that PrCa risk is decreased beginning with moderate-intense physical activity. Some studies have even shown a dose–response relationship between increasing levels of physical activity and a decreasing incidence of PrCa.

The exact means by which exercise helps reduce the risk of PrCa is unknown, but several plausible mechanisms exist. These include changes in endogenous hormones, energy balance, and immune function. Physical activity may suppress dihydrotestosterone

(DHT) activity, which causes development of prostate cells and benign prostatic hypertrophy. DHT is also thought to promote the development of PrCa. Physically active men have lower levels of these hormones and are, hypothetically, at a decreased risk of PrCa.

Research indicates that regular physical activity could decrease the risk of cancer by changing the production of SHBG and circulating sex hormones and their bioavailability with aging. Research shows that exercise causes serum hormone and growth factor changes that include reductions in insulin, IGF-I, estradiol, and free testosterone, as well as increases in SHBG and IGF-binding protein I (IGFBP-I). These changes result in reduced growth and induced apoptosis (cell death) and are associated with increases of p53 and p21 proteins in the tumor cells. Protein p53 responds to DNA damage and activates other genes or factors to cause cell cycle arrest, DNA repair, or apoptosis in response to DNA damage. Protein p21 is a down stream effector of p53 and induces cell cycle. IGF-I is known to stimulate degradation of the p53 protein and inhibit apoptosis. Results also show that exercise helps stabilize p53 by reducing IGF-I and increasing IGFBP-I and activating p21, causing cell cycle arrest and inducing apoptosis in the prostate tumor cell.

Physical activity and its role in the enhancement of the immune system are similar to that of breast cancer. Research shows that physical activity lowers levels of biologically available sex hormones, such as testosterone, which is a steroid hormone from the androgen group. Increased levels of testosterone are linked with an increased risk of PrCa. Physical activity may decrease the production of androgens, such as testosterone. Physical activity also increases the amount of circulating SHBG, which binds to testosterone and other sex hormones, reducing testosterone's availability to influence tumor tissues or cause PrCa.

OVARIAN CANCER

Ovarian cancer is the sixth most common cancer among women and the seventh leading cause of death from cancer in women. Ovarian cancer is known as one of the estrogen-related cancers, which also includes cancers of the breast and endometrium (corpus uteri). Ovarian cancer is the leading cause of death among the estrogen-related cancers, with a 61 percent mortality rate worldwide. The much higher survival rate of those afflicted with breast cancer over ovarian and endometrial cancers is likely a result of the increased attention given to breast cancer in the recent past and of better adherence to procedures for early detection. Because ovarian cancer is less likely to be detected early, prevention is of utmost importance. It has been shown that reduced risk of ovarian cancer is strongly associated with parity and oral contraceptive use.

Physical activity has been demonstrated as a useful means of protection against certain types of cancers and has promising potential as a protective activity for ovarian cancer. Current and past research has shown that leisure-time, or recreational, physical activity is inversely associated with the occurrence of epithelial ovarian cancer. Although the exact frequency, intensity, duration, and mode of exercise needed to have an effect are not certain, the evidence appears to favor a high frequency of high-intensity activity (as defined by more than 60 percent of the maximum heart rate) as being the most beneficial. Lower frequencies of high-intensity and moderate-intensity activity may also positively affect ovarian cancer risk. It is also possible that different levels of physical activity may be required to affect ovarian cancer risk for women of different menopausal status. Higher-intensity activity may be more beneficial for premenopausal women, and postmenopausal women may obtain more risk protection from moderate-intensity activity.

Similarities in the biological mechanisms of reduced risk exist for the mechanisms of physical activity and for those of parity and oral contraceptive use. Both parity and the use of oral contraceptives decrease the absolute number of menstrual cycles. In a similar fashion, physical activity decreases the number of lifetime ovulatory cycles; evidently, physical activity delays menarche, and in a few cases it is known to cause amenorrhea and anovulatory cycles. Ovarian cancer is possibly caused by follicular rupture over repeated ovulatory cycles; thus, if physical activity reduces ovulation frequency—as does parity and oral contraceptive use—then it is reasonable to expect physical activity to reduce ovarian cancer risk.

Participation in regular physical activity may improve body composition. Being overweight or obese alters the function of several hormones in the body—and estrogen in particular. Physical activity is known to decrease the concentration of estrogen; in addition, physical activity targets excess visceral fat (i.e., the fat stores surrounding internal organs) in a preferential manner. This type of fat has been implicated as being the most detrimental to health. Because ovarian cancer is an estrogen-dependent cancer, it is likely that any effect of physical activity on body composition would affect overall risk for developing ovarian cancer.

LUNG CANCER

Lung cancer is currently the most common and the most deadly cancer worldwide; out of 1.35 million cases reported, 1.10 million, or 87 percent, were fatal. Because of the highly deadly nature of lung cancers, primary prevention is of utmost importance. Although 80–90 percent of lung cancer cases are attributable to cigarette smoking, many smokers do not develop lung cancer, even with prolonged use. Therefore, researchers are investigating the effects of other environmental and biological agents that may factor significantly into the etiology of lung cancer.

Several studies have explored the relationship between lung cancer and physical activity. One study surveyed a large group of Harvard University alumni for health history, using health questionnaires sent in 1962 and 1966, participation in physical activity with a questionnaire in 1977, and incidence of lung cancer with questionnaires in 1988 and 1993. The investigators concluded that participation in activities of at least moderate intensity is inversely associated with lung cancer risk. Similar trends in the study were apparent for nonsmokers and those who smoked fewer than 20 cigarettes per day.

A study conducted in Norway followed a large cohort of both men and women across a similar time period (1972–91). In this study, men who exercised at least 4 hours a week showed a decrease in lung cancer risk. The decrease in risk was more strongly associated with types of lung cancer common to the deeper periphery of the lung—small-cell carcinomas and adenocarcinomas. Although the physically active men in this study showed this decreased risk, the same association was not seen among the women. Another study substantiates the histological data, demonstrating a decrease in risk of small-cell carcinoma in men; in this study, however, there was a decrease of lung cancer risk in physically active women as well as men.

Although some studies have shown a decrease in risk, others have indicated no risk association at all or an increase in risk with occupational physical activity. The researchers, however, postulated that the increase in risk associated with occupational physical activity indicated that exposure to environmental risk factors was at work, and not a negative effect of physical activity itself. Approximately half of the studies available indicate that an inverse association is present, although there is a relative dearth of information concerning lung cancer specifically as compared to the wealth of literature concerning breast or colon cancer.

There are several plausible biological mechanisms for a relationship between physical activity and lung cancer risk. These include, first, enhanced pulmonary function defined by greater ventilation and perfusion. Increasing these two variables may reduce the amount of time potential carcinogenic agents have to interact with cells in the airways and also potentially reduce the concentration of those agents. This particular mechanism, however, may be more important when considering small-cell carcinomas and adenocarcinomas, because these are located more peripherally in the lung tissue and particle deposition is favored in the larger airways.

The second mechanism for a relationship between physical activity and lung cancer risk is reduced oxidative stress via reduced production of free radicals, as well as increased activity of free radical scavenger enzymes, such as the glutathione system. The final mechanism is altered levels of IGF and IGFBP, which are associated with many site-specific cancers, including lung cancer. High levels of IGF-1 increase the risk of lung cancer, and high levels of IGFBP-3—proteins that reduce the bioavailability of IGF-1 and thus inhibit the growth of non-small-cell carcinomas—are associated with decreased risk.

A significant component of the immune system present in the lungs is that of resident macrophages in and around individual alveoli. If physical activity enhances the function of macrophages systemwide, then it is likely that this is a mechanism for any protective effect of physical activity on lung cancer risk. Furthermore, physical activity has been shown to most strongly reduce risk for cancers present in the periphery of the lung tissue; alveoli, along with their macrophages, make up the peripheral lung tissue.

Physical activity is shown to have potential beneficial effects on reducing the risk of most cancer types. However, the relationship between the biological mechanisms of cancer and physical activity is still poorly understood. Therefore, further research is needed to determine the relationship between physical activity and the risk of developing cancer.

SEE ALSO: Exercise (Lack of); Obesity.

BIBLIOGRAPHY. J. Kruk and H. Y. Aboul-Enein, "Physical Activity and the Prevention of Cancer," *Asian Pacific Journal of Cancer Prevention* (v.7, 2006); A. McTiernan, C. Ulrich, S. Slate, and J. Potter, "Physical Activity and Cancer Etiology: Associations and Mechanisms," *Cancer Causes and Control* (v.9, 1998); C. M. Friedenreich and M. R. Orenstein, "Physical Activity and Cancer Prevention: Etiologic Evidence and Biological Mechanisms," *Journal of Nutrition* (v.132, 2002); J. L. Durstine and G. E. Moore, *ACSM's Exercise Management for Persons with Chronic Disease and Disabilities* (2nd ed.) (Human Kinetics, 2002); C. M. Schneider, C. A. Dennehy, and S. D. Carter, *Exercise and Cancer Recovery* (Human Kinetics, 2003); A. McTiernan, *Cancer Prevention and Management through Exercise and Weight Control*, (CRC Press, 2006).

G. William Lyerly
Jonathan A. Moore
Gregory A. Hand
University of South Carolina

Prostate Cancer

PROSTATE CANCER IS the most frequently diagnosed cancer and also the second leading cause of cancer-related deaths in American men, with an estimated 218,890 cases and 27,050 deaths expected in 2007. The only known risk factors for prostate cancer are age, family history, and ethnicity. The occurrence of prostate cancer increases in men with age of 45 years and above and with a family history of prostate cancer in first-degree relatives. In the United States, prostate cancer is more common in African-American men than in whites or any other ethnic population. The most common form of prostate cancer is adenocarcinoma, which arises from the prostate secretory epithelium. The choice and the response to cancer therapy depend on the site and the anatomical event of the tumor.

The development of hormone-dependent prostate cancer (HDPC) is associated with the epithelium's response to androgen signaling. The testis produces testosterone, which is converted to dihydrotestosterone in the prostate, and this substance binds to the androgen receptors and is further metabolized to 3α-androstanediol glucuronide. A study has found a correlation between reduced serum 3α-androstanediol glucuronide levels and low rates of prostate cancer in Japanese men. The second group of hormone-resistant prostate cancers (HRPC) arise from neuroendocrine elements within the prostate and produce neuropeptides or NE factors.

SCREENING AND DIAGNOSIS

Early asymptomatic prostate cancers are detected by digital rectal exam (DRE) and prostate-specific antigen (PSA). PSA, a protease secreted by the prostate for aiding fertilization, increases in prostate cancer from a normal level of 4 ng/ml to 10 ng/ml or higher. The American Cancer Society recommends annual prostate cancer screening for men at age 50 years and above who have at least a 10-year life expectancy. Men at high risk, such as African Americans and those with a strong family history, should be screened from age 45 years onward.

A prostate biopsy may be carried out under the guidance of a transrectal ultrasonography or by fine-needle aspiration. The Gleason score is the sum of two most common scores that grade the specimen's histopathological appearance and predict the behavior and the aggressiveness of the disease on a scale from 1 to 5, where 5 indicates worst prognosis. The tumor-node-metastasis system decides the tumor stage on the gross appearance and the tumor invasiveness, detected by imaging techniques such as magnetic resonance imaging.

TREATMENT AND RESEARCH

Treatment options depend on factors such as age, tumor grade, and stage. Young or slow-growing tumors may be monitored every 6 months for growth by screening tests, or the surgical option of radical prostatectomy, which is the excision of the tumor and parts of the surrounding tissue, may be used. Advanced diseases (including bone metastasis) require therapies involving X-rays or external beam radiation and brachytherapy, in which radioactive pellets are seeded into the tumor. HDPC respond to androgen-deprivation therapy almost always (90 percent), whereas chemotherapy (e.g., docetaxel, estramustine) is effective in HRPC. Minimal invasive therapies employ different energy sources such as cryotherapy and high-intensity focused ultrasound to target focal lesions in older patients or in cases of relapse. The treatment can result in side effects such as urinary incontinence or increased frequency, diarrhea, impotence, and infertility. Survival rates are better for low-grade tumors, but the relativity of survival and recurrence depends on the age, grade, and stage to begin with. HRPC and relapses have a far graver prognosis than HDPC.

Various studies have assessed the role of selenium and vitamins A, C, D, and E in prostate carcinogenesis. Gene *HPC1* has a possible role in hereditary prostate cancers. Genetic studies involving oncogenes, tumor suppressor genes, and growth factors that are implicated in tumor development and different therapeutic options such as gene therapy, antiangiogenetic agents, and immunotherapeutics are also being investigated.

SEE ALSO: Alternative Therapy: Herbs; Chemotherapy; National Cancer Institute; Radiation Therapy.

BIBLIOGRAPHY. American Urological Association Education and Research, *Prostate Cancer Topics*, www.urology-health.org (cited 2002).

Sheetal Bajaj, M.D.
University of Southern California

Proton Therapy

PROTONS ARE AN example of particle radiotherapy and are produced by a cyclotron or synchrotron. Proton beam therapy has become of interest because of its ability to accurately target and kill tumors that are either near the surface or deep seated within the body. Unlike more conventional radiotherapy treatment techniques, which employ the use external beams of electrons or X-rays, proton beam therapy offers the potential for providing an improved distribution of radiation dose such that normal, healthy tissue surrounding a tumor is spared, thereby reducing collateral side effects from radiotherapy.

Protons were first proposed to have a role in the treatment of human malignancies in 1946 by Robert

Rathbun Wilson, Ph.D., while working at the Harvard cyclotron laboratory. Soon after, the use of proton beam radiotherapy for cancer treatment was pursued at select centers in the United States, Russia, and Sweden.

The first treatments were for patients with pituitary disorders and were performed in the mid-1950s by a cyclotron built for physics research at the Berkeley Radiation laboratory. The use of protons to treat the pituitary was of particular interest because the well-defined beam of a proton made it possible to deliver a large dose to the pituitary without causing excessive damage to nearby structures in the central nervous system.

After the initial success of this treatment, similar endeavors were undertaken at the Massachusetts General Hospital by a neurosurgeon by the name of Dr. Ray Kjellberg in the 1960s. Dr. Kjellberg began treating small intracranial targets with radiosurgical techniques at the Harvard cyclotron laboratory. Together with the physics group at the Harvard cyclotron laboratory, Dr. Kjellberg was able to develop instrumentation, methodology, and techniques for radiosurgical beam delivery, using protons. The treatments by Kjellberg have evolved into an active proton therapy program at the Massachusetts General Hospital, now known as the Northeast Proton Therapy Center, which is still active today.

In the 1960s and 1970s, while work continued at Harvard and Berkeley cyclotron facilities, further research in proton therapy was undertaken at several different physics research facilities around the world, most notably in Russia. Most of the work in Russia was done at the Joint Institute Nuclear Research and the Moscow Institute for Theoretical and Experimental Physics and in St. Petersburg. Soon after, treatment with proton beams was also begun at the National Institute for Radiobiological Sciences in Chiba, Japan, which is where a spot-scanning system for proton therapy was first developed.

The work from such institutions and others around the world has laid the foundation for proton radiation treatment as it is delivered today at active hospital centers. The first hospital-based proton therapy program in the United States was built in Loma Linda, California, in the 1980s. The first patient was treated at the Loma Linda Medical Center in October 1990. Since the inception of the center, nearly 12,000 patients have been treated at the Loma Linda cancer center. Worldwide, almost 45,000 patients have been treated with proton beam radiotherapy since its first use at the Berkeley Radiation laboratory.

Today, there are six active proton therapy centers across the United States. In addition to the Loma Linda cancer center, proton therapy treatment is carried out at the Northeast Proton Therapy Center at Massachusetts General Hospital, which was recently renamed the Francis H. Burr Proton Therapy Center. Treatment is also available in Sacramento at the University of California, Davis, Proton Facility, a facility that is dedicated to proton therapy for ocular tumors, and at the Midwest Proton Radiotherapy Institute at Indiana University. Most recently, two new proton treatment facilities were started in Houston, Texas, at the University of Texas M.D. Anderson Cancer and at the University of Florida Proton Therapy Institute in Jacksonville, Florida.

HOW IT WORKS

Protons are hydrogen atoms whose electrons have been removed. Proton beams used in radiation therapy are produced by a cyclotron, which accelerates protons to nearly the speed of light. Protons are extracted from the cyclotron and directed with magnetic fields toward a target, usually a tumor. Like conventional forms of radiotherapy, proton beam therapy works by aiming an energetic particle, in this a case, a proton, onto a target, which is usually a tumor. These charged protons induce DNA damage and ultimately lead to the cell's death. Cancer cells are particularly sensitive to this type of attack on their DNA because of their high rate of cell division coupled with their diminished ability to repair any damaged DNA.

The physical properties of proton beams are much different from those of the X-ray beams used in conventional forms of radiotherapy. Protons are large particles that possess a positive charge that penetrate matter to a fixed depth, which varies depending on the energy of the beam. X-rays, in contrast, are electromagnetic rays that possess no charge or mass and that penetrate completely through tissue. Despite the differences between the physical properties of proton and X-ray beams, the radiobiological properties of the two are indistinguishable from each other. For instance, the relative biological effect, a standard measure used to compare the biologic effects of various radiation sources, of X-rays is 1; it is only 1.1 for protons, meaning that the biological effects of the two are nearly identical.

However, the dose distribution of protons is significantly different, which makes protons an attractive alternative for use in modern radiation therapy. When a fast, charged particle such as a proton moves through matter, it ionizes particles and deposits a dose along its path. As the charged particle's energy decreases, the interaction cross section increases, resulting in a peak. This peak correlates with the depth at which maximum dose is delivered and is referred to as the Bragg Peak.

With the use of protons, the dose deposited by a beam of monoenergetic protons increases slowly with depth until it reaches a sharp maximum, near the end of the particle's range in the Bragg Peak. The depth of the Bragg Peak varies with the energy of the proton beam. As the energy of the proton beam increases, so does the depth of the Bragg Peak.

Unlike the beam with X-rays or electrons, however, a proton beam has sharp edges that produce little scatter. Moreover, the dose delivered by a proton beam immediately falls to zero after the Bragg Peak. In other words, the entrance dose of a proton beam is relatively low, meaning that little energy is lost as protons enter the body. However, as the beam penetrates deeper into the tissue, there is a sharp rise in dose deposited at the depth that correlates with the beam's Bragg Peak. This is followed by a sudden end

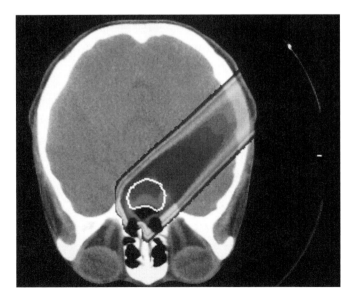

Proton beam therapy has the ability to accurately target and kill tumors that are near the surface or deep seated within the body.

in dose deposition; this is the point where the beam stops. Thus, no tissue is irradiated beyond the Bragg Peak. This property can be exploited to maximize the dose delivered to a particular depth of tissue while minimizing any dose delivered to tissue beyond that depth, thereby decreasing any unwanted irradiation to normal, healthy tissue surrounding a tumor.

To make proton beams clinically useful, the Bragg peak needs to be spread out such that the entire width of a tumor can be targeted. This is accomplished through the use of a modulator, which is a special wheel placed in the beam to spread out the Bragg Peak of the beam to fit the entire width of the desired target.

INDICATIONS

Proton beam therapy is useful in treating a variety of cancers. The ideal tumor for treatment with proton radiotherapy should be one that is localized, requires high doses of radiation for control, and is located near sensitive normal tissues. Various studies have been performed to investigate the potential of proton beam therapy in the treatment of pediatric tumors, head-and-neck tumors, prostate cancer, lung cancer, gastrointestinal tumors, and ocular cancer.

One area in which proton beam radiotherapy has been of particular interest is in the treatment of choroidal malignant melanomas. This is a type of eye cancer for which the only known treatment, before radiation therapy, was enucleation, or complete removal of the eye. Recent studies have established that proton radiotherapy provides similar long-term survival rates as enucleation in the treatment of small choroidal melanomas. Most recently, researchers have also shown that proton irradiation is also effective in the treatment of medium-sized choroidal melanomas, which are traditionally treated by enucleation. Local tumor control, rate of metastases, and survival rates with proton radiotherapy are comparable when seen with enucleation. Thus, proton radiotherapy provides an effective method of treating choroidal melanomas without severely compromising the function of the eye or visual acuity or causing unwanted cosmetic side effects that are typically seen after enucleation.

Proton radiotherapy has also been shown to have a beneficial effect in the treatment of several pediatric tumors. For example, tumors that arise at the base of the skull in children have traditionally been a considerable challenge for the treating radiation oncologist. Radiation treatment, traditionally performed with photons, aimed at tumors in this location has a great risk of damaging surrounding structures such as cranial nerves, arteries, brain parenchyma, and brainstem. Sequelae from photon radiation therapy to this region include intellectual and sociobehavioral deficits after treatment, as well as cosmetic defects as a result of impaired development of facial structures following irradiation. In recent studies, proton radiotherapy has been shown to provide an effective and safe alternative to photon radiation in the treatment of these tumors because of its ability to deliver higher radiation doses to these radioresistant tumors while also decreasing the sequelae from treatment. Thus, although further clinical trials need to be done, proton radiation therapy can offer children with aggressive, recurrent, or unresectable skull base tumors the prospect of lasting tumor control and survival without significantly impairing the function of the surrounding central nervous system. Other pediatric tumors that may benefit from proton radiotherapy include medulloblastomas, astrocytomas, ependymomas, optic gliomas, rhabdomyosarcomas, sarcomas, optic gliomas, and primitive neuroectodermal tumors.

Proton therapy may also provide an effective means of treating prostate cancer, the most common noncutaneous skin cancer afflicting men in the United States. Traditional treatment modalities for prostate cancer include external beam radiotherapy, prostate brachytherapy, or radical prostatectomy. All of these treatment modalities have been shown to be excellent methods for achieving high survival rates and biochemical disease control. With all of the current advances in prostate cancer treatment, a man diagnosed with prostate cancer today will most likely die with—rather than of—prostate cancer. However, unwanted side effects from traditional radiation treatment can severely decrease a patient's quality of life. For example, following prostate irradiation patients may become impotent or develop multiple urinary or rectal problems given the close proximity of the prostate to the bladder and rectum. For this reason, proton therapy provides a possible alternative for delivering an effective dose to the prostate while also avoiding any radiation-induced damage to the surrounding bladder and rectum. Recent data from studies done at Loma Linda have

supported the potential role of proton therapy in the treatment of early prostate cancer.

Proton radiotherapy also has the potential for use in the treatment of various head and neck tumors. Similar to prostate cancer, the treatment of head and neck tumors with traditional radiotherapy is effective and provides promising survival rates. However, side effects from head and neck irradiation include dry mouth, sore throat, difficulty swallowing, and loss of taste. The dry mouth, also known as xerostomia, can be permanent in some cases. Many other structures may also be damaged by radiotherapy to the head and neck, such as the jawbone, eyes, and spinal cord. In the future, proton radiotherapy may be used, alone or in combination with traditional radiation therapy, to further reduce the dose received by normal tissues. Proton radiotherapy may be particularly useful for treating cancers arising in the nasopharynx, nasal cavity, and paranasal sinuses. Proton therapy may also be used to treat moderate to advanced oropharyngeal malignancies. Thus, proton radiotherapy may play an important part in the treatment of head and neck cancer in the future. However, the exact role of proton therapy in head and neck cancers remains to be evaluated in a clinical trial.

FUTURE OF PROTON THERAPY

Proton radiotherapy, either alone or in combination with conventional radiation therapy, will likely play an increasing role in the treatment of various malignancies. It is important to note that proton therapy is still considerably more expensive than conventional radiotherapy. In the long run, overall treatment costs with proton therapy may, however, diminish because the incidence of short- and long-term side effects will potentially be lower. Nationwide, widespread usage of proton beam therapy has been hindered by the high cost associated with this type of treatment. The equipment needed to generate a proton beam and the facilities necessary to house the equipment are quite expensive. The price to equip a facility with the equipment needed to generate a proton beam can range from US$40–100 million by itself.

A group of physicists, clinicians, and accelerator physicists have now formed an organization called the Particle Therapy Cooperative Group. Members of this organization meet twice a year and have a strong influence in the development of proton therapy. Recently, several sessions at Particle Therapy Cooperative Group meetings have been devoted to discussions of clinical protocols involving the use of proton beam therapy. Before proton beam radiation can become a mainstay therapy for certain types of cancer, the effectiveness of proton therapy must be first determined through various clinical trials. In the meantime, some radiation physicists are already looking past protons and into possibility of using antiprotons for radiation therapy. Data examining the biological effectiveness of these particles are preliminary at this point but have suggested that the role antiprotons play warrants further investigation.

SEE ALSO: Brain Tumor, Ependymoma, Childhood; Brain Tumor, Medulloblastoma, Childhood; Prostate Cancer; Radiation Therapy; Radiation, Gamma; Radiation, Ionizing.

BIBLIOGRAPHY. Martin Fuss, Lilia N. Loredo, Paul A. Blacharski, Roger I. Grove, and Jerry D. Slater, "Proton Radiation Therapy for Medium and Large Choroidal Melanoma: Preservation of the Eye and Its Functionality," *International Journal of Radiation Oncology Biology Physics* (v.49, 2001); Eric J. Hall and Amato J. Giaccia, *Radiobiology for the Radiologist* (6th ed.) (Lippincott Williams & Wilkins, 2006); William R. Hendee, Geoffrey S. Ibbott, and Eric G. Hendee, *Radiation Therapy Physics* (3rd ed.) (Wiley-Liss, 2005); M. Holzscheiter, N. Bassler, N. Agazaryan, et al., "The Biological Effectiveness of Antiproton Irradiation," *Radiotherapy and Oncology* (v.81, 2006); Eugen B. Hug, Reinhart A. Sweeney, Pamela M. Nurre, et al., "Proton Radiotherapy in Management of Pediatric Base of Skull Tumors," *International Journal of Radiation Oncology Biology Physics* (v.52, 2002); Bengt Johansson, Mona Ridderheim, and Bengt Glimelius, "The Potential of Proton Beam Radiation Therapy in Prostate Cancer, Other Urological Cancers and Gynaecological Cancers," *Acta Oncologica* (v.44, 2005); Alfred R. Smith, "Proton Therapy," *Physics in Medicine and Biology* (v.51, 2006).

MARK VIKAS MISHRA
NATIONAL CANCER INSTITUTE

Psychosocial Issues and Cancer

THE EXPERIENCE OF cancer, like many medical conditions, is not limited to the physical aspects of the illness. The physical sequelae of symptoms, treatments, and side effects associated with cancer can potentially pervade emotional, social, occupational, and recreational functioning, and ultimately impact the quality of life of patients and their loved ones. Patients must learn to cope with a host of life changes that are often dramatic and overwhelming, including changes to their body and physical functioning, roles, relationships, and overall lifestyle, all within the context of a looming potential threat to their life. Psychosocial issues can emerge at any point in the cancer experience, including diagnosis, treatment, end of life, and survivorship. In recent years, there has been increased recognition of the importance of providing comprehensive cancer care that addresses not only the medical, but also the psychosocial issues associated with cancer. Knowledge of the psychosocial impact of cancer can benefit patients, family members, and cancer treatment providers by increasing understanding of the potential issues that may arise and the need for referral for interventions that can help patients cope effectively with these issues.

EMOTIONAL DISTRESS

Cancer and its treatment can effect a heavy impact on emotional well-being. Although cancer is now more openly acknowledged and discussed than in the past, when it was commonly referred to in whispered and veiled tones (i.e., as "The 'C' word"), its reputation of being linked to suffering, disability, and death remains. Not surprisingly, a diagnosis of cancer is often received with great distress. This is compounded by the fact that there can be minimal, vague, or lack of symptoms leading up to diagnosis, rendering the news of a cancer diagnosis an unexpected shock. Although emotional distress in response to the diagnosis and treatment of cancer is to some degree expected, it is important to not simply dismiss emotional reactions as "normal," because many cancer patients do in fact meet diagnostic criteria for clinical disorders. Therefore, it is crucial to accurately assess and diagnose psychiatric disorders among patients with cancer, particularly because these can complicate treatment adherence and outcomes.

The multiple stressors associated with cancer can lead to the development or exacerbation of existing depression. Prevalence rates of depression spectrum syndromes vary widely, but it is estimated that up to one half of adults and one quarter of children/adolescents are affected. Physiological causes of cancer-related depression may include increased pain and the direct effects of treatments such as chemotherapy, radiation, and specific medications (e.g., steroids). Psychosocial contributions may include prior history of depression, poor coping skills, and social isolation. The themes underlying depression in cancer patients may revolve around issues of sadness, loss, and decreased self-esteem related to changes in/loss of control over health, physical appearance (i.e., disfigurement), physical functioning, and role functioning (i.e., work and relationships). Hopelessness about the future can be significant for patients who are confronting an uncertain medical course, as well as for patients with terminal disease, who face additional grief associated with anticipation of and preparation for the end of life. Suicidal ideation may emerge around desires to end physical and emotional suffering and control the time of death, and should be monitored carefully.

In addition to depression, the experience of cancer can trigger multiple anxieties, encompassing practical (e.g., maintaining work and household responsibilities while feeling ill and juggling medical appointments), medical (e.g., fears of needles and painful treatments), and existential (e.g., uncertainties about health status and survival) concerns. Anxiety might be particularly expected around the time of diagnosis, and may increase as patients anticipate treatments and think about the future course of their illness. As with depression, some patients might develop new diagnoses of anxiety disorders, whereas others might experience an exacerbation of pre-existing anxiety disorders in reaction to the specific threats of cancer and its treatments.

Prevalence rates for anxiety disorders in cancer populations have ranged as high as 77 percent. Fears can be focused on very specific issues, such as cancer-related procedures (e.g., needle aspirations, MRI tests) and treatments (e.g., chemotherapy, radiation, surgery), or can be more generalized in nature (e.g., posttraumatic stress). Many patients experience emotional distress around medical visits, anniversaries related to their diagnosis or treatment, and even when going off treatment (for fear that there will now be nothing to protect them from cancer). As with depression, causes of cancer-related anxiety can be due to physiological factors such as pain and medical treatments, as well as psychosocial risk factors such as coping styles and belief systems.

SOCIAL FUNCTIONING

In addition to aforementioned emotional issues, cancer can also significantly impact patients social functioning in a number of domains. First, patients might not be able to maintain their usual social roles and activities, due to feeling ill from the disease itself and treatment-related side-effects, or from lack of time due to numerous medical appointments. They might not be able to engage in their regular recreational activities (which often involve others). It might be a challenge just to keep up with usual conversations and social pursuits, such as spending time with family and friends. Cancer can present a number of challenges for patients who are single and interested in dating, including how and when to tell a prospective partner about their diagnosis and how to manage shame and fear of rejection around physical disfigurement/dysfunction.

Caregiver stress and burnout is another phenomenon that affects many families in which a member has cancer. As a result of chronic psychological, social and physical demands of caring for a loved one with cancer, family members of cancer patients may experience anxiety, depression, interpersonal and work-related disruption, physical symptoms, and financial stress. On the other hand, care giving may also provide positive rewards such as enriched purpose or meaning in life and improved self-esteem. Another important variable related to patients' social life is social support. Some members of patients' social networks will rally to help, while others might distance themselves, perhaps out of fear, or lack of knowledge of how best to respond.

EXISTENTIAL/SPIRITUAL THEMES

Among the most pervasive of the psychosocial issues associated with cancer are the existential and spiritual concerns that may arise throughout the course of the illness. Initially, patients might grapple with the shock of a cancer diagnosis as they attempt to come to terms with this potential threat to their very existence. Questions such as "Why me?" and "Why is there suffering?" and associated themes of punishment/guilt can present as tests of faith, which may ultimately result in crises of faith as people question long-held religious beliefs. Alternatively, patients may turn to spirituality or religion to help them cope with these existential challenges. A continual existential challenge that can occur includes maintaining one's identity in the face of a new role as a "cancer patient." As time goes on, and patients try to integrate the illness into their life, they may focus on how to find meaning and purpose in their illness.

Recent research and clinical interest in the increased psychological growth that can result after cancer illustrates growing attention to such existential issues. Existential and spiritual issues can be particularly salient for patients with terminal cancer, who may reflect upon on how they have lived their life (i.e., "life review") and want to take care of "unfinished business," and face questions such as what happens after death. Existential/spiritual themes may also be prominent for those who survive cancer. Patients often face the challenge of rebuilding their lives which have been disrupted by cancer. Although some may approach this with new energy of wanting to "re-invent themselves" stemming from a feeling of receiving "a new lease on life," the practical realities of life after cancer can be daunting, including needing to re-establish life goals, including those in occupational, financial, personal, and relationship areas.

Perhaps the most significant existential issue for cancer survivors is how to focus on living as the threat of cancer recurrence looms, commonly referred to as the Damocles Syndrome. In addition, as a result of advances in treatments that have now rendered cancer as more of a chronic than acute disease, many people now live with a disease that is associated with a constant and unpredictable threat to stability of health and quality of life.

OVERALL QUALITY OF LIFE (QOL)

In addition to the specific psychosocial issues that can result from a cancer diagnosis, the cumulative psychosocial effects of cancer are often referred to in terms of an overall impact on patients' quality of life (QOL). Even in the absence of clinical levels of emotional distress or impairment in social functioning, many patients report significant decrements in their overall quality of life as a result of cancer. Physically, patients might experience a range of side effects and long-term physical disability due to cancer treatments. In particular, pain and fatigue, commonly reported by patients, can hamper overall ability to engage in typical tasks and can disrupt QOL long after treatment has ended. In addition, patients might experience treatment-related early menopause and sexual difficulties, which can significantly diminish physical, emotional, and social quality of life. Im-paired cognitive functioning due to cancer treatment can also significantly alter their quality of life. Patients with cancer have reported problems with attention, concentration, and memory; for some, these issues reportedly can last for years after completion of treatment. Such cognitive deficits can interfere with occupational, social, and general daily functioning. Social quality of life, as alluded to above, can also receive a significant blow due to cancer.

The severe disruption in patients' daily routines due to numerous medical appointments and loss of physical strength, can affect their social relationships, and impact longer-term goals and plans. Finally, these effects on quality of life can ultimately take their toll on patients' emotional quality of life, particularly when they serve not only as consequences of cancer, but also as additional stressors. For example, the cognitive impairments experienced can trigger frustration and worry and present as obstacles to daily functioning, and the loss of important social activities may be associated with decreased enjoyment that is usually gained from social contact.

In sum, patients with cancer must simultaneously contend with a host of physical and psychosocial issues while coping with cancer. The psychosocial adjustment trajectory can be as variable as the disease itself. Comprehensive cancer care will ideally include attention to both the physical and psychosocial issues, with the ultimate goal of improving the functioning of patients with cancer and helping them cope effectively with the challenges of cancer.

SEE ALSO: Survivors of Cancer; Survivors of Cancer Families; Sex and Cancer; Pain and Pain Management; Daily Life.

BIBLIOGRAPHY. Jimmie C. Holland, Psycho-oncology (Oxford, 1998); Annette L. Stanton "Psychosocial Concerns and Interventions for Cancer Survivors", *Journal of Clinical Oncology* (v.24/32, November 2006). Michael Stefanek, Paige McDonald, & Stephanie Hess "Religion, Spirituality and Cancer: Current Status and Methodological Challenges", *Psycho-Oncology* (v.14/6, June 2005).

MELANIE S. HARRIS, PH.D.
TOURO COLLEGE: LANDER COLLEGE FOR WOMEN
ALYSON B. MOADEL, PH.D.
ALBERT EINSTEIN COLLEGE OF MEDICINE

Purdue Cancer Center

BASIC CANCER RESEARCH centers are dedicated to the research of cancer and of its causes, preventions, and cures. These centers do not provide clinical care but, rather, focus all their efforts onto investigations into cancer. The Purdue Cancer Center (PCC) at Purdue University in West Lafayette, Indiana, is a basic cancer research center, as designated by the National Cancer Institute (NCI).

The PCC has a slogan of being "committed to helping cancer patients by identifying new molecular targets and designing future agents and drugs for effectively detecting and treating cancer." It was established in 1978 to address this commitment via the collaboration of research in engineering, chemistry, and biology. The PCC's goals are "to prevent cancer, to ease its detection, and to cure it."

Purdue University was founded in 1869. Benefactor John Purdue gave his name to the new institution. The initial mission of the university was to provide an education in agriculture and mechanic arts. The main campus is at West Lafayette, where the PCC is located; in addition, there are four other campuses.

Ideas for the formation of the PCC began after the U.S. government established the NCI in an initiative against cancer, the second-leading cause of death at the time. Thus, in the early 1970s, members of the Purdue University scientific faculty began to hold monthly meetings. They called themselves the Cancer Discussion Group and held seminars and workshops to highlight their research on cancer. In 1975, their efforts were formalized into the University Cancer Research Committee, aided by a 2-year grant from the NCI. Separately, the PCC was opened in 1976. Two years later, the PCC received its first NCI Cancer Center Support Grant. This grant has stayed with the PCC ever since.

Funding from the NCI as well as from Purdue University sponsored the construction of the Hansen Life Sciences Research Building, four floors of which are dedicated to the PCC. Researchers at the PCC strive to reach the challenge goal of the NCI, which is to end the suffering and death from cancer by the year 2015.

The PCC is managed by an Executive Committee, which holds monthly meetings. Members of the committee are the PCC director, the Oncological Sciences Center director, three other scientific program leaders, and a veterinary oncology representative. There is also a Director's Advisory Board, which meets annually to advise the PCC, as well as to secure funding for the center's research. This Board was established in 2002. Finally, there is an External Advisory Council, which has met annually since 1993. This council serves the PCC by giving advice on its scientific program and mission. Council members are distinguished cancer scientists from across the nation.

The center recognizes the need for extensive and effective collaboration among research institutions. It is therefore partnered with three cancer organizations, the Indiana University Cancer Center, the Oncological Sciences Center at Discovery Park, and the Walther Cancer Institute. The Oncological Sciences Center is a multidisciplinary research center at Purdue University. Researchers there bring together engineering, life sciences, and the studies of communication and human behavior to study cancer. The Oncological Sciences Center investigates the use of nanotechnology, drug delivery, imaging, and blood protein analysis as methods to detect cancer early on, as well as the use of natural substances that can prevent cancer. The Walther Cancer Institute is based in Indianapolis, Indiana; it is a nonprofit research institute for basic cancer research.

Researchers at the PCC benefit from a comprehensive selection of shared resources and facilities for analytical cytology, DNA sequencing, drug discovery, macromolecular crystallography, mass spectrometry, nuclear magnetic resonance, and transgenic mice. At the analytical cytometry facility, researchers have access to flow cytometry for analytical and sorting use, as well as confocal microscopy imaging. Confocal microscopy allows researchers to image in a single plane of focus, thereby eliminating noise signals from matter above or below the plane of focus. This facility can also aid scientists with data analysis. The DNA sequencing facility also offers microarray analysis assistance. The Drug Discovery facility aids in evaluation of potential drug candidates for inhibiting cell division, because tumors result from uncontrolled cell division. Macromolecular crystallography signifies the use of X-ray diffraction or macromolecule crystallization to analyze the structure of the tumor. Four rooms are available for crystallization at four temperatures minus 20, 12, 4, and minus 5 degrees Celsius, with a variability of only one-half of a degree. Experiments can also be performed at other temperatures.

Mass spectrometry allows scientists to determine the identity of an unknown molecule, based on the size ratios of its component molecules or fragments. Nuclear magnetic resonance also can be used to identify the atomic and structural composition of a molecule, typically based on the magnetic properties of its hydrogen atoms. Transgenic mice can be used to investigate the roles of specific genes and their interactions in cancer development, therapy, or prevention.

Researchers in scientific departments on the Purdue University campus also conduct investigations related to cancer. For example, in the Department of Food and Nutrition, scientists examine the links between nutrition and cancer. Specifically, research focuses on how nutritional elements can help to prevent cancer.

Funding for research at the PCC comes from numerous sources such as governmental grants, private foundation funds, corporate sponsorship, individual contributions, and fundraising events. One annual event is the Purdue Cancer Benefit Concert. Special funding sources are available for young investigators, to encourage bright scientists to enter the area of cancer research. For example, the Jim and Diann Robbers Cancer Research Grant for New Investigators is a fund established in 1998 and converted to an endowed fund 5 years later. The Cancer Center Executive Committee determines the recipients of these grants, which total $20,000 for 2 years. Jim Robbers has been on the faculty of Purdue University since 1966 and has worked with carcinogenic mycotoxins. In additional, the Indiana Elks sponsor Innovative Grants, which support novel, unique ideas that may seem too risky for other funding sources. Proposals for Innovative Grants are peer reviewed by faculty at Purdue University.

SEE ALSO: Chemical Industry; Chemoprevention; Chemotherapy; Experimental Cancer Drugs; Gene Therapy; Genetics; Indiana University Cancer Center; MIT Center for Cancer Research; National Cancer Institute.

BIBLIOGRAPHY. Chad Boutin, "Cancer Research Careers Will Get Head Starts from Gifts to Purdue," *Purdue University News* (October 12, 2005), new.uns.purdue.edu (cited December 2006); Michael Kahn and Stella Pelengaris, *The Molecular Biology of Cancer* (Blackwell Publishing Professional, 2006); Razelle Kurzrock and Moshe Talpaz, *Molecular Biology in Cancer Medicine* (2nd ed.) (Taylor and Francis, 1999); Lauren Pecorino, *Molecular Biology of Cancer: Mechanisms, Targets, and Therapeutics* (Oxford University Press, 2005); D. Rusciano, M. M. Burger, and D R. Welch, *Cancer Metastasis: Experimental Approaches (Laboratory Techniques in Biochemistry and Molecular Biology)* (Elsevier Science, 2000); D. R. Welch, ed., *Cancer Metastasis—Related Genes (Cancer Metastasis—Biology and Treatment, Vol. 3)* (Springer, 2002).

Claudia Winograd
University of Illinois at Urbana-Champaign

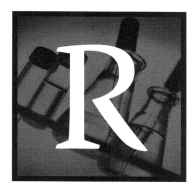

Radiation

RADIATION REFERS TO the transmission of energy, either as a stream of particles or as a wave, away from a radioactive source. In a medical context, the term *radiation* is generally used synonymously to mean ionizing radiation, which is any form of radiation with enough energy to ionize a target atom. Common examples of ionizing radiation include X-rays, gamma-rays, and ultraviolet light, all of which are higher in energy than nonionizing forms of radiation like radio waves, microwaves, and visible light. In high enough doses, ionizing radiation can be harmful to any biological system, causing tissue death and DNA mutations that can lead to cancer. However, at closely regulated doses, the unique properties of radiation have been harnessed for a variety of different medical uses including diagnostic imaging and cancer treatment.

DISCOVERY

Naturally occurring radiation was first discovered by Henri Becquerel (1852–1908) in 1896. He noted that when placed next to an unexposed photographic plate, uranium had the ability to somehow expose the plate through its light-proof wrapping. Becquerel's work was advanced by Marie Currie (1867–1934) and her husband Pierre Currie (1859–1906), who isolated new radioactive compounds and deter-mined that the source of natural radiation was the decay of large, unstable nuclei. By 1898, Ernest Rutherford (1871–1937) had discovered that natural radiation could be divided into three categories based on charge and penetrating ability. Alpha particles, now known to be the nuclei of helium atoms, were positively charged and could be stopped by a sheet of paper. Beta particles, now known to be high-energy electrons, were negatively charged and stopped by aluminum. Gamma particles, now known to be not particles but high-energy photons, were not charged and could penetrate even through lead.

A year before Becquerel discovered naturally occurring radiation, W. C. Roentgen (1845–1923) discovered the first artificially created form of ionizing radiation, which he called X-rays. Roentgen had been working with cathode ray tubes, which use electricity to form a stream of electrons inside a vacuum tube, when he observed that even when covered, his cathode ray tube could expose a photographic plate. Roentgen also observed that the penetration of X-rays differed depending on the target substance and theorized that they could therefore be used to examine an object's internal structure. Famously testing this idea by shooting X-rays through his wife's hand and onto a photo plate, Roentgen produced an image of the bony structure of the hand. Producing such an image is still formally known as a roentgenogram, although it is much more commonly referred to simply as an X-ray.

RADIATION EXPOSURE AND HARMFUL EFFECTS

Ionizing radiation is known to be harmful, and in high enough doses it can be lethal to humans. Ionization, the removal of an electron from an atom, produces highly energetic and therefore highly reactive radical compounds. When ionizing radiation passes through living tissue, the process of ionization can break apart chemical bonds in molecules needed by the cell to maintain its shape, the integrity of its membrane, and proper biological function. The radical compounds also participate in unusual reactions that disrupt cellular function. Normally, a cell can recover from damage to its machinery, made up of proteins, by degrading the damaged protein and replacing it with a new copy. However, if the radiation dose is large enough, the cell will be overwhelmed and die, leading to acute radiation sickness. Common symptoms include anemia and loss of immune function, resulting from destruction of the cells of the bone marrow; diarrhea and gastrointestinal bleeding from loss of the cells lining of the gastrointestinal tract; nausea; seizures; and ataxia from destruction of the nervous system, as well as blindness as a result of the death of retinal cells and burns on skin as a result of its being exposed to the radiation.

Damage to a cell's DNA is particularly harmful because, unlike protein, the cell cannot readily replace its DNA. Radiation can produce mutations in cellular

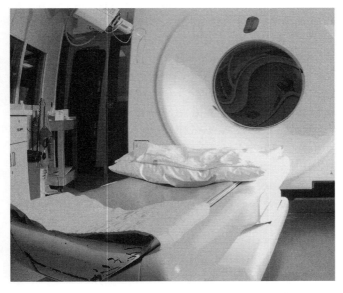

It is unknown precisely what is a "safe" upper limit of radiation exposure and to what degree exposure increases cancer.

DNA that can either up- or downregulate how much of a certain protein is produced, or it can change its function by slightly altering its shape. Most such changes will simply cause the cell to die. However, mutations in certain regulatory regions that control a cell's ability to divide, known as tumor suppressor genes, or mutations that promote unregulated cell proliferation, known as oncogenes, can trigger a cancerous transformation. Because all of the daughter cells of the initial mutant also contain the same mutation, they too will proliferate, eventually resulting in a distinct tumor mass.

Exposure to radiation is usually measured in either the unit rad or gray, abbreviated Gy, which is a measure of how much energy is absorbed by the exposed material (100 rad = 1 Gy). However, because certain forms of radiation, particularly alpha radiation, are much more harmful to biological systems than X-ray or gamma rays, the dose in rads is multiplied by the relative biological effectiveness of the radiation source to determine the effective dose, measured in rem (rem is an abbreviation for rad equivalent man). The general U.S. population receives an average dose of 0.3 rem, or 300 mrem, per year, 80 percent of which comes from naturally occurring sources, and the rest from man-made sources. The radioactive gas radon accounts for most of the natural radiation exposure. Other natural sources include cosmic and solar radiation, which are experienced most at high altitudes because the Earth's atmosphere and magnetic field act to filter out such radiation. Medical imaging studies such as X-rays and computed tomography (CT) scans and radiation therapy account for the majority of radiation from man-made sources.

Because cancers that arise as a result of radiation exposure are indistinguishable from those that occur spontaneously in the general population, it is unknown precisely what a "safe" upper limit of radiation exposure would be and to what degree radiation exposure increases the rate of cancer. Therefore, to limit additional exposure as much as possible, the U.S. government requires that the general population be exposed to less than 100 mrem of radiation per year from man-made sources. Adults working in radiation-related fields, such as nuclear power and X-ray technicians, are allowed to receive a dose of 5 rem (5,000 mrem) per year. Airline crews have the highest occupation exposure, because of the increased cosmic radiation they encounter at high altitudes. For comparison, a dose of 1,000 rem delivered in a short period of time is nearly always fatal, and a concentrated dose of 400 rem is fatal half of the time. However, because of the body's ability to repair radiation damage, the same 400-rem dose would almost never be fatal if it were spread out over a period of weeks or months.

RADIOLOGICAL IMAGING FOR MEDICAL DIAGNOSIS

As noted by Roentgen, X-rays can be used to image the internal structures of the body because some tissues, like bone, absorb much more of the radiation than others. This technique, often referred to as a "plain film," is widely used in modern medical practice to evaluate the lungs, teeth, bones, and foreign objects. Computerized axial tomography scans, commonly called CT scans, were developed in the mid-1970s and provided the first three-dimensional images of the body. CT scans work by taking X-ray images at many different angles in a 180-degree arc around the patient. The X-rays are detected by an electronic detector, and the information from multiple angles is reconstructed into a three-dimensional image that is viewed one slice of the body at a time. The ability of CT scans to look into the body before an invasive procedure has revolutionized the management of many diseases, including cancer, for which CT scans are used to look for tumor metastasis, lymph node involvement, response to chemotherapy, or reoccurrence after surgery.

In addition to X-ray and CT scans, which direct radiation from an outside source through the body, radioactive compounds can be injected into or ingested by a patient to produce a functional image. By adding a radioactive element to a molecule with a known biological function, like glucose, the movement of the molecule can be tracked. This technique is known as nuclear medicine. Normally such scans are performed with a stationary gamma ray detector to produce a two-dimensional image, but similar to with CT scans, it is possible to create a three-dimensional reconstruction using a single photon emission CT, or SPECT, scan. Positron emission tomography, or PET, scans are similar in principle to nuclear medicine scans, but they generate radiation via a different mechanism. They are commonly conducted with radiolabeled glucose to scan for cancer metastasis,

as cancer cells import glucose at a faster rate than normal cells.

SEE ALSO: Neutrons; Nuclear Industry; Proton Therapy; Radiation Therapy; Radiation, Gamma; X-Rays.

BIBLIOGRAPHY. Douglas C. Giancoli, *Physics: Principles with Applications* (Prentice-Hall, 2006); Lee Goldman and Dennis Ausiello, *Cecil Textbook of Medicine* (W.B. Saunders, 2004); Leonard Gunderson and Joel Tepper, *Clinical Radiation Oncology* (Elsevier Churchill Livingstone, 2007).

JOHN PAUL SHEN
WASHINGTON UNIVERSITY SCHOOL OF MEDICINE

Radiation, Gamma

GAMMA RADIATION, A form of electromagnetic energy, has been shown to damage the DNA of human cells, causing cell death or cancer. Cells that rapidly divide are most susceptible to the harmful effects of gamma rays. Rapidly-diving cancer cells are also susceptible to these effects, providing the basis for the use of gamma radiation in the treatment of cancer. Gamma radiation is used in a wide range of clinical settings to treat patients with cancer.

Gamma radiation is emitted by the radioactive isotope decay of naturally radioactive elements, such as radium-226, or artificially radioactive elements, such as cobalt-60. During a decay reaction, the nucleus of an unstable atom rearranges to a state of lower energy, releasing the excess energy as electromagnetic waves, or *photons*. Gamma radiation has the shortest wavelength and highest energy of any form of light in the electromagnetic radiation spectrum.

The high energy of gamma rays are damaging to human cells, causing cell death or mutations in the cells' genetic material. Breaks in the double stranded DNA is perhaps the most significant mechanism by which gamma radiation causes disease in humans. The skin, an important functional barrier to infectious material, does not protect against the harmful effects of gamma radiation. Thus, every cell in the body is susceptible to the effects of gamma rays.

Following a break in a cell's DNA, the cell will attempt to repair the damaged DNA. If the damage is

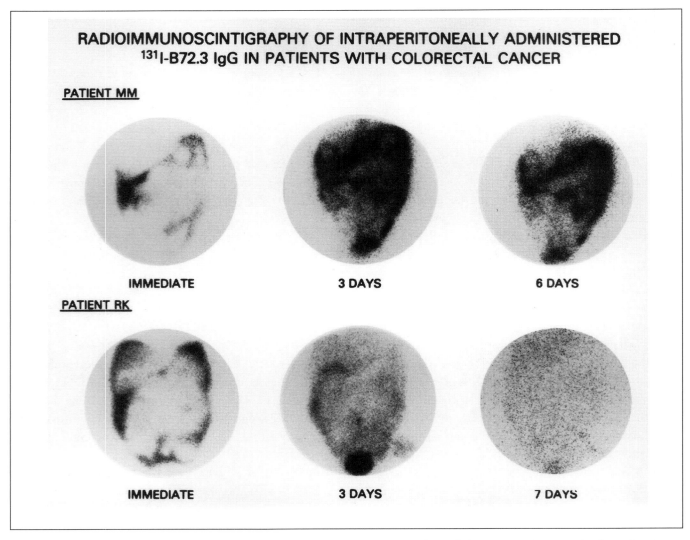

RADIOIMMUNOSCINTIGRAPHY OF INTRAPERITONEALLY ADMINISTERED ¹³¹I-B72.3 IgG IN PATIENTS WITH COLORECTAL CANCER

Gamma camera scans of the abdomens (colons) of two patients. Gamma radiation, a form of electromagnetic energy, has been shown to damage the DNA of human cells, causing cell death. Cells that rapidly divide are most susceptible to the harmful effects of gamma rays.

excessive, and the cell is unable to repair the damage, the cell will die. The radiation often produces mutations in the cell's DNA that are passed on to future generations of the cell. This is especially true of rapidly-dividing cells, which don't have enough time to correctly repair the damaged DNA. The effects that result from the damaged DNA may only be obvious to a person after several years.

Even in small doses, gamma radiation has long been known to cause cancer in humans. Exposure to gamma rays exerts perhaps its most immediate effects on the rapidly-dividing cells produced in the bone marrow, including blood cells. Current evidence suggests that within 3 to 10 years after acute radiation exposure, the risk of developing leukemia, especially of myelogenous origin, greatly increases. The risk of developing solid cancerous tumors is increased as well after exposure to gamma radiation, although it often takes several decades before the effects of the radiation is apparent. Several cancers have been linked to gamma radiation exposure, including those of skin, breast, lung, thyroid, bone, and lymph tissue.

The ability of gamma rays to penetrate tissue and damage cells' DNA has allowed for the use of radiation to treat, and often cure, various types of cancer. Radiation therapy is targeted directly to rapidly-dividing cancer cells, killing the cells or halting their ability to divide. Cancer cells, which divide rapidly without regulation, are especially susceptible to the harmful effects of gamma radiation. Although targeted to cancer cells, the radiation still has the potential to damage and cause further cancer in surrounding healthy tissue. The healthy cells, however, grow at a slower rate and are better able to repair the damage than are cancer cells.

Radiation therapy is the primary treatment modality for a number of different types of cancer. Radiation therapy has been shown, in some cases, to cure a wide range of cancers, including Hodgkin's and certain non-Hodgkin's lymphomas, head and neck carcinomas, limited-stage prostate carcinomas, gynecological tumors, central nervous system tumors, and some forms of skin cancer. In some studies, radiation therapy in conjunction with chemotherapy has been shown to increase survival rates more than either treatment alone.

Radiation therapy is used to treat cancer in a wide range of clinical settings. Radiation therapy is often used in conjunction with surgery to ensure that all the malignant cells are removed from the body. Radiation may be used preoperatively to shrink a tumor, making it easier to remove, intraoperatively, or postoperatively. Radiation therapy has also been used to reduce pain and improve patients' quality of life by shrinking inoperable tumors.

The use of mobile devices in *Intra-operative Radiotherapy* (IORT) is a relatively recent advancement in radiation treatments. Mobile devices allow the surgeon to use radiotherapy while the tissues are still exposed during surgery. After removal of the tumor surgically, the radiation targets the area surrounding the tumor. Currently, Mobile IORT units have been shown to successfully increase survival in patients with a wide range of cancers, including early-stage breast cancer and rectal cancer.

In *external radiation therapy*, the most common type of radiation therapy, a machine emits gamma rays targeted to a specific site in the body. External radiation therapy is usually an outpatient procedure, in which patients visit a hospital or clinic five days a week for several weeks. Patients are not radioactive during or after treatments. Each plan of radiation treatment is individualized and unique to the patient. Many factors, including the type of cancer, location of the cancer, grade and stage of the cancer,

and coexistent therapies are important in planning radiation treatments.

In *internal radiation therapy* (also known as brachytherapy, implant therapy, interstitial radiation, or intravacitary radiation), gamma rays are emitted from a small container of radioactive material implanted directly into, or near the tumor. These implants, known as *seeds* or *capsules*, may be temporary or permanent and emit a continuous, controlled amount of radiation. The radiation is concentrated near the cancer, with minimal exposure to the surrounding, healthy cells. Patients usually remain in the hospital for a few days after the treatment. While the patient is in the hospital, the implant emits its highest level of radiation. During this time, patients are limited in their exposure to visitors. Once the implant is removed, there is no longer any radioactivity present in the body. In permanent implants, the amount of radiation emitted is decreased to a safe level before the patients are discharged from the hospital. Many different types of radioactive materials can be used in the implant, including cesium, iridium, iodine, phosphorus, and palladium.

Stereotactic radiosurgery, a therapy that has been increasing greatly in use over the past few decades, has been shown to be successful in treating brain cancers and other neurological conditions. In stereotactic radiosurgery, a single high-level dose of precisely directed gamma rays are focused directly at the tumor without damaging any surrounding healthy tissue. Currently, the use of stereotactic radiosurgery is limited to the head and neck, because the structures contained within are likely to remain static during the procedure. A patients' treatment plan is typically prepared by a team of medical physicists, radiation oncologists, and neurosurgeons, with the aid of three-dimensional computer analysis of Computed Tomography (CT) scans and Magnetic Resonance Imaging (MRI) scans. During the procedure, the patient's head and neck are held stationary in a fixation device. Stereotactic radiosurgery, in which no skin incision or skull opening is required, offers patients a safe and effective alternative to brain surgery. The procedure is also especially attractive in treating brain cancers that are not accessible to standard surgical techniques.

Currently two forms of stereotactic radiosurgery are in use. The *Leksell Gamma Knife*, originally defined and developed by Lars Leksell in the 1950s and

60s, is a stationary machine most useful in the treatment of small tumors and blood vessels. The Gamma Knife, which typically requires one treatment session in a single hospital stay, contains 201 cobalt-60 sources in a spherical housing. The sources are arranged in a way that the gamma rays emitted are precisely focused and intersect at a common point. The second method of stereotactic radiosurgery utilizes a moveable linear accelerator based machine, or *LINAC*. In LINAC radiosurgery, patients are given several small doses of gamma radiation over several weeks. Overall, the total dose a patient receives with a LINAC machine is typically higher than with the Gamma Knife, and there is great controversy over which method is preferred for specific cancers.

Radioimmunotherapy is showing great promise in the treatment of cancers that have spread beyond their primary origin (i.e. metastasized). Immune system proteins called *antibodies*, which recognize and bind to specific target cells, are being tested to bind to particular proteins on cancer cells. The man-made antibodies are injected and travel in the bloodstream until they reach the cancer cells, to which they bind. Radiation then targets and kills these antibody-labeled cells. Although still for the most part in its experimental stages, radioimmunotherapy has shown therapeutic potential for treating a wide of cancers, including those of the central nervous system, blood, skin, and colon.

SEE ALSO: American College of Radiation Oncology; American Society for Therapeutic Radiation & Oncology; Radiation, Ionizing; Radiation Therapy; X-Rays.

BIBLIOGRAPHY. Michael L. Goodman, "Gamma Knife Radiosurgery: Current Status and Review", *Southern Medical Journal* (v. 83, 1990); Stephen M. Hahn and Eli Glatstein, "Principles of Radiation Therapy", *Harrison's Principles of Internal Medicine* (16th ed., 2005); McGraw-Hill Companies, Inc., "Radiation Therapy", www.answers.com/topic/radiation-therapy (cited April 2007).

SHAUN E. GRUENBAUM
MEDICAL SCHOOL FOR INTERNATIONAL HEALTH
BEN-GURION UNIVERSITY OF THE NEGEV AND
COLUMBIA UNIVERSITY MEDICAL CENTER
BENJAMIN F. GRUENBAUM
UNIVERSITY OF CONNECTICUT

Radiation, Ionizing

EXPOSURE TO IONIZING radiation is a well-quantified cancer risk factor, based on information gained from epidemiological and experimental studies over the past half-century or so. The evidence indicates that cancer risk is increased by exposure in rough proportion to the amount of energy deposited in tissue (radiation dose, usually quantified in units of gray [Gy] or milligray [mGy], where 1 Gy corresponds to 1 joule of energy per kilogram of tissue). However, organs and tissues differ in their sensitivity to radiation carcinogenesis, and organ-specific, radiation-related excess cancer risk for a given radiation dose may vary by type of ionizing radiation as well by gender, age at exposure, age and time following exposure, and lifestyle factors such as reproductive history and exposure to other carcinogens such as tobacco smoke. On average, the bulk of radiation dose to individuals comes from natural background sources that have changed little over the span of human existence, and to which perhaps as much as 10 percent of human cancer risk may be attributable.

Our extensive knowledge of the carcinogenic effects of ionizing radiation comes from studies involving the irradiation of cells and experimental animals, from epidemiological studies of populations that have experienced unusually high levels of radiation exposure for medical or occupational reasons, or from catastrophic events such as the 1986 Chernobyl reactor accident and the atomic bombings in 1945 of Hiroshima and Nagasaki, Japan.

Ionizing radiation includes the more energetic end of the electromagnetic spectrum (X-rays and gamma rays) and subatomic particles such as electrons, neutrons, and alpha particles (helium nuclei each comprising two protons and two neutrons). These types of radiation can disrupt molecular bonds by displacing electrons (ionization). A characteristic type of DNA damage produced by ionizing radiation, even by a single radiation track through a cell, involves closely spaced, multiple lesions that can compromise cellular DNA repair mechanisms. Although most of the cells sustaining such radiation-induced damage may be eliminated by damage response pathways, some cells are capable of escaping these pathways, propagating, and eventually undergoing malignant transformation, a crucial step in cancer development.

SOURCES AND TYPES OF IONIZING RADIATION

We live, and have always lived, in a sea of ionizing radiation produced by the radioactive decay of unstable isotopes of elements in rocks, soil, and our own bodily tissues and by nuclear reactions occurring in the sun and distant stars. A major part of all exposure to such background radiation exposure is attributable to the inhalation of radon gas, which is produced by the radioactive decay of radium in rocks and soil and that, as it seeps out into the atmosphere, can become trapped and concentrated in poorly ventilated environments such as dwellings and underground mines. Radiation from radon and its radioactive decay products consists of mainly alpha particles, which have very limited ability to penetrate tissue but can damage cellular DNA in the lung if the radioactive source is inhaled and deposited in the airways. Gamma and X-rays, in contrast, are highly penetrating and can affect cells even when the radiation source is outside the body. Electrons are only somewhat more penetrating than alpha particles, but the immediate cause of most radiation-related damage to DNA is believed to be interactions with secondary electrons energized by transfer from electromagnetic or particle radiation originating outside the cell.

Different types of radiation differ somewhat in biological effectiveness per unit of dose. For example, alpha particle radiation absorbed in tissue is considered to be about 20 times more effective as a carcinogen than the same dose of gamma rays. The concept of equivalent dose, expressed in units of Sievert (Sv), was introduced for purposes of radiation protection. For gamma radiation, 1 mGy dose corresponds to 1 mSv dose equivalent, whereas for alpha radiation, 1 mGy dose corresponds to 20 mSv dose equivalent.

During the past century, following the discovery of X-rays by Roentgen in 1895 and Becquerel's discovery of radioactivity a year later, human population exposure to ionizing radiation has been increased by medical, industrial, and military uses of radiation technology. Such man-made radiation currently contributes about 18 percent of the total annual radiation exposure to the population of the United States, according to a recent, authoritative report by a committee of the U.S. National Academy of Sciences (NAS). However, radiation dose to individuals can vary widely, and most of our information on radiation-related, human cancer risk has been obtained during the past half-century, from studies of fairly large, and well-defined, human populations with documented radiation exposures at unusually high doses (e.g., dose equivalent in excess of 100 mSv). Such doses may be compared to background radiation, from which the yearly exposure is thought to be biologically comparable to about 1.15 mSv to the whole body from gamma radiation, 10.4 mSv to the lung and bronchus from inhaled radon and its decay products, and an additional 0.6 mSv to the whole body from man-made sources of radiation including medical X-rays, nuclear medicine, consumer products, occupational exposures, radioactive fallout, and the nuclear fuel cycle. As a further reference point, whole-body exposures in excess of 4 Sv (4,000 mSv) are usually fatal in the absence of medical intervention, whereas much higher doses, limited to single organs or restricted parts of the body, are often used safely for treatment of cancer.

RADIATION EFFECTS

The use of X-rays and radioactive materials in science, medicine, and industry led to the recognition, documented by reports of radiation burns, that radiation exposure, although helpful for the diagnosis and treatment of disease, might also be harmful, and protective measures were taken to limit exposure. It took somewhat longer for the carcinogenic potential of ionizing radiation to be recognized, but today the relationship between radiation dose and cancer risk is well characterized and well quantified, probably more so than for any other common environmental carcinogen. This is largely because extensive work in radiation physics and radiation biology and medicine has led to a good understanding of the relationship between radiation exposure, which is the energy impinging on an organism, and radiation dose, which is the amount per unit mass absorbed by a selected bit of tissue. Thus, radiation dose is relatively easy to estimate compared to a chemical dose to the same tissue, which requires understanding of the pathways by which a given intake of the chemical carcinogen results in absorption of the chemical by the tissue of interest.

An early study comparing cancer mortality among British radiologists who had registered with a radiological society before 1921 with that among radiologists who began their practice later, and who were therefore likely to have received lower radiation doses because of protective practices introduced over time, is an example of an influential study in which the fact of exposure was related to risk but individual dose estimates were not available. However, experimental studies of radiation effects such as cell inactivation, mutation, and cancer have taken advantage of the experimenters' ability to regulate, with precision, radiation doses to target cells or tissues. Similarly, epidemiological investigations of exposed populations have benefited enormously from information enabling scientists to reconstruct individual, and even organ-specific, radiation doses. Benefits include the estimation of dose–response relationships and of the modification of such relationships by individual properties such as sex, age, lifestyle, and perhaps genetic inheritance.

Leukemia was the first human cancer for which risk was unequivocally demonstrated to increase with radiation dose. This increase was shown among atomic bomb survivors and among a series of British patients treated by X-ray for ankylosing spondylitis, a painful form of arthritis of the spine. The thyroid gland was the first solid cancer site for which radiation dose was strongly implicated as a risk factor, based on the screening of atomic bomb survivors and of patients treated by radiation for diseases of the head and neck. Today, radiation dose responses to gamma-ray and X-ray radiation in the under-4-Sv range are very well established for all solid cancers as a group and for cancers of the female breast, the thyroid gland, stomach, colon, liver, lung, bladder, and ovary in particular. The evidence for a radiation-related risk is also persuasive for cancers of the oral cavity as a group and for salivary glands in particular, for esophageal cancer, for nonmelanoma skin cancer in general and basal cell skin cancer in particular, and for malignant and benign tumors of the brain and central nervous system as a whole and for glioma and meningioma in particular among malignant brain tumors, as well as schwannoma among benign brain tumors. As mentioned earlier, increased lung cancer risk is also associated with internal exposure to radon and its decay products. Bone sarcoma risk is associated with radiation dose from ingested or injected radium.

From cancer data with a statistically highly significant radiation dose–response, much can be learned about the functional form of the dose–response relationship and about modification of radiation-related risk by other factors like gender, age at exposure,

age at observation for risk, reproductive history, and smoking history. For example, there is a general tendency, with some exceptions, for dose-specific risk of radiation-related cancer to be inversely associated with exposure age. Both radiation-related and baseline cancer risk tend to increase with increasing age following exposure, but the age-related increase for radiation-related risk may not be as steep as that for baseline cancer risk. We know that a first full-term pregnancy at a relatively young age (e.g., before age 25 years) is protective against radiation-related breast cancer risk, even if the radiation exposure preceded the first full-term pregnancy. The interaction between smoking and radiation exposure as lung cancer risk factors is less clear, with some evidence indicating that radon-related excess risk, as distinguished from smoking-related risk, among uranium miners is higher for smokers than for nonsmokers, and some evidence indicating that radiation-related excess risk among atomic bomb survivors exposed to gamma radiation did not differ by smoking level.

The intriguing possibility that human beings may differ in their sensitivity to radiation carcinogenesis because of genetic variation is difficult to address given the rarity in human populations of genes strongly associated with increased cancer risk and the present difficulty of investigating more common genes that may be weakly associated with risk, but it can be expected to receive continuing research attention.

Radiation-related cancer risk estimates, based mainly on information from populations exposed to up to 2 Sv or more, are relevant to decisions involving actual or potential exposures at 100 mSv or less, a range that includes nearly all nonmedical exposures. Present radiation protection practice is to assume that risk in this range is proportional to radiation dose equivalent in Sv. Using estimates prepared by the NAS committee mentioned earlier, the sex-averaged lifetime excess cancer incidence following a whole-body exposure to 100 mSv at age 20 years would be about 13 per thousand, in addition to a baseline population lifetime rates of 440 per thousand. Estimated excess mortally would be about 6 compared to 300 baseline cancer deaths per thousand.

On the basis of the risks estimated in the NAS report, annual average exposure from natural background and human activities as discussed above, and current U.S. life tables, it appears that about 7 percent of all cancers, and 10 percent of all cancer deaths, mostly from radon-related lung cancer in association with tobacco smoking, may be attributable to natural background radiation, and that another 1 percent of the total is associated with man-made radiation exposure, which is dominated by medical uses.

SEE ALSO: Doll, Richard; Radiation; Radiation, Gamma; Radiation Therapy; X-Rays.

BIBLIOGRAPHY. National Research Council of the National Academy of Sciences, Committee to Assess Health Risks from Exposure to Low Levels of Ionizing Radiation, *Health Risks from Exposure to Low Levels of Ionizing Radiation, BEIR VII Phase 2* (National Academy Press, 2006).

CHARLES LAND
NATIONAL INSTITUTES OF HEALTH

Radiation Therapy

RADIATION THERAPY (RT; also called ionizing radiation, X-ray therapy, or irradiation) is used for treating cancer by focusing high-energy radiation beams into specific locations in the body. This high-energy radiation, when focused on cancer cells, breaks up genetic material and interferes with the growth of the tumor. The term *tumor* is a Latin word for swelling and describes the way that cancer presents itself in the body. The rapid growth of cells that cause this swelling can be slowed or stopped by using RT. Radiation beams are delivered specifically to the area of cancerous cells and therefore minimize the effect on neighboring, normal cells. Radiation oncologists are doctors who train specifically in using RT, and they work together with other physicians to treat patients with cancer. According to the American Cancer Society, more than 50 percent of patients with cancer currently receive this treatment in the United States.

GOALS OF THERAPY

The goals of RT have changed significantly over the years. In the 1960s, RT was used as an empirical strategy for shrinking tumors, with relatively low success rates and high potential for adverse effects. Negative effects such as damage of normal, healthy neighbor-

ing tissue are undesirable and lead to poor treatment outcomes. At present, application of this technology has become part of a multidisciplinary approach for treatment of patients with cancer. The aim of RT is to provide a precise dose of radiation to a specific volume of tumor, avoiding damage to surrounding healthy tissue. As a result, precision in the use of RT has improved quality of life, prolonged survival, and decreased the cost of care for many patients undergoing treatment for cancer.

Before beginning therapy, the goals of treatment are determined as curative or palliative. Curative means that there is a high probability of long-term survival after treatment. A few side effects of adequate dose of therapy are accepted as part of the treatment. Palliative care, or easing of symptoms from incurable cancer, means that even with treatment, there is no hope for long-term survival because of the extent of tumor growth. Treatment is performed to control tumor growth to increase the time of survival of the patient as well as to prevent potential discomfort from further tumor growth. Palliative treatment is especially important in dealing with the effects of extensive metastases (spreading of cancer to other locations). Metastases can cause pain, which can be significantly reduced by irradiating them.

On the whole, the goals of RT are to decrease the size of the tumor or to completely eliminate it. Oftentimes RT is used in conjunction with surgical removal and chemotherapy treatments. RT treatment before surgery is done to reduce a tumor mass that is too great to be removed surgically. Sometimes RT is used together with chemotherapy to improve the chances of shrinking and eliminating the person's cancer. Each patient requires an individualized approach for his or her particular form of cancer. Members of the healthcare team, in conjunction with a radiation oncologist, make the decisions for whom to prescribe irradiation treatment.

METHODS OF THERAPY

The way that RT works and is able to reduce or eliminate tumors is through altering the cell cycle in the cells that are treated. The cell cycle is the process of growth and division that most cells in the body undergo. Cancerous cells are ones that are typically growing and dividing faster than normal body cells, and RT takes advantage of this. The cell cycle is important in cancer treatments because cells that are actively dividing are the ones most affected by therapy. Radiosensitivity is used to describe those rapidly or quickly dividing cells that are susceptible to radiation damage. RT attacks dividing cancer cells, but it can also affect the dividing cells of normal tissues. RTs side effects are the result of this damage to normal cells. Each time RT is given, it becomes a balance between destroying the cancer cells and sparing normal cells.

There are few places in the body where a cancer could not originate in or reach via metastases. RT provides a specific and focused treatment option for tumors that cannot be treated surgically. Treatment planning and simulation are important first steps in the RT process. Planning and simulation ensure that the treatment is more effective and precise and less damaging to surrounding tissues. Simulation involves preparing and positioning the patient just like during therapy sessions, but without delivering radiation. This practice allows the patient to feel more knowledgeable about the procedure as well as giving the physician a chance to make sure that each treatment will be replicable.

Previously, it was thought that once an area was treated with radiation, it could not be irradiated again because of the too-high risk of damage to the normal cells in the treatment area. However, recent research shows that in some treatments, a second course of RT can be given.

There are two broad categories of RT: external and internal. External RT involves high-energy beams directed at the affected area. The procedure is painless and performed once per day for a period of several weeks. Through the duration of therapy, small pinpoint tattoos are used to mark the treatment area to ensure that the beam is directed in the same place with each dose. Internal radiation, also called brachytherapy, is delivery of the radiation treatment by placing small amounts of a radioactive material in the area next to where cancer is localized. The implanted material stays in the small area next to the cancerous cells for the duration of the treatment. In brachytherapy, higher doses of radiation are delivered over a shorter period of time. The implants are adapted to the placement site and could include seeds, wires, or plates specially made from the radioactive material.

Just as there is more than one way of delivering radiation, there are also different sources of ionizing radiation that can be used for external therapy and that have more energy than others. In the case of external therapy, the more energetic the source, the more deeply the radiation can penetrate into tissues. In planning treatments and attempting to minimize risk to healthy tissues, it is important to consider the types of radiation to be used. A radiation oncologist (a doctor specially trained to treat cancer patients with radiation) selects the type and energy of radiation that is most suitable for each patient's cancer.

The most commonly used radiation treatment involves high-energy photons. These are the same photons that are used to form an image for an X-ray.

Alternatively, electron beams produced by a linear accelerator are used for tumors that are near the surface of the body. These beams do not penetrate as deeply into tissues and could be used on structures close to the surface.

Proton beams are a more recent addition in radiation treatments. Protons are the central parts of atoms (along with neutrons). On their own, they do not cause much damage while passing through tissues, but they are very effective at damaging cells at which they are targeted. This type of treatment is being developed to reduce normal tissue damage. Proton therapy is covered for most indications by Medicare and is used routinely for numerous aggressive cancers. More research is required to determine other applications. Some of the techniques used in proton treatment can also expose the patient to neutrons (see below). The downsides to proton therapy are the relative expense of setting up all of the required equipment, which is only available at certain centers and may require patients to travel or move to the area.

Neutrons make up the other part of an atom's nucleus. They are used for some cancers of the head, neck, and prostate. Neutron therapy is used when other forms of RT have failed. Use of neutrons in RT has declined because of the more severe long-term side effects that have been reported with its use.

COMPLICATIONS OF THERAPY

Complications are highly dependent on the site where irradiation is being applied, as well as the dose.

Area of Treatment	Complications
Brain	Earache, headache, dizziness, hair loss
Head and neck	Dry mouth, hoarseness, weight loss
Lung	Cough, fibrosis
Breast	Cough, skin redness, lung irritation
Abdomen	Nausea, vomiting, diarrhea, urinary frequency
Extremities, skin	Redness, dryness

The most common side effects of RT are to the skin at the site of application, where redness and soreness often occur a week or more into the treatment. Swelling is another common symptom at the site of treatment. The body's immune system responds to RT by recruiting lymphoid cells to the site of tumor and normal cell destruction. Genital organs are very sensitive to radiation, and their direct exposure to high doses will potentially cause infertility in both male and female patients.

Continued work in radiation oncology has given us more information about the short- and long-term effects of RT. For each organ, the maximum safe and tolerable doses of radiation have been worked out. It is becoming clear that when combining RT with other treatment options, these same doses could lead to severe late effects in different organs. Tolerance doses for different organs are useful as guides, but the emphasis has shifted to considering all of the other treatments that a patient is undergoing. It is now important to consider the volume of an organ that is being irradiated, as well as what other concurrent treatments have an effect on this same organ.

Because radiation oncologists work as part of a multidisciplinary team of physicians, care for patients with cancer can be coordinated to improve outcomes and decrease immediate as well as late side effects. Treatment for children requires dose adjustment as well as closer monitoring for long-term side effects.

SPECIFIC EXAMPLES OF LATE EFFECTS OF TREATMENT

Normal tissues vary in how they respond to radiation in the long term. Tissues and organs in which cells are more rapidly dividing, for instance, in the intestine or immune system, are more likely to be affected in the short term, whereas tissues whose cells divide slowly or not at all could show a slower onset of effects from RT. In general, prevention is key. Radiation oncologists carefully plan and execute treatments to minimize exposure of other tissues in the treatment of tumors.

Following are some examples of how various organs manifest damage, as well as how this damage is detected and treated by the physicians.

In the brain, damage is detected by the presence of a headache, somnolence (sleepiness), and losses in memory. The cause of these changes is alteration in blood flow as well as changes in the myelin sheaths (an insulating layer around certain nerve fibers). Typically, damage takes 6–12 months to develop. The patient is seen every day or every week until relief from symptoms is achieved. With the spinal cord, damage is detected through the presence of shooting pains, tingling sensations, numbness, or weakness in the muscles. The shooting pains (or specifically Lhermitte's sign), occur 2–4 months after irradiation treatment and are persistent for 6–9 months. Numbness takes 6–12 months to progress. Treatment includes rehabilitative care.

In the lungs, detection of lung damage occurs on the appearance of a cough, pink sputum production, and fibrosis, which manifests as progressive decrease in lung function. It takes 1–3 months after a single dose of RT for these radiation reactions to occur. The patient showing these symptoms is treated with high-dose steroids for lung inflammation, and the dose is tapered as the symptoms diminish.

For the heart, changes caused by irradiation are not detectable on an electrocardiogram (a test to monitor heart function). Most commonly, the pericardium (or tissue lining the heart) is damaged. Symptoms of pericardial effusion appear within 6 months to a year after irradiation. Coronary artery disease seems to appear 10–15 years after treatment and is associated with the usual risk factors of obesity, smoking, and high blood pressure.

In the liver, vague or sometimes intense abdominal pain in the region, followed by retention of fluid in the abdomen (ascites), is the primary sign of late liver damage. Ascites take 2–4 months to develop, and there is no effective treatment once they are formed, so the emphasis should be on careful radiation dose monitoring and prevention.

For the kidneys, numerous clinical presentations exist for the signs and symptoms of kidney damage, depending on the exposure to radiation. Prevention and minimizing damage to healthy tissue are the key to successful RT treatment near the kidney.

Finally, for the small and large intestine, increased frequency of bowel movements and black, tarry stools and weight loss are common symptoms of intestinal damage from RT; they present 6 months to 2 years after treatment.

NEWER METHODS OF RT

Radiopharmaceuticals are a different way of delivering radioactive materials, similar to brachytherapy. These drugs can be given intravenously (in the vein), by mouth, or be placed into a body cavity. Depending on the actual drug used, these capsules hew to various parts of the body and deliver radiation specifically at the site of cancer. One way that the radioactivity is delivered to the correct location is by the use of antibodies. Antibodies are protein substances normally found in the body and normally used for differentiating between materials that are self and those that are foreign. In radiopharmaceutical applications, antibodies are used like Zip codes or postal codes to specify where the radioactive drug needs to be delivered. Attaching antibodies to the drugs makes sure that they is delivered exactly to the target cells. Prerequisite to this therapy is knowing where the cancer is found and having antibodies that recognize it.

This approach is reasonable to use in situations in which cancerous cells have spread to numerous locations where it may not be feasible to focus beams and irradiate the tissues separately. Combining radiopharmaceuticals with irradiation is another approach that can be used in certain types of cancer with metastases. For instance, late-stage prostate cancer in men typically metastasizes to the bone. In this case, irradiation of the prostate can be combined with radiopharmaceutical therapy to relieve bone pain in these patients. Introduction of radioactive substances into the bloodstream is not without risk. These capsules of high-energy compounds are able to decrease blood cells and put patients at risk for infections. More specific information is found in the safety section.

A neat application of radiopharmaceuticals is in the treatment of thyroid cancer. Normal thyroid is the location where iodine is taken up in the body, and a cancer of the thyroid is composed of dividing cells that require iodine. Giving radioactive iodine through the vein directly targets it to be delivered in the thyroid gland and to act on the rapidly dividing cancer cells there. The fact that iodine is preferentially taken up in the thyroid gland makes sure that giving radioiodine (iodine 131) has minimal effects on the rest of the body and destroys only the thyroid gland cells.

SAFETY CONCERNS

Whenever receiving RT, patients should be notified of the safety concerns that affect them and those around them. When receiving external RT, one is not radioactive, and no special precautions are required. When undergoing treatment with internal RT, such as with an implant or with radiopharmaceuticals, however, there are special safety precautions that are important to keep in mind. For high-dose, short-term radioactive implants, typically patients will be required to stay at the hospital to minimize exposure to friends and relatives. With permanent low-dose (seed) implants, it is recommended that the patient avoid close contact with people for a few days while the radiation dose is at its highest.

Patients are instructed to avoid prolonged contact with children and pregnant women for a few months. Use of condoms during intercourse is also recommended for a short period of time. Radiopharmaceuticals leave the body within a few weeks, and during that time, doctors and nurses give specific instructions to the patient to minimize exposures. Because the radioactive component of these drugs may be cleared through numerous routes, good personal hygiene is recommended for the duration of the treatment. This includes good handwashing technique, multiple toilet flushes, using separate utensils, and avoiding contact with infants, children, and pregnant women.

SEE ALSO: AIDS-Related Cancers; American Cancer Society; Association of Cancer Online Resources; Childhood Cancers.

BIBLIOGRAPHY. K. S. Clifford Chao, Carlos Perez, and Luther Brady, *Radiation Oncology: Management and Decisions* (Lippincott-Raven, 1999); W. Schlegel, T. Bortfeld, and A.-L. Grosu, *New Technologies in Radiation Oncology* (Springer-Verlag, 2006); American Cancer Society, www.cancer.org/ (cited February 2007); William Small, Jr. and

Gayle E. Woloschak, eds., *Radiation Toxicity: A Practical Guide* (Springer, 2006); L. Dewit, J. K. Anninga, and C. A. Hoefnagel, "Radiation Injury in the Human Kidney: A Prospective Analysis Using Specific Scintigraphic and Biochemical Endpoints," *International Journal of Radiation Oncology, Biology, Physics* (v.19, 1990); Cancer Treatment Centers of America, *Brachytherapy* www.brachytherapy.com/ (cited February 2007).

Anna Gushchin
University of Pittsburgh School of Medicine

Radon

RADON IS A naturally occurring noble radioactive gas that tends to reach higher, or enhanced, concentrations inside a structure as compared to the outside. Radon generally enters a building through cracks or at penetration sites in the substructure of a home or building. Radon has many attributes that tend to minimize the public's risk perception. For example, it is invisible, odorless, and tasteless, and thus presents no sensory reminders to stimulate taking action to test or follow-up with mitigation.

Radon is a known Class A carcinogen and has been shown to be a major occupational lung carcinogen in radon-exposed underground miners. Extrapolations from pooled miners' studies have indicated that radon is also a major environmental carcinogen. More recently, large-scale pooled epidemiologic case–control studies examining the relationship between residential radon exposure and lung cancer have provided direct evidence that prolonged exposure to radon, even at or below the U.S. Environmental Protection Agency's (EPA) action guideline of 4 pCi/L (150 Bq/m3), increases lung cancer risk. In fact, radon is considered to be the second leading cause of lung cancer overall and the primary cause of lung cancer in individuals who never smoked.

Radon is a chemical element found on the periodic table at atomic weight 86. Radon is a radioactive noble gas formed in the uranium-238 radioactive decay chain. The direct parent of 222Rn is radium-226 (226Ra). Similar to other noble gasses, radon is colorless, odorless, and tasteless and is relatively chemically inert. Radon's radioactive isotopes have mass numbers ranging from 204 to 224. Radon-222 (222Rn) has the longest half-life (3.82 days) of the radon isotopes formed in the 238U decay chain and presents the greatest health risk. The major contributors of indoor 222Rn are soil gas emanations from soils and rocks; off-gassing of waterborne radon from groundwater sources into the indoor air during showering, dishwashing, and so on; emanation from construction materials; and outdoor air. In most geographic locations, ground source (soils, rocks, etc.) radon represents the major contributor to indoor radon concentrations. Since 1986, the EPA has recommended an indoor radon action level of 4 pCi/L. Although the EPA proposed a waterborne radon standard of 300 pCi/L in 1991, there are currently no nationwide standards for 222Rn in public or private drinking water supplies. The average indoor air radon concentration in the United States is approximately 1.4 pCi/L, and outdoor radon concentrations average around 0.4 pCi/L.

The short-lived solid alpha-, beta-, and gamma-emitting radon daughter products (progeny) achieve secular equilibrium with 222Rn within 4 hours. If inhaled and deposited in the lungs, these solid decay products can initiate lung cancer. Polonium-218 (218Po) and polonium-214 (214Po), two of the immediate alpha particle emitting decay products, present the greatest radiogenic risk to the lung. In 1998, the National Research Council analyzed data

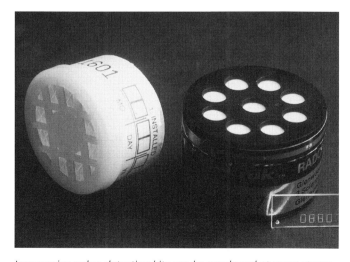

Inexpensive radon detection kits can be purchased at many stores and are often provided at reduced costs by health departments.

compiled from studies of radon-exposed underground miners and projected that 18,600 (range: 3,000–32,000) lung cancer deaths each year in the United States are attributable to residential 222Rn (progeny) exposure.

Large-scale case–control epidemiologic studies using enhanced dosimetry and pooled epidemiologic studies both in North America and Europe have demonstrated that prolonged exposure to radon decay products, even at or below the EPA's action level of 4 pCi/L, significantly increases lung cancer risk. The EPA estimates that approximately 21,000 lung cancer deaths in the United States each year are attributable to prolonged residential radon exposure. Inexpensive radon detection kits can be purchased at many hardware or discount stores and are often provided at reduced costs by local health departments. The most cost-effective approach of preventing radon-induced lung cancer is installation of radon-resistant construction at the time of new home construction. Radon concentrations can also be reduced in existing building through subslab depressurization.

SEE ALSO: Lung Cancer, Small Cell; Lung Cancer, Non-Small Cell; Radiation; Radiation, Ionizing.

BIBLIOGRAPHY. Sarah Darby, D. Hill, A. Auvinen, et al., "Radon in Homes and Risk of Lung Cancer: Collaborative Analysis of Individual Data from 13 European Case-Control Studies," *British Medical Journal* (v.330, 2005); R. William Field, D. J. Steck, B. J. Smith, et al., "Residential Radon Gas Exposure and Lung Cancer: The Iowa Radon Lung Cancer Study," *American Journal of Epidemiology* (v.151/11, 2000); Daniel Krewski, J. H. Lubin, J. M. Zielinski, et al., "Residential Radon and Risk of Lung Cancer: A Combined Analysis of 7 North American Case-Control Studies," *Epidemiology* (v.16/2, 2005); Jay Lubin, J. Boice, Jr., C. Edling, et al., "Radon and Lung Cancer Risk: A Joint Analysis of 11 Underground Miner Studies," NIH Publication No. 94-3644 (U.S. Department of Health and Human Services, 1994); National Research Council, "Risk Assessment of Radon in Drinking Water" (National Academy Press, 1998); National Research Council, "Health Effects of Exposure to Radon, BEIR VI" (National Academy Press, 1998).

R. FIELD
UNIVERSITY OF IOWA

Raloxifene

BREAST CANCER IS a common disease both in the United States and worldwide. Advances in breast cancer treatment in terms of surgery, radiation, and chemotherapy/hormonal therapy have resulted in improvements in survival for those diagnosed with breast cancer. However, in terms of eradicating breast cancer, efforts focused on prevention can be just as important as those focused on treatment. Raloxifene, a U.S. Food and Drug Administration (FDA)–approved medication that has been used for the treatment of osteoporosis, has been found to decrease the risk of developing invasive breast cancer. However, raloxifene has also been associated with a small increased risk of developing blood clots in the legs or lungs. The decision of whether to take raloxifene for breast cancer prevention should only be made in conjunction with a healthcare provider who can identify whether someone is at high enough risk for breast cancer to justify the rare but potentially harmful side effects.

IMPORTANCE OF BREAST CANCER PREVENTION

The American Cancer Society estimated that among women in the United States, roughly 210,000 new cases of invasive breast cancer will be diagnosed each year, with approximately 40,000 deaths attributable to breast cancer. Among U.S. women, this makes breast cancer the most common cancer and the second most common cause of cancer death (lung cancer is the most common cause of cancer death among U.S. women). The median age at breast cancer diagnosis is around 60 years, with 95 percent of breast cancers found in women aged 40 years or older at the time of diagnosis. Breast cancer among men is rare and makes up less than 1 percent of breast cancers diagnosed in the United States. Breast cancer incidence varies widely globally, with the highest rates found in the United States and Western Europe and the lowest rates found in Asia.

DESCRIPTION OF RALOXIFENE

Raloxifene belongs to a class of medications called selective estrogen receptor modulators (SERMs). Estrogens are hormones, the main actions of which are to help regulate reproductive functions, such as menstruation and pregnancy. In addition, estrogens help maintain bone density. To influence cellular functions, estrogen must first attach to estrogen receptors, which are proteins in the nuclei of cells with binding sites for estrogen. After estrogen binds to its receptor, the receptor complex can then activate or inhibit various genes. Before menopause, the main source of estrogen is the ovary; after menopause, estrogens are mainly produced in fat tissue. The principal circulating estrogens in women are called estradiol and estrone.

Medications that compete with estrogen for binding at the estrogen receptor or that affect the interaction of the estrogen receptor with estrogen and target genes can be important in preventing and treating estrogen-sensitive (also called estrogen receptor positive) breast cancers. Raloxifene binds at the estrogen receptor but is considered to be selective because in some tissues it has estrogen-like activity, whereas in other tissues its actions are antiestrogenic (i.e., opposite that of estrogen). For example, raloxifene has estrogen-like effects in bone but is antiestrogenic in breast tissue. Other examples of SERMs are tamoxifen, which is effective for both the prevention and treatment of breast cancer, and clomiphene, which is used to induce ovulation in the management of infertility.

RALOXIFENE'S EFFECTS

The majority of the data on the effects of raloxifene on cancer were derived from four large randomized clinical trials: MORE (Multiple Outcomes of Raloxifene Evaluation), CORE (Continuing Outcomes Relevant to Evista), STAR (Study of Tamoxifen and Raloxifene), and RUTH (Raloxifene Use for the Heart). The study designs are summarized below.

BENEFITS: BREAST CANCER PREVENTION

All three placebo-controlled studies (MORE, CORE, and RUTH) demonstrated a statistically significant decrease in the risk of invasive breast cancer, ranging from 44 percent (RUTH) to 72 percent (MORE) in women without a prior history of invasive breast cancer. The relative decrease in breast cancer risk was observed regardless of the subjects' risk of breast cancer, predicated by the Gail model (an epidemiologic model that predicts a person's 5-year risk of breast cancer using age, family history of breast cancer, reproductive history, and history of benign breast disease).

The STAR trial provided additional confirmatory evidence for raloxifene as a cancer prevention agent by demonstrating that raloxifene was as effective as tamoxifen in decreasing the incidence of invasive breast cancer. Tamoxifen was already FDA approved for both the treatment and prevention of estrogen-sensitive breast cancer. Similar to tamoxifen, raloxifene decreased the incidence only of estrogen receptor positive cancer, not estrogen receptor negative cancers. However, in contrast to tamoxifen, which also decreased the risk of in situ (noninvasive) breast cancer, raloxifene had no effect on the incidence of in situ cancers.

The ideal duration for raloxifene is still not known. Tamoxifen is generally used for only 5 years because data from the breast cancer treatment setting indicate that over time, the increasing risks of uterine cancer and thromboembolic events began to outweigh the benefits. In addition, the benefits of tamoxifen appear to last longer than 5 years, with continued benefit observed in the treatment trials of tamoxifen even when the drug stopped being administered. In the prevention setting, the CORE trial was the only trial that

Name of trial	First results published	Raloxifene compared to	Number of subjects	Length of planned treatment (years)	Median follow-up (years)
MORE	1999	Placebo	7705	4	4
CORE*	2004	Placebo	4011	8	7.9
STAR	2006	Tamoxifen	19747	5	3.9
RUTH	2006	Placebo	10101	N/A	5.6

* Please note that CORE participants represent a subgroup of subjects from MORE who chose to continue treatment for an additional four years.

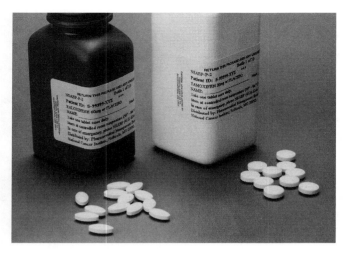

Raloxifene, an FDA–approved medication has been found to decrease the risk of developing invasive breast cancer.

examined a longer period of treatment (8 years), and it found continued benefit after 8 years of treatment compared to 4 years of treatment. However, it is possible that, similar to with raloxifene, the additional benefit of tamoxifen observed at 8 years simply represents a carryover effect from the first 4 years, rather than true continued benefit for 8 years of use. For the purposes of osteoporosis prevention or treatment, raloxifene should be continued indefinitely.

Estrogen deficiency is one of the main causes of osteoporosis after menopause. Raloxifene clearly increases bone density in postmenopausal women and is FDA approved for the treatment and prevention of osteoporosis. Several large, randomized trials have supported this indication, with raloxifene decreasing the incidence of vertebral fractures (fractures of the spine) by about one-third, though raloxifene had less of an effect on fractures outside of the spine.

Although raloxifene's effect on bone density was greater than that of placebo or tamoxifen, it was lesser in magnitude than the improvements observed with hormone replacement therapy or bisphosphonates. In premenopausal women, raloxifene decreased bone density, which is opposite to its effects in postmenopausal women. Nevertheless, raloxifene remains a reasonable option for the prevention and treatment of early osteoporosis in postmenopausal women.

Similar to tamoxifen, raloxifene has been associated with a significant decrease in low-density lipoprotein

(LDL) cholesterol. For example, in one multicenter randomized trial involving 601 women, those taking raloxifene had a 6.4 percent decrease in total cholesterol and 10.1 percent decrease in LDL cholesterol, compared to 1.2 percent and 1.0 percent, respectively, in those women taking the placebo. Although these changes were significant, they were relatively modest in magnitude compared to the effects of lipid-lowering agents, such as lovastatin or simvastatin. A few studies have also observed an increase in high-density lipoprotein (HDL) cholesterol with raloxifene, although this increase has not been consistently seen across all studies. Raloxifene does not affect triglycerides. However, despite these favorable effects on lipid profiles, there has been no effect of raloxifene on coronary events.

RISKS: THROMBOEMBOLIC EVENTS (BLOOD CLOTS AND STROKES)

In the placebo-controlled trials, raloxifene increased the risk of thromboembolic events, defined as either a pulmonary embolus (a blood clot within one of the blood vessels of the lung) or a deep venous thrombosis (a blood clot within one of the deep major veins of the leg). The risk of developing some type of thromboembolic event is about 50–100 percent higher in women on raloxifene compared to those on placebo. Although raloxifene clearly has a higher risk of thromboembolic events than placebo, the risk appears lower that that associated with tamoxifen and is still quite small overall (about one to two excess cases per 1,000 women per year on raloxifene).

Although tamoxifen has been clearly associated with an increased risk of stroke, the associations of this risk with raloxifene have been less clear. The RUTH trial did not observe any difference in the incidence of stroke between the placebo and raloxifene groups, but it did see a higher incidence of fatal stroke in the raloxifene group. Compared to tamoxifen in STAR, the risk of stroke appeared similar. Therefore, it appears that raloxifene may be associated with a small increase in stroke, although it is not clear whether this increase is the same or less than the stroke risk seen with tamoxifen.

OTHER SIDE EFFECTS

Women taking raloxifene were more likely to experience hot flushes, leg cramps, and peripheral edema (leg swelling) compared to those on placebo, although the overall occurrence of these symptoms in the raloxifene group was still low (less than 15 percent). In general, these side effects were not severe enough to prevent women from taking raloxifene as directed and usually resolved with continued use of the medication. For example, in the CORE study, during the second 4 years of raloxifene treatment, there was no difference in the incidence of hot flashes, leg cramps, or edema between the raloxifene and placebo groups despite the significant differences noted during the first 4 years of treatment. In addition, the more time elapsed since menopause, the lower the risk of hot flashes in women.

NO EFFECT: UTERINE CANCER
Estrogens stimulate the growth of uterine cells, which can lead to hyperplasia and cancer. Because of its estrogen-like effects in the uterus, tamoxifen can increase uterine cancer risk by about two- to three-fold. Unlike tamoxifen, raloxifene does not have a stimulatory effect on the uterus. Several studies evaluated serial uterine ultrasounds in women taking raloxifene and showed no increase in the thickness or proliferative activity of the endometrium (uterine lining). Confirming this, none of the placebo-controlled trials of raloxifene showed an increase in uterine cancer risk.

When compared directly to tamoxifen in STAR, the rates of uterine cancer showed a trend toward being lower in the raloxifene arm (36 cases with tamoxifen and 23 cases in raloxifene), although the difference did not reach statistical significance ($p = 0.07$). However, there was a statistically significant lower incidence of uterine hyperplasia (84 percent decrease) and lower hysterectomy rates for noncancer reasons in the raloxifene compared to the placebo arm (244 on tamoxifen compared to 111 on raloxifene). In summary, raloxifene does not appear to have a significant effect on uterine cancer risk.

HEART DISEASE AND CATARACTS
None of the randomized placebo-controlled trials of raloxifene demonstrated any difference in the incidence of coronary events between the raloxifene and placebo arms.
Tamoxifen has been associated with an increased risk of cataracts, but no such increase has been seen with raloxifene when compared to placebo. When directly

compared to tamoxifen in STAR, raloxifene had a lower risk of cataracts and cataract surgery.

ADVANCED BREAST CANCER
Although animal models of breast cancer suggested that raloxifene had antitumor activity, clinical studies in patients with metastatic (advanced) breast cancer were disappointing. No complete responses were observed, and the partial response rate was much lower than that for tamoxifen or other hormonal agents. Therefore, there is no role for raloxifene in the treatment of advanced breast cancer or for prevention of recurrence in women with a personal history of invasive or noninvasive breast cancer.

ROLE OF RALOXIFENE IN CANCER PREVENTION
Although raloxifene has not yet been approved by the FDA for breast cancer prevention, raloxifene can be considered a reasonable option, given the data from the randomized placebo controlled trials and its statistical equivalence to tamoxifen, a FDA-approved breast cancer prevention agent. Raloxifene can only be used in postmenopausal women. Scant data exist on raloxifene in premenopausal women, but its effects seem to differ compared to those in postmenopausal women, and it may also cause birth defects.

To decide who should consider raloxifene, the entry criteria for the clinical trials should be used, which include postmenopausal women older than 35 with a 5-year risk of breast cancer of at least 1.67 percent, calculated using the Gail model, or a history of lobular carcinoma in situ. Raloxifene is only available by prescription and should only be taken after consultation with a healthcare provider. Raloxifene is not indicated in women with a personal history of invasive breast cancer.

CONTROVERSIAL AREAS
It is unclear why raloxifene only decreased the risk of invasive breast cancer but not that in situ, whereas tamoxifen decreased the risk of both invasive and noninvasive breast cancers. The majority of the subjects in the clinical trials evaluating raloxifene were Caucasian, so it is not known whether raloxifene would have the same effects in other populations.

Given that primary breast cancer is postulated to develop over many years and the majority of the trials evaluated treatment durations of less than 5 years, it is not clear whether raloxifene truly prevents the development of new breast cancer or simply suppresses the growth or development of subclinical breast cancer.

Although tamoxifen was approved by the FDA in 1998 as a breast cancer prevention agent, use has been limited because of concerns regarding tamoxifen's risk (mainly uterine cancer and thromboembolic events) and also because of the unfamiliarity of primary care providers with tamoxifen, which has primarily been used by oncologists. However, accumulating data have supported the use of raloxifene as a breast cancer prevention agent. Although raloxifene can increase the risk of uncommon adverse events such as thromboembolic events, it can also decrease the risk of both invasive breast cancer and vertebral fractures, so it should be considered as a possible cancer prevention agent in women at higher risk for breast cancer but lower risk for thromboembolic events.

SEE ALSO: Breast Cancer.

BIBLIOGRAPHY. American Cancer Society, *Breast Cancer Facts & Figures 2005–2006* (American Cancer Society, 2006); E. Barrett-Connor, L. Mosca, P. Collins, et al., "Effects of Raloxifene on Cardiovascular Events and Breast Cancer in Postmenopausal Women," *New England Journal of Medicine* (v.355/2, 2006); J. A. Cauley, L. Norton, M. E. Lippman, et al., "Continued Breast Cancer Risk Reduction in Postmenopausal Women Treated with Raloxifene: 4-Year Results from the MORE Trial. Multiple Outcomes of Raloxifene Evaluation," *Breast Cancer Research and Treatment* (v.65/2, 2001); P. D. Delmas, N. H. Bjarnason, B. H. Mitlak, et al., "Effects of Raloxifene on Bone Mineral Density, Serum Cholesterol Concentrations, and Uterine Endometrium in Postmenopausal Women," *New England Journal of Medicine* (v.337/23, 1997); S. Martino, J. A. Cauley, E. Barrett-Connor, et al., "Continuing Outcomes Relevant to Evista: Breast Cancer Incidence in Postmenopausal Osteoporotic Women in a Randomized Trial of Raloxifene," *Journal of the National Cancer Institute* (v.96/23, 2004); V. G. Vogel, J. P. Costantino, D. L. Wickerham, et al., "Effects of Tamoxifen vs Raloxifene on the Risk of Developing Invasive Breast Cancer and Other Disease Outcomes: The NSABP Study of Tamoxifen and Raloxifene (STAR) P-2 trial," *Journal of the American Medical Association* (v.295/23, 2006).

Wendy Chen
Harvard University

Rectal Cancer

RECTAL CANCER IS one of the most fatal forms of cancer, ranking second to lung cancer in men and third after lung and breast cancer in women. Genetics plays an important role in the development of rectal cancer; a genetic link to the disease is present in more than half of all cases. Other factors include alcohol intake and a diet high in animal fats and proteins. Viruses, especially retroviruses, play a role is about 15 percent of rectal cancer cases. Dietary fiber, retinoids, selenium, and calcium, in contrast, may be protective. In the United States, 135,000 new cases of rectal cancer appear each year.

DISEASE PROGRESSION

Rectal cancer develops in a multistep path. The first sign is often a polyp—a small, benign growth in the colon lining, with fast-dividing cells. Through gradual accumulation of mutations that activate oncogenes and knock out tumor-suppressor genes, this polyp can develop into a malignant tumor. About six DNA changes must occur for a cell to become fully cancerous. These usually include the appearance of at least one active oncogene, the mutation or loss of several tumor-suppressor genes, and chromosome abnormalities. In many malignant tumors, the gene for telomerase is activated, removing a natural limit on the number of times the cell can divide.

Rectal cancer occurs in five main steps. First, a loss of tumor-suppressor gene *APC* occurs in the normal rectal epithelial cells. Following this, a small benign growth (polyp) develops. Second, the *Ras* oncogene becomes activated, causing abnormal cell growth. Third, loss of tumor-suppressor gene *DCC* follows, giving new cancer cells more freedom to grow and resulting in the formation of a much larger benign growth (adenoma). Fourth, there is a loss of tumor-suppressor gene *p53*. Finally, additional mutations result in the transition from a benign to a malignant tumor (carcinoma). Signs and symptoms of rectal cancer may include diarrhea, cramping, constipation, abdominal pain, and rectal bleeding, which may be visible or occult.

DIAGNOSIS AND TREATMENT

Screening of rectal cancer may involve testing the blood in feces, digital rectal examination, colonoscopy, sigmoidoscopy, and barium enema. A newer approach to detecting rectal cancer is a positron emission tomography (PET) scan. During a PET scan, a radioactive sugar is first injected into the patient; the sugar will collect in rectal tissues with high metabolic activity, such as cancer cells. Using three-dimensional scanning technology, an image is obtained by measurements involving emission of radiation from the sugar. This image fits the exact contours of rectal cancer cells. PET scans are not, however, used on a regular basis for screening rectal cancers.

The primary treatment for rectal cancer is surgery, followed by chemotherapy or radiotherapy. The type of treatment chosen depends on the stage of the disease at the time of diagnosis. Rectal cancer is fully treatable in early stages; however, fewer treatment options are available in later stages. Patients with hereditary rectal cancer, such as hereditary nonpolyposis colorectal cancer or familial adenomatous polyposis may be referred for genetic counseling and genetic testing.

SEE ALSO: American Association for Cancer Education; Colon Cancer.

BIBLIOGRAPHY. National Cancer Institute, "Genetics of Colorectal Cancer (PDQ)," www.cancer.gov/ (cited October 2006); Robert L. Nussbaum, Roderick R. McInnes, and Huntington F. Willard, *Thompson & Thompson Genetics in Medicine* (6th ed.) (Saunders, 2001); Gerard J. Tortora and Sandra R. Grabowski, *Principles of Anatomy & Physiology* (Wiley, 2003).

RAHUL GLADWIN
UNIVERSITY OF HEALTH SCIENCES ANTIGUA—
SCHOOL OF MEDICINE

Religion

DESPITE INCREASING CANCER survival rates, because of high mortality rates, cancer is still perceived as a life-threatening disease. As a consequence, a cancer diagnosis may immediately evoke existential apprehension not only for those diagnosed but also for those close to them. An acute awareness of the possibility of dying is likely to raise questions about the ultimate meaning of existence and the nature of reality. When people with religious beliefs or a spiritual orientation to life are faced with a serious stressor, they often use religion/spirituality to cope. Not surprisingly, religious/spiritual coping is one of the most common coping strategies used by cancer patients and their families. How an individual appraises the cancer experience from a religious/spiritual viewpoint affects whether religious/spiritual coping is beneficial or harmful. Many studies, although not all, have found a positive association between religious/spiritual coping and quality of life.

Although no consensus has emerged, a distinction between religion and spirituality has been made. Religion is usually understood to involve a formal system of religious beliefs and practices intended to facilitate a relationship with a deity and promote a person's relationship to self and others. Spirituality is generally understood to involve an individual's search for purpose, meaning, inner peace, and direction in life, which may or may not include belief in a deity or religious practices. Spirituality is a component of religion, but religion is not necessarily a component of spirituality.

Social support may be an important component of this more formal system of religious beliefs. Whereas spiritual support is perceived as support from God or Powerful Other, which deals with the individual's personal relationship with God or Powerful Other, social (congregational) support deals with interpersonal support from clergy or members of an individual's religious/spiritual community. These categories (spiritual and social support) may overlap, for example, in prayers for healing by clergy or by others in the religious/spiritual community.

FACING CANCER: RELIGIOUS/ SPIRITUAL COPING

As the cancer patient and family struggle to understand why they or their loved one has been diagnosed with cancer, an existential or religious/spiritual crisis may be triggered. Their most basic assumptions about the world may be challenged. They may fear that God or Powerful Other has abandoned them or that the illness is a divine judgment. Some may abandon their faith or conclude that life is meaningless. Alternatively, they may find that their faith or spirituality helps them cope with cancer. Many survivors report that cancer has deepened their faith, given them a closer relationship with God or others, or changed their values for the better, or that they have found new meaning in life.

Studies examining religious/spiritual coping in medically ill patients have found that 34–84 percent used religion/spirituality to cope with their illness. In general, religious/spiritual coping refers to the use of cognitive and behavioral efforts that arise out of one's religion or spirituality to manage specific external or internal demands. Religious/spiritual coping methods are multidimensional and can span the range from active to passive, from emotional to cognitive, from inner to interpersonal, and from positive to negative. Religious/spiritual coping assists in the search for meaning and purpose as well as providing comfort and a sense of personal control. Religious/spiritual coping is prominent among advanced stage cancer patients and those socially disenfranchised, including the elderly, immigrants, and racial/ethnic minorities.

The literature on posttraumatic growth or benefit finding in response to cancer has highlighted the potential for beneficial changes, such as finding meaning in life and spiritual growth as a result of cancer. Some studies have found that religious/spiritual coping promotes long-term adjustment to cancer by maintaining the patient's self-esteem; providing a sense of meaning, purpose, and hope in life; and giving the patient emotional comfort. The use of religious/spiritual coping has been related to greater life satisfaction, happiness, and positive affect. Individuals can reframe the cancer experience either positively or negatively based on their belief system. Religious/spiritual practices such as prayer and meditation can provide inner peace as well as a sense of control over events in medical situations likely to induce feelings of helplessness. Religious/spiritual belief systems can provide a framework for understanding and facing mortality.

In contrast, all studies examining the role of religious/spiritual coping have not produced positive outcomes. For example, a recent survey conducted by Gallup found that church attendance and seeking support from a priest/minister was associated with greater distress among Catholics, which was not the case among Evangelicals. Similarly, the beneficial effect of service attendance in lowering depressive symptoms was found only for black participants. Furthermore, studies have also found religious/spiritual coping to be harmful. Certain kinds of religious/spiritual coping, such as questioning or avoiding, have been associated with greater levels of general as well as cancer-specific distress and with diminished life satisfaction and emotional and social well-being. Although these studies are quite limited, they do indicate the possibility that whether the use of religious/spiritual coping has beneficial or detrimental effects depends on the individual's personality, religious denominations, and sociocultural context.

FAMILY AND FRIENDS

As the number of cancer survivors increases, the number of family members and friends who provide care or support also increases. Family members often assume the role of primary caregivers of cancer patients after hospital discharge. Provision of cancer care is a unique and specific type of stress because of the threat of death, and family and friend caregivers may use religion/spirituality to cope. Surprisingly little is known about family members' use of religious/spiritual coping or experiences in finding faith and meaning from the challenge of cancer in a close relative.

A few studies examined the role of spirituality among spousal cancer caregivers and found that maintaining faith and finding meaning in cancer caregiving buffered the adverse effects of caregiving stress on mental health, whereas it aggravated the caregiving stress effects on physical health. Efforts to encourage caregivers to attend to their own needs, seek health services, and manage stress effectively are particularly important for highly spiritual cancer caregivers, who are prone to neglect themselves. Improved self-care, however, may pose significant challenges for these caregivers, because they may have to lessen the intensity of the care they provide. They may then feel guilty, thereby increasing stress and potentially reducing the stress-buffering effects for mental health. How best to maintain the balance between mental and physical health while providing care is a complex issue, particularly for highly spiritual caregivers, and deserves further investigation.

SPIRITUAL SUPPORT INTERVENTIONS

The importance of teamwork in cancer care among patients, their family caregivers, medical professionals, community volunteers, and spiritual counselors has been acknowledged in various disciplines. An increasing number of institutions are including religion/spirituality in the curriculum for healthcare students, particularly in oncology. Understanding the perspective of patients and their family on illness, death, and dying from diverse religious and philosophical orientations is the key for the most effective spiritual support, particularly at the end of life.

Harvey Chochinov and colleagues have developed a promising novel intervention, Dignity Therapy, for reducing suffering and distress at the end of life. Dignity Therapy, which is designed to address psychosocial and existential distress, has been tailored to address the psychosocial and existential needs of terminally ill cancer patients. This therapy is intended to help the patient develop heightened senses of dignity and meaning, an increased sense of purpose and will to live, and reduced suffering and depressive symptoms, leading to a better quality of life for both patient and family members. Brenda Cole and Kenneth Pargament have developed "Re-Creating Your Life," a psychotherapeutic intervention for cancer patients that addresses existential concerns related to control, identity, relationships, and meaning.

A few interventions focusing on spirituality or religious coping have been developed to help family and friends not only during cancer treatment and survivorship but also in coping with bereavement. These programs identify families at risk of complicated bereavement through screening and then help them to achieve better family functioning, thus improving psychosocial adjustment.

SEE ALSO: Survivors of Cancer Families.

BIBLIOGRRAPHY: Gallup International Millennium Survey (2000); I. C. Thuné-Boyle, J. A. Stygall, M. R. Keshtgar, and S. P. Newman. "Do Religious/Spiritual Coping Strategies Affect Illness Adjustment in Patients with Cancer? A Systematic Review of the Literature," *Social Science and Medicine* (v.63, 2006); H. M. Chochinov, T. Hack, T. Hassard, L. J. Kristjanson, S. McClement, and M. Harlos, "Dignity Therapy: A Novel Psychotherapeutic Intervention for Patients Near the End of Life," *Journal of Clinical Oncology* (v.23, 2005); M. Stefanek, P. G. McDonald, and S. A. Hess, "Religion, Spirituality and Cancer: Current Status and Methodological Challenges," *Psycho-Oncology* (v.14, 2005).

YOUNGMEE KIM, PH.D.
CORINNE CRAMMER, PH.D.
MICHAEL STEFANEK, PH.D.
AMERICAN CANCER SOCIETY

Religion, Jewish Women and Cancer

FAMILY HISTORY IS an extremely important risk factor for cancers of the breasts, ovaries, colon, and prostate. As patients are being empowered to become more active in their own healthcare, it becomes increasingly important to develop detailed records of familial health history, both past and present. This past decade has produced many profound changes in the understanding of how certain cancers follow familial lines. One of the most dramatic findings is the significantly higher incidence of Ashkenazi women developing breast and ovarian cancers as compared to non-Jewish women and non-Ashkenazi (Sephardic) Jewish women.

The correlation between Jewish women of Ashkenazi (Eastern European) descent and higher risk for breast and certain other cancers has been attributed to inherited alterations or mutations in the BRCA1 and BRCA2 genes. BRCA1 and BRCA2 refer to the breast cancer 1 and breast cancer 2 genes, respectively. The specific mutation appears to be a shortened protein, which may result in that protein's inability to function properly in its role of repairing mutations in other genes. Over time, this malfunction may cause uncontrolled cell growth, resulting in tumor formation.

POPULATION ANALYSIS

Within the general population of families with histories significant for breast cancer, over 100 alterations have been identified in each of the BRCA genes.

In Ashkenazi families with histories of hereditary cancer, three specific alterations in these genes have been identified as being associated with an increased risk of breast and ovarian cancers in women and prostate cancer in men.

Two of these three gene alterations occur in BRCA1, and one occurs in BRCA2. These two specific BRCA1 alterations can be found in approximately 1.1 percent of the Ashkenazi Jewish population. In the general U.S. population, however, the percentage of people with any mutation in BRCA1 is estimated to be between 0.1 and 0.6 percent.

Women with an inherited BRCA1 or BRCA2 mutation reportedly not only have up to an 80 percent chance of developing breast cancer during their life-time but also have a significantly higher chance of developing it at a younger age (premenopause) than women who are not born with one of these gene mutations. Ashkenazi Jews are reported to be five times more likely than the general population to have an altered BRCA1 or BRCA2 gene. This translates into approximately 23 people out of 1,000 Ashkenazi Jews with the mutation.

DEFINING ASHKENAZI

Ashkenazi Jews can be defined in the context of multiple perspectives including religious, cultural, linguistic, and ethnic. For the purpose of evaluating the inherited genetic traits and mutations as described above, Ashkenazi Jews, also called Ashkenazim, are defined as Jews whose ancestry contains descendants of Jews from Germany, Poland, Austria, and Eastern Europe.

With a history of approximately 1,000 years of reproductive isolation, the Ashkenazim genome is relatively well defined. In fact, in 2006, a study of the DNA passed from mother to child, mtDNA (mitochondrial DNA), indicated a maternal lineage that traced nearly 40 percent of the current Ashkenazi population's population to just four women.

As with other populations with largely endogamous (marriage within a specific group) histories, Ashkenazim have a greater probability of inheriting and passing on ethnospecific genes. Other historically endogamous ethnic groups with newly discovered, potentially significant, genetic alterations include Icelandic, Norwegian, and Dutch.

GENETIC TESTING

The highest probabilities of a linkage between breast and ovarian cancers and BRCA1 or BRCA2 genes occurs within families with multiple cases of breast cancer, within families with histories of both breast and ovarian cancer, within families where one or more family members developed two separate primary cancers, and within families of Ashkenazi Jewish heritage.

Both men and women with altered BRCA1 or BRCA2 genes can pass it down to both their male and female children. It is important to note, however, that parents who do possess alterations in BRCA1 or BRCA2 do not necessarily produce offspring who will

inherit the mutated genes. Further, inheriting altered BRCA1 or BRCA2 genes does not mean that the person will get cancer, it just means they are at higher risk. In addition, even if the mutations are inherited and cancer develops, not every cancer in these families will be linked to alterations in these genes.

Genetic testing can be used to detect such gene mutations, and thus the risk of developing certain cancers, and is often recommended in high-risk families. Again, it is important to keep in mind that positive test results (i.e., results indicating that inherited mutations in BRCA1 or BRCA2 are present) indicate an increased risk of developing certain cancers—they do not predict whether cancer will develop. Conversely, having a negative test result does not mean the person will not get cancer, it just means that the person's risk of cancer is the same as that of the general population.

For women who do test positive for the gene mutations, there are evolving levels of cancer risk management including, but not limited to, monitoring techniques, prophylactic surgeries, behavioral modifications, chemoprevention, and potentially gene therapy.

MONITORING AND TREAMENTS

Diligent monitoring of the breasts and ovaries is key for early detection of breast and ovarian cancers. The earlier the detection, the greater the possibility of successful treatments. Breast surveillance procedures, especially when used in combination with each other, are very effective for discovering early signs of breast cancer. The best current breast monitoring and early detection techniques are, in order of efficacy, mammograms, clinical exams, and breast self-exams.

Ovarian cancers, in contrast, notoriously escape early detection, in large part because of the ambiguous nature of the symptoms, such as leg or back pain, gas, bloating, off-cycle bleeding, and indigestion. Contributing further to delayed detection of ovarian cancers is the lack of sufficient screening options. Current screening methods include transvaginal sonography, the CA-125 blood test, and clinical exams. Transvaginal ultrasound, although generally reliable for detecting tumorous growths, is not effective at distinguishing between cancerous and benign growths.

CA-125 blood tests are designed to determine the levels of CA-125 protein in the blood. It developed as an evaluation tool because many women with ovarian cancer display higher levels of this protein. Unfortunately, the CA-125 blood test is an inconsistent measure at best because some noncancerous conditions can increase the blood levels of CA-125 for a false-positive effect, and some ovarian cancers do not produce enough CA-125 to test positive, resulting in a false-negative effect.

Prophylactic surgeries are radical preventative measures that involve the removal of healthy tissues that are most at risk for developing cancer. Although preventative mastectomy (removal of healthy breasts) and preventative salpingo-oophorectomy (removal of healthy fallopian tubes and ovaries) procedures do remove much of the tissue at risk, some tissue remnants are invariably still present in the body, and thus these surgeries are not a 100 percent guarantee against developing breast or ovarian cancers.

Chemoprevention, also called chemoprophylaxis, is the administration of substances intended to reduce the risk of developing cancer. Clinical chemoprevention trials are currently being conducted to evaluate intervention techniques incorporating the use of diet, vitamins, and hormone therapies.

SEE ALSO: Chemoprevention; Surgery.

BIBLIOGRAPHY. Doron M. Behar, E. Metspalu, T. Kivisild, et al., "The Matrilineal Ancestry of Ashkenazi Jewry: Portrait of a Recent Founder Event," *American Journal of Human Genetics* (v.78/3, 2006); American Cancer Society, *Detailed Guide: Ovarian Cancer*, www.cancer.org/ (cited May 2006); National Institutes of Health, *Questions and Answers for Estimating Cancer Risk in Ashkenazi Jews*, rex.nci.nih.gov/ (cited May 1997); National Institutes of Health, National Human Genome Institute, www.genome.gov (cited September 2006).

JILLIAN CIPA-TATUM
INDEPENDENT SCHOLAR

Religion, Meditation and Risk

MEDITATION IS THE practice of freeing the mind from conscious thought and becoming aware only of the individual within the universe. It is believed by practitioners that meditation enables the individual to reach elevated states of consciousness associated with spiritual understanding that is superior to that of people who are unable to achieve these states. Many, if not all, major religions have some form of meditative tradition, and they are often related to an ascetic movement within the larger body of religious thought. Nevertheless, the most well-known and perhaps most commonly practiced forms of meditation are those associated with the south and east Asian religions of Hinduism, and particularly Buddhism.

Buddhist meditation is aimed deliberately at helping to free the mind from samsara, which is the endless wheel of suffering in which the soul is constantly reborn into a new existence, with all the pain that entails, until such time as it is able to grasp the message of the Lord Buddha—that it is desire that links the soul to the physical universe. If the mind can be trained to release its grasp on the desire for physical things, for which the first step is to understand the nature and extent of that desire, then it can move toward the state of enlightenment, in which no further rebirth is necessary. As a consequence, the one who would wish to meditate is taught to become mindful of the body, of breathing in and out, and of the interaction between the body and the surrounding world. As this mindfulness increases, the various forms of desire that the body exhibits become more apparent, and consequently, steps may be taken to conquer and eradicate those forms of desire. There are many stories of famous monks and other advanced practitioners of meditation who are able to demonstrate superhuman detachment from physical appetites and even display abilities such as levitation. Some scientific experiments do indicate that deep forms of meditation can bring about different patterns of brainwave activity, although it is not yet clear what the implications of this meditation might be.

Meditation in the Western tradition tends to focus on the reduction of the distractions to the mind that arise from manifestations of the physical world, which will assist the mind in freeing itself from mundane considerations and then be free to pursue advanced intellectual or religious truths. This form of meditation is evident in the work of the philosopher Rene Descartes. It is a form of quietism in which the trivialities of the physical world are recognized for the vanities that they are, which in turn enables the mind to concentrate on the eternal verities that should be the main interest of the soul and on its desire to travel to heaven. This form of meditation is well known from the thoughts of Marcus Aurelius and Boethius.

Meditation is advocated by some people as a possible treatment against cancer. There is no clinical evidence to indicate that it can be an effective treatment, although it does appear that individuals who are able to use meditation to achieve a calm and positive frame of mind sometimes respond better to treatment in some cases. However, this is likely to be because of the positive nature of the mindset, which can arise from a number of causes. The various forms of yoga, for example, which are derived from south Asian religious practices, commonly have as a stated aim the improvement of physical as well as mental health through breathing exercises and through training the body to become more disciplined and resistant to external stimuli.

It is also possible that east Asian martial arts and practices such as Tai Chi are also part of meditation, in that they encourage the mind to enter a Zen-like state in which, by concentrating entirely on a well-practiced and repetitive set of physical exercises, the mind enters a state equivalent to meditation. Insofar as meditation is able to bring the mind and body into a more relaxed state, at least partially freeing a patient from anxiety and stress, it will have a positive effect on receptivity to cancer treatments (and, indeed, all forms of medical intervention). The American Cancer Society, for example, observes that, "Meditation is a mind-body process that uses concentration or reflection to relax the body and calm the mind." The society lists meditation, along with Tai Chi, yoga, music therapy, and other activities, as "helpful complementary approach[es]."

SEE ALSO: Religion.

BIBLIOGRAPHY. Boethius Ancius, *The Consolation of Philosophy* (Penguin Classics, 2000); Rael B. Cahn, and John Polich, "Meditation States and Traits: EEG, ERP, and Neuroimaging Studies," *Psychological Bulletin* (v.132/2, 2006); Rene Descartes, *Meditations on First Philosophy: In Which the Existence of God and the Distinction of the Soul are Demonstrated* (Hackett Publishing Company, 1993); Marcus Aurelius, *Meditations* (Penguin Classics, 2006); Alan B. Wallace, *Genuine Happiness: Meditation as the Path to Fulfillment* (Wiley, 2005); American Cancer Society, www.cancer.org/

JOHN WALSH
SHINAWATRA UNIVERSITY

Religion, Preventability vs. Preordained

CULTURE AND RELIGION have long been known to play a vital role in influencing one's health beliefs and health-seeking behaviors. The effect of religion on one's health-seeking behaviors varies between religions with different belief systems. The conviction that disease may be prevented through medicine, prayer, or repentance may have an entirely different effect on one's health than the belief that one's disease is preordained by a higher force. Although the role of religion in the prevention or course of cancer is often underaddressed by healthcare professionals, research has demonstrated that behaviors related to cancer screening, coping with cancer, seeking treatment for cancer, and overall quality of life can be greatly influenced by one's religious beliefs.

Over the past several years, the importance of religious beliefs in the context of health, illness, and clinical practice has played an increasing role. The use of religion and spirituality in coping is particularly prevalent in patients with cancer, given the potentially life-threatening nature of the illness. Failure to understand the culture and religious beliefs of a target group can significantly hinder health professionals' efforts to promote health activities and services to that group.

Fatalism, or the belief that all of human destiny is predetermined by a higher power, was present in the beliefs of the ancient Stoics and still pervades much of Hindu, Buddhist, and Islam thought today. According to fatalism, human behavior cannot change future events, which are preordained and absolute. Fate is a cosmic determinism, irrational and impersonal in nature. As such, disease and suffering are considered a natural part of life, which can not be prevented.

Fatalistic beliefs have been shown to decrease participation in cancer-screening activities. Studies have shown that routine mammography, for example, is an uncommon practice in Chinese women raised in the teachings of Buddhism, Taoism, and Confucianism. One study has demonstrated that only 32 percent of Chinese-American immigrant women have ever undergone a mammography, compared to 86 percent of white Americans. According to another study, twice as many Chinese-American women as white Americans had never heard of a mammography or breast examination.

In interviews with Chinese women who immigrated to Australia, the women expressed dismissal of Western paradigms of health promotion and prevention. They felt the Western notions were irrelevant, as most of the women viewed disease as something associated with the unchanging cycle in the Chinese philosophy of birth, aging, sickness, and death. Some women believed that negative thoughts, such as thinking about cancer, could possibly bring about a negative outcome and affect one's health. Many of these women did not discuss cancer in their communities because it was an unpleasant topic, and they were therefore unlikely to recommend screening to their friends. Other women did not see any point to breast cancer screening, as they felt that it would in no way change the likelihood that they could develop cancer.

Divine Providence, in contrast to fatalism, is considered to be supremely personal and rational. According to Divine Providence, which dominates much of Jewish and Christian thought, God plays a significant role in guiding and supporting earthly events, although free will can ultimately affect one's future. Believers in Divine Providence argue that disease can be prevented by physical, cognitive, and spiritual actions and that one's behavior may even alter the course of disease.

Many people who believe that disease can be prevented feel the need to respect their body, because it's God's creation, by participating in healthy behaviors. Furthermore, many stress the importance of positive hopes despite a grave diagnosis, and others even offer prayers asking God to intervene and heal the sick.

Statistics show that over half of American adults attend religious services at least once per month; this rate is even higher among African-American adults (67 percent). As such, the church is serving as a powerful channel for health promotion and educa-tion efforts by incorporating religious aspects of the church into behavior-changing programs.

In recent years, the church has been used effectively to include a wide range of health programs, including prostate cancer education, cervical cancer control, and mammography screening. These church-based interventions have been especially successful in African-American communities, in large part because of the central role of the church and the strong link between faith and health in the African-American community.

Although many African Americans have low health-seeking behaviors because of a lack of awareness, fear of doctors or disease, and previous negative experiences with the screening processes, most view cancer as a preventable disease. In one study, African-American men and women expressed affirmative thoughts that prostate cancer could be prevented by healthy behaviors and cancer-screening methods, and it was demonstrated that strong faith encouraged adherence to health promotion practices. The study participants also expressed the attitude that the body is God's temple and should be cared for properly.

Some African-American men still expressed somewhat fatalistic attitudes, which often resulted in decreased screening for prostate cancer. Many of these men, however, still felt that they should encourage others to actively fight the disease and hope for a cure with God's help. Other religious beliefs in the African-American community, such as the belief that disease is a punishment for sin, may discourage active participation in health promotion and cancer prevention activities.

COPING WITH RELIGION

Religious activities have been shown to be among the highest coping strategies. Religious coping with disease, although usually thought of as an emotional process, has cognitive (i.e., attributing disease to God's master plan) and behavioral (i.e., going to church) components. Studies have demonstrated that between 34 and 86 percent of patients with a serious medical illness use religious cognitions or activities to help cope. Religious coping has been shown to be typically more helpful than hindering to one's health, particularly when God is seen as compassionate and a willing collaborator.

Religious coping has been shown to have a strong effect on the quality of life in patients with cancer. Positive religious coping, such as benevolent religious appraisals, has been shown to significantly improve patients' quality of life, whereas negative religious coping, such as feelings of anger toward God, has been shown to decrease patients' quality of life. Fatalistic beliefs have often been shown to correlate with an increased quality of life, presumably because patients accept death and disease as an inevitable component to the circle of life.

Studies have further demonstrated that the belief that developing a disease is preordained certainty greatly affects whether patients will seek treatment for cancer and remain compliant with that treatment. One study showed that fatalistic beliefs were among the highest contributors for refusing the diagnosis for, or treatment of, lung cancer. Physicians need to be aware of one's cultural beliefs when diagnosing cancer and proposing a treatment strategy.

The role of religion in health beliefs and health-seeking behaviors has been gaining increasing attention over the years. Many physicians, particularly those serving minority populations, are currently being educated in cross-cultural awareness. An approach by healthcare professionals that is understanding and sensitive toward patients' belief systems, combined with effective patient education, is essential to ensuring that patients participate in screening activities for disease and adhere to treatment strategies.

SEE ALSO: Religion; Religion, Use of Interventions; Psychosocial Issues and Cancer; Screening, Access to.

BIBLIOGRAPHY. Deborah E. Blocker, LaHoma Smith Romocki, Kamilah B. Thomas, et al., "Knowledge, Beliefs and Barriers Associated with Prostate Cancer Prevention and Screening Behaviors among African-American Men," *Journal of the National Medical Association* (v.98, 2006); Cannas Kwok and Gerard Sullivan, "Influence of Traditional Chinese Beliefs on Cancer Screening Behaviour among Chinese-Australian Women," *Journal of Advanced Nursing* (v.54, 2006); Alicia K. Matthews, Nerida Berrios, Julie S. Darnell, and Elizabeth Calhoun, "A Qualitative Evaluation of a Faith-Based Breast and Cervical Cancer Screening Intervention for African American Women," *Health Education and Behavior* (v.33, 2006); Barbara F. Sharp, Linda A. Steljes, and Howard S. Gordon, "A Little Bitty Spot and I'm a Big Man: Patients' Perspectives on Refusing Diagnosis or Treatment for Lung Cancer," *Psycho-Oncology* (v.14, 2005).

SHAUN E. GRUENBAUM
COLUMBIA UNIVERSITY MEDICAL CENTER
BENJAMIN F. GRUENBAUM
UNIVERSITY OF CONNECTICUT

Religion, Use of Interventions

RELIGION AND SPIRITUALITY are often highly involved in individuals' processes of coping with the stresses of cancer, from diagnosis through treatment and into long-term survivorship. Although religion and spirituality exert multiple influences on well-being, their effects are generally regarded as helpful. Because of these common and salutary roles of religion and spirituality in the context of cancer, a number of psychosocial interventions centered on religion and spirituality have been developed; such approaches are typically classified as complementary and alternative medicine interventions. Although research on these interventions is still in its early stages, there is evidence that interventions based on a religious or spiritual framework can be effective in increasing physical, emotional, and spiritual well-being for those living with or recovering from cancer.

DESCRIPTION OF RELIGIOUS/ SPIRITUAL INTERVENTIONS

Religious/spiritual interventions for those with cancer vary widely in terms of structure and content. Such interventions can be conducted in a group or a one-on-one format, and often involve cognitive-behavioral techniques, along with sharing, ritual, prayer, affirmation, imagery, reading and contemplation, and meditation. Pastoral counseling approaches are also common religious/spiritual interventions for cancer patients and survivors. A variety of topics commonly targeted for exploration in religious and spiritual interventions includes the implications of the cancer for one's life and how it may be integrated into one's identity; issues of meaning and purpose in life; emotions such as fear, anger, and grief; control over cancer and over one's life, and the role of God in this control; spiritual doubt or struggle; forgiveness; and one's relationship with other people and with God.

One central component of most religious/spiritual interventions is the process of coping with the cancer, including the religious and nonreligious meanings that patients may assign to their cancer, the resources that religiousness and spirituality may provide, and the various coping strategies that draw on religion and spirituality and that may be brought to bear in dealing with the myriad stressors of diagnosis and treatment. Regarding the meaning of cancer, religious and spiritual interventions encourage patients and survivors to explore their understanding of why and how the cancer occurred and what it represents for them in the context of their lives. Regarding resources, religious and spiritual interventions typically encourage cancer patients to examine the previous and current roles of religion and spirituality in their lives and to identify aspects that may provide strength and comfort as they deal with treatment and its aftermath. Religious and spiritual resources may include specific traditions, teachings, and beliefs; group, congregational, and clergy support; and one's personal relationship with God or a deity. Religious coping strategies that have been shown to be helpful in dealing with illness include relying on religious spiritual and social support resources, praying or meditating, drawing strength and comfort from one's religion or spirituality, relying on God as a collaborator in facing problems, and using religious and spiritual perspectives to reframe situations in more positive ways.

EFFECTIVENESS OF RELIGIOUS/SPIRITUAL INTERVENTIONS

Because the many complexities of individuals' cancer situations, including prognosis, length and type of treatment, time since diagnosis and treatment, iatrogenic effects, and other factors, studies on the effectiveness of religious and spiritual interventions for those dealing with cancer or its aftermath are difficult to conduct. Nonetheless, research is accumulating that documents the effectiveness of religious and spiritual interventions in the context of cancer. Such interventions have been shown to have positive effects on physical, emotional, and spiritual aspects of well-being. Aspects of cancer patients' physical well-being shown to be positively influenced by religious and spiritual interventions include reported suffering resulting from

treatment side effects, frequency and severity of pain, physical functioning, quality of life, and even mortality. Emotional aspects of cancer patients' well-being shown to improve following religious and spiritual interventions include depression, anxiety, hopelessness, isolation, and fear. Perhaps most important, spiritual outcomes of cancer patients, such as a sense of peace and a sense of meaning in life, appear to be positively influenced by religious and spiritual interventions.

MECHANISMS OF EFFECT

Although research has documented the beneficial effects of religious and spiritual interventions on a variety of indices of well-being, the mechanisms through which these interventions exert their positive effects are less clear. First, it appears that religious and spiritual interventions can increase cancer patients' sense of hope and optimism. This may allow them to experience higher levels of positive emotion and to be more resilient over time as they face the vicissitudes of cancer treatment and recovery. In addition, these interventions may help individuals to maintain a sense of self-esteem and emotional peace and comfort, as well as to strengthen their emotional bonds with others. In turn, these positive emotions may enhance cancer patients' motivation to survive and recover, leading them to be more engaged in their treatment and to adhere better to their treatment and perform health behaviors that may enhance their physical as well as psychological recovery. In addition, drawing on religious and spiritual resources and coping strategies may reduce cancer patients' stress levels, allowing them to direct their energies toward healing.

In addition, religious and spiritual interventions explore issues of control, a central concern of most cancer patients. Because much of the cancer experience is beyond the patient's control, feelings of being overwhelmed and helpless can arise. Religious and spiritual approaches to issues of control can help patients to find a more comfortable balance between taking active control over some aspects of their treatment and accepting more comfortably those aspects that they cannot control, perhaps by "giving it up to God" or trusting that their God will take care of things that they cannot. Such balance between activity and acceptance provides for inner peace and can be useful in directing patients' energies toward those aspects of their cancer experience more amenable to direct control.

Perhaps the most powerful aspects of religious and spiritual interventions are their focus on meaning: Both the meaning of the cancer and the broader sense of meaning in life are core aspects of all religious and spiritual interventions. These interventions help patients to explore questions such as "Why me?" and "Why now?" as well as their struggles and doubts, contrasting their stressful cancer experience with their larger views of the fairness, justice, and benevolence of God and the universe. Ultimately, these explorations can result in more satisfactory integration of the cancer experience into their larger system of beliefs, resulting in a sense of peace and acceptance. In addition, as patients proceed through treatment, attempts at understanding the cancer experience may give way to larger concerns about significance and about how their cancer may inform or influence the meaning of their lives. Patients often report a stronger sense of purpose in their lives as well as more appreciation of daily experiences and a deepened sense of spirituality. These positive outcomes may be facilitated by religious and spiritual interventions.

As noted, evidence on the effectiveness of religious/ spiritual interventions is still accumulating, and much remains to be learned. Further, it is clear that religious and spiritual interventions may not be appropriate for all cancer patients and survivors. Not everyone is religious or spiritual, and those individuals who are not would likely not benefit from these interventions. In addition, because many individuals identify themselves as spiritual but not religious, some interventions may be adapted to focus on spirituality without including explicit religious content. Further, most religious and spiritual interventions for cancer patients and survivors have been developed and studied within the United States; much work remains to be done for cancer patients and survivors in other cultures and countries.

SEE ALSO: Alternative Therapy: Mind, Body, and Spirit; Psychosocial Issues and Cancer; Religion.

BIBLIOGRAPHY. Mary E. Kaplar, Amy B. Wachholtz, and William H. O'Brien, "The Effect of Religious and Spiritual Interventions on the Biological, Psychological, and Spiritual Outcomes of Oncology Patients: A Meta-Analytic Review," *Journal of Psychosocial Oncology* (v.22, 2004); Ernest H. Rosenbaum and Isadora Rosenbaum, *Everyone's Guide to Cancer Supportive Care: A Comprehensive Handbook for Patients and Their Families* (Somerville House, 1998) *Facing Forward Series: Life After Cancer Treatment* (National Cancer Institute, 2002).

CRYSTAL L. PARK, PH.D.
UNIVERSITY OF CONNECTICUT

Rhabdomyosarcoma, Childhood

CANCER IN CHILDREN and adolescents is uncommon. There are approximately 150 new cases of cancer per 1 million children in the United States each year. According to the National Cancer Institute, only about 2 percent of cancers in Western industrialized nations occur in children; however, cancer is the second most common cause of death in children. Cancer is responsible for 10 percent of childhood deaths. Sarcomas are cancers of the connective tissue in the body. There are two types of sarcoma: soft tissue sarcomas and bone sarcomas. Soft tissue sarcomas can develop in muscle, fat, fibrous tissue, or blood vessels. These tumors affect the tissues that support, surround, and protect the body organs.

Rhabdomyosarcoma is the most common soft tissue sarcoma in children. It is a cancer of muscle or fibrous tissue. Rhabdomyosarcoma is the fifth most common form of childhood cancer overall and accounts for approximately 5 percent of all childhood cancers. It is most frequently diagnosed in children between the ages of 2 and 6 years. Roughly 70 percent of patients with rhabdomyosarcoma are children under the age of 10 years. The disease is more common among males and the white population.

Rhabdomyosarcoma can occur in any area of the body containing striated (skeletal, voluntary) muscle. The most common sites are the head and neck, the bladder, the testes, and the extremities. Roughly 25 percent of these tumors are located in the genitourinary system. Rhabdomyosarcoma can also be found in the chest or in the abdominal wall. The most common presentation is a mass, although the symptoms differ on the basis of the cancer's location and its effect on surrounding structures. For instance, genitourinary tumors may present with blood in the urine (hematuria), vaginal bleeding, difficulty voiding, or constipation. Parameningeal tumors in the head can cause symptoms that mimic sinusitis, including ear discharge, headache, and facial pain. They can also disturb the function of cranial nerves. Tumors around the eye, known as orbital rhabdomyosarcomas, can lead to protrusion of the eye and vision deficits. Tumors of the neck, abdomen, or extremities may present as painless swellings or rapidly enlarging, firm growths.

CAUSES AND RISK FACTORS

The cause of rhabdomyosarcoma is unknown. Most cases are thought to be sporadic, meaning that they are not linked with a particular risk factor or another diagnosis. However, associations have been postulated with a few conditions, including neurofibromatosis type 1, Beckwith-Wiedemann syndrome, Costello syndrome, cardiofaciocutaneous syndrome, and multiple congenital anomalies. Use of cocaine and marijuana by the mother during pregnancy may also be a risk factor for rhabdomyosarcoma in a child. Children with rare genetic disorders have a higher risk of developing rhabdomyosarcoma. This includes children with Li-Fraumeni syndrome, a disease considered when maternal breast cancer, adrenocorticocarcinoma, and childhood sarcoma are diagnosed in the same family.

EVALUATION AND TREATMENT

Complete evaluation for rhabdomyosarcoma includes a comprehensive physical examination and a variety of diagnostic tests. This includes computed tomography (CT) or magnetic resonance imaging (MRI) scans of the primary area suspected of having cancer to verify the extent of the tumor. A chest CT, bone scan, bone marrow biopsy, and lumbar puncture make up the metastatic workup—a series of tests done to evaluate the possible spread of cancer to regional lymph nodes or to more distant sites. The most common sites of metastasis are the lungs, bones, and bone marrow. The most definitive test for rhabdomyosarcoma is a biopsy of the tumor. The tissue is examined with light and electron microscopy, immunohistologic staining, and molecular studies. Malignant changes in the skeletal muscle cells are characteristic of rhabdomyosarcoma.

The size, location, and spread of the tumor determine the course of treatment. Physicians use these characteristics of the tumor to identify the particular type and stage of cancer. Staging is based on the results of the diagnostic tests listed above. These tests will detect metastasis in only 15–20 percent of patients; to decrease the chance of missing metastatic cancer it is

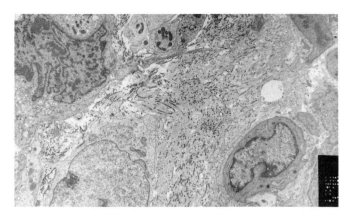

Rhabdomyosarcoma is the most common soft tissue sarcoma in children. It is a cancer of muscle or fibrous tissue.

assumed that all patients have micrometastatic disease. Therefore, systemic chemotherapy is recommended for all patients with rhabdomyosarcoma. A typical chemotherapeutic regimen includes the use of vincristine, actinomycin D, and cyclophosphamide (known as VAC therapy). These are powerful medications that are given to kill cancer cells or to at least decrease the size of large tumors that cannot be removed surgically.

On the basis of the cancer's stage, physicians can tell whether it is appropriate to try and remove the tumor. Surgery is not recommended if the procedure will cause of significant loss of function; for example, the removal of a large section of bladder, resulting in the loss of bladder control. Rhabdomyosarcoma of an extremity may require amputation to remove the part of the arm or leg affected by cancer. Prosthetic limbs are often used for children to allow them to eventually regain function of their extremity. However, it may take months to adapt to the prosthesis. Radiation therapy is also used to treat rhabdomyosarcoma, especially in cases where the tumor cannot be completely excised. High-energy radiation is aimed specifically at cancer cells to kill them while minimizing the amount of damage done to normal cells in the surrounding area. The larger the amount of tumor left after an attempted excision, the larger the area targeted by radiotherapy, and thus the greater amount of normal tissue subjected to radiation to eradicate any remaining cancer.

PROGNOSIS AND FOLLOW-UP

Approximately two-thirds of children treated for rhabdomyosarcoma are cured after treatment. Complete surgical removal of the tumor is associated with better survival rates. Children with localized cancer have roughly an 80 percent chance of long-term survival. Only about one-third of patients with metastatic disease will survive. After all forms of treatment, follow-up testing (MRI, CT, bone scan) is done to confirm complete tumor excision. This testing is also done to monitor for cancer recurrence. Unfortunately, the majority of patients who have a relapse will die from the disease. Although chemotherapy, radiation, and surgery have been quite effective in treating childhood rhabdomyosarcoma, considerable side effects are associated with their use. Early effects include nausea, diarrhea, vomiting, hair loss, bruising, and increased risk of infection. Long-term side effects include impaired muscle and bone growth, hemorrhagic cystitis, secondary leukemia, infertility, hearing impairment, and heart and kidney problems.

SEE ALSO: Sarcoma, Soft Tissue, Childhood; Childhood Cancers.

BIBLIOGRAPHY. Philip Breitfeld and Holcombe Grier, "Rhabdomyosarcoma," *Rudolph's Pediatrics* (McGraw-Hill, 2002); National Cancer Institute, *Childhood Rhabdomyosarcoma (PDQ): Treatment,* www.cancer.gov (cited April 2006); "Rhabdomyosarcoma," *Holland-Frei Cancer Medicine* (BC Decker, 2003).

STACY FRYE
MICHIGAN STATE UNIVERSITY
COLLEGE OF HUMAN MEDICINE

Richmond, Julius B.

THE SURGEON GENERAL of the United States from 1977 until 1981, Julius Richmond was active in campaigning against the smoking lobby, trying to reduce smoking in the young. Trying to promote a healthier lifestyle, the reduction in smoking coincided with a decrease in coronary heart disease cases, and some preventable illnesses.

Julius Benjamin Richmond was born on September 26, 1916, in Chicago, Illinois, the son of Jacob and Anna (née Dayno) Richmond, both of whom were born in Russia. Julius Richmond went to school at Lake Villa Township. He earned his Bachelor of Science from the University of Illinois at Urbana in 1937 and a Master's in Science from the College of Medicine in Chicago, graduating as an M.D. from the same school in 1939. He spent 18 months as an intern at Cook County Hospital, Chicago, before working at Chicago's Municipal Contagious Disease Hospital in 1941–42 and then returning to Cook County Hospital. Following the outbreak of World War II, in February 1942 Richmond enlisted in the army and was a flight surgeon with the Air Force's Flying Training Command until 1946.

Returning to the medical school at the University of Illinois as a professor in pediatrics from 1946 until 1953, Richmond was a Markle Foundation scholar in medical science for the last five of those years, becoming active in the Institute for Psychoanalysis in Chicago. He then moved to the Syracuse College of Medicine (now the Upstate Medical Center) at the State University of New York. There his work interested Sargent Shriver, head of the Kennedy Foundation. The newly established Office of Economic Opportunity (OEO) had been recently established by President Lyndon Johnson, and Shriver persuaded Richmond to take a leave of absence to work at the OEO. In 1966, Richmond was awarded the Agnes Bruce Greig Award. In the following year he left the OEO, after being given the Distinguished Service Award, and returned to the Syracuse College of Medicine as dean of the medical faculty. In 1971, Richmond moved to Harvard University to be a professor in the Harvard Medical School, working in child psychiatry and human development from 1971 until 1973 and in preventative and social medicine from 1971 until 1979.

In July 1977 President Jimmy Carter invited Richmond to become the Assistant Secretary for Health, which post Richmond accepted on the condition that it be combined with that of the Surgeon General. In that position, Richmond tried to implement many of the ideas of the OEO and of the Great Society programs of Johnson.

In the areas of cancer, Richmond worked with Secretary of Health Joseph Califano, in particular being inspired by the 1964 *Report on Smoking and Health* of former Surgeon General Luther Terry to establish the Office of Disease Prevention and Health Promotion in 1979, under Assistant Surgeon General Michael McGinnis.

This new office attempted to set specific targets for different age groups to try to reduce the amount of smoking in the United States. This smoking-reduction program was attacked by the tobacco lobby, especially after Califano spoke openly of cigarette smoking as being a major contributor to preventable disease. Richmond was most struck by the disparity in smoking rates between the poor and the affluent and between the different races, which discrepancies he highlighted in many speeches.

When his term in office ended, Richmond returned to Harvard as a professor of health policy from 1981 until 1988 and was the John D. MacArthur Professor of Management and the director of the Division of Health Policy Research and Education from 1987 to the present day. He received honorary degrees from Indiana University and Rush Presbyterian St. Luke Medical Center in 1978; the University of Illinois in 1979; the Medical College of Pennsylvania, the National College of Education at Evanston, and Georgetown University in 1980; Tufts University and the State University of New York (Syracuse) in 1986; and the University of Arizona in 1991. He is Fellow of the American Orthopsychiatric Association (winning the Ittleson Award in 1994) and the American Psychiatric Association and is an honorary member of the American Academy of Child Psychiatry and an associate member of the New England Council of Child Psychiatry.

In 1937 Richmond married Rhee Chidekel, and they had three children: Barry J., Charles Allen, and Dale Keith (deceased). Rhee Richmond died in 1985, and 2 years later Julius Richmond married Jean Rabow.

SEE ALSO: Smoking and Society.

BIBLIOGRAPHY. *American Men and Women of Science* (R.R. Bowker/Gale Group, 1971–2003); *Contemporary Authors* (Gale Group, 1978); *International Who's Who* (Europa Publications, 1989–2000); *Who's Who in America* (Marquis Who's Who, 1974–2004); *Who's Who in the East* (Marquis Who's Who, 1974–1995); *Who's Who in Medicine and Healthcare* (Marquis Who's Who, 1996–1999); *Who's Who in Science and Engineering* (Marquis Who's Who, 1994–2002).

JUSTIN CORFIELD
GEELONG GRAMMAR SCHOOL, AUSTRALIA

Robert H. Lurie Comprehensive Cancer Center

THE ROBERT H. Lurie Comprehensive Cancer Center is the focus of cancer research, treatment, and education at Northwestern University, a private university whose main campus is located in Evanston, Illinois, near Chicago. The Cancer Center was founded at Northwestern in 1974. In 1989, Ann and Robert Lurie committed to a major endowment for an institution dedicated to cancer research, and in 1991 the Robert H. Lurie Cancer Center was adopted as the name.

In 1998, the name was modified to the "Robert H. Lurie Comprehensive Cancer Center" after the National Cancer Institute (NCI) granted the center its "comprehensive" designation. The Lurie Center is a founding member of the National Comprehensive Cancer Network, a not-for-profit alliance of 20 of the nation's leading cancer centers

The Lurie Center is located in Chicago, Illinois, and is affiliated with a number of institutions in Chicago and Evanston, including (in Chicago) the Northwestern Memorial Hospital, the Rehabilitation Institute of Chicago, the Jesse Brown Veteran's Administration (VA) Medical Center, Northwestern's Feinberg School of Medicine, the Dominick DiMattero Cancer Research Laboratories, the Robert H. Lurie Medical Research Center, the Children's Memorial Hospital and Children's Memorial Research Center, and (in Evanston) the Arthur and Gladys Pancoe Evanston Northwestern Healthcare Life Sciences Pavilion and Evanston Northwestern Healthcare.

RESEARCH

Research at the Lurie Center is organized into three areas: basic sciences, clinical sciences, and cancer prevention and control. Research activities are supported by 14 shared research core facilities: bioinformatics, biostatistics, cell imaging, the clinical pharmacy core, the clinical research office, the flow cytometry facility, the genomics core facility, the Keck biophysics facility, the monoclonal antibody facility, the mouse phenotyping facility, the outcomes measurement and survey core, the pathology core facility, the structural biology facility, and the transgenic and targeted mutagenesis laboratory.

Research in the Basic Sciences Division is organized into five research programs, each including several themes. The Viral Oncogenesis program includes studies in the mechanisms of viral oncogenesis, viral replication strategies, host pathogenesis and immune modulation, and therapeutic intervention and animal models of viral infection and oncogenesis. The Tumor Invasion, Metastasis, and Angiogenesis program includes studies regarding cell–cell and cell–matrix interaction, adhesion receptor signaling, matrix structure, assembly and remodeling, mechanisms and regulation of motility, and vascular biology. The Hormone Action and Signal Transduction program includes research projects in the mechanism of ligand–receptor interaction, signal transduction pathways, cellular responses to tumor-derived hormones and growth factors, and the effect of anticancer agents on signal transduction pathways.

The Cancer Genes and Molecular Targeting program includes studies on the mechanisms and pathways controlling cell growth differentiation and oncogenesis, the discovery of new classes of therapeutic agents, and the development of new methods of early cancer detection. The Cancer Cell Biology program includes studies in posttranscriptional regulation, subcellular localization of proteins and DNA, control of cell fate determination, and animal models of cancer and therapeutics.

The Clinical Sciences Division includes three research programs. The Breast Cancer program includes studies in methods of signaling and disease progression, animal models for treatment and prevention, and clinical studies in prevention, early detection, and treatment. The Prostate Cancer program includes studies in the cellular and molecular biology of prostate cancer, the epidemiology of prostate cancer, therapeutics, and quality-of-life and outcomes research in prostate cancer. The Hematological Malignancies program includes studies that characterize normal hematopoiesis and study genetic alterations associated with hematologic malignancies and that identify molecular targets and evaluate the efficacy of novel therapeutic compounds.

The Cancer Prevention and Control Division is organized into two research programs. The Cancer Prevention program includes studies in epidemiology, chemoprevention, biomarkers and early detection, and behavioral science. The Cancer Control

program includes studies on the costs and patterns of cancer treatment; measuring, analyzing, and interpreting quality of life; and palliative and rehabilitation oncology.

The Lurie Center holds two Specialized Program of Research Excellence (SPORE) grants from the NCI. The Breast Cancer SPORE focuses on improved genetic screening; more accurate prognosis and prediction of response to chemotherapy; more effective therapy for patients with HER2-positive, metastatic disease; and mitigation of the side effects of taxane-based chemotherapy. The Prostate Cancer SPORE focuses on identification of cellular and molecular alterations in prostate cancer, prevention and risk factors in prostate cancer development, innovative prostate cancer therapeutics and rehabilitation, and quality-of-life and outcomes research in prostate cancer.

SPECIAL PROGRAMS

Comprehensive cancer screening, prevention, and treatment services are offered at the Lurie Center and affiliated institutions. In addition, a number of specialty services are available. The Bluhm Family Breast Cancer Early Detection and Prevention Program offers comprehensive risk assessment for breast cancer for women, as well as referral to specialized services such as genetic counseling and ductal lavage for those judged to be at high risk. The Cancer Chemoprevention Program is a nationwide effort headed by the Lurie Center to treat cancer in persons at high risk before it is detectable.

The Center for Genetic Medicine is a collaborative project of Northwestern University, Northwestern Memorial Hospital, Children's Memorial Hospital, and Evanston Northwestern Healthcare, which aims to establish genetically based diagnostic tools and therapies and to expand genetics-based research. The Familial Prostate Cancer Screening Program provides men with a family history of prostate cancer with up-to-date clinical testing and allows scientists to collect materials to advance the field of prostate cancer research.

The Fertility Preservation Program informs cancer patients of their options in preserving their fertility; the Lurie Center is one of five institutions in the United States that has been designated a Center of Excellence in fertility preservation by the Fertile Hope Organization. The Geriatric Oncology Consultation Service was established to meet the needs of senior citizens with cancer, and assessments and interventions are available in many areas, including social supports, cognitive and functional ability, gait assessment, chronic medical conditions, medications, nutrition, and financial concerns. The Lynn Sage Breast Cancer Program provides a multidisciplinary team approach to meeting the needs of breast cancer patients and their families. The Lurie Center participates in the National Ovarian Cancer Early Detection Program, an international collaborative effort to improve understanding and early detection and treatment of ovarian cancer.

The Pigmented Lesion Clinic provides patient education and state-of-the-art medical care for persons with irregular moles, dysplastic moles, and melanoma. The Psychosocial Oncology Program includes a team of physicians, psychologists, social workers, nutritionists, and a clinical care nurse that assists patients in dealing with the social, psychological, emotional, physical, functional, and practical aspects of cancer and cancer treatment. The Survivors Taking Action and Responsibility (STAR) Program provides services to adult survivors of childhood cancers, including education and patient care, and conducts research concerning their medical and psychological status. The Hematopoietic Stem Cell Transplant Program conducts research and provides treatment based on stem cell transplantation.

SEE ALSO: Breast Cancer; Disparities, Issues in Cancer; Education, Cancer; Prostate Cancer; Survivors of Cancer; Survivors of Cancer Families.

BIBLIOGRAPHY. The Robert H. Lurie Comprehensive Cancer Center of Northwestern University, www.cancer.northwestern.edu (cited December 2006).

Sarah Boslaugh
Washington University School of Medicine

Roche Group (Switzerland)

ROCHE IS A global healthcare company headquartered in Basel, Switzerland, that operates under two major divisions: pharmaceuticals and diagnostics. It has major operations in the United States, United Kingdom, Germany, Austria, and China and is active in more than 150 countries worldwide. Roche's prescription drugs include cancer therapies Avastin, Tarceva, Herceptin, Rituxan, and Xeloda.

Founded in 1896 by Fritz Hoffmann-La Roche, the company was initially known for producing vitamin preparations and derivatives. However, after it was embroiled in illegal price-fixing controversies with vitamins in the 1990s, it sold this part of the business in 2002. In addition to the development and manufacture of cancer therapeutics, the company is also known for manufacturing drugs for obesity, AIDS, acne, hepatitis, and influenza. Roche markets many of its bestselling drugs with affiliates Genentech and Chugai Pharmaceuticals. Descendants of the founding Hoffmann and Oeri families own half of the company, and fellow Swiss pharmaceutical giant Novartis owns another 33 percent. The company reported record high sales of over $28,969 million during fiscal year 2005.

In collaboration with Genetech, Roche markets Avastin (bevacizumab), a humanized monoclonal antibody that targets vascular endothelial growth factor (VEGF), the key mediator of tumor blood vessel formation. By inhibiting VEGF, Avastin causes regression of tumor vasculature; reduces intratumoral pressure, improving the delivery of cytotoxic agents to the tumor; and inhibits formation of new tumor blood vessel, thus restricting tumor growth. Avastin is the first U.S. Food and Drug Administration (FDA)–approved therapy that combats tumor blood vessel formation, and it is currently being used in combination with other drugs for advanced colorectal and nonsquamous non-small cell lung cancer.

Tarceva (erlotinib) is an orally administered small molecule drug that inhibits the human epidermal growth factor receptor (EGFR or HER1) pathway that promotes tumor growth by intracellular signaling. It is currently FDA approved for patients with advanced non-small cell lung cancer after failure of at least one prior chemotherapy regimen, and for advanced pancreatic cancer in combination with gemcitabine. Herceptin (trastuzumab) is a monoclonal antibody that blocks the function of HER2 receptor, another member of the EGFR pathway that is implicated in breast cancer. It has received FDA approval for patients with metastatic breast cancer whose tumors overexpress HER2.

In collaboration with Genentech, Roche is also commencing the launch of clinical trials for Omnitarg (pertuzumab), a new monoclonal antibody that blocks the ability of HER2 to dimerize with other HER receptors. Rituxan (rituximab), Roche's top selling product in 2005, is a humanized monoclonal antibody that binds to the CD20 protein on the surface of normal and cancerous B-lymphocytes. It then activates the body's natural defences, which attack and kill these cells. Given as an infusion on an outpatient basis, the drug is approved for relapsed or refractory low-grade or follicular, B-cell non-Hodgkin's lymphoma.

Finally, Xeloda (capecitabine) is an orally administered fluoropyrimidine that is approved for use in metastatic colorectal and breast cancers.

Roche's diagnostics arm offers centralized and molecular diagnostic tools and services, as well as point-of-care diagnostics used in a variety of healthcare settings. It bought the patents for the important polymerase chain reaction technique in 1992. In collaboration with Affymetrix, Roche developed the AmpliChip CYP450 Genotyping test, which received FDA approval in late 2004. This test employs DNA microarray technology to detect mutations in the CYP2D6 and CYP 2C19 genes, which play major roles in metabolism of approximately 25 percent of all prescription drugs. It is intended to be an aid for physicians in individualizing treatment selection and dosing for drugs metabolized through these genes. Similar AmpliChip platforms for leukemia and the p53 gene, mutation of which is implicated in several cancers, are currently under development.

Roche prides itself in pioneering the development of integrated packages teaming complementary diagnostic and therapeutic products and services. The Roche 2006 Half-Year report stated that the company foresees its sales growing ahead of the market in both divisions in the recent future.

SEE ALSO: Drugs; Genentech; Pharmaceutical Companies.

BIBLIOGRAPHY. Roche website, www.roche.com (cited January 2007).

Anirban P. Mitra
University of Southern California, Los Angeles

Romania

THIS EASTERN EUROPEAN country was formed as a kingdom in 1881, and although it was on the side of Germany during World War I, after the war it was given Transylvania, previously occupied by Hungary. After World War II it lost Bessarabia, which became Moldavia (later Moldova), which was incorporated into the Soviet Union. It has a population of 22,303,000 (2006) with 184 doctors and 409 nurses per 100,000 people.

Prior to the 19th century most of the treatment of cancer and tumors in Romania relied on herbal medicines with some evidence that the Scythians who ruled the region from the 7th–3rd centuries B.C.E. did use some surgical procedures. Indeed during the medieval period barber-surgeons who worked in towns and operated from stalls in markets also cut away tumors. During the 19th century medical treatments in Romania began to be influenced by changes in surgical procedures in Russia, Germany, and Turkey.

Until 1912 the same methods of dealing with the various forms of cancers in Romania was surgery. In 1912 the first radiotherapy unit was established in Bucharest, Romania's capital. During the 1920s oncologist Aurel Babes developed a cytological diagnoses for vaginal smears for cervical cancer, and in 1929 the Institute for the Study and Prophylaxis of Cancer was established in Cluj, in north-central Romania. Initially run by I. Moldovan, it quickly emerged as one of the major treatment and research centers in Romania for neoplastic disease, with much work there on malignant tumors in the 1970s by K. Gross, Monique Crisan and Doina Ionescu; and also by Doina Ionescu, G. Simu, and Draga Nestor into hystogenesis of non-tumoral changes in hosts inoculated with Rous Sarcoma viruses.

After World War II, the medical facilities throughout Romania were massively increased in size. In 1949 the Ministry of Health established the Institutul Oncologic Bucuresti (Institute of Oncology, Bucharest). There are also centers for oncology throughout Romania which date from this period. One of these which runs an effective registry is the Institutul de Igiena Sanatate Publica si Cercetari Medicale (Institute of Public Health and Medical Research) at Iasi, which specializes in radiation hygiene.

During the 1960s and 1970s researchers and doctors in Romania developed many cancer treatment techniques which have proved effective to varying degrees. As a result, Romanian doctors and medical researchers were prominent at medical conferences around the world. Most of the research in Romania took place at the Institutul Oncologic Bucuresti. Gabriela Dinescu worked on Zone Electrophoresis of Normal and Tumoral Mitochondria; Dr. A. Lupu researched into the genetic resistance to some specific rat tumors; Maria Nedelea and V. Dobra studied the immunological reaction and morphologic modifications of the lymphoid organs tested on treated and resistant-rendered rats; and G. Sandru and E. Repciuc produced important results from tests on cellular soluble products with migration inhibitory properties.

Tereza Rusanescu and Rodica Murgoci also from the Oncological Institute in Bucharest worked on the Modifications of Tumoral Development with Glycolitic Inhibition and Antigenic Stimulation. Other projects include Maria Furnica and Adriana Ganea working on radiobiology; Nicolae Voiculetz and Marilena Sbenghe who researched into common features of repair processes for some DNA-damages induced by gamma-rays and alkylating agents; and Tr. Blaga and Ecaterina Anghel who studied local perimetastatic conjunctive reactions produced in young rats by irradiation.

Also in Bucharest research was carried out at the University Clinic Carol Davila Hospital, where D. Gavruiliu, A. Cohn, E. Albu, and I. Fagarasanu worked on analyzing the late results in carcinoma of the oseophagus; and I. Fagarasani, A. Bucar, and V. Bratu worked on the detection of liver and pacreas tumors by radioisotope scanning. The Victor Babes Institute of Morbid Anatomy has also seen some important cancer research by Maria Zaharia, Alexandru Cristea, and Emil C. Cracium into pathological regenerations and intraepithelial of microcancer of the collum uteri. There was also research by I. Birzu from the St, Grigorescu Clinique de Radiologie-Oncologie de l'Hopital Dr. I. Cantacuzino who worked on radiobiology for experimental tumors.

There has also been much work carried out at Cluj-Napoca (formerly Cluj) in north-west Romania (formerly in Hungary). Constantin Nistor, Elisabeta David, Kurt Gross, and Elena Bebesel from the On-cological Institute at Cluj worked on biochemistry modifications produced by Haloacetyl-Amino-N and Benzene Sulfonamides used in the treatment of malignant tumors. Mention should also be made of projects by Otilia Bojan, I. Kiricuta, and I. Mustea who since 1968 studied the ability of tumors to function as nitrogen traps.

Mititelu Grigore from the Department of Veterinary Medicine at the Ministry of Agriculture, studied the distribution of lung cancer, grouped according to the Kreyberg system; I. Krepsz, L. Vincze, and F. P. Gyergyay from the Department of Radiology at the Institute of Medicine and Pharmacy at Tirgu-Mures worked on the combined actions of radiotherapy and pertussis vaccine tumor growth; and Z. Szecsei, A. Kertesz, E. Lax, and St. Darvas who studied clinical chemotherapy.

Such was the reputation of Romania's anticancer program, that numbers of foreigners came to the country to seek treatment. The most famous of these was Kwame Nkrumah, president of Ghana, who died of cancer in Bucharest in 1972.

The main cause of cancer in Romanian men is in lung cancer. The relatively high rates come not only from heavy levels of smoking cigarettes, but also exposure of workers to asbestos and other carcinogens. Breast cancer remains the most common form of cancer for women in Romania, with 2,000 dying in 2002, and a further 6,000 being diagnosed.

Nowadays there are faculties of medicine in many universities in Romania. The main center of research and treatment in the country remains the Institutul Oncologic Bucuresti, which is a member of the International Union Against Cancer (U.I.C.C.). Located in Bulvardul 1 Mai, and affiliated with the Academia de Stiinte Medicale, it has research facilities dealing with environmental and clinical oncology, surgery, radiobiology, chemotherapy, and immunotherapy. It publishes the quarterly journal *Oncologia*.

SEE ALSO: Cervical Cancer; Lung Cancer, Non-Small Cell; Lung Cancer, Small Cell.

BIBLIOGRAPHY. Ruxandra Carmen Artenie, "Current Asbestos Issues in Romania," www.btinternet.com/~ibas/eas_ra_romania.htm (cited November 2006); O. Costachel, "Cancer Treatment Facilities in Romania," *Oncology: Proceedings of the Tenth International Cancer Congress*

(v. 3, 1970), p427-33; L. E. Douglass, "A Further Comment on the Contributions of Aurel Babes to Cytology and Pathology," *Acta Cytologica* (v. 11, 1967); S. Izsak. "L'institut pour L'étude et la Prophylaxie du Cancer de Cluj (1929): Premier Institute Oncologique de Roumanie," *International Congress of the History of Medicine* (1974), p.1563-66; O. Luchian, A. Todea, and A. Ferencz. *Study regarding the occupational morbidity in Romania in 2000* (Institute of Public Health, Bucharest, Romania, 2001).

JUSTIN CORFIELD
GEELONG GRAMMAR SCHOOL, AUSTRALIA

Rosenberg, Barnett

AN AMERICAN CHEMIST, Barnett Rosenberg was the winner of the Charles F. Kettering Prize of the General Motors Cancer Foundation in 1984 for "the discovery of cisplatin and the significant role of platinum coordination complexes in the treatment of human cancer. Cisplatin-based combination chemotherapy has proven especially effective against testicular cancer, ovarian cancer and head and neck cancer." The discovery of cisplatin also won Rosenberg the Harvey prize from Technion-Israel Institute of Technology.

Barnett Rosenberg was born in 1926 and gained his doctorate from Graduate School of Arts and Science, New York University, in 1956, with his thesis entitled *Persistent Internal Polarization.* In 1961, Rosenberg joined Michigan State University and taught there until his retirement in 1997. He has published many academic papers including one, co-authored with J. H. Burness, M. J. Bandurski, and L. J. Passman, on the interaction of platinum-containing polycations and polyanions with biomacromolecules, published in the *Journal of Clinical Hematology and Oncology* in 1977.

During research in 1965, Rosenberg and his colleagues were able to prove that certain platinum-containing compounds inhibited cell division and thereby cured solid tumors. The discovery took place when Rosenberg was looking into the effects of an electric field on the growth of bacteria and noticed that the bacteria ceased to divide when they were placed within an electric field. Rosenberg per-formed this experiment many times and eventually discovered that this phenomenon only took place when he was using a platinum electrode. The next stage in this research was the development of a chemotherapy drug called cisplatin, which obtained approval from the U.S. Food and Drug Administration in 1978. In 1979, Rosenberg was named as Michiganian of the Year, and 5 years later, was awarded the Charles F. Kettering Prize. In 1982, Rosenberg founded the Barros Institute in Holt, Michigan. He was also awarded the second Bennett J. Cohen Award in 1998.

SEE ALSO: Head and Neck Cancer; Testicular Cancer.

BIBLIOGRAPHY. *American Men and Women of Science* (Gale Group, 2003).

JUSTIN CORFIELD
GEELONG GRAMMAR SCHOOL, AUSTRALIA

Roswell Park Cancer Institute

LOCATED IN BUFFALO, New York, the Roswell Park Cancer Institute (RPCI) is the only Comprehensive Cancer Center in upstate New York, as designated by the National Cancer Institute (NCI).

The RPCI goal is simple: "To banish cancer." Its mission is a dedication to "providing total care to the cancer patient; to conducting research into the causes, treatment and prevention of cancer; and to educating the public and the next generation of those who study and treat cancer." Thus, the principle focus of the RPCI is to provide a caring environment for patients, loved ones, and faculty.

In 1897, Dr. Roswell Park and Mr. Edward H. Butler, publisher of the *Buffalo Evening News*, requested funds from the State of New York to build a cancer research laboratory at the University of Buffalo School of Medicine. In 1898, the New York State Pathological Laboratory of the University of Buffalo opened its doors as the world's first institution dedicated entirely to the research of cancer. This facility would later become the RPCI. In 1990, the RPCI, the Fox Chase Cancer Center, and the Yale University Comprehensive Cancer Center were the first three cancer centers approved by the National Cancer Advisory Board as NCI-designated Comprehensive Cancer Centers.

To earn the designation as a Comprehensive Cancer Center from the NCI, several criteria must be met. First, the cancer center must hold a P30 Cancer Center Support Grant (CCSG) award. CCSGs are intended for two types of cancer centers: specialized and comprehensive. The term *comprehensive* signifies that care is provided in a multidisciplinary environment dedicated to long-term cancer care.

The disciplines involved should include research in biomedical and clinical therapies as well as community efforts toward education and prevention. A focus on epidemiology of cancer is also required. The NCI investigates the cancer center and determines whether the provided care and research have sufficient breadth to be considered comprehensive. Community efforts of the cancer center are also considered. Finally, the NCI has defined three major areas of care, basic research, clinical research, and "prevention, control, and population/behavioral sciences." How well these three areas of a cancer center collaborate affect the NCI's decision to grant Comprehensive Cancer Care status.

The RPCI recognizes that excellent cancer treatment extends beyond just the physical treatment of the cancer; therefore, a holistic approach to a patient's medical and psychosocial needs is practiced. In effecting this holistic approach, the RPCI has outlined several visions, which are to undertake innovative research into cancer prevention, control, causes, and cures; provide access to recently advanced treatments to its patients; offer unique cancer treatments to individuals with cancer; offer unique cancer treatments with the goal of improving the patient's quality of life; support education resources for all providers of cancer care; emphasize community outreach programs, focusing on underserved and at-risk populations in Western New York; and support prevention techniques in an effort to reduce the public burden of the costs of cancer research and care for preventable cancers and their related illnesses. In addition, the institute offers cancer support groups, psychosocial oncology services, physical therapy, interpreter services, and several other social services to its patients.

The clinicians at the RPCI specialize in many types of cancer, including those of the brain, pituitary, and spine; breast; esophagus; gastrointestinal system; gynecologic system; head and neck; lung; and prostate, as well as leukemia, lymphoma, melanoma, myeloma, sarcoma, and pediatric cancers such as retinoblastoma.

A critical method of evaluating the effectiveness and safety of a novel potential cancer therapy is the clinical trial. Patients are extensively screened to determine their eligibility for a clinical trial; furthermore, they are thoroughly counseled to aid their decision process, which involves weighing the risks against the potential benefits.

Patients at the RPCI have access to many specialized services in cancer therapy and care. These services include blood and marrow transplantation, cancer pain management, clinical genetics and genetic counseling, diagnostic radiology, the gamma knife, interleukin 2 therapy, minimally invasive surgery, Mohs surgery (a specialized technique for skin cancer surgery), photodynamic therapy, radiation therapy, robotic surgery, and supportive care.

In an effort to keep its clinicians abreast of the most recent updates in the fields of cancer prevention, treatment, and other cancer research, the RPCI supports the Continuing Medical Education program. In addition, at its medical center, the RPCI offers fellowships in oncology for physicians and dentists, as well as a faculty forum lecture series, grand rounds, a course to help patients quit smoking, and other education opportunities.

Six research programs take place at the RPCI. The programs are in biophysical therapies, cancer prevention, genetics, targeted therapeutics, tumor immunology, and prostate cancer. In addition, researchers may belong to Disease-Site Research Groups, which are breast, gastrointestinal, genitourinary, gynecological, head and neck, lung, neurooncology, pediatrics, sarcoma and melanoma, and hematologic oncology. Faculty members in the RPCI research sector are based in eight departments: biostatistics, cancer biology, cancer genetics, cancer prevention and population sciences, cell stress biology, immunology, molecular and cellular biology, and pharmacology and therapeutics.

The RPCI is managed by a board of directors consisting of professionals from cancer organizations, pharmaceutical companies, and other fields involved with cancer. The Roswell Park Alliance Community Advisory Board leads the RPCI fundraising events. These events include a black-tie gala, a golf tournament, a bike ride, and an auction. In addition, pediatric patients at RPCI design holiday cards, which are sold in the winter holiday season as a fundraising initiative. Furthermore, the Roswell Park Alliance Foundation Trustees manage the funds received by the RPCI in forms of donations and contributions. This foundation was established in 1991.

The institute is affiliated with several other cancer organizations, including the NCI and the National Comprehensive Cancer Network. In 1952, the RPCI established the Summer Research Participation Program, the first of its kind in the nation. High school and university juniors in the program conduct summer research in cancer. As of 2006, the entire RPCI campus became smoke-free. An office of commercial development serves RPCI faculty members in legal affairs such as patents and copyrights, acting as a corporate liaison for licenses to products and technology developed at the RPCI and otherwise supporting these products and technologies.

SEE ALSO: Fox Chase Cancer Center; Memorial Sloan-Kettering Cancer Center; National Cancer Institute; Yale Cancer Center.

BIBLIOGRAPHY. James S. Gordon and Sharon Curtin, *Comprehensive Cancer Care: Integrating Alternative, Complementary, and Conventional Therapies* (HarperCollins, 2001); Michael Kahn and Stella Pelengaris, *The Molecular Biology of Cancer* (Blackwell Publishing Professional, 2006); Razelle Kurzrock and Moshe Talpaz, *Molecular Biology in Cancer Medicine* (2nd ed.) (Taylor and Francis, 1999).

CLAUDIA WINOGRAD
UNIVERSITY OF ILLINOIS AT URBANA-CHAMPAIGN

Russia

THE LARGEST COUNTRY in the world, the Russian Federation had a population of 142,400,000 in 2006, with 421 doctors and 821 nurses per 100,000 people. The Russian Empire lasted until 1917, when it was replaced by a series of republics that later joined to form the Union of Soviet Socialist Republics. In 1991, the republics split again to form 15 different countries.

Surgery and some herbal pastes were used by the Russians to treat tumors until the 18th century. During that period, the advances in cancer surgery saw the emergence of many of the structures that formed the Russian medical system until the 1917 revolution. The main Russian medical faculty was the Russian School of Therapeutics in Moscow, which was destroyed in 1812 and restored by Dr. M. I. Mudrov (1776–1831).

During the 19th century, G. A. Zakharin (1829–97) helped establish a new era in clinical medicine in Russia with great emphasis on diagnosis at an early stage. Another major advance in cancer treatment occurred in 1875–76, when Mistislav Alexandrovich Novinsky (1841–1914), a graduate student at the Medical-Surgery Academy of St. Petersburg, was able to successfully transplant a nasal carcinoma from one dog to another, proving that tumors could be transplanted between animals of the same species.

After the Russian Revolution in 1917, there was an increased focus on providing healthcare for everybody. This proved impossible during the Russian Civil War, but when this conflict ended in 1922, hospitals were built in many parts of the Soviet Union. However, it was not until the end of World War II that the Soviet Union was able to establish a complete cancer registry. This registry quickly showed a rise in people suffering from cancer during the 1950s and 1960s, largely because there were more people seeking treatment through better diagnosis and awareness. In 1950, there were 5,915 beds for cancer patients in the Russian Federation, rising to 12,781 in 1960 and 13,861 in the following year. Initially, most of the cancer efforts were directed at mass prophylactic examinations and increased health education.

There were a large number of cancers prevalent in the Soviet Union, including lung cancer from heavy smoking, cancers from pollution and later from nuclear power plants, stomach cancer in the Russian Far East and in polluted areas of the country, and breast cancer and cervical cancer in women. In 1960, stomach cancer made up one-third of all cancer cases, with uterine and cervical cancer forming 16 percent, skin cancer, 12 percent, mouth 7.5 percent, cancer of the lungs and bronchi 7 percent, breast cancer 6 percent, cancer of the oesophagus 5 percent, rectal cancer 2 percent, cancer of the larynx 1.5 percent, and cancer of other organs 10 percent. In 1962, the 8th International Cancer Congress was held in Moscow from July 22 to 28, with the Soviet postal authorities issuing a stamp on July 16 to commemorate the holding of the congress in the Soviet Union.

ONCOLOGY RESEARCH

The Oncology Research Center (usually known as the "Oncology Center") in Moscow is the largest in the world and has a long record of pioneering anticancer research. Located in Kashirskoe shosse, Moscow, the center is affiliated with the Russian Academy of Medical Sciences. It was responsible for the coordination of cancer research throughout the Soviet Union, and now in Russia, and is involved in collaborative research with other countries. It has extensive research commitments throughout the Russian Federation and provides treatment in inpatient accommodation with 1,000 beds and in policlinics for adults and children. The main areas of research are into the origins and mechanisms of the development of tumors, the improvement of existing and the development of new methods of diagnosing and treating malignant tumors, the development of new antitumor preparations, and improvement in the control of cancer. As well as its base in Moscow, the center also has a Siberian branch located in Tomsk.

A. I. Ageenko, I. S. Bashkayev, and L. M. Myriem from the Moscow Oncological Institute worked on the investigation of virus carcinogenesis, and V. V. Gorodilova, V. Y. Rogalsky, S. F. Malysheva, Z. M. Sarayeva, and I. G. Silina worked on immunological investigations of human tumors.

The P.A. Gersten Oncological Research Institute in Moscow has also been at the forefront of cancer research in Russia, especially in the area of clinical use of nuclear medicine, including the use of diagnostic radioisotopes. During the 1970s, the institute developed using radiotherapy, chemotherapy, and immunotherapy and also established clinical stations dealing with gynecology, head and neck, urology, neurology, heart and lung, circulation, and bone cancer.

L. A. Zilber of the Gamaleya Institute of Epidemiology and Microbiology in Moscow worked on the possible participation of latent viruses in neoplastic processes induced by carcinogenic agents, and Dr. Zilber also researched with a colleague, V. Y. Schevljaghyn, on the morphological transformation of human embryonic tissue by the Rous Sarcoma virus. Others at the institute included I. N. Kryukova, I. R. Obuch, and T. I. Birulina, who worked on the study of antigens induced by the Rous Sarcoma virus; G. I. Abelev, who prepared an analysis of antigenic structures of tumors based on heteroimmune sera; and O. M. Lejneva, E. C. Ievleva, and N. V. Engelhardt from the department of Tumor Virology and Immunology at the institute, whose research was into specific antigens of mouse leukemias detected in the syngeneic system. N. G. Blokhina and N. N. Blokhin, also from the institute, studied the treatment of gastric cancer with 5-fluoruracil.

The P.A. Herzen Moscow Oncological Institute has seen much research into cancer. V. M. Bergolz and V. V. Dementyeva worked on the application of surviving tissue culture for the detection of leukosogenic agents in human leukemic material; and I. P. Tereshchenko, I. K. Podzev, C. G. Shehitkov, V. I. Boykova, N. I. Bolonina, and E. V. Mandryk all worked on the questions concerning host resistance in the course of experimental carcinogenesis. V. A. Kochetkova and A. P. Bajenova also researched the prolongation of some antiblastomatous preparations' action with the help of polyvinylpyrrolidone. In addition, V. P. Demidov, also from the institute, worked on the surgical and combined treatment of mediastinal malignant tumors. Mention should also be made of the Sklifovsky Institute in Moscow, where B. A. Petrov studied the resection of the thoracic part of the esophagus for cancer treatment.

ABRIKOSOV'S TUMOR

Moscow University's Aleksei Ivanovich Abrikosov (1875–1955) wrote about myoblastoma myomas, a soft tissue sarcoma now known as Abrikosov's Tumor. During the 1970s, research was carried out by Tamilla D. Esakova and Boris K. Semin from Moscow State University into the metabolism of chemical carcinogenesis.

Other recent Russian specialists include N. A. Kraevsky and N. T. Raikhlin, both of the Institute of Experimental and Clinical Oncology, Academy of Medical Sciences of the U.S.S.R., Moscow. J. M. Olenov and V. J. Fell, from the Laboratory of Cancer Cell Genetics at the Institute of Cytology, Academy of Sciences of the U.S.S.R., worked on the heteroantigens of rat tumors. N. P. Pal'mina, V. D. Gaintseva, and E.

V. Burlakova, from the Institute of Chemical Physics at the Academy of Sciences in Moscow, were involved in work on the combined action of ionizing radiation and radical reaction inhibitors on tumor and tumor–host organisms.

In 1926, the Leningrad Institute of Oncology was founded by Nikolai Petrov, and from its opening until 1965 the institute treated 55,000 patients. It also published the premier Soviet oncology journal, *Voprosy Onkologii*, beginning in 1955. There was also important work done at the 1st Leningrad Pavlov Medical Institute by V. I. Kolesov and A. O. Levin on the significance of perfusion chemotherapy in the complex treatment of malignant tumors of the limbs. Chemotherapy began in 1950, when it was originally used by L. F. Larionov of the Leningrad Institute of Oncology. Two years later, the Institute of Experimental and Clinical Oncology was created to promote chemotherapy research, leading to, in 1966, the All-Union Antitumor Chemotherapeutic Center.

At the Gorky Medical Institute, V. I. Kukosh, A. A. Chernavsky, and E. M. Budarina studied cancer in the operated stomach and possible surgical treatments. N. M. Emanuel, V. A. Barsel, L. S. Evseenko, and V. V. Disvetova, of the Institute of Chemical Physics, Academy of Sciences of the U.S.S.R., worked on the Dibunol as a new antitumor agent. In addition, A. A. Demin, from the Medical Institute of Novsibirsk, worked on the effect of RNA and DNAse on Leucemia.

In Kazan, the capital of the Republic of Tartarstan, research into cancer was also performed. During the 1960s, M. I. Belyaeva, N. I. Vylegzanin, V. G. Winter, and N. P. Balaban all worked on the secretion of nucleic acids by cancer cells. Vylegzanin also worked on a clinical and experimental study of carcinoma with A. P. Starostin, and M. Z. Sigal researched the structural analysis of the stomach with cancerous affection. Y. A. Ratner worked on the experience of surgical treatment of malignant intestinal tumors, and Z. S. Gilyasutdinova researched the condition of neuroelements of uterine fibromyoma in women who were pregnant and in those who were not.

Other regional oncology centers that have been important in cancer treatment studies have been at Tyumen, where N. A. Zubov worked at the Tyumen Research Institute of Regional Infectional Pathology on opisthorchiasis and primary cancers of the liver; at Orenburg, where G. M. Mnuhina at the Orenburg Medical Institute researched histogenesis and morphogenesis of laryngeal cancer; at Kuibyshev, where Alexander Aminev and Solomon Rodkin worked at the local medical institute on arteriography in rectal cancer; and at Kalinin, where A. B. Hillerson and L. A. Solovyeva at the Department of Obstetrics and Gynecology worked on thecomatosis and thecablastoma of the ovary.

Throughout other parts of the Soviet Union before 1992, there had been much research undertaken that was used in parts of Russia. This included pioneering work at the Institute of Organic Synthesis at the Academy of Sciences of the Latvian S.S.R., and also research in Belarus, Georgia, Kazakhstan, and the Ukraine, in particular. The well-known story *Cancer Ward* (1968) by Alexander Solzhenitsyn was actually set in an imaginary hospital in Uzbekistan, but the author felt his work could have easily applied to many parts of Russia.

Boris Pasternak (1890–1960), who won the Nobel Prize in 1950 for his book *Doctor Zhivago*, suffered from cancer during his latter years, and Chaim Weizmann (1874–1952), born in Russia and President of Israel from 1948 to 1952, suffered from cancer. Mention should also be made of Llewellyn E. Thompson, Jr. (1904–72), the U.S. Consul to Moscow in 1943 and Ambassador to the Soviet Union from 1957 to 1962 and from 1966 to 1969, and Charles Eustis Bohlen (1904–74), U.S. Ambassador from 1953 to 1957, who both subsequently died from cancer.

The All-Union Oncological Society of the Soviet Union was the major body in the country until 1991 but has now been replaced by the Russian All-Union Oncological Society. The N.N. Blokhin Cancer Research Centre and the N.N. Petrov Research Institute of Oncology are both members of the International Union Against Cancer.

SEE ALSO: Belarus; Ukraine.

BIBLIOGRAPHY. Gordon Hyde, *The Soviet Health Service: A Historical and Comparative Study* (Lawrence & Wishart, 1974); A. Y. Ivanyuskhin and A. K. Khetagurova, "Palliative Care in Russia," *Journal International de Bioethique* (v.16.3/4, 2005); N. I. Perevodchikovo, "Brief Historical Statement: Chemotherapy of Malignant Tumors in the U.S.S.R.," *National Cancer Institute Monographs* (v.45, 1977); *Report of the VIII International Cancer Congress* (International Cancer Congress, 1962); Henry E. Sigerist,

Medicine and Health in the Soviet Union (Citadel Press, 1947); S. Syrjanen, I. P. Shabalova, N. Petrovichev, et al., "Human Papillomavirus Testing and Conventional Pap Smear Cytology as Optional Screening Tools of Women at Different Risks for Cervical Cancer in the Countries of the Former Soviet Union," *Journal of Lower Genital Tract Disease* (v.6/2, 2002).

JUSTIN CORFIELD
GEELONG GRAMMAR SCHOOL, AUSTRALIA

Rwanda

RWANDA, A LANDLOCKED central African republic, was controlled by the Germans as a part of German East Africa until World War I. It was then administered by Belgium under a League of Nations mandate, and after 1946 it was a U.N. trusteeship, as a part of Ruanda-Urundi, being split in 1959 to form Rwanda and Burundi. On July 1, 1962, Rwanda became independent as the Republic of Rwanda. It had a population of 9,038.000 in 2005 and has a chronically underfunded health service.

During the German period of occupation, healthcare, except that for Europeans and the small local elite, was primitive, with most people relying on herbal cures. Even during the Belgian rule under the mandate of the League of Nations, medical care was not extensive and was largely focused in Kigali, the country's capital, with clinics located in a few large townships. After independence, there were attempts to improve healthcare services, and with longer life expectancies, there a higher prevalence of cancer has been seen, especially skin cancer.

There have been few studies of cancer in Rwanda, but one by P. Ngendahayo and D. M. Parkin, conducted from 1982 until 1984 at the main pathology department of Rwanda, showed that in males, excluding skin cancers, the most frequent concerns were Kaposi's sarcoma (11.5 percent), stomach cancer (9.9 percent), non-Hodgkin's lymphoma (8.1 percent), and primary carcinoma of the liver (6.6 percent). For women, uterine cervical cancer accounted for 21.4 percent, breast cancer 16.8 percent, and stomach cancer 6.5 percent of cases. Lung cancer is relatively uncommon in Rwanda, as few people smoke, and colorectal and breast cancer are also prevalent at much lower rate than in developed countries.

In a follow-up study, Parkin and others worked on statistics from the cancer registry in Butare in southern Rwanda. They had access to the figures from May 1991 until February 1994—2 months before the outbreak of civil war.

The statistics there showed that people in Rwanda had similar types of cancer as in other parts of sub-Saharan Africa, with liver cancer and cervical cancer being the most common (12 percent each), followed by stomach cancer (9 percent). It also showed that there was a heavier prevalence of cancers associated with HIV, such as Kaposi's sarcoma (6 percent) and non-Hodgkin's lymphoma (3 percent). The relatively high rates of these and some other types of cancer resulted from the high rates of HIV in the country and from many people having had multiple sexual partners. The Institut National de Recherche Scientifique, located in Butare, runs an official registry, and there is also a faculty of medicine at the Université Nationale du Rwanda, at which much cancer treatment takes place.

SEE ALSO: AIDS-Related Cancers; Lung Cancer; Sarcoma, Kaposi's.

BIBLIOGRAPHY. R. Newton, P. J. Ngilimana, A. Grulich, V. Beral, B. Sindikuwabo, A. Nganyira, and D. M. Parkin, "Cancer in Rwanda," *International Journal of Cancer* (v.66/1, 1996); P. Ngendahayo and D. M. Parkin, "Cancer in Rwanda: Study of Relative Frequency [in French]," *Bulletin du Cancer* (v.73/2, 1986).

JUSTIN CORFIELD
GEELONG GRAMMAR SCHOOL, AUSTRALIA

Resource Guide

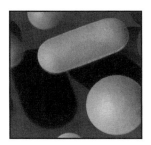

BOOKS

Abbruzzese, J. and Ebrahimi, B. *Myths & Facts About Pancreatic Cancer* (PRR, 2002)

Alliance for Lung Cancer Advocacy, Support, and Education. *The Lung Cancer Manual* (Alliance for Lung Cancer Advocacy, Support, and Education, 2003)

American Cancer Society. *Cancer Facts & Figures 2007* (ACS, 2007)

American Cancer Society. *Cancer Facts and Figures 2006* (American Cancer Society, 2006)

American Cancer Society. *Good for You: Reducing Your Risk of Developing Cancer* (American Cancer Society, 2002)

American Institute for Cancer Research. *Stopping Cancer Before It Starts* (St. Martin's Press, 2000)

Austoker, Joan. *A History of the Imperial Cancer Research Fund 1902–1986* (Oxford University Press, 1988)

Beauchamp, Thomas and Childress, James. *Principles of Biomedical Ethics* (Oxford University Press, 2001)

Branverman, Debra. *Heal Your Heart with EECP* (Celestial Arts, 2005)

Buckman, Robert. *What You Really Need to Know About Cancer.* (John Hopkins University Press, 1995)

Burtis, Carl and Ashwood, Edward. *Tietz Textbook of Clinical Chemistry* (Saunders, 1999)

Cancer Care. *A Helping Hand: The Resource Guide for People With Cancer* (Cancer Care, 2002)

Castleman, Michael. *Nature's Cures* (Rodale Books, 1996)

Cefrey, H. *Coping with Cancer, Its Side Effects, or Other Serious Illness* (Rosen, 2000)

Chabner, Bruce. *Cancer Chemotherapy and Biotherapy: Principles and Practice* (Lippincott Williams and Wilkins, 2006)

Chine Map Press. *Atlas of Cancer Mortality in the People's Republic of China* (China Map Press, 1979)

Cicala, R. *The Cancer Pain Sourcebook* (Contemporary Books, 2001)

Colditz, Graham A. and Hunter, David, eds. *Cancer Prevention: The Causes and Prevention of Cancer, Volume I* (Kluwer Academic, 2000)

Colditz, Graham A. and Stein, C.J. *Handbook of Cancer Risk Assessment and Prevention.* (Jones and Bartlett, 2004).

Committee on Cancer Survivorship: Improving Care and Quality of Life. *From Cancer Patient to Cancer Survivor: Lost in Transition*, Maria Hewitt, Sheldon Greenfield, and Ellen Stovall, eds. (National Academies Press, 2006)

Cukier, D. and McCullough, V. *Coping With Radiation Therapy* (Lowell House, 2000)

Devita, V. T., Hellman, S., Rosenberg, S. A., eds. *Cancer: Principles and Practice of Oncology* (Lippincott-Raven Publishers, 1997)

Dollinger, M. *Everyone's Guide to Cancer Therapy* (Andrews McMeel, 2002)

Dooley, J. and Betancourt, M. *The Coming Cancer Breakthroughs: What You Need to Know About the Latest Cancer Treatment Options* (Kensington Books, 2002)

Eyre, H., Lange, D., and Morris L. *Informed Decisions: The Complete Book of Cancer Diagnosis, Treatment, and Recovery* (American Cancer Society, 2002)

Fanco, Eduardo L., and Rohan, Thomas E., eds. *Cancer Precursors: Epidemiology, Detection and Prevention* (Springer-Verlag, 2002)

Fincannon, J. and Bruss, K. *Couples Confronting Cancer: Keeping Your Relationship Strong* (American Cancer Society, 2003)

Finn, R. *Cancer Clinical Trials: Experimental Treatments & How They Can Help You* (O'Reilly & Associates, 1999)

Fischer, David, and Durivage, Henry M. Tish Knobf and Nancy Beaulieu, *The Cancer Chemotherapy Handbook* (Mosby, 2003)

Foley, Kathleen M. and Gelband, Hellen. *National Cancer Policy Board/Institute of Medicine, Improving Palliative Care for Cancer* (National Academy Press, 2001)

Fromer, M. *The Journey to Recovery: A Complete Guide to Cancer Chemotherapy* (Adams Media, 2001)

Glemser, Bernard. *Man Against Cancer: Research & Progress* (Bodley Head, 1969)

Greenwald, P., Kramer, B.F., Weed, D.L. eds. *Cancer Prevention and Control* (Marcel Dekker, 1995)

Harpham, W. *When a Parent has Cancer: A Guide for Caring for Your Children* (HarperCollins, 1997)

Hartwell, Leland H., Hood, Leroy, Goldberg, Michael L, Reynolds, Ann E., Silver, Lee M. and Veres, Ruth C., *Genetics: From Genes to Genomes* (McGraw-Hill, 2000)

Hirshaut, Y. and Pressman, P. *Breast Cancer: The Complete Guide* (Bantam Books, 2000)

Hofrichter, Richard ed. *Health and Social Justice: Politics, Ideology and Inequity in the Distribution of Disease* (Jossey-Bass, 2003)

Holick M, ed. *Vitamin D: Molecular Biology, Physiology, and Clinical Applications* (Humana, 1999)

Howe, D. *His Prostate and Me: A Couple Deals With Prostate Cancer* (Winedale, 2002)

Dos Santos Silva, I., ed. *Cancer Epidemiology: Principals and Methods* (IARC, 1999)

IARC. *Tobacco Smoke and Involuntary Smoking* (International Agency for Research on Cancer, 2004)

Iver, Knud and Secher, Assens. *The Danish Cancer Researcher, Johannes Fibiger: Professor in the University of Copenhagen* (Nyt Nordisk Forlag, 1947)

Johnston, L. *Colon & Rectal Cancer: A Comprehensive Guide for Patients & Families* (O'Reilly & Associates, 2000)

Johnston, L. *Lung Cancer: Making Sense of Diagnosis, Treatment & Options* (O'Reilly & Associates, 2001)

Johnston, L. *Non-Hodgkin's Lymphomas: Making Sense of Diagnosis, Treatment & Options.* (O'Reilly & Associates, 1999)

Kaplan, Henry S. and Jones, Patricia T. eds. *Cancer in China* (A.R. Liss, 1978)

Keough, Carol. *The Complete Book of Cancer Prevention* (Rodale Books, 1988)

Kluger, R. *Ashes to ashes: America's hundred-year cigarette war, the public health, and the unabashed triumph of Philip Morris* (Alfred A. Knopf, Inc, 1996)

Kneece, J. *Your Breast Cancer Treatment Handbook* (EdcuCare Publishing, 2001)

Lackritz, B. *Adult Leukemia; A Comprehensive Guide for Patients and Families* (O'Reilly & Associates, 2001)

Langford, L. *Ovarian Cancer: Your Guide to Taking Control* (O'Reilly & Associates, Inc, 2003)

Levin, B. *American Cancer Society: Colorectal Cancer, a thorough and compassionate resource for patients and their families* (Random House; 1999)

Love, S. *Dr. Susan Love's Breast Book* (Perseus Publishing, 2000)

Lydiatt, W. *Cancers of the Mouth & Throat: A Patient's Guide to Treatment* (Addicus Books, 2001)

Marks, S. *Prostate & Cancer, a Family Guide to Diagnosis, Treatment & Survival* (Perseus Publishing, 2003)

National Cancer Policy Board. *Childhood Cancer Survivorship: Improving Care and Quality of Life*, Hewitt, M., Weiner, SL., and Simone, JV., eds. (National Academy of Sciences, 2003)

New York Cancer Committee. *History of the American Society for the Control of Cancer, 1913-1943* (Westchester Cancer Committee, 1943)

Olson, James S., *The History of Cancer: An Annotated Bibliography* (Greenwood Press, 1989)

Parkin, D.M., Whelan, S.L., J., Raymond, Ferlay and Young, J. eds. *Cancer Incidence in Five Continents Vol VII* (International Agency for Research on Cancer and International Association of Cancer Registries, 1997)

Parkin, DM., Ferlay, J., Hamdi-Cherif, M., Sitas, F., Thomas, JO., Wabinga H. and Whelan, SL., eds., *Cancer in Africa: Epidemiology and Prevention* (IARC, 2003)

Patterson, James T. *The Dread Disease: Cancer and Modern American Culture* (Harvard University Press, 1987)

Raven, Ronald W. *The Theory and Practice of Oncology* (Parthenon Publications, 1990)

Rettig, Richard A., *Cancer Crusade: The Story of the National Cancer Act of 1971* (Authors Choice Press, 2005)

Rosenberg, Steve and Barry, John. *The Transformed Cell —Unlocking the Mysteries of Cancer* (G.P. Putman's Sons, 1992)

Ross, W. *Crusade: The Official History of the American Cancer Society* (Arbor House, 1987)

Rushing, L. and Joste, N. *Abnormal Pap Smears: What Every Woman Needs To Know* (Prometheus, 2001)

Schoenberg, M. *The Guide to Living with Bladder Cancer* (Johns Hopkins University Press, 2000)

Schofield, J. and Robinson, W. *What You Really Need to Know About Moles and Melanoma.* (Johns Hopkins University Press, 2000)

Smedley, Howard and Sikora, Karol. *Cancer What It Is and How Its Treated* (Basil Blackwell Ltd., 1985)

Spence, Alexander. *Biology of Human Aging* (Prentice Hall, 1989)

Stewart, S. *Autologous Stem Cell Transplants: A Handbook for Patients* (Blood & Marrow Transplant Information Network, 2000)

Stewart, S. *Bone Marrow and Blood Stem Cell Transplants: A Guide for Patients* (Blood & Marrow Transplant Information Network, 2002)

The International Agency for Research on Cancer (IARC), *Volume 67: Human Immunodeficiency Viruses And Human T-Cell Lymphotropic Viruses* (IARC, 1996)

Tollison, CD., Satterthwaithe, J. R., Tollison, J.W., eds. *Practical Pain Management* (Lippincott Williams and Wilkins, 2002)

Turow, Joseph, *Playing Doctor* (Oxford University Press, 1989)

US DHHS. *The Health Consequences of Involuntary Exposure to Tobacco Smoke: A Report of the Surgeon General* (U.S. Department of Health and Human Services, Centers for Disease Control and Prevention, National Center for Chronic Disease Prevention and Health Promotion, Office On Smoking and Health, 2006)

Weed, Douglas L. and Coughlin, Steven S. "Ethics in Cancer Prevention and Control" in *Weight Control* (CRC Press, 2006)

INTERNET

www.iarc.fr – International Agency for Research on Cancer

www.ahrq.gov – Agency for Healthcare Research and Quality

www.cancer.ca – Canadian Cancer Society

www.cancer.gov – National Cancer Institute

www.cancer.org – American Cancer Society

www.chemotherapy.com – Chemotherapy Online

www.clinicaltrials.gov – Developed by the National Library of Medicine

www.mdsupport.org – Harvard Support Group

www.nia.nih.org – National Institute of Aging

www.pnas.org – Proceedings of the National Academy of Sciences

www.who.int – World Health Organization

www.yourdiseaserisk.wustl.edu – Sitemann Cancer Center, Washington University School of Medicine

JOURNALS

American Journal of Clinical Pathology
American Journal of Medicine
American Journal of Preventive Medicine
Angiogenesis Weekly
Anticancer Research
British Journal of Cancer
British Medical Journal
CA: A Cancer Journal for Clinicians
Cancer Biology and Therapy
Cancer Causes and Control
Cancer Cell
Cancer Epidemiology Biomarkers Prevention
Cancer Immunology Immunotherapy
Cancer Journal
Cancer Research
Carcinogenesis
Carotenoids in Health and Disease
Cell
Clinical Cancer Research
Environmental Health Perspective
European Journal of Cancer Prevention
Journal of Biological Chemistry
Journal of Clinical Instigation
Journal of Clinical Medicine and Research
Journal of Clinical Oncology
Journal of Mammary Gland Biology and Neoplasia
Journal of Medical Sciences Monitor
Journal of Molecular Diagnostics
Journal of Nutrition
Journal of Physical Anthropology
Journal of the American Medical Association
Journal of the National Cancer Institute
Molecular Aspects of Medicine
Molecular Cancer Research
Nature Reviews Cancer
New England Journal of Medicine
Nucleic Acids Research
Nutrition and Cancer
Oncology Reporters
Oncology Research
Perspectives in Biology and Medicine
Pharmacogenetics
Protein Nucleic Acid
Science
Science and Medicine
Stat Med
The Medical Clinics of North America
Toxicology Science

Glossary

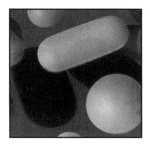

Adapted from the National Cancer Institute online glossary
by the University of Texas M.D. Anderson Cancer Center.

Abdomen (AB-do-men): The part of the body that contains the pancreas, stomach, intestines, liver, gallbladder, and other organs.

Accelerated phase (ak-SEL-er-ay-ted): Refers to chronic myelogenous leukemia that is progressing. The number of immature, abnormal white blood cells in the bone marrow and blood is higher than in the chronic phase, but not as high as in the blast phase.

Achlorhydria (a-klor-HY-dree-a): A lack of hydrochloric acid in the digestive juices in the stomach. Hydrochloric acid helps digest food.

Acoustic (ah-KOOS-tik): Related to sound or hearing.

Actinic keratosis (ak-TIN-ik ker-a-TO-sis): A precancerous condition of thick, scaly patches of skin; also called solar or senile keratosis.

Acute leukemia: Leukemia that progresses rapidly.

Adenocarcinoma (AD-in-o-kar-sin-O-ma): Cancer that begins in cells that line certain internal organs.

Adenoma (AD-in-o-ma): A noncancerous tumor.

Adjuvant therapy (AD-joo-vant): Treatment given in addition to the primary treatment to enhance the effectiveness of the primary treatment.

Adrenal glands (a-DREE-nal): A pair of small glands, one located on top of each kidney. The adrenal glands produce hormones that help control heart rate, blood pressure, the way the body uses food, and other vital functions.

Aflatoxin (AF-la-TOK-sin): A substance made by a mold that is often found on poorly stored grains and nuts. Aflatoxins are known to cause cancer in animals.

Agranulocyte (A-gran-yoo-lo-SITE): A type of white blood cell; monocytes and lymphocytes are agranulocytes.

Allogeneic bone marrow transplantation (AL-o-jen-AY-ik): A procedure in which a patient receives bone marrow from a compatible, though not genetically identical, donor.

Alpha-fetoprotein (AL-fa FEE-to-PRO-teen): A protein often found in abnormal amounts in the blood of patients with liver cancer.

Alveoli (al-VEE-o-lye): Tiny air sacs at the end of the bronchioles.

Amputation (am-pyoo-TAY-shun): Surgery to remove all or some of a body part.

Amylase (AM-il-aze): An enzyme that helps the body digest starches.

Anal cancer: Anal cancer, an uncommon cancer, is a disease in which cancer (malignant) cells are found in the anus. The anus is the opening at the end of the rectum (the end part of the large intestine) through which body waste passes.

Anaplastic (an-ah-PLAS-tik): A term used to describe cancer cells that divide rapidly and bear little or no resemblance to normal cells.

Anastamosis (an-AS-ta-MO-sis): A procedure to connect healthy sections of the colon or rectum after the diseased portion has been surgically removed.

Androgen (AN-dro-jenz): A hormone that promotes the development and maintenance of male sex characteristics.

Anemia (a-NEE-mee-a): A decrease in the normal amounts of red blood cells.

Anesthesia (an-es-THEE-zha): Loss of feeling or awareness. A local anesthetic causes loss of feeling in a part of the body. A general anesthetic puts the person to sleep.

Anesthetic (an-es-THET-ik): A substance that causes loss of feeling or awareness. A local anesthetic causes loss of feeling in a part of the body. A general anesthetic puts the person to sleep.

Angiogenesis (an-gee-o-GEN-e-sis): Blood vessel formation, which usually accompanies the growth of malignant tissue.

Angiogram (AN-jee-o-gram): An X-ray of blood vessels; the patient receives an injection of dye to outline the vessels on the X-ray.

Angiography (an-jee-O-gra-fee): A procedure to X-ray blood vessels. The blood vessels can be seen because of an injection of a dye that shows up in the X-ray pictures.

Angiosarcoma (AN-jee-o-sar-KO-ma): A type of cancer that begins in the lining of blood vessels.

Antiandrogen (an-tee-AN-dro-jen): A drug that blocks the action of male sex hormones.

Antibiotics (an-ti-by-AH-tiks): Drugs used to treat infection.

Antibody (AN-ti-BOD-ee): A protein produced by certain white blood cells in response to a foreign substance (antigen). Each antibody can bind only to a specific antigen. The purpose of this binding is to help destroy the antigen. Antibodies can work in several ways, depending on the nature of the antigen. Some antibodies disable antigens directly. Others make the antigen more vulnerable to destruction by white blood cells.

Anticonvulsant (an-ti-kon-VUL-sant): Medicine to stop, prevent, or control seizures (convulsions).

Antigen: Any foreign or "non-self" substance that, when introduced into the body, causes the immune system to create an antibody.

Antithymocyte globulin (anti-THIGH-moe-site GLA-bu-lin): A protein preparation used to prevent and treat graft-versus-host disease.

Anus (AY-nus): The opening of the rectum to the outside of the body.

Aplastic anemia: A deficiency of certain parts of the blood caused by a failure of the bone marrow's ability to generate cells.

Apoptosis (ay-paw-TOE-sis): A normal cellular process involving a genetically programmed series of events leading to the death of a cell.

Areola (a-REE-oe-la): The area of dark-colored skin that surrounds the nipple.

Arterial embolization (ar-TEE-ree-al EM-bo-lih-ZAY-shun): Blocking an artery so that blood cannot flow to the tumor.

Arteriogram (ar-TEER-ee-o-gram): An X-ray of blood vessels, which can be seen after an injection of a dye that shows up in the X-ray pictures.

Asbestos (as-BES-tus): A natural material that is made up of tiny fibers. If the fibers are inhaled, they can lodge in the lungs and lead to cancer.

Ascites (a-SYE-teez): Abnormal buildup of fluid in the abdomen.

Aspiration (as-per-AY-shun): Removal of fluid from a lump, often a cyst, with a needle and a syringe.

Astrocytoma (as-tro-sye-TOE-ma): A type of brain tumor that begins in the brain or spinal chord in small, star-shaped cells called astrocytes.

Asymptomatic: Presenting no symptoms of disease.

Ataxic gait (ah-TAK-sik): Awkward, uncoordinated walking.

Atypical hyperplasia (hy-per-PLAY-zha): A benign (noncancerous) condition in which tissue has certain abnormal features.

Autologous bone marrow transplantation (aw-TAHL-o-gus): A procedure in which bone marrow is removed from a patient and then is given back to the patient following intensive treatment.

Axilla (ak-SIL-a): The underarm.

Axillary (AK-sil-air-ee): Pertaining to the lymph nodes under the arm.

Axillary dissection (AK-sil-air-ee): Surgery to remove lymph nodes under the arm.

B cells: White blood cells that develop in the bone marrow and are the source of antibodies. Also known as B lymphocytes.

Barium enema: A series of X-rays of the lower intestine. The X-rays are taken after the patient is given an enema with a white, chalky solution that contains barium. The barium outlines the intestines on the X-rays.

Barium solution: A liquid containing barium sulfate that is used in X-rays to highlight parts of the digestive system.

Barrett's esophagus: A change in the cells of the tissue that lines the bottom of the esophagus. The esophagus may become irritated when the contents of the stomach back up (reflux). Reflux that happens often over a long period of time can lead to Barrett's esophagus.

Basal cell carcinoma (BAY-sal sel kar-sin-O-ma): A type of skin cancer that arises from the basal cells.

Basal cells: Small, round cells found in the lower part, or base, of the epidermis, the outer layer of the skin.

Basophil: A type of white blood cell. Basophils are granulocytes.

BCG (Bacillus Calmette-Guerin): A substance that activates the immune system. Filling the bladder with a solution of BCG is a form of biological therapy for superficial bladder cancer.

Benign (beh-NINE): Not cancerous; does not invade nearby tissue or spread to other parts of the body.

Benign prostatic hyperplasia (hy-per-PLAY-zha): A noncancerous condition in which an overgrowth of prostate tissue pushes against the urethra and the bladder, blocking the flow of urine. Also called benign prostatic hypertrophy or BPH.

Benign tumor (beh-NINE): A noncancerous growth that does not spread to other parts of the body.

Beta-carotene: A substance from which vitamin A is formed; a precursor of vitamin A.

Bilateral: Affecting both the right and left side of body.

Bile: A yellow or orange fluid made by the liver. Bile is stored in the gallbladder. It passes through the common bile duct into the duodenum, where it helps digest fat.

Bioimmunotherapy: Treatment to stimulate or restore the ability of the immune system to fight infection and disease.

Biological response modifiers (by-o-LOJ-i-kal): Substances that stimulate the body's response to infection and disease. The body naturally produces small amounts of these substances. Scientists can produce some of them in the laboratory in large amounts and use them in cancer treatment. Also called BRMs.

Biological therapy (by-o-LOJ-i-kul): The use of the body's immune system, either directly or indirectly, to fight cancer or to lessen side effects that may be caused by some cancer treatments. Also known as immunotherapy, biotherapy, or biological response modifier therapy.

Biopsy (BYE-ahp-see): The removal of a sample of tissue, which is then examined under a microscope to check for cancer cells.

Bladder: The hollow organ that stores urine.

Bladder cancer: Bladder cancer is a disease in which cancer (malignant) cells are found in the bladder. The bladder, a hollow organ in the lower part of the abdomen, stores urine.

Blast phase: Refers to advanced chronic myelogenous leukemia. In this phase, the number of immature, abnormal white blood cells in the bone marrow and blood is extremely high. Also called blast crisis.

Blasts: Immature blood cells.

Blood-brain barrier: A network of blood vessels with closely spaced cells that makes it difficult for potentially toxic substances (such as anticancer drugs) to penetrate the blood vessel walls and to enter the brain.

Bone marrow: The soft, spongy tissue in the center of large bones that produces white blood cells, red blood cells, and platelets.

Bone marrow aspiration (as-per-AY-shun) or biopsy (BY-op-see): The removal of a small sample of bone marrow (usually from the hip) through a needle for examination under a microscope to see whether cancer cells are present.

Bone marrow biopsy (BYE-ahp-see): The removal of a sample of tissue from the bone marrow with a large needle. The cells are checked to see whether they are cancerous. If cancerous plasma cells are found, the pathologist estimates how much of the bone marrow is affected. Bone marrow biopsy is usually done at the same time as bone marrow aspiration.

Bone marrow transplantation (trans-plan-TAY-shun): A procedure in which doctors replace marrow destroyed by treatment with high doses of anticancer drugs or radiation. The replacement marrow may be taken from the patient before treatment or may be donated by another person.

Bone scan: A technique to create images of bones on a computer screen or on film. A small amount of radioactive material is injected and travels through the bloodstream. It collects in the bones, especially in abnormal areas of the bones, and is detected by a scanner.

Bowel: Another name for the intestine. There is both a small and a large bowel.

Brachytherapy (BRAK-i-THER-a-pee): Internal radiation therapy using an implant of radioactive material placed directly into or near the tumor.

Brain stem: The stemlike part of the brain that is connected to the spinal cord.

Brain stem glioma (glee-O-ma): A type of brain tumor that occurs in the lowest, stemlike part of the brain.

Brain tumor:

  astrocytoma: Astrocytomas are tumors that start in brain cells called astrocytes. There are different kinds of astrocytomas, which are defined by how the cancer cells look under a microscope.

  ependymoma: Ependymal tumors are tumors that begin in the ependyma, the cells that line the passageways in the brain where special fluid that protects the brain and spinal cord (called cerebrospinal fluid) is made and stored. There are different kinds of ependymal tumors, which are defined by how the cells look under a microscope.

  glioblastoma: Glioblastoma multiformes are tumors that grow very quickly and have cells that look very different from normal cells. Glioblastoma multiforme is also called grade IV astrocytoma.

  medulloblastoma: Medulloblastomas are brain tumors that begin in the lower part of the brain. They are almost always found in children or young adults. This type of cancer may spread from the brain to the spine.

BRCA1: A gene located on chromosome 17 that normally helps to restrain cell growth. Inheriting an altered version of BRCA1 predisposes an individual to breast, ovary, and prostate cancer.

Breast reconstruction: Surgery to rebuild a breast's shape after a mastectomy.

Bronchi (BRONK-eye): Air passage that leads from the windpipe to the lungs.

Bronchioles (BRON-kee-ols): The tiny branches of air tubes in the lungs.

Bronchitis (BRON-KYE-tis): Inflamation (swelling and reddening) of the bronchi.

Bronchoscope (BRON-ko-skope): A flexible, lighted instrument used to examine the trachea and bronchi, the air passages that lead into the lungs.

Bronchoscopy (bron-KOS-ko-pee): A test that permits the doctor to see the breathing passages through a lighted tube.

Buccal mucosa (BUK-ul myoo-KO-sa): The inner lining of the cheeks and lips.

Burkitt's lymphoma: A type of non-Hodgkin's lymphoma that most often occurs in young people between the ages of 12 and 30. The disease usually causes a rapidly growing tumor in the abdomen.

Bypass: A surgical procedure in which the doctor creates a new pathway for the flow of body fluids.

Calcium (KAL-see-um): A mineral found mainly in the hard part of bones.

Cancer: A term for diseases in which abnormal cells divide without control. Cancer cells can invade nearby tissues and can spread through the bloodstream and lymphatic system to other parts of the body.

Cancer screening: Different tests may show whether a person has a higher than normal risk for getting certain types of cancer. The person's family history and medical history are also key parts of the cancer screening process.

Carcinogen (kar-SIN-o-jin): Any substance that is known to cause cancer.

Carcinogenesis: The process by which normal cells are transformed into cancer cells.

Carcinoma (kar-sin-O-ma): Cancer that begins in the lining or covering of an organ.

Carcinoma in situ (kar-sin-O-ma in SY-too): Cancer that involves only the cells in which it began and has not spread to other tissues.

Cartilage (KAR-ti-lij): Firm, rubbery tissue that cushions bones at joints. A more flexible kind of cartilage connects muscles with bones and makes up other parts of the body, such as the larynx and the outside of the ears.

Catheter (KATH-et-er): A tube that is placed in a blood vessel to provide a pathway for drug or nutrients.

Cauterization (KAW-ter-i-ZAY-shun): The use of heat to destroy abnormal cells.

CEA assay: A laboratory test to measure the level of carcinoembryonic antigen (CEA), a substance that is sometimes found in an increased amount in the blood of patients with certain cancers.

Cell: The basic unit of any living organism.

Cell differentiation: The process during which young, immature (unspecialized) cells take on individual characteristics and reach their mature (specialized) form and function.

Cell motility: The ability of a cell to move.

Cell proliferation: An increase in the number of cells as a result of cell growth and cell division.

Cellular adhesion: The close adherence (bonding) to adjoining cell surfaces.

Central nervous system: The brain and spinal cord. Also called CNS.

Cerebellum (sair-uh-BELL-um): The portion of the brain in the back of the head between the cerebrum and the brain stem.

Cerebral hemispheres (seh-REE-bral HEM-iss-feerz): The two halves of the cerebrum.

Cerebrospinal fluid (seh-REE-bro-spy-nal): The watery fluid flowing around the brain and spinal cord. Also called CSF.

Cerebrum (seh-REE-brum): The largest part of the brain. It is divided into two hemispheres, or halves.

Cervical cancer: Cancer of the cervix, a common kind of cancer in women, is a disease in which cancer (malignant) cells are found in the tissues of the cervix. The cervix is the opening of the uterus (womb).

Cervical intraepithelial neoplasia (SER-vih-kul in-tra-eh-pih-THEEL-ee-ul NEE-o-play-zha): A general term for the growth of abnormal cells on the surface of the cervix. Numbers from 1 to 3 may be used to describe how extensive the abnormal cells are and how deeply they penetrate through the epithelium. Also called CIN.

Cervix (SER-viks): The lower, narrow end of the uterus that forms a canal between the uterus and vagina.

Chemoprevention (KEE-mo-pre-VEN-shun): The use of natural or laboratory made substances to prevent cancer.

Chemotherapy (kee-mo-THER-a-pee): Treatment with anticancer drugs.

Cholangiosarcoma (ko-LAN-jee-o-sar-KO-ma): A type of cancer that begins in the bile ducts.

Chondrosarcoma (KON-dro-sar-KO-ma): A cancer that forms in cartilage, occurring mainly in the pelvis, femur, and shoulder areas.

Chordoma (kor-DO-ma): A form of bone cancer that usually starts in the lower spinal column.

Chromosome (KRO-mo-soam): Part of a cell that contains genetic information. Normally, human cells contain 46 chromosomes that appear as a long thread inside the cell.

Chronic leukemia (KRON-ik): Leukemia that progresses slowly.

Chronic phase (KRON-ik): Refers to the early stages of chronic myelogenous leukemia or chronic lymphocytic leukemia. The number of immature, abnormal white blood cells in the bone marrow and blood is higher than normal, but lower than in the accelerated or blast phase.

Clinical trials: Research studies that involve patients. Each study is designed to find better ways to prevent, detect, diagnose, or treat cancer and to answer scientific questions.

CNS (central nervous system): The brain and the spinal cord.

CNS prophylaxis (pro-fi-LAK-sis): Chemotherapy or radiation therapy to the central nervous system (CNS). This is preventive treatment. It is given to kill cancer cells that may be in the brain and spinal cord, even though no cancer has been detected there.

Colectomy (ko-LEK-to-mee): An operation to remove all or part of the colon. In a partial colectomy, the surgeon removes only the cancerous part of the colon and a small amount (called a margin) of surrounding healthy tissue.

Colon (KO-lun): The long, coiled, tubelike organ that removes water from digested food. The remaining material, solid waste called stool, moves through the colon to the rectum and leaves the body through the anus.

Colon cancer: Cancer of the colon, a common form of cancer, is a disease in which cancer (malignant) cells are found in the tissues of the colon. The colon is part of the body's digestive system. The last 6 feet of intestine is called the large bowel or colon.

Colonoscope (ko-LON-o-skope): A flexible, lighted instrument used to view the inside of the colon.

Colonoscopy (ko-lon-OS-ko-pee): An examination in which the doctor looks at the colon through a flexible, lighted instrument called a colonoscope.

Colony-stimulating factors: Substances that stimulate the production of blood cells. Treatment with colony-stimulating factors (CSF) can help the blood-forming tissue recover from the effects of chemotherapy and radiation therapy.

Colorectal (ko-lo-REK-tul): Related to the colon and/or rectum.

Colostomy (ko-LOS-to-mee): An opening created by a surgeon into the colon from the outside of the body. A colostomy provides a new path for waste material to leave the body after part of the colon has been removed.

Colposcopy (kul-POSS-ko-pee): A procedure in which a lighted magnifying instrument (called a colposcope) is used to examine the vagina and cervix.

Combination chemotherapy: Treatment in which two or more chemicals are used to obtain more effective results.

Common bile duct: Bile ducts are passageways that carry bile. Two major bile ducts come together into a "trunk," the common bile duct, which empties into the upper part of the small intestine (the part next to the stomach).

Computed tomography (tom-OG-rah-fee): An X-ray procedure that uses a computer to produce a detailed picture of a cross section of the body; also called CAT or CT scan.

Condylomata acuminata (kon-di-LOW-ma-ta a-kyoo-mi-NA-ta): Genital warts caused by certain human papillomaviruses.

Conization (ko-ni-ZAY-shun): Surgery to remove a cone-shaped piece of tissue from the cervix and cervical canal. Conization may be used to diagnose or treat a cervical condition. Also called cone biopsy.

Continent reservoir (KAHN-tih-nent RES-er-vwar): A pouch formed from a piece of small intestine to hold urine after the bladder has been removed.

Corpus: The body of the uterus.

Craniopharyngioma(KRAY-nee-o-fah-rin-jee-O-ma): A type of brain tumor that develops in the region of the pituitary gland near the hypothalamus, the area of the brain that controls body temperature, hunger, and thirst. These tumors are usually benign but are sometimes considered malignant because they can press on or damage the hypothalamus and affect vital functions.

Craniotomy (kray-nee-OT-o-mee): An operation in which an opening is made in the skull so the doctor can reach the brain.

Cryosurgery (KRY-o-SER-jer-ee): Treatment performed with an instrument that freezes and destroys abnormal tissues.

Cryptorchidsm (kript-OR-kid-izm): A condition in which one or both testicles fail to move from the abdomen, where they develop before birth, into the scrotum; also called undescended testicles.

CT (or CAT) scan: A series of detailed pictures of areas inside the body; the pictures are created by a computer linked to an X-ray machine. Also called computed tomography scan or computed axial tomography scan.

Curettage (kyoo-re-TAHZH): Removal of tissue with a curette.

Curette (kyoo-RET): A spoon-shaped instrument with a sharp edge.

Cutaneous (kyoo-TAY-nee-us): Related to the skin.

Cutaneous T-cell lymphoma: Cutaneous T-cell lymphoma is a disease in which certain cells of the lymph system (called T lymphocytes) become cancer (malignant) and affect the skin. Lymphocytes are infection-fighting white blood cells that are made in the bone marrow and by other organs of the lymph system. T-cells are special lymphocytes that help the body's immune system kill bacteria and other harmful things in the body.

Cyst (sist): A sac or capsule filled with fluid.

Cystectomy (sis-TEK-to-mee): Surgery to remove the bladder.

Cystoscope (SIS-to-skope): An instrument that allows the doctor to see inside the bladder and remove tissue samples or small tumors.

Cystoscopy (sist-OSS-ko-pee): A procedure in which the doctor inserts a lighted instrument into the urethra (the tube leading from the bladder to the outside of the body) to look at the bladder.

Dermatologist (der-ma-TOL-o-jist): A doctor specializing in the diagnosis and treatment of skin problems.

Dermis (DER-mis): The lower or inner layer of the two main layers of cells that make up the skin.

Diabetes (dye-a-BEE-teez): A disease in which the body does not use sugar properly. (Many foods are converted into sugar, a source of energy for cells.) As a result, the level of sugar in the blood is too high. This disease occurs when the body does not produce enough insulin or does not use it properly.

Diagnosis: The process of indentifying a disease by the signs and symptoms.

Dialysis (dy-AL-i-sis): The process of cleansing the blood by passing it through a special machine. Dialysis is necessary when the kidneys are not able to filter the blood.

Diaphanography (DY-a-fan-OG-ra-fee): An exam that involves shining a bright light through the breast to reveal features of the tissues inside. This technique is under study; its value in detecting breast cancer has not been proven. Also called transillumination.

Diaphragm (DY-a-fram): The thin muscle below the lungs and heart that separates the chest from the abdomen.

Diathermy (DIE-a-ther-mee): The use of heat to destroy abnormal cells. Also cauterization or electrodiathermy.

Diethylstilbestrol (die-ETH-ul-stil-BES-trol): A drug that was once widely prescribed to prevent miscarriage. Also called DES.

Differentiation: In cancer, refers to how mature (developed) the cancer cells are in a tumor. Differentiated tumor cells resemble normal cells and grow at a slower rate than undifferentiated tumor cells, which lack the structure and function of normal cells and grow uncontrollably.

Digestive system: The organs that take in food and turn it into products that the body can use to stay healthy. Waste products the body cannot use leave the body through bowel movements. The digestive system includes the salivary glands, mouth, esophagus, stomach, liver, pancreas, gallbladder, intestines, and rectum.

Digestive tract (dye-JES-tiv): The organs through which food passes when we eat. These are the mouth, esophagus, stomach, small and large intestines, and rectum.

Digital rectal exam: An exam to detect cancer. The doctor inserts a lubricated, gloved finger into the rectum and feels for abnormal areas. Also called DRE.

Dilation and curettage (di-LAY-shun and KYOO-re-tahzh): A minor operation in which the cervix is expanded enough (dilation) to permit the cervical canal and uterine lining to be scraped with a spoon-shaped instrument called a curette (curettage). This procedure also is called D and C.

Dilator (DIE-lay-tor): A device used to stretch or enlarge an opening.

DNA: The protein that carries genetic information; every cell contains a strand of DNA (deoxyribonucleic acid).

Douching (DOO-shing): Using water or a medicated solution to clean the vagina and cervix.

Dry orgasm: Sexual climax without the release of semen.

Duct (dukt): A tube through which body fluids pass.

Ductal carcinoma in situ (DUK-tal kar-sin-O-ma in SY-too): Abnormal cells that involve only the lining of a duct. The cells have not spread outside the duct to other tissues in the breast. About 15–20 percent of breast cancers are sometimes called carcinoma in situ. They may be either ductal carcinoma in situ (sometimes called intraductal carcinoma) or lobular carcinoma in situ. Even though it is referred to as a cancer, it is not actually cancer. However, patients with this condition have a 25 percent chance of developing breast cancer in either breast in the next 25 years. Also called DCIS or intraductal carcinoma.

Dumping syndrome: A group of symptoms that occur when food or liquid enters the small intestine too rapidly. These symptoms include cramps, nausea, diarrhea, and dizziness.

Duodenum (doo-o-DEE-num): The first part of the small intestine.

Dysplasia (dis-PLAY-zha): Abnormal cells that are not cancer.

Dysplastic nevi: (dis-PLAS-tik NEE-vye): Atypical moles; moles whose appearance is different from that of common moles. Dysplastic nevi are generally larger than ordinary moles and have irregular and indistinct borders. Their color often is not uniform, and ranges from pink or even white to dark brown or black; they usually are flat, but parts may be raised above the skin surface.

Edema (eh-DEE-ma): Swelling; an abnormal buildup of fluid.

Ejaculation: The release of semen through the penis during orgasm.

Electrodesiccation (e-LEK-tro-des-i-KAY-shun): Use of an electric current to destroy cancerous tissue and control bleeding.

Electrolarynx (e-LEK-tro-LAR-inks): A battery-operated instrument that makes a humming sound to help laryngectomees talk.

Embolization (EM-bo-li-ZAY-shun): Blocking an artery so that blood cannot flow to the tumor.

Encapsulated (en-KAP-soo-lay-ted): Confined to a specific area; the tumor remains in a compact form.

Endocervical curettage (en-do-SER-vi-kul kyoo-re-TAZH): The removal of tissue from the inside of the cervix using a spoon-shaped instrument called a curette.

Endocrinologist (en-do-kri-NOL-o-jist): A doctor that specializes in diagnosing and treating hormone disorders.

Endometrial cancer: Cancer of the endometrium, a common kind of cancer in women, is a disease in which cancer (malignant) cells are found in the lining of the uterus (endometrium). The uterus is the hollow, pear-shaped organ where a baby grows. Cancer of the endometrium is different from cancer of the muscle of the uterus, which is called sarcoma of the uterus.

Endometriosis (en-do-mee-tree-O-sis): A benign condition in which tissue that looks like endometrial tissue grows in abnormal places in the abdomen.

Endometrium (en-do-MEE-tree-um): The layer of tissue that lines the uterus.

Endoscope (EN-do-skope): A thin, lighted tube through which a doctor can look at tissues inside the body.

Endoscopic retrograde cholangiopancreatography (en-do-SKAH-pik RET-ro-grade ko-LAN-jee-o-PAN-kree-a-TAW-gra-fee): A procedure to X-ray the common bile duct. Also called ERCP.

Endoscopy (en-DOS-ko-pee): An examination of the esophagus and stomach using a thin, lighted instrument called an endoscope.

Ependymoma (eh-PEN-dih-MO-ma): A type of brain tumor that usually develops in the lining of the ventricles but may also occur in the spinal chord.

Enterostomal therapist (en-ter-o-STO-mul): A health professional trained in the care of urostomies and other stomas.

Environmental tobacco smoke: Smoke that comes from the burning end of a cigarette and smoke that is exhaled by smokers. Also called ETS or second-hand smoke. Inhaling ETS is called involuntary or passive smoking.

Enzyme: A substance that affects the rate at which chemical changes take place in the body.

Ependymoma (eh-PEN-di-MO-ma): Ependymal tumors are tumors that begin in the ependyma, the cells that line the passageways in the brain where special fluid that protects the brain and spinal cord (called cerebrospinal fluid) is made and stored. There are different kinds of ependymal tumors, which are defined by how the cells look under a microscope.

Epidermis (ep-i-DER-mis): The upper or outer layer of the two main layers of cells that make up the skin.

Epidermoid carcinoma (ep-i-DER-moyd): A type of lung cancer in which the cells are flat and look like fish scales. Also called squamous cell carcinoma.

Epiglottis (ep-i-GLOT-is): The flap that covers the trachea during swallowing so that food does not enter the lungs.

Epithelial carcinoma (ep-i-THEE-lee-ul kar-si-NO-ma): Cancer that begins in the cells that line an organ.

Epithelium (EP-i-THEE-lee-um): A thin layer of tissue that covers organs, glands, and other structures in the body.

ERCP (endoscopic retrograde cholangiopancreatography) (en-do-SKOP-ik RET-ro-grade ko-LAN-gee-o-PAN-kree-a-TOG-ra-fee): A procedure to X-ray the common bile duct.

Erythrocytes (e-RITH-ro-sites): Cells that carry oxygen to all parts of the body. Also called red blood cells (RBCs).

Erythroleukemia (e-RITH-ro-loo-KEE-mee-a): Leukemia that develops in erythrocytes. In this rare disease, the body produces large numbers of abnormal red blood cells.

Erythroplakia (eh-RITH-ro-PLAY-kee-a): A reddened patch with a velvety surface found in the mouth.

Esophageal (e-soff-a-JEE-al): Related to the esophagus.

Esophageal cancer: Cancer of the esophagus is a disease in which cancer (malignant) cells are found in the tissues of the esophagus. The esophagus is the hollow tube that carries food and liquid from the throat to the stomach.

Esophageal speech (e-SOF-a-JEE-al): Speech produced with air trapped in the esophagus and forced out again.

Esophagectomy (e-soff-a-JEK-to-mee): An operation to remove a portion of the esophagus.

Esophagoscopy (e-soff-a-GOSS-ko-pee): Examination of the esophagus using a thin, lighted instrument.

Esophagram (e-SOFF-a-gram): A series of X-rays of the esophagus. The X-ray pictures are taken after the patient drinks a solution that coats and outlines the walls of the esophagus. Also called a barium swallow.

Esophagus (e-SOF-a-gus): The muscular tube through which food passes from the throat to the stomach.

Estrogen (ES-tro-jin): A female hormone.

Etiology: The study of the causes of abnormal condition or disease.

Ewing's sarcoma (YOO-ingz sar-KO-ma): Ewing's sarcoma/primitive neuroepithelial tumor is a rare disease in which cancer (malignant) cells are found in the bone. The most common areas in which it occurs are the pelvis, the thigh bone (femur), the upper arm bone (humerus), and the ribs. Ewing's sarcoma/primitive neuroepithelial tumor most frequently occurs in teenagers.

External radiation: Radiation therapy that uses a machine to aim high-energy rays at the cancer.

Fallopian tubes (fa-LO-pee-in): Tubes on each side of the uterus through which an egg moves from the ovaries to the uterus.

Familial polyposis (pol-i-PO-sis): An inherited condition in which several hundred polyps develop in the colon and rectum.

Fecal occult blood test (FEE-kul o-KULT): A test to check for hidden blood in stool. (Fecal refers to stool. Occult means hidden.)

Fertility (fer-TIL-i-tee): The ability to produce children.

Fetus (FEET-us): The unborn child developing in the uterus.

Fiber: The parts of fruits and vegetables that cannot be digested. Also called bulk or roughage.

Fibroid (FY-broid): A benign uterine tumor made up of fibrous and muscular tissue.

Fibrosarcoma: A type of soft tissue sarcoma that begins in fibrous tissue, which holds bones, muscles, and other organs in place.

Fluoroscope (FLOOR-o-skope): An X-ray machine that makes it possible to see internal organs in motion.

Fluoroscopy (Floor-OS-ko-pee): An X-ray procedure that makes it possible to see internal organs in motion

Fluorouracil (floo-ro-YOOR-a-sil): An anticancer drug. Its chemical name is 5-fluorouracil, commonly called 5-FU.

Follicles (FAHL-ih-kuls): Shafts through which hair grows.

Fractionation: Dividing the total dose of radiation therapy into several smaller, equal doses delivered over a period of several days.

Fulguration (ful-gyoor-AY-shun): Destroying tissue using an electric current.

Gallbladder (GAWL-blad-er): The pear-shaped organ that sits below the liver. Bile is stored in the gallbladder.

Gamma knife: Radiation therapy in which high-energy rays are aimed at a tumor from many angles in a single treatment session.

Gastrectomy (gas-TREK-to-mee): An operation to remove all or part of the stomach.

Gastric (GAS-trik): Having to do with the stomach.

Gastric atrophy (GAS-trik AT-ro-fee): A condition in which the stomach muscles shrink and become weak. It results in a lack of digestive juices.

Gastric cancer: Cancer of the stomach, also called gastric cancer, is a disease in which cancer (malignant) cells are found in the tissues of the stomach.

Gastroenterologist (GAS-tro-en-ter-OL-o-jist): A doctor who specializes in diagnosing and treating disorders of the digestive system.

Gastrointestinal tract (GAS-tro-in-TES-ti-nul): The part of the digestive tract where the body processes food and eliminates waste. It includes the esophagus, stomach, liver, small and large intestines, and rectum.

Gastroscope (GAS-tro-skope): A thin, lighted instrument to view the inside of the stomach.

Gastroscopy (gas-TROS-ko-pee): An examination of the stomach with a gastroscope, an instrument to view the inside of the stomach.

Gene: The biological or basic unit of heredity found in all cells in the body.

Gene deletion: The total loss or absence of a gene.

Gene therapy: Treatment that alters genes (the basic units of heredity found in all cells in the body). In stud-ies of gene therapy for cancer, researchers are trying to improve the body's natural ability to fight the disease or to make the tumor more sensitive to other kinds of therapy.

Genetic: Inherited; having to do with information that is passed from parents to children through DNA in the genes.

Genetic testing: Specific tests can be done to see whether a person has changes in certain genes that are known to be associated with cancer.

Genitourinary system (GEN-i-toe-YOO-rin-air-ee): The parts of the body that play a role in reproduction, in getting rid of waste products in the form of urine, or in both.

Germ cells: The reproductive cells of the body specifically, either egg or sperm cells.

Germ cell tumors: A type of brain tumor that arises from primitive (developing) sex cells, or germ cells.

Germinoma (jer-mih-NO-ma): The most frequent type of germ cell tumor in the brain.

Germline mutation: See hereditary mutation.

Gestational trophoblastic disease: Gestational trophoblastic tumor, a rare cancer in women, is a disease in which cancer (malignant) cells grow in the tissues that are formed following conception (the joining of sperm and egg). Gestational trophoblastic tumors start inside the uterus, the hollow, muscular, pear-shaped organ where a baby grows. This type of cancer occurs in women during the years when they are able to have children.

Gland: An organ that produces and releases one or more substances for use in the body. Some glands produce fluids that affect tissues or organs. Others produce hormones or participate in blood production.

Glioblastoma multiforme (glee-o-blast-TO-ma mul-tih-FOR-may): A type of brain tumor that forms in the nervous (glial) tissue of the brain. They grow very quickly and have cells that look very different from normal cells. Glioblastoma multiforme is also called grade IV astrocytoma.

Glioma (glee-O-ma): A name for brain tumors that begin in the glial cells, or supportive cells, in the brain. "Glia" is the Greek word for glue.

Glottis (GLOT-is): The middle part of the larynx; the area where the vocal cords are located.

Grade: Describes how closely a cancer resembles normal tissue of its same type, and the cancer's probable rate of growth.

Grading: A system for classifying cancer cells in terms of how malignant or aggressive they appear microscopically. The grading of a tumor indicates how quickly cancer cells are likely to spread and plays a role in treatment decisions.

Graft: Healthy skin, bone, or other tissue taken from one part of the body to replace diseased or injured tissue removed from another part of the body.

Graft-versus-host disease: A reaction of donated bone marrow against a patient's own tissue. Also called GVHD.

Granulocyte (GRAN-yoo-lo-site): A type of white blood cell. Neutrophils, eosinophils, and basophils are granulocytes.

Groin: The area where the thigh meets the hip.

GVHD (graft-versus-host disease): A reaction of donated bone marrow against a patient's own tissue.

Gynecologic oncologists (guy-ne-ko-LA-jik on-KOL-o-jists): Doctors who specialize in treating cancers of the female reproductive organs.

Gynecologist (guy-ne-KOL-o-jist): A doctor specializing in treating diseases of the female reproductive organs.

Hair follicles (FOL-i-kuls): The sacs in the scalp from which hair grows.

Hairy cell leukemia: A rare type of chronic leukemia in which the abnormal white blood cells appear to be covered with tiny hairs.

Helicobacter pylori (HEEL-i-ko-BAK-ter pie-LOR-ee): Bacteria that cause inflammation and ulcers in the stomach.

Hematogenous: Orginating in the blood, or disseminated by the circulation or through the bloodstream.

Hematologist (hee-ma-TOL-o-jist): A doctor who specializes in treating diseases of the blood.

Hepatitis (hep-a-TYE-tis): Inflammation of the liver.

Hepatitis B: A type of hepatitis that is carried and passed on through the blood. It can be passed on through sexual contact or through the use of "dirty" (bloody) needles.

Hepatoblastoma (HEP-a-to-blas-TO-ma): A type of liver tumor that occurs in infants and children.

Hepatocellular carcinoma (HEP-a-to-SEL-yoo-ler kar-si-NO-ma): The most common type of primary liver cancer.

Hepatocyte (HEP-a-to-site): A liver cell.

Hepatoma (HEP-a-TO-ma): A liver tumor.

Hereditary mutation: A gene change in the body's reproductive cells (egg or sperm) that becomes incorporated into the DNA of every cell in the body of offspring; hereditary mutations are passed on from parents to offspring.

Herpes virus (HER-peez-VY-rus): A member of the herpes family of viruses. One type of herpesvirus is sexually transmitted and causes sores on the genitals.

HER-2/neu: Oncogene found in some breast and ovarian cancer patients that is associated with a poor prognosis.

Hodgkin's disease: Hodgkin's disease is a type of lymphoma. Lymphomas are cancers that develop in the lymph system, part of the body's immune system.

Hormonal therapy: Treatment of cancer by removing, blocking, or adding hormones.

Hormone receptor test: A test to measure the amount of certain proteins, called hormone recptors, in breast cancer tissue. Hormones can attach to these proteins. A high level of hormone receptors means hormones probably help the cancer grow.

Hormone therapy: Treatment that prevents certain cancer cells from getting the hormones they need to grow.

Hormones: Chemicals produced by glands in the body and circulate in the bloodstream. Hormones control the actions of certain cells or organs.

Human papillomaviruses (pap-i-LOW-ma VY-rus-ez): Viruses that generally cause warts. Some papillomaviruses are sexually transmitted. Some of these sexually transmitted viruses cause wartlike growths on the genitals, and some are thought to cause abnormal changes in cells of the cervix.

Humidifier (hyoo-MID-ih-fye-er): A machine that puts moisture in the air.

Hydrocephalus (hy-dro-SEF-uh-lus): The abnormal buildup of cerebrospinal fluid in the ventricles of the brain.

Hypercalcemia (hy-per-kal-SEE-mee-a): A higher-than-normal level of calcium in the blood. This condition can cause a number of symptoms, including loss of appetite, nausea, thirst, fatigue, muscle weakness, restlessness, and confusion.

Hyperfractionation: A way of giving radiation therapy in smaller-than-usual doses two or three times a day.

Hyperplasia (hye-per-PLAY-zha): A precancerous condition in which there is an increase in the number of normal cells lining the uterus.

Hyperthermia (hy-per-THER-mee-a): Treatment that involves heating a tumor.

Hypothalamus (hy-po-THAL-uh-mus): The area of the brain that controls body temperature, hunger, and thirst.

Hysterectomy (hiss-ter-EK-to-mee): An operation in which the uterus and cervix are removed.

Ileostomy (il-ee-OS-to-mee): An opening created by a surgeon into the ileum, part of the small intestine, from the outside of the body. An ileostomy provides a new path for waste material to leave the body after part of the intestine has been removed.

Imaging: Tests that produce pictures of areas inside the body.

Immune system (im-YOON): The complex group of organs and cells that defends the body against infection or disease.

Immunodeficiency: A lowering of the body's ability to fight off infection and disease.

Immunology: A science that deals with the study of the body's immune system.

Immunosuppression: The use of drugs or techniques to suppress or interfere with the body's immune system and its ability to fight infections or disease. Immunosuppression may be deliberate, such as in preparation for bone marrow or other organ transplantation to prevent rejection by the host of the donor tissue, or incidental, such as often results from chemotherapy for the treatment of cancer.

Immunotherapy (IM-yoo-no-THER-a-pee): Treatment that uses the body's natural defenses to fight cancer. Also called biological therapy.

Implant (or internal) radiation: Internal radiation therapy that places radioactive materials in or close to the cancer.

Impotent (IM-po-tent): Inability to have an erection and/or ejaculate semen.

Incidence: The number of new cases of a disease diagnosed each year.

Incision (in-SI-zhun): A cut made in the body during surgery.

Incontinence (in-kON-ti-nens): Inability to control the flow of urine from the bladder.

Infertility: The inability to produce children.

Infiltrating cancer: See invasive cancer.

Inflammatory breast cancer: A rare type of breast cancer in which cancer cells block the lymph vessels in the skin of the breast. The breast becomes red, swollen, and warm, and the skin of the breast may appear pitted or have ridges.

Inguinal orchiectomy (IN-gwin-al or-kee-EK-to-mee): Surgery to remove the testicle through the groin.

Insulin (IN-su-lin): A hormone made by the islet cells of the pancreas. Insulin controls the amount of sugar in the blood.

Interferon (in-ter-FEER-on): A type of biological response modifier (a substance that can improve the body's natural response to disease). It stimulates the growth of certain disease-fighting blood cells in the immune system.

Interleukin (in-ter-LOO-kin): A substance used in biological therapy. Interleukins stimulate the growth and activities of certain kinds of white blood cells.

Interleukin 2 (in-ter-LOO-kin): A type of biological response modifier (a substance that can improve the body's natural response to disease). It stimulates the growth of certain blood cells in the immune system that can fight cancer. Also called IL-2.

Internal radiation (ray-dee-AY-shun): Radiation therapy that uses radioactive materials placed in or near the tumor.

Intestine (in-TES-tin): The long, tube-shaped organ in the abdomen that completes the process of digestion. It consists of the small and large intestines.

Intraepithelial (in-tra-eh-pih-THEEL-ee-ul): Within the layer of cells that forms the surface or lining of an organ.

Intrahepatic (in-tra-hep-AT-ik): Within the liver.

Intrahepatic bile duct (in-tra-hep-AT-ik): The bile duct that passes through and drains bile from the liver.

Intraoperative radiation therapy: Radiation treatment given during surgery. Also called IORT.

Intraperitoneal chemotherapy (IN-tra-per-i-to-NEE-al): Treatment in which anticancer drugs are put directly into the abdomen through a thin tube.

Intrathecal chemotherapy (in-tra-THEE-cal KEE-mo-THER-a-pee): Chemotherapy drugs infused into the thin space between the lining of the spinal cord and brain to treat or prevent cancers in the brain and spinal cord.

Intravenous (in-tra-VEE-nus): Injected in a vein. Also called IV.

Intravenous pyelogram (in-tra-VEE-nus PIE-el-o-gram): A series of X-rays of the kidneys and bladder. The X-rays are taken after a dye that shows up on X-ray film in injected into a vein. Also called IVP.

Intravenous pyelography (om-tra-VEE-nus py-LOG-ra-fee): X-ray study of the kidneys and urinary tract. Structures are made visible by the injection of a substance that blocks X-rays. Also called IVP.

Intravesical (in-tra-VES-ih-kal): Within the bladder.

Invasion: As related to cancer, the spread of cancer cells into healthy tissue adjacent to the tumor.

Invasive cancer: Cancer that has spread beyond the layer of tissue in which it developed. Invasive breast cancer is also called infiltrating cancer or infiltrating carcinoma.

Invasive cervical cancer: Cancer that has spread from the surface of the cervix to tissue deeper in the cervix or to other parts of the body.

IORT (intraoperative radiation therapy): Radiation treatment given during surgery.

Islet cell cancer (EYE-let): Cancer arising from cells in the islets of Langerhans.

Islets of Langerhans (EYE-lets of LANG-er-hanz): Hormone-producing cells in the pancreas.

IV (intravenous) (in-tra-VEE-nus): Injected in a vein.

IVP (intravenous pyelogram) (in-tra-VEE-nus PYE-el-o-gram): X-ray study of the kidneys, uterus, and urinary tract. Structures are made visible by the injection of a substance that blocks X-rays.

Jaundice (JAWN-dis): A condition in which the skin and the whites of the eyes become yellow and the urine darkens. Jaundice occurs when the liver is not working properly or when a bile duct is blocked.

Kaposi's sarcoma (KAP-o-seez-sar-KO-ma): A relatively rare type of cancer that develops on the skin of some elderly persons or those with a weak immune system, including those with acquired immune deficiency syndrome (AIDS).

Kidney cancer: Renal cell cancer (also called cancer of the kidney or renal adenocarcinoma) is a disease in which cancer (malignant) cells are found in certain tissues of the kidney. Renal cell cancer is one of the less common kinds of cancer. It occurs more often in men than in women.

Kidneys (KID-neez): A pair or organs in the abdomen that remove waste from the blood. The waste leaves the blood as urine.

Krukenberg tumor (KROO-ken-berg): A tumor of the ovary caused by the spread of stomach cancer.

Laparoscopy (lap-a-ROS-ko-pee): A surgical procedure in which a lighted instrument shaped like a thin tube is inserted through a small incision in the abdomen. The doctor can look through the instrument and see inside the abdomen.

Laparotomy (lap-a-ROT-o-mee): An operation that allows the doctor to inspect the organs in the abdomen.

Large cell carcinomas: A group of lung cancers in which the cells are large and look abnormal.

Laryngeal (lair-IN-jee-al): Having to do with the larynx.

Laryngectomee (lair-in-JEK-toe-mee): A person who has had his or her voice box removed.

Laryngectomy (lair-in-JEK-toe-mee): An operation to remove all or part of the larynx.

Laryngoscope (lair-IN-jo-skope): A flexible lighted tube used to examine the larynx.

Laryngoscopy (lair-in-GOS-ko-pee): Examination of the larynx with a mirror (indirect laryngoscopy) or with a laryngoscope (direct laryngoscopy).

Larynx (LAIR-inks): An organ in the throat used in breathing, swallowing, and talking. It is made of cartilage and is lined by a mucous membrane similar to the lining of the mouth. Also called the "voice box."

Larynx cancer: Cancer of the larynx (or voice box) is a disease in which cancer (malignant) cells are found in the tissues of the larynx. Your larynx is a short passageway shaped like a triangle that is just below the pharynx in the neck. The pharynx is a hollow tube about 5 inches long that starts behind the nose and goes down to the neck to become part of the tube that goes to the stomach (the esophagus).

Laser (LAY-zer): A powerful beam of light used in some types of surgery to cut or destroy tissue.

Leiomyosarcoma: Leiomyosarcoma is a tumor of smooth muscle tissue. This cancer affects the uterus, lower abdomen, and extremities (hands and feet) most often.

Lesion (LEE-zhun): An area of abnormal tissue change.

Leukemia (loo-KEE-mee-a): Cancer of the blood cells.

> **acute lymphoblastic:** Acute lymphocytic leukemia (also called acute lymphoblastic leukemia or ALL) is a disease in which too many infection-fighting white blood cells called lymphocytes are found in the blood and bone marrow.

> **acute myeloblastic:** Acute myeloid leukemia (AML) is a disease in which cancer (malignant) cells are found in the blood and bone marrow. Normally, the bone marrow makes cells called blasts that develop (mature) into several different types of blood cells that have specific jobs to do in the body. AML affects the blasts that are developing into white blood cells called granulocytes. In AML, the blasts do not mature and become too numerous.

> **chronic myelogenous:** Chronic myelogenous leukemia (also called CML or chronic granulocytic leukemia) is a disease in which too many white blood cells are made in the bone marrow. CML affects the blasts that are developing into white blood cells called granulocytes.

Leukocytes (LOO-ko-sites): Cells that help the body fight infections and other diseases. Also called white blood cells (WBCs).

Leukoplakia (loo-ko-PLAY-kee-a): A white spot or patch in the mouth

Li-Fraumeni Syndrome: A rare family predisposition to multiple cancers, caused by an alteration in the p53 tumor suppressor gene.

Ligation (lye-GAY-shun): The process of tying off blood vessels so that blood cannot flow to a part of the body or to a tumor.

Limb perfusion (per-FYOO-zhun): A chemotherapy technique that may be used when melanoma occurs on an arm or leg. The flow of blood to and from the limb is stopped for a while with a tourniquet, and anticancer drugs are put directly into the blood of the limb. This allows the patient to receive a high dose of drugs in the area where the melanoma occurred.

Liver: A large, glandular organ, located in the upper abdomen, that cleanses the blood and aids in digestion by secreting bile.

Liver cancer: Liver cancer is a disease in which cancer (malignant) cells start to grow in the tissues of the liver. The liver is one of the largest organs in the body, filling the upper right side of the abdomen and protected by the rib cage.

Liver scan: An image of the liver created on a computer screen or on film. For a liver scan, a radioactive substance is injected into a vein and travels through the bloodstream. It collects in the liver, especially in abnormal areas, and can be detected by the scanner.

Lobe: A portion of the liver, lung, breast, or brain.

Lobectomy (lo-BEK-to-mee): The removal of a lobe.

Lobular carcinoma in situ (LOB-yoo-lar-sin-O-ma in SY-too): Abnormal cells in the lobules of the breast. This condition seldom becomes invasive cancer. However, having lobular carcinoma in situ is a sign that the woman has an increased risk of developing breast cancer. Also called LCIS.

Lobule (LOB-yule): A small lobe.

Local: Reaching and affecting only the cells in a specific area.

Local therapy: Treatment that affects cells in the tumor and the area close to it.

Lower GI series: A series of X-rays of the colon and rectum that is taken after the patient is given a barium enema. (Barium is a white, chalky substance that outlines the colon and rectum on the X-ray.)

Lubricant (LOO-brih-kant): An oily or slippery substance. A vaginal lubricant may be helpful for women who feels pain during intercourse because of vaginal dryness.

Lumbar puncture: The insertion of a needle into the lower part of the spinal column to collect cerebrospinal fluid or to give intrathecal chemotherapy. Also called a spinal tap.

Lumpectomy (lump-EK-toe-mee): Surgery to remove only the cancerous breast lump; usually followed by radiation therapy.

Luteinizing hormone-releasing hormone (LHRH) **agonist** (LOO-tin-eye-zing ... AG-o-nist): A substance that closely resembles LHRH, which controls the production of sex hormones. However, LHRH agonists affect the body differently than does LHRH. LHRH agonists keep the testicles from producing hormones.

Lymph (limf): The almost colorless fluid that travels through the lymphatic system and carries cells that help fight infection and disease.

Lymph nodes: Small, bean-shaped organs located along the channels of the lymphatic system. The lymph nodes store special cells that can trap bacteria or cancer cells traveling through the body in lymph. Clusters of lymph nodes are found in the underarms, groin, neck, chest, and abdomen. Also called lymph glands.

Lymphangiogram (lim-FAN-jee-o-gram): An X-ray of the lymphatic system. A dye is injected to outline the lymphatic vessels and organs.

Lymphangiography (imf-an-jee-OG-ra-fee): X-ray study of lymph nodes and lymph vessels made visible by the injection of a special dye.

Lymphatic system (lim-FAT-ik): The tissues and organs that produce, store, and carry white blood cells that fight infection and disease. This system includes the bone marrow, spleen, thymus, and lymph nodes and a network of thin tubes that carry lymph and white blood cells. These tubes branch, like blood vessels, into all the tissues of the body.

Lymphedema (LIMF-eh-DEE-ma): A condition in which excess fluid collects in tissue and causes swelling. It may occur in the arm or leg after lymph vessels or lymph nodes in the underarm or groin are removed.

Lymphoma: Cancer that arises in cells of the lymphatic system.

Lymphocytes (LIMF-o-sites): White blood cells that fight infection and disease.

Lymphocytic (lim-fo-SIT-ik): Referring to lymphocytes, a type of white blood cell.

Lymphoid (LIM-foyd): Referring to lymphocytes, a type of white blood cell. Also refers to tissue in which lymphocytes develop.

M proteins: Antibodies or parts of antibodies found in unusually large amounts in the blood or urine of multiple myeloma patients.

Magnetic resonance imaging (mag-NET-ik REZ-o-nan IM-a-jing): A procedure in which a magnet linked to a computer is used to create detailed pictures of areas inside the body. Also called MRI.

Maintenance therapy: Chemotherapy that is given to leukemia patients in remission to prevent a relapse.

Malignant (ma-LIG-nant): Cancerous; can invade nearby tissue and spread to other parts of the body.

Mammogram (MAM-o-gram): An X-ray of the breast.

Mammography (mam-OG-ra-fee): The use of X-rays to create a picture of the breast.

Mastecomy (mas-TEK-to-mee): Surgery to remove the breast (or as much of the breast as possible).

Mediastinoscopy (MEE-dee-a-stin-AHS-ko-pee): A procedure in which the doctor inserts a tube into the chest to view the organs in the mediastinum. The tube is inserted through an incision above the breastbone.

Mediastinotomy (MEE-dee-a-stin-AH-toe-mee): A procedure in which the doctor inserts a tube into the chest to view the organs in the mediastinum. The tube is inserted through an incision next to the breastbone.

Mediastinum (mee-dee-a-STY-num): The area between the lungs. The organs in this area include the heart and its large veins and arteries, the trachea, the esophagus, the bronchi, and lymph nodes.

Medical oncologist (on-KOL-o-jist): A doctor who specializes in treating cancer. Some oncologists specialize in a particular type of cancer treatment. For example, a radiation oncologist specializes in treating cancer with radiation.

Medulloblastoma (MED-yoo-lo-blas-TOE-ma): A type of brain tumor that recent research suggests develops from primitive (developing) nerve cells that normally do not remain in the body after birth. Medulloblastomas are sometimes called primitive neuro-ectodermal tumors. They are almost always found in children or young adults.

Melanin (MEL-a-nin): A skin pigment (substance that gives the skin its color). Dark-skinned people have more melanin than light-skinned people.

Melanocytes (mel-AN-o-sites): Cells in the skin that produce and contain the pigment called melanin.

Melanoma: Cancer of the cells that produce pigment in the skin. Melanoma usually begins in a mole.

Membrane: A thin layer of tissue that covers a surface.

Meninges (meh-NIN-jeez): The three membranes that cover the brain and spinal cord.

Meningioma (meh-nin-jee-O-ma): A type of brain tumor that develops in the meninges. Because these tumors grow very slowly, the brain may be able to adjust to their presence; meningiomas often grow quite large before they cause symptoms.

Menopause (MEN-o-pawz): When a woman's menstrual periods permanently stop. Also called "change of life."

Menstrual cycle (MEN-stroo-al): The hormone changes that lead up to a woman's having a period. For most women, one cycle takes 28 days.

Mesothelioma: Malignant mesothelioma, a rare form of cancer, is a disease in which cancer (malignant) cells are found in the sac lining the chest (the pleura) or abdomen (the peritoneum). Most people with malignant mesothelioma have worked on jobs where they breathed asbestos.

Metastasize (meh-TAS-ta-size): To spread from one part of the body to another. When cancer cells metastasize and form secondary tumors, the cells in the metastatic tumor are like those in the original (primary) tumor.

Microcalcifications (MY-krow-kal-si-fi-KA-shunz): Tiny deposits of calcium in the breast that cannot be felt but can be detected on a mammogram. A cluster of these very small specks of calcium may indicate that cancer is present.

Mole: An area on the skin (usually dark in color) that contains a cluster of melanocytes.

Monoclonal antibodies (MON-o-KLO-nul AN-ti-BOD-eez): Substances that can locate and bind to cancer cells wherever they are in the body. They can be used alone, or they can be used to deliver drugs, toxins, or radioactive material directly to tumor cells.

Monocyte: A type of white blood cell.

Morphology: The science of the form and structure of organisms (plants, animals, and other forms of life).

MRI (magnetic resonance imaging): A procedure in which a magnet linked to a computer is used to create detailed pictures of areas inside the body.

Mucus: A thick fluid produced by the lining of some organs of the body.

Multiple myeloma (mye-eh-LO-ma): Cancer that affects plasma cells. The disease causes the growth of tumors in many bones, which can lead to bone pain and fractures. In addition, the disease often causes kidney problems and lowered resistance to infection.

Mutations: Changes in the way cells function or develop, caused by an inherited genetic defect or an environmental exposure. Such changes may lead to cancer.

Mycosis fungoides (my-KO-sis fun-GOY-deez): A type of non-Hodgkin's lymphoma that first appears on the skin. Also called cutaneous T-cell lymphoma.

Myelin (MYE-eh-lin): The fatty substance that covers and protects nerves.

Myelodysplastic syndrome (MYE-eh-lo-dis-PLAS-tik SIN-drome): Myelodysplastic syndromes, also called pre-leukemia or "smoldering" leukemia, are diseases in which the bone marrow does not function normally and not enough normal blood cells are made. (See Preleukemia)

Myelogenous (mye-eh-LAH-jen-us): Referring to myelocytes, a type of white blood cell. Also called myeloid.

Myelogram (MYE-eh-lo-gram): An X-ray of the spinal cord and the bones of the spine.

Myeloid (MYE-eh-loyd): Referring to myelocytes, a type of white blood cell. Also called myelogenous.

Myometrium (my-o-MEE-tree-um): The muscular outer layer of the uterus.

Nasopharynx cancer: Cancer of the nasopharynx is a disease in which cancer (malignant) cells are found in the tissues of the nasopharynx. The nasopharynx is behind the nose and is the upper part of the throat (also called the pharynx). The pharynx is a hollow tube about 5 inches long that starts behind the nose and goes down to the neck to become part of the tube that goes to the stomach (the esophagus).

Neck dissection (dye-SEK-shun): Surgery to remove lymph nodes and other tissues in the neck.

Neoplasia (NEE-o-play-zha): Abnormal new growth of cells.

Neoplasm: A new growth of tissue. Can be referred to as benign or malignant.

Nephrectomy (nef-REK-to-mee): Surgery to remove the kidney. Radical nephrectomy removes the kidney, the adrenal gland, nearby lymph nodes, and other surrounding tissue. Simple nephrectomy removes just the affected kidney. Partial nephrectomy removes the tumor, but not the entire kidney.

Nephrotomogram (nef-ro-TOE-mo-gram): A series of special X-rays of the kidneys. The X-rays are taken from different angles. They show the kidneys clearly, without the shadows of the organs around them.

Neuroblastoma: Neuroblastoma is a disease in which cancer (malignant) cells are found in certain nerve cells in the body. Neuroblastoma most commonly starts in the abdomen, either in the adrenal glands (located just above the kidney in back of the upper abdomen) or around the spinal cord. Neuroblastoma can also start around the spinal cord in the chest, neck, or pelvis.

Neurologist (noo-ROL-o-jist): A doctor who specializes in the diagnosis and treatment of disorders of the nervous system.

Neuroma (noo-RO-ma): A tumor that arises in nerve cells.

Neurosurgeon (NOO-ro-SER-jun): A doctor who specializes in surgery on the brain and other parts of the nervous system.

Neutrophil (NOO-tro-fil): A type of white blood cell.

Nevus (NEE-vus): The medical term for a spot on the skin, such as a mole. A mole is a cluster of melanocytes that usually appears as a dark spot on the skin. The plural of nevus is nevi (NEE-vye).

Nitrosoureas (nye-TRO-so-yoo-REE-ahz): A group of anticancer drugs that can cross the blood–brain barrier. Carmustine (BCNU) and lomustine (CCNU) are nitrosoureas.

Non-Hodgkin's lymphoma: Adult non-Hodgkin's lymphoma is a disease in which cancer (malignant) cells are found in the lymph system. There are many types of non-Hodgkin's lymphomas. Some types spread more quickly than others. The type is determined by how the cancer cells look under a microscope.

Nonmelanoma skin cancer: Skin cancer that does not involve melanocytes. Basal cell cancer and squamous cell cancer are nonmelanoma skin cancers.

Nonseminoma (non-sem-i-NO-ma): A classification of testicular cancers that arise in specialized sex cells called germ cells. Nonseminomas include embryonal carcinoma, teratoma, choriocarcinoma, and yolk sac tumor.

Non-small cell lung cancer: A form of lung cancer associated with smoking, exposure to environmental tobacco smoke, or exposure to radon. Non-small cell lung cancer is classified as squamous cell carcinoma, adenocarcinoma, and large cell carcinoma depending on what type of cells are in the cancer.

Oat cell cancer: A type of lung cancer in which the cells look like oats. Also called small cell lung cancer.

Oligodendroglioma (OL-ih-go-den-dro-glee-O-ma): A rare, slow-growing type of brain tumor that occurs in the cells that produce myelin, the fatty covering that protects nerves.

Ommaya reservoir (o-MYE-a REZ-er-vwahr): A device implanted under the scalp and used to deliver anticancer drugs to the fluid surrounding the brain and spinal cord.

Oncogene: The part of the cell that normally directs cell growth, but which can also promote or allow the uncontrolled growth of cancer if damaged (mutated) by an environmental exposure to carcinogens, or damaged or missing because of an inherited defect.

Oncologist (on-KOL-o-jist): A doctor who specializes in treating cancer. Some oncologists specialize in a particular type of cancer treatment. For example, a radiation oncologist specializes in treating cancer with radiation.

Oncology: The study of tumors encompassing the physical, chemical, and biologic properties.

Oophorectomy (oo-for-EK-to-mee): The removal of one or both ovaries.

Ophthalmoscope (off-THAL-mo-skope): A lighted instrument used to examine the inside of the eye, including the retina and the optic nerve.

Optic nerve: The nerve that carries messages from the retina to the brain.

Oral cavity cancer: Cancer of the lip and oral cavity is a disease in which cancer (malignant) cells are found in the tissues of the lip or mouth. The oral cavity includes the front two-thirds of the tongue, the upper and lower gums (the gingiva), the lining of the inside of the cheeks and lips (the buccal mucosa), the bottom (floor) of the mouth under the tongue, the bony top of the mouth (the hard palate), and the small area behind the wisdom teeth (the retromolar trigone).

Oral surgeon: A dentist with special training in surgery of the mouth and jaw.

Orchiectomy (or-kee-EK-to-mee): Surgery to remove the testicles.

Organisms: Plants, animals, and other forms of life that are made up of complex and interconnected systems of cells and tissue.

Oropharynx (or-o-FAIR-inks): The area of the throat at the back of the mouth.

Osteosarcoma (OSS-tee-o-sar-KO-ma): A cancer of the bone that is most common in children. Also called osteogenic sarcoma. It is the most common type of bone cancer.

Ostomy (AHS-toe-mee): An operation to create an opening from an area inside the body to the outside. See Colostomy.

Otolaryngologist (AH-toe-lar-in-GOL-o-jist): A doctor who specializes in treating diseases of the ear, nose, and throat.

Ovarian cancer: Cancer of the ovary is a disease in which cancer (malignant) cells are found in the ovary. Approximately 25,000 women in the United States are diagnosed with this disease each year. The ovary is a small organ in the pelvis that makes female hormones and holds egg cells that, when fertilized, can develop into a baby.

Ovaries (O-var-eez): The pair of female reproductive glands in which the ova, or eggs, are formed. The ovaries are located in the lower abdomen, one on each side of the uterus.

p53: A gene in the cell that normally inhibits the growth of tumors, which can prevent or slow the spread of cancer.

Palate (PAL-et): The roof of the mouth. The front portion is bony (hard palate), and the back portion is muscular (soft palate).

Palliative treatment: Treatment that does not alter the course of a disease but improves the quality of life.

Palpation (pal-PAY-shun): A technique in which a doctor presses on the surface of the body to feel the organs or tissues underneath.

Pancreas: A gland located in the abdomen. It makes pancreatic juices, and it produces several hormones, including insulin. The pancreas is surrounded by the stomach, intestines, and other organs.

Pancreatic cancer: Cancer of the pancreas is a disease in which cancer (malignant) cells are found in the tissues of the pancreas. The pancreas is about 6 inches long and is shaped something like a thin pear, wider at one end and narrowing at the other. The pancreas lies behind the stomach, inside a loop formed by part of the small intestine.

Pancreatectomy (pan-kree-a-TEK-to-mee): Surgery to remove the pancreas. In a total pancreatectomy, the duodenum, common bile duct, gallbladder, spleen, and nearby lymph nodes also are removed.

Pancreatic juices: Fluids made by the pancreas. Pancreatic juices contain proteins called enzymes that aid in digestion.

Papillary tumor (PAP-i-lar-ee): A tumor shaped like a small mushroom with its stem attached to the inner lining of the bladder.

Papilledema (pap-il-eh-DEE-ma): Swelling around the optic nerve, usually caused by pressure on the nerve by a tumor.

Pap test: Microscopic examination of cells collected from the cervix. It is used to detect changes that may be cancer or may lead to cancer, and it can show noncancerous conditions, such as infection or inflammation. Also called Pap smear.

Paralysis (pa-RAL-ih-sis): Loss of ability to move all or part of the body.

Paraneoplastic syndrome (pair-a-nee-o-PLAS-tik): A group of symptoms that may develop when substances released by some cancer cells disrupt the normal function of surrounding cells and tissue. Such symptoms do not necessarily mean that the cancer has spread beyond the original site.

Parotid cancer: Cancer of the salivary gland is a disease in which cancer (malignant) cells are found in the tissues of the salivary glands. Your salivary glands make saliva, the fluid that is released into your mouth to keep it moist and to help dissolve your food. Major clusters of salivary glands are found below your tongue (sublingual glands), on the sides of your face just in front of your ears (parotid glands), and under your jawbone (submaxillary glands).

Pathologist (pa-THOL-o-jist): A doctor who identifies diseases by studying cells and tissues under a microscope.

Pediatric (pee-dee-AT-rik): Pertaining to children.

Pelvis: The lower part of the abdomen, located between the hip bones.

Penile cancer: Cancer of the penis, a rare kind of cancer in the United States, is a disease in which cancer (malignant) cells are found on the skin and in the tissues of the penis.

Percutaneous transhepatic cholangiography (per-kyoo-TAN-ee-us trans-heh-PAT-ik ko-LAN-jee-AH-gra-fee): A test sometimes used to help diagnose cancer of the pancreas. During this test, a thin needle is put into the liver. Dye is injected into the bile ducts in the liver so that blockages can be seen on X-rays.

Perfusion: The process of flooding fluid through the artery to saturate the surrounding tissue. In regional perfusion, a specific area of the body (usually an arm or a leg) is targeted, and high doses of anticancer drugs are flooded through the artery to reach the surrounding tissue and kill as many cancer cells as possible. Such a procedure is performed in cases in which the cancer is not thought to have spread past a localized area.

Perineal prostatectomy (pe-ri-NEE-al): Surgery to remove the prostate through an incision made between the scrotum and the anus.

Peripheral blood stem cell transplantation (per-IF-er-al): A procedure that is similar to bone marrow transplantation. Doctors remove healthy immature cells (stem cells) from a patient's blood and store them before the patient receives high-dose chemotherapy and possibly radiation therapy to destroy the leukemia cells. The stem cells are then returned to the patient, where they can produce new blood cells to replace cells destroyed by the treatment.

Peripheral stem cell support (per-IF-er-ul): A method of replacing blood-forming cells destroyed by cancer treatment. Certain cells (stem cells) in the blood that are similar to those in the bone marrow are removed from the patient's blood before treatment. The cells are given back to the patient after treatment.

Peristalsis (pair-ih-STAL-sis): The rippling motion of muscles in the digestive tract. In the stomach, this motion mixes food with gastric juices, turning it into a thin liquid.

Peritoneal cavity: The lower part of the abdomen that contains the intestines (the last part of the digestive tract), the stomach, and the liver. It is bound by thin membranes.

Peritoneum (PAIR-i-to-NEE-um): The large membrane that lines the abdominal cavity.

Pernicious anemia (per-NISH-us a-NEE-mee-a): A blood disorder caused by a lack of vitamin B12. Patients who have this disorder do not produce the substance in the stomach that allows the body to absorb vitamin B12.

Petechiae (peh-TEE-kee-a): Tiny red spots under the skin; often a symptom of leukemia.

Pharynx (FAIR-inks): The hollow tube about 5 inches long that starts behind the nose and ends at the top of the trachea (windpipe) and esophagus (the tube that goes to the stomach).

Photodynamic therapy (fo-to-dy-NAM-ik): Treatment that destroys cancer cells with lasers and drugs that become active when exposed to light.

Pigmemt: A substance that gives color to tissue. Pigments are responsible for the color of skin, eyes, and hair.

Pineal gland (PIN-ee-al): A small gland located in the cerebrum.

Pineal region tumors: Types of brain tumors that occur in or around the pineal gland, a tiny organ near the center of the brain. The pineal region is very difficult to reach therefore these tumors often cannot be removed.

Pineoblastoma (PIN-ee-o-blas-TOE-ma): A fast-growing type of brain tumor that occurs in or around the pineal gland, a tiny organ near the center of the brain.

Pineocytoma (PIN-ee-o-sye-TOE-ma): A slow-growing type of brain tumor that occurs in or around the pineal gland, a tiny organ near the center of the brain.

Pituitary cancer: Pituitary tumors are tumors found in the pituitary gland, a small organ about the size of a pea in the center of the brain just above the back of the nose. Your pituitary gland makes hormones that affect your growth and the functions of other glands in your body. Most pituitary tumors are benign. This means that they grow very slowly and do not spread to other parts of the body.

Pituitary gland (pih-TOO-ih-tair-ee): The main endocrine gland; it produces hormones that control other glands and many body functions, especially growth.

Plasma: The liquid part of the blood.

Plasma cells: Special white blood cells that produce antibodies.

Plasmacytoma: A tumor that is made up of cancerous plasma cells.

Plasmapheresis (plas-ma-fer-EE-sis): The process of removing certain proteins from the blood. Plasmapheresis can be used to remove excess antibodies from the blood of multiple myeloma patients.

Plastic surgeon: A surgeon who specializes in reducing scarring or disfigurement that may occur as a result of accidents, birth defects, or treatment for diseases (such as melanoma).

Platelets (PLAYT-lets): Blood cells that help clots form to help control bleeding. Also called thrombocytes.

Pleura (PLOOR-a): The thin covering that protects and cushions the lungs. The pleura is made up of two layers of tissue that are separated by a small amount of fluid.

Pleural cavity: A space enclosed by the pleura, thin tissue covering the lungs and lining the interior wall of the chest cavity. It is bound by serous membranes.

Pneumatic larynx (noo-MAT-ik): A device that uses air to produce sound to help a laryngectomee talk.

Pneumonectomy (noo-mo-NEK-to-mee): An operation to remove an entire lung.

Pneumonia (noo-MONE-ya): An infection that occurs when fluid and cells collect in the lung.

Polyp (POL-ip): A mass of tissue that projects into the colon.

Positron emission tomography scan: For this type of scan, a person is given a substance that reacts with tissues in the body to release protons (parts of an atom). Through measuring the different amounts of protons released by healthy and cancerous tissues, a computer creates a picture of the inside of the body. Also called PET scan.

Postremission therapy: Chemotherapy to kill leukemia cells that survive after remission induction therapy.

Precancerous (pre-KAN-ser-us): A term used to describe a condition that may or is likely to become cancer.

Precancerous polyps: Growths in the colon that often become cancerous.

Prednisone: A drug often given to multiple myeloma patients along with one or more anticancer drugs. Prednisone appears to act together with anticancer drugs in helping to control the effects of the disease on the body.

Preleukemia (PREE-loo-KEE-mee-a): A condition in which the bone marrow does not function normally. It does not produce enough blood cells. This condition may progress and become acute leukemia. Preleukemia also is called myelodysplastic syndrome or smoldering leukemia.

Primitive neuroectodermal tumors (NOO-ro-ek-toe-DER-mul): A type of brain tumor that recent research suggests develops from primitive (developing) nerve cells that normally do not remain in the body after birth. Primitive neuroectodermal tumors are often called medulloblastomas.

Proctoscopy (prok-TOS-ko-pee): An examination of the rectum and the lower end of the colon using a thin lighted instrument called a sigmoidoscope.

Proctosigmoidoscopy (PROK-toe-sig-moid-OSS-ko-pee): An examination of the rectum and the lower colon using a thin, lighted instrument called a sigmoidoscope.

Progesterone (pro-JES-ter-own): A female hormone.

Prognosis (prog-NO-sis): The probable outcome or course of a disease; the chance of recovery.

Prophylactic cranial irradiation (pro-fi-LAK-tik KRAY-nee-ul ir-ray-dee-AY-shun): Radiation therapy to the head to prevent cancer from spreading to the brain.

Prostatectomy (pros-ta-TEK-to-mee): An operation to remove part or all of the prostate.

Prostate cancer: Cancer of the prostate, a common form of cancer, is a disease in which cancer (malignant) cells are found in the prostate. The prostate is one of the male sex glands and is located just below the bladder (the organ that collects and empties urine) and in front of the rectum (the lower part of the intestine). The prostate is about the size of a walnut. It surrounds part of the urethra, the tube that carries urine from the bladder to the outside of the body. The prostate makes fluid that becomes part of the semen, the white fluid that contains sperm.

Prostate gland (PROS-tate): A gland in the male reproductive system just below the bladder. It surrounds part of the urethra, the canal that empties the bladder. It produces a fluid that forms part of semen.

Prostate-specific antigen: A protein whose level in the blood goes up in some men who have prostate cancer or benign prostatic hyperplasia. Also called PSA.

Prostatic acid phosphatase (FOS-fa-tase): An enzyme produced by the prostate. Its level in the blood goes up in some men who have prostate cancer. Also called PAP.

Prosthesis (pros-THEE-sis): An artificial replacement for a body part.

Prosthodontist (pros-tho-DON-tist): A dentist with special training in making replacements for missing teeth or other structures of the oral cavity to restore the patient's appearance, comfort, and/or health.

Proteins (PRO-teenz): Substances that are essential to the body's structure and proper functioning.

PTC (percutaneous transhepatic cholangiography) (per-kyoo-TAN-ee-us trans-heh-PAT-ik ko-LAN-jee-AH-gra-fee): A test sometimes used to help diagnose cancer of the pancreas. During this test, a thin needle is put into the liver. Dye is injected into the bile ducts in the liver so that blockages can be seen on X-rays.

Radiation fibrosis (ray-dee-AY-shun-fye-BRO-sis): The formation of scar tissue as a result of radiation therapy to the lung.

Radiation therapy (ray-dee-AY-shun): Treatment with high-energy rays to kill cancer cells.

Radiation oncologist (ray-dee-AY-shun on-KOL-o-jist): A doctor who specializes in using radiation to treat cancer.

Radiation therapy (ray-dee-AY-shun): Treatment with high-energy rays (such as X-rays) to kill cancer cells. The radiation may come from outside the body (external radiation) or from radioactive materials placed directly in the tumor (implant radiation). Also called radiotherapy.

Radical cystectomy (RAD-i-kal sis-TEK-to-mee): Surgery to remove the bladder as well as nearby tissues and organs.

Radical prostatectomy: Surgery to remove the entire prostate. The two types of radical prostatectomy are retropubic prostatectomy and perineal prostatectomy.

Radioactive (RAY-dee-o-AK-tiv): Giving off radiatiion.

Radiologist: A doctor who specializes in creating and interpreting pictures of areas inside the body. The pictures are produced with X-rays, sound waves, or other types of energy.

Radionuclide scanning: An exam that produces pictures (scans) of internal parts of the body. The patient is given an injection or swallows a small amount of radioactive material. A machine called a scanner then measures the radioactivity in certain organs.

Radiosensitizers: Drugs that make cells more sensitive to radiation.

Radon (RAY-don): A radioactive gas that is released by uranium, a substance found in soil and rock. When too much radon is breathed in, it can damage lung cells and lead to lung cancer.

Rectal cancer: Cancer of the rectum, a common form of cancer, is a disease in which cancer (malignant) cells are found in the tissues of the rectum. The rectum is part of the body's digestive system. The last 6 feet of intestine is called the large bowel or colon. The last 8 to 10 inches of the colon is the rectum.

Rectum: The last 8 to 10 inches of the large intestine. The rectum stores solid waste until it leases the body through the anus.

Recur: To occur again. Recurrence is the reappearance of cancer cells at the same site or in another location.

Red blood cells: Cells that carry oxygen to all parts of the body. Also called erythrocytes.

Reed-Sternberg cell: A type of cell that appears in patients with Hodgkin's disease. The number of these cells increases as the disease advances.

Reflux: The term used when liquid backs up into the esophagus from the stomach.

Regional chemotherapy: Treatment with anticancer drugs that affects mainly the cells in the treated area.

Relapse: The return of signs and symptoms of a disease after a period of improvement.

Remission: Disappearance of the signs and symptoms of cancer. When this happens, the disease is said to be "in remission." A remission can be temporary or permanent.

Remission induction therapy: The initial chemotherapy a patient with acute leukemia receives to bring about a remission.

Renal capsule: The fibrous connective tissue that surrounds each kidney.

Renal cell cancer: Cancer that develops in the lining of the renal tubules, which filter the blood and produce urine.

Renal pelvis: The area at the center of the kidney. Urine collects here and is funneled into the ureter.

Reproductive cells: Egg and sperm cells. Each mature reproductive cell carries a single set of 23 chromosomes.

Reproductive system: The group of organs and glands involved with having a child. In women, these are the uterus (womb), the fallopian tubes, the ovaries, and the vagina (birth canal). The reproductive system in men includes the testes, the prostate, and the penis.

Resection (ree-SEK-shun): Surgical removal of part of an organ.

Respiratory system (RES-pi-ra-tor-ee): The organs that are involved in breathing. These include the nose, throat, larynx, trachea, bronchi, and lungs.

Respiratory therapy (RES-pi-ra-tor-ee): Exercises and treatments that help patients recover lung function after surgery.

Retinoblastoma: An eye cancer caused by the loss of both gene copies of the tumor-suppressor gene RB; the inherited form typically occurs in childhood, because one gene is missing from the time of birth.

Retropubic prostatectomy (re-tro-PYOO-bik): Surgical removal of the prostate through an incision in the abdomen.

Rhabdomyosarcoma: Rhabdomyosarcoma is a disease in which cancer (malignant) cells begin growing in muscle tissue somewhere in the body. Rhabdomyosarcoma is a type of a sarcoma, which means a cancer of the bone, soft tissues, or connective tissue (e.g., tendon or cartilage). Rhabdomyosarcoma begins in the soft tissues in a type of muscle called striated muscle. It can occur anywhere in the body.

Risk factor: Something that increases the chance of developing a disease.

RNA (ribonucleic acid): One of the two nucleic acids found in all cells. The other is DNA (deoxyribonucleic acid). RNA transfers genetic information from DNA to proteins produced by the cell.

Salivary glands (SAL-i-vair-ee): Glands in the mouth that produce saliva.

Salpingo-oophorectomy (sal-PING-o-OO-for-EK-to-mee): Surgical removal of the fallopian tubes and ovaries.

Sarcoma (sar-KO-ma): A malignant tumor that begins in connective and supportive tissue.

Scans: Pictures of organs in the body. Scans often used in diagnosing, staging, and monitoring patients include liver scans, bone scans, and computed tomography (CT) or computed axial tomography (CAT) scans. In liver scanning and bone scanning, radioactive substances that are injected into the bloodstream collect in these organs. A scanner that detects the radiation is used to create pictures. In CT scanning, an X-ray machine linked to a computer is used to produce detailed pictures of organs inside the body.

Schiller test (SHIL-er): A test in which iodine is applied to the cervix. The iodine colors healthy cells brown; abnormal cells remain unstained, usually appearing white or yellow.

Schwannoma (shwah-NO-ma): A type of benign brain tumor that begins in the Schwann cells, which produce the myelin that protects the acoustic nerve the nerve of hearing.

Screening: Checking for disease when there are no symptoms.

Scrotum (SKRO-tum): The external pouch of skin that contains the testicles.

Sebum (SEE-bum): An oily substance produced by certain glands in the skin.

Seizures (SEE-zhurz): Convulsions; sudden, involuntary movements of the muscles.

Semen: The fluid that is released through the penis during orgasm. Semen is made up of sperm from the testicles and fluid from the prostate and other sex glands.

Seminal vesicles (SEM-in-al VES-i-kulz): Glands that help produce semen.

Seminoma (sem-in-O-ma): A type of testicular cancer that arises from sex cells, or germ cells, at a very early stage in their development.

Shunt: A catheter (tube) that carries cerebrospinal fluid from a ventricle in the brain to another area of the body.

Side effects: Problems that occur when treatment affects healthy cells. Common side effects of cancer treatment are fatigue, nausea, vomiting, decreased blood cell counts, hair loss, and mouth sores.

Sigmoidoscope (sig-MOY-da-skope): An instrument used to view the inside of the colon.

Sigmoidoscopy (sig-moid-OSS-ko-pee): A procedure in which the doctor looks inside the rectum and the lower part of the colon (sigmoid colon) through a lighted tube. The doctor may collect samples of tissue or cells for closer examination. Also called proctosigmoidoscopy.

Sinus cancer: Cancer of the paranasal sinus and nasal cavity is a disease in which cancer (malignant) cells are found in the tissues of the paranasal sinuses or nasal cavity. Your paranasal sinuses are small hollow spaces around your nose. The sinuses are lined with cells that make mucus, which keeps the nose from drying out; the sinuses are also a space through which your voice can echo to make sounds when you talk or sing.

Skin cancer: Skin cancer is a disease in which cancer (malignant) cells are found in the outer layers of your skin. The skin has two main layers and several kinds of cells. The top layer of skin is called the epidermis. It contains three kinds of cells: flat, scaly cells on the surface called squamous cells; round cells called basal cells; and cells called melanocytes, which give your skin its color.

Skin graft: Skin that is moved from one part of the body to another.

Small cell lung cancer: A type of lung cancer in which the cells are small and round. Also called oat cell lung cancer.

Small intestine: The part of the digestive tract that is located between the stomach and the large intestine.

Smoldering leukemia: (See Preleukemia.)

Soft tissue sarcoma: A sarcoma that begins in the muscle, fat, fibrous tissue, blood vessels, or other supporting tissue of the body.

Somatic cells: All the body cells except the reproductive cells.

Somatic mutations: See mutation.

Speech pathologist: A specialist who evaluates and treats people with communication and swallowing problems. Also called a speech therapist.

Speculum (SPEK-yoo-lum): An instrument used to widen the opening of the vagina so that the cervix is more easily visible.

Sperm banking: Freezing sperm before cancer treatment for use in the future. This procedure can allow men to father children after loss of fertility.

SPF (Sun protection factor): A scale for rating sunscreens. Sunscreens with an SPF of 15 or higher provide the best protection from the sun's harmful rays.

Spinal tap: A test in which a fluid sample is removed from the spinal column with a thin needle. Also called a lumbar puncture.

Spleen: An organ that produces lymphocytes, filters the blood, stores blood cells, and destroys those that are aging. It is located on the left side of the abdomen near the stomach.

Splenectomy (splen-EK-toe-mee): An operation to remove the spleen.

Sputum (SPYOO-tum): Mucus from the lungs.

Squamous cell carcinoma (SKWAY-mus): Cancer that begins in squamous cells, which are thin, flat cells resembling fish scales. Squamous cells are found in the tissue that forms the surface of the skin, the lining of the hollow organs of the body, and the passages of the respiratory and digestive tracts.

Squamous cells (SKWAY-mus): Flat cells that look like fish scales; they make up most of the epidermis, the outer layer of the skin.

Squamous intraepithelial lesion (SKWAY-mus in-tra-eh-pih-THEEL-ee-ul LEE-zhun): A general term for the abnormal growth of squamous cells on the surface of the cervix. The changes in the cells are described as low grade or high grade, depending on how much of the cervix is affected and how abnormal the cells are. Also called SIL.

Stage: The extent of a cancer, especially whether the disease has spread to other parts of the body.

Staging: Doing exams and tests to learn the extent of the cancer, especially whether it has spread from its original site to other parts of the body.

Stem cells: The cells from which all blood cells develop.

Stereotaxis (stair-ee-o-TAK-sis): Use of a computer and scanning devices to create three-dimensional pictures. This method can be used to direct a biopsy, external radiation, or the insertion of radiation implants.

Sterile: The inability to produce children.

Steroids (STEH-roidz): Drugs used to relieve swelling and inflammation.

Stoma: An opening in the abdominal wall; also called an ostomy or urostomy.

Stool: The waste matter discharged in a bowel movement; feces.

Stool test: A test to check for hidden blood in the bowel movement.

Subglottis (SUB-glot-is): The lowest part of the larynx; the area from just below the vocal cords down to the top of the trachea.

Sun Protection Factor (SPF): A scale for rating sunscreens. Sunscreens with an SPF of 15 or higher provide the best protection from the sun's harmful rays.

Sunscreen: A substance that blocks the effect of the sun's harmful rays. Using lotions or creams that contain sunscreens can protect the skin from damage that may lead to cancer.

Supportive care: Treatment given to prevent, control, or relieve complications and side effects and to improve the patient's comfort and quality of life.

Supraglottis (SOOP-ra-GLOT-is): The upper part of the larynx, including the epiglottis; the area above the vocal cords.

Surgery: A procedure to remove or repair a part of the body or to find out if disease is present.

Systemic (sis-TEM-ik): Reaching and affecting cells all over the body.

Systemic therapy (sis-TEM-ik): Treatment that uses substances that travel through the bloodstream, reaching and affecting cancer cells all over the body.

Systemic treatment (sis-TEM-ik): Treatment using substances that travel through the bloodstream, reaching and affecting cancer cells all over the body.

T-cell lymphoma (lim-FO-ma): A cancer of the immune system that appears in the skin; also called mycosis fungoides.

Testicles (TES-ti-kuls): The two egg-shaped glands that produce sperm and male hormones.

Testicular cancer: Cancer of the testicle (also called the testis), a rare kind of cancer in men, is a disease in which cancer (malignant) cells are found in the tissues of one or both testicles. The testicles are round and a little smaller than golf balls. Sperm (the male germ cells that can join with a female egg to develop into a baby) and male hormones are made in the testicles. There are two testicles located inside of the scrotum (a sac of loose skin that lies directly under the penis).

Testosterone (tes-TOS-ter-own): A male sex hormone.

Thermography (ther-MOG-ra-fee): A test to measure and display heat patterns of tissues near the surface of the breast. Abnormal tissue generally is warmer than healthy tissue. This technique is under study; its value in detecting breast cancer has not been proven.

Thoracentesis (thor-a-sen-TEE-sis): Removal of fluid in the pleura through a needle.

Thoracic (thor-ASS-ik): Pertaining to the chest.

Thoracotomy (thor-a-KOT-o-mee): An operation to open the chest.

Thrombocytes (THROM-bo-sites): See Platelets.

Thrombophlebitis (throm-bo-fleh-BYE-tis): Inflammation of a vein that occurs when a blood clot forms.

Thymoma: Malignant thymoma is a disease in which cancer (malignant) cells are found in the tissues of the thymus. The thymus is a small organ that lies under the breastbone. It makes white blood cells called lymphocytes, which travel through your body and fight infection. People with malignant thymoma often have other diseases of their immune system. The most common disease in people with thymoma is one in which the muscles are weak, called myasthenia gravis.

Thymus: An organ in which lymphocytes mature and multiply. It lies behind the breastbone.

Thyroid cancer: Cancer of the thyroid is a disease in which cancer (malignant) cells are found in the tissues of the thyroid gland. Your thyroid gland is at the base of your throat. It has two lobes, one on the right side and one on the left. Your thyroid gland makes important hormones that help your body to function normally.

Tissue (TISH-oo): A group or layer of cells that together perform specific functions.

Tonsils: Small masses of lymphatic tissue on either side of the throat.

Topical chemotherapy (kee-mo-THER-a-pee): Treatment with anticancer drugs in a lotion or cream.

Total pancreatectomy (pan-cree-a-TEK-to-mee): Surgery to remove the entire pancreas.

Toxins: Poisons produced by certain animals, plants, or bacteria.

Trachea (TRAY-kee-a): The airway that leads from the larynx to the lungs. Also called the windpipe.

Tracheoesophageal puncture (TRAY-kee-o-eh-SOF-a-JEE-al PUNK-chur): A small opening made by a surgeon between the esophagus and the trachea. A valve keeps food out of the trachea but lets air into the esophagus for esophageal speech.

Tracheostomy (TRAY-kee-AHS-toe-mee): Surgery to create an opening (stoma) into the windpipe. The opening itself may also be called a tracheostomy.

Tracheostomy button (TRAY-kee-AHS-toe-mee): A small plastic tube placed in the stoma to keep it open.

Tracheostomy tube (TRAY-kee-AHS-toe-mee): A 2- to 3-inch-long metal or plastic tube that keeps the stoma and trachea open. Also called a trach ("trake") tube.

Transformation: The change that a normal cell undergoes as it becomes malignant.

Transfusion (trans-FYOO-zhun): The transfer of blood or blood products from one person to another.

Transitional cell carcinoma: Cancer that develops in the lining of the renal pelvis. This type of cancer also occurs in the ureter and the bladder.

Transitional cells: Cells lining some organs.

Transplantation (trans-plan-TAY-shun): The replacement of an organ with one from another person.

Transrectal ultrasound: The use of sound waves to detect cancer. An instrument is inserted into the rectum. Waves bounce off the prostate and the pattern of the echoes produced is converted into a picture by a computer.

Transurethral resection (TRANZ-yoo-REE-thral ree-SEK-shun): Surgery performed with a special instrument inserted through the urethra. Also called TUR.

Transurethral resection of the prostate (TRANZ-yoo-REE-thral): The use of an instrument inserted through the penis to remove tissue from the prostate. Also called TUR or TURP.

Transvaginal ultrasound: Sound waves sent out by a probe inserted in the vagina. The waves bounce off the ovaries, and a computer uses the echoes to create a picture called a sonogram. Also called TVS.

Tumor (TOO-mer): An abnormal mass of tissue that results from excessive cell division. Tumors perform no useful body function. They may either be benign (not cancerous) or malignant (cancerous).

Tumor debulking: Surgically removing as much of the tumor as possible.

Tumor marker: A substance in blood or other body fluids that may suggest that a person has cancer.

Tumor necrosis factor (ne-KRO-sis): A type of biological response modifier (a substance that can improve the body's natural response to disease). Scientists are still learning how this substance causes cancer cells to die.

Tumor-suppressor gene: Genes in the body that can suppress or block the development of cancer.

Tumors of unknown primary origin: This is a disease in which cancer (malignant) cells are found somewhere in the body, but the place where they first started growing (the origin or primary site) cannot be found.

Ulcerative colitis: A disease that causes long-term inflammation of the lining of the colon.

Ultrasonography: A test in which sound waves (called ultrasound) are bounced off tissues and the echoes are converted into a picture (sonogram).

Ultrasound: A test that bounces sound waves off tissues and internal organs and changes the echoes into pictures (sonograms). Tissues of different densities reflect sound waves differently.

Ultraviolet (UV) radiation (ul-tra-VYE-o-let ray-dee-AY-shun): Invisible rays that are part of the energy that comes from the sun. UV radiation can burn the skin and cause melanoma and other types of skin cancer. UV radiation that reaches the earth's surface is made up of two types of rays, called UVA and UVB rays. UVB rays are more likely than UVA rays to cause sunburn, but UVA rays pass further into the skin. Scientists have long thought that UVB radiation can cause melanoma and other types of skin cancer. They now think that UVA radiation also may add to skin damage that can lead to cancer. For this reason, skin specialists recommend that people use sunscreens that block or absorb both kinds of UV radiation.

Upper GI series: A series of X-rays of the upper digestive system that are taken after a person drinks a barium solution, which outlines the digestive organs on the X-rays.

Ureter (yoo-REE-ter): The tube that carries urine from the kidney to the bladder.

Urethra (yoo-REE-thra): The tube that empties urine from the bladder.

Urinalysis: A test that determines the content of the urine.

Urinary tract (YUR-in-air-ee): The organs of the body that produce and discharge urine. These include the kidneys, ureters, bladder, and urethra.

Urine (YUR-in): Fluid containing water and waste products. Urine is made by the kidneys, stored in the bladder, and leaves the body through the urethra.

Urologist (yoo-RAHL-o-jist): A doctor who specializes in diseases of the urinary organs in females and the urinary and sex organs in males.

Urostomy (yoo-RAHS-toe-mee): An operation to create an opening from inside the body to the outside, making a new way to pass urine.

Uterine cancer: Cancer of the endometrium, a common kind of cancer in women, is a disease in which cancer (malignant) cells are found in the lining of the uterus (endometrium). The uterus is the hollow, pear-shaped organ where a baby grows. Cancer of the endometrium is different from cancer of the muscle of the uterus, which is called sarcoma of the uterus. Sarcoma of the uterus, a very rare kind of cancer in women, is a disease in which cancer (malignant) cells start growing in the muscles or other supporting tissues of the uterus.

Uterus (YOO-ter-us): The small, hollow, pear-shaped organ in a woman's pelvis. This is the organ in which an unborn child develops. Also called the womb.

Vagina (vah-JYE-na): The muscular canal extending from the uterus to the exterior of the body.

Vaginal cancer: Cancer of the vagina, a rare kind of cancer in women, is a disease in which cancer (malignant) cells are found in the tissues of the vagina. The vagina is the passageway through which fluid passes out of the body during menstrual periods and through which a woman has babies. It is also called the "birth canal."

Vasectomy (vas-EK-to-mee): An operation to cut or tie off the two tubes that carry sperm out of the testicles.

Ventricles (VEN-trih-kulz): Four connected cavities (hollow spaces) in the brain.

Vinyl chloride (VYE-nil KLO-ride): A substance used in manufacturing plastics. It is linked to liver cancer.

Viruses (VYE-rus-ez): Small living particles that can infect cells and change how the cells function. Infection with a virus can cause a person to develop symptoms. The disease and symptoms that are caused depend on the type of virus and the type of cells that are infected.

Vital: Necessary to maintain life. Breathing is a vital function.

Vocal cords: Two small bands of muscle within the larynx. They close to prevent food from getting into the lungs, and they vibrate to produce the voice.

Waldenstrom's macroglobulinemia: This is a rare, chronic cancer that affects white blood cells called B lymphocytes, or B cells. These cells form in the lymph nodes and the bone marrow, the soft, spongy tissue inside bones, and are an important part of the body's immune (defense) system. Some B cells become plasma cells, which make, store, and release antibodies. Antibodies help the body fight viruses, bacteria, and other foreign substances. In Waldenstrom's macroglobulinemia, abnormal B cells multiply out of control. They invade the bone marrow, lymph nodes, and spleen and produce excessive amounts of an antibody called IgM.

Wart: A raised growth on the surface of the skin or other organ.

Whipple procedure: A type of surgery used to treat pancreatic cancer. The surgeon removes the head of the pancreas, the duodenum, a portion of the stomach, and other nearby tissues.

White blood cells: Cells that help the body fight infection and disease. These cells begin their development in the bone marrow and then travel to other parts of the body.

Wilms' tumor: Wilms' tumor is a disease in which cancer (malignant) cells are found in certain parts of the kidney. The kidneys are a "matched" pair of organs found on either side of the backbone. Inside each kidney are tiny tubes that filter and clean the blood, taking out unneeded products, and making urine. Wilms' tumor occurs most commonly in children under the age of 15 and is curable in the majority of affected children.

Xerogram: An X-ray of soft tissue.

Xeroradiography (ZEE-roe-ray-dee-OG-ra-fee): A type of mammography in which a picture of the breast is recorded on paper rather than on film.

X-ray: High-energy radiation used in low doses to diagnose diseases and in high doses to treat cancer.

Index

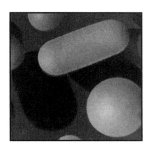

Note: Page numbers in **boldface** refer to volume numbers and major topics. Article titles are in **boldface**.

Basler IG, **2:**624

Basombrío, Miguel Angel, **1:**57

Bates, Phyllis, **3:**1049

Batma, Laarbi, **2:**587

Batra, B.K., **2:**455

batteries, history of, **1:**88

battery acid, **1:**88-90

bayberry wax, **3:**1020

Bayer Schering Pharma A.gG., **3:**770

BCG vaccine, **1:**109, **1:**145, **3:**880–881

Bcl-2, **1:**340

Beatty, Sir Chester, **3:**940, **3:**1047–1048

Bebesel, Elena, **2:**749

Beckman Research Institute, **1:**207

Beckwith-Wiedemann syndrome, **1:**6, **3:**1025

becquerel (unit), **2:**626

Becquerel, Henri, **2:**715, **2:**721

beeswax, **3:**1020

Behbudov, S.M., **1:**81

Belarus, **1:**91

Belarusian State Cancer Registry, **1:**91

Belgian Congo. *See* Congo

Belgian Federation against Cancer, **1:**92

Belgium, **1:**91-92

    assisted suicide, **1:**66

      UCB, **3:**921–922

Belinsky, Steven A., **3:**961

Bellil, Samira, **1:**21

Bellocco, R., **3:**863

Belqola, Said, **2:**587

Belyaeva, M.I., **2:**754

Ben-Zvi, Isaac, **2:**488, **3:**924

Benacerraf, Baruj, **2:**587–588, **3:**989

Benedeczky, Istvan, **2:**450

Bener, A., **3:**938

benign teratomas, **2:**395

Benigno, Teodoro, **2:**678

Benin, **1:**92-93

Benitez-Bribiesca, Luis, **2:**581

Bennett, M.B., **3:**828

Benz, Karl, **1:**80, **2:**374

Benz, M., **2:**662

benzaldonium chloride, **1:**281

benzene, carcinogenicity of, **1:**80, **3:**825

benzidine, **1:**297, **1:**300

benzidine-based dyes, **1:**297, **3:**890

benzopyrene, **3:**903

benzopyrone, **2:**541

benzotrichloride, **1:**282

benzoyl chloride, **1:**297

Bercovitz, Nathaniel, **1:**200

Berg, John, **3:**861

Berg, Paul, **3:**942

Bergolz, V.M., **2:**753

beriberi, **3:**1003, **3:**1004

Berlinguet, Louis, **1:**155

Berrigan, Daniel, **3:**944

Bertagnolli, M.M., **1:**237

bertholite, **1:**203

Berwick, Marianne, **3:**961

beryllium, **1:**93-94

beryllium dust, chemical pneumonitis, **1:**93

beryllium lung disease, **1:**93

Best Practices in Colorectal Carcinoma (BP-CRC), **1:**159

beta-benzene-hexachloride, **2:**466

beta-carotene, **1:**94-99

    as antioxidant, **1:**98

    cancer and, **1:**94–96

    dietary sources of, **1:**94

    metabolism of, **1:**96–97

    pro-oxidant activity, **1:**98–99

Beta-Carotene and Retinol Efficacy Trial. *See* CARET Study

beta-catenin pathway. *See* CTNNB1 pathway

beta-lactam antibiotics, coatulation abnormalities in cancer patients and, **1:**52

beta particles, **2:**715

betel nuts, **2:**459, **2:**515, **2:**590, **2:**661, **3:**832, **3:**993

bevacizumab, **1:**104, **1:**106, **1:**339, **2:**380

Bevan, Silvanus, **2:**401

Beveridge, Charles E.G., **3:**844

Bexxar, **1:**104

BHA, **1:**354

Bhide, S.V., **2:**455

BHT, **1:**354

Bhumibol (Prince), **3:**890

bicalutamide, **1:**292

Bichat, Xavier, **1:**363

Bichel, P., **1:**259

glass industry, **2**:399–401

hair dye, **1**:299, **2**:414–416

herbicides, **2**:426–429

insecticides, **2**:464–467

lead, **2**:375, **2**:520–523

nickel compounds, **2**:616–618

paint, **2**:650–652

paper industry, **2**:657–660

perfume, **2**:667–668

pesticides, **2**:670–672, **2**:695

plastics industry, **1**:3–5, **2**:685–687, **3**:933–996

polishes, **2**:690–692

protective clothing, **1**:215

selenium, **3**:784–786

solvents, **3**:825–827

sulfuric acid, **1**:89–90

textile dyes, **1**:299, **3**:888–890

vinyl, **3**:994–996

war gases, **3**:1013–1014

water treatment, **3**:1016–1018

See also aerospace industry; air pollution; carcinogens; drugs; pharmaceutical industry; water pollution

chemical milling, **1**:10

chemical modifiers, **1**:261

chemical pneumonitis, beryllium dust, **1**:93

chemical wastes, **2**:460

chemical weapons, **3**:1014

See also weapons

Chemical Weapons Convention of 1993, **3**:1014

chemolabeled monoclonal antibodies, **1**:104–105

chemoprevention, 1:185-187

See also anticancer drugs; chemotherapy

chemotherapeutic drugs. *See* anticancer drugs; chemoprevention; chemotherapy

chemotherapy, 1:185–186, **1:187-195**, **1**:290

antibiotic use concurrent with, **1**:52

before bone marrow transplantation, **1**:118

for brain tumors in children, **1**:124, **1**:125–126, **1**:128, **1**:129

for breast cancer, **1**:136, **1**:139

breastfeeding and, **1**:138

Burkitt's lymphoma, **2**:543

carcinogenicity of anticancer drugs, **1**:53–55

clinical trials, **1**:186–187

for colon cancer, **1**:223

for colorectal cancer, **1**:339

combination chemotherapy, **1**:185, **1**:193

cost of therapy, **1**:194, **1**:234–235

during pregnancy, **1**:137, **1**:192–193

of germ cell tumors, **2**:393

hepatocellular carcinoma, **2**:425

history of, **1**:38, **1**:188

Hodgkin's disease, **2**:544, **2**:546

for hypothalamic and visual pathway gliomas, **2**:454

indications for, **1**:188–189

liposomal therapy, **1**:194

method of delivery, **1**:186, **1**:191

for multiple myeloma, **1**:177, **2**:594

for myelodysplastic syndromes, **1**:177

pancreatic cancer, **2**:654

premature menopause, **1**:136–137

side effects, **1**:186, **1**:191–193

side effects of, **1**:252, **2**:393–394

signs of clinical improvement, **1**:193–194

targeted therapies, **1**:292, **3**:881

treatment modes, **1**:190–191

See also anticancer drugs; experimental cancer drugs; monoclonal antibodies; vaccines

chemotherapy drugs. *See* anticancer drugs

Chen, Dr. Suzie, **1**:165

Chen, T.Y., **3**:868

Cherd Songsri, **3**:891

Chernavsky, A.A., **2**:754

Chernobyl disaster, **1**:91, **2**:627, **2**:628, **2**:720, **3**:924

See also radiation disasters

Chernozemski, I., **1**:144

Cherry, Dr. Simon, **2**:676

Chester Beatty Research Institute, **3**:940, **3**:1048

chewing tobacco, **1**:287, **3**:810–812

Chi, C.H., **3**:830

Chiang Ching-kuo, **3**:869

Chiang Hsiao-ping, **3**:869

Chichester, Sir Francis, **2**:661

Chiesa, Dr. Gerardo, **1**:57

childhood and cancer risk, 1:195-197

Childhood Brain Tumor Foundation (CBTF), 1:197-198

Childhood Cancer Ombudsman Program, **1**:170